Advances in
perinatal medicine

Advances in perinatal medicine

The Proceedings of the XV European Congress
of Perinatal Medicine,
Glasgow, September 1996

Edited by
Forrester Cockburn

Emeritus Professor of Child Health,
University of Glasgow, Scotland
and
President of the European Association
of Perinatal Medicine, 1994–96

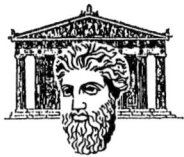

The Parthenon Publishing Group
International Publishers in Medicine, Science & Technology

NEW YORK   LONDON

Library of Congress Cataloging-in-Publication Data
Advances in perinatal medicine/edited by Forrester
  Cockburn.
       p.   cm.
  Proceedings of the 15th European Congress of
     Perinatal Medicine, held 10–13 Sept. 1996, Glasgow,
     Scotland.
     Includes bibliographical references and index.
     ISBN 1-85070-944-0
     1. Perinatology—Congresses. I. Cockburn,
     Forrester. II. European Congress of Perinatal
     Medicine (15th: 1996: Glasgow, Scotland).
     [DNLM: 1. Perinatology—congresses. WQ 210
A2438 1997]
     RG600.A353 1997
     618.3′2—dc21
     DNLM/DLC
     for Library of Congress   97-23209
                                                              CIP

British Library Cataloguing-in-Publication Data
Advances in perinatal medicine: the proceedings of the
  XVth European Congress of Perinatal Medicine,
  Glasgow, Scotland, 10–13 September 1996
     1. Perinatology
  I. Cockburn, Forrester II. European Congress of
     Perinatal Medicine (15th: 1996: Glasgow, Scotland)
     618.3′2
     ISBN 1-85070-944-0

Published in the USA by
The Parthenon Publishing Group Inc.
One Blue Hill Plaza
PO Box 1564, Pearl River
New York 10965, USA

Published in the UK and Europe by
The Parthenon Publishing Group Limited
Casterton Hall, Carnforth
Lancs. LA6 2LA, UK

Copyright © 1997 The Parthenon Publishing Group

First published 1997

*No part of this book may be reproduced in any form without
permission from the publishers, except for the quotation of brief
passages for the purposes of review.*

Typeset by AMA Graphics Ltd., Preston, UK
Printed and bound by
Butler & Tanner Ltd., Frome and London, UK

Contents

List of principal contributors

E. N. Adamson-Macedo
42 Showell Road
Bushbury
Wolverhampton WV10 9LT
UK

S. Bambang Oetomo
Division of Neonatology
Beatrix Children's Hospital
University Hospital of Groningen
Hanzeplein 1, PO Box 30.001
9700 RB Groningen
The Netherlands

M. J. Brodie
Department of Medicine and Therapeutics
Epilepsy Unit
Western Infirmary
Glasgow G11 6NT
UK

F. Cockburn
Department of Child Health
Royal Hospital for Sick Children
Yorkhill
Glasgow G3 8SJ
UK

E. V. Cosmi
2nd Institute of Obstetrics and Gynecology
University La Sapienza
Policlinico Umberto 1
Viale Regina Elena 324
00161 Roma
Italy

C. Davis
Yorkhill NHS Trust
Yorkhill
Glasgow G3 8SJ
UK

J. M. Davison
Department of Obstetrics and Gynaecology
4th Floor, Leazes Wing
Royal Victoria Infirmary
Queen Victoria Road
Newcastle upon Tyne NE1 4LP
UK

J. A. Deprest
Gynecologie en Verloskunde
UZ Leuven
Herestraat 49
B-3000 Leuven
Belgium

H. Dolk
Environmental/Epidemiology Unit
Department of Public Health and Policy
London School of Hygiene and Tropical
    Medicine
Keppel Street
London WC1E 7HT
UK

P. M. Dunn
Department of Child Health
University of Bristol
Southmead Hospital
Bristol BS10 5NB
UK

W. Endres
Department of Pediatrics
University of Innsbruck
Anichstrasse 35
A-6020 Innsbruck
Austria

T. K. A. B. Eskes
Institute for the Prevention of Birth Defects
Department of Obstetrics and Gynecology
University Hospital Nijmegen
PO Box 9101
6500 HB Nijmegen
The Netherlands

J. E. E. Fleming
Department of Obstetrics and Gynaecology
University of Glasgow
The Queen Mother's Hospital
Glasgow G3 8SJ
UK

E. Gilland
Department of Anatomy and Cell Biology
Medicinaregatan 3–5
S 413 90 Göteborg
Sweden

A. Green
Clinical Chemistry Department
The Birmingham Children's Hospital
Ladywood Middleway
Ladywood
Birmingham B16 8ET
UK

I. A. Greer
Department of Obstetrics and Gynaecology
University of Glasgow
Glasgow Royal Infirmary
10 Alexandra Parade
Glasgow G31 2ER
UK

A. Günther
Department of Internal Medicine
Justus-Liebig University Giessen
Klinikstrasse 36
35392 Giessen
Germany

H. L. Halliday
Regional Neonatal Unit
Royal Maternity Hospital
Grosvenor Street
Belfast BT12 6BB
UK

E. Halmesmäki
Helsinki University Central Hospital
Department of Obstetrics and Gynecology
Haartmaninkatu 2
00290 Helsinki
Finland

M. Hepburn
Department of Obstetrics and Gynaecology
    and of Social Policy & Social Work
Glasgow Royal Maternity Hospital
Rottenrow
Glasgow G4 0NA
UK

D. James
Division of Fetomaternal Medicine
Queen's Medical Centre
Floor C East Block
Nottingham NG7 2UH
UK

R. J. Johnson
Southmead NHS Trust
Westbury on Trym
Bristol BS10 5NB
UK

P. Jouppila
Department of Obstetrics and Gynecology
University of Oulu
90220 SF Oulu
Finland

J. G. Koppe
Department of Neonatology
EKZ.AMC
Meibergdreef 9
1105 AZ Amsterdam Z.O.
The Netherlands

A. Kurjak
Department of Obstetrics and Gynecology
University of Zagreb, School of Medicine
Sveti Duh Hospital
64 Sveti Duh
10000 Zagreb
Croatia

R. N. Laurini
Division of Developmental Pathology and
    Autopsies
Institute of Pathology, University of Lausanne
Rue du Bugnon 25
CH-1011 Lausanne
Switzerland

J. Le Bidois
Institut de Puericulture de Paris
Unite d' Explorations Cardiologiques
26 Boulevard Brune
75014 Paris
France

O. Linderkamp
Division of Neonatology
University of Heidelberg
Im Neuenheimer Feld 150
D-69120 Heidelberg
Germany

Y. W. Loke
Research Group in Human Reproductive
    Immunobiology
Department of Pathology
University of Cambridge
Tennis Court Road
Cambridge CB2 1QP
UK

L. Ludman
Institute of Child Health
University of London
30 Guilford Street
London WC1N 1EH
UK

A. Marini
Clinica Mangiagalli
via Commenda 12
20122 Milano
Italy

H. E. McHaffie
Institute of Medical Ethics
University of Edinburgh
Department of Medicine
Royal Infirmary
Lauriston Place
Edinburgh EH3 9YW
UK

N. McIntosh
Department of Child Life & Health
The University of Edinburgh
2 Sylvan Place
Edinburgh EH9 1UW
UK

J. C. Möller
Kinderklinik der Medizinischen Universität
Kahlhorstrasse 31–35
23538 Lübeck
Germany

C. J. Morley
Department of Paediatrics
Box 226 Addenbrooke's Hospital
Cambridge CB2 2QQ
UK

K. Nicolaides
Harris Birthright Research Centre for Fetal
    Medicine
King's College School of Medicine
Denmark Hill
London SE5 8RX
UK

C. Niven
Department of Nursing and Midwifery
University of Stirling
Stirling
FK9 4LA
UK

J. Norman
Department of Obstetrics and Gynaecology
Royal Infirmary
10 Alexandra Parade
Glasgow G3 2ER
UK

E. Perks
University of Southampton
School of Nursing and Midwifery
Level F
Coxford Road
Southampton SO16 5YA
UK

B. Persson
Helsingborg Hospital
Department of Pediatrics
25187 Helsingborg
Sweden

P. A. M. Raine
Royal Hospital for Sick Children
Yorkhill
Glasgow G3 8SJ
UK

J.-P. Relier
Maternité de Port-Royal
123 Boulevard de Port-Royal
75014 Paris
France

J. S. Robinson
Department of Obstetrics and Gynaecology
University of Adelaide
Adelaide
South Australia 5005

J. S. Robinson
Department of Nursing and Midwifery Studies
University of Nottingham
B50 Medical School
Queen's Medical Centre
Nottingham NG7 2UH
UK

E. Saling
Institute of Perinatal Medicine
Mariendorfer Weg 28
D 12051 Berlin-Neukölln
Germany

P. J. J. Sauer
Department of Pediatrics
Division of Neonatology
Erasmus University – Academic Hospital
    Rotterdam
Sophia Children's Hospital Rotterdam
PO Box 2060
3000 CB Rotterdam
The Netherlands

O. D. Saugstad
Department of Pediatric Research
University of Oslo
Rikshospitalet
Pilestredet 32
N-0027 Oslo
Norway

K. Selke
Marderweg 9
51109 Köln
Germany

H. L. Spohr
Kinderklinik des Rittberg Krankenhaus
Carstennstrasse 58
D 1000 Berlin 45
Germany

P. J. Steer
Department of Obstetrics and Gynaecology
Charing Cross and Westminster Medical
    School
Chelsea & Westminster Hospital
369 Fulham Road
London SW10 9NH
UK

P. Temesvári
Department of Pediatrics
Dr Sámuel Diósszilágyi Hospital
PO Box 72
H-6901 Makó
Hungary

J. Thorburn
5 Queensbury Avenue
St Bearsden
Glasgow G61 3LR
UK

C. Trevarthen
Department of Psychology
University of Edinburgh
7 George Square
Edinburgh EH7 9JZ
UK

A. Valls-i-Soler
Departamento de Pediatria
Hospital de Cruces
Universidad del Pais Vasco
Plaza de Cruces, s/n
48903 Barakaldo-Vizcaya
Spain

F. A. Van Assche
Department of Obstetrics and Gynecology
University Hospital Leuven
Herestraat 49
B-3000 Leuven
Belgium

V. C. H. von Loewenich
Department of Neonatology
University Children's Hospital
D-60590 Frankfurt AM
Germany

M. Wagner
Nyhausen 40
1051 Copenhagen K
Denmark

J. J. Walker
Department of Obstetrics and Gynaecology
St James' University Hospital
Beckett Street
Leeds LS9 7GF
UK

L. T. Weaver
Department of Child Health
Yorkhill Hospital
University of Glasgow
Glasgow G3 8SJ
UK

M. F. Whitfield
Newborn Services
BC's Children's Hospital Room E405
University of British Columbia
4480 Oak Street
Vancouver V6H 3V4
British Columbia
Canada

M. J. Whittle
Academic Department of Obstetrics and
   Gynaecology
Birmingham Maternity Hospital
University of Birmingham
Edgbaston
Birmingham B15 2TG
UK

D. Wolke
Department of Psychology
University of Hertfordshire
Hatfield Campus
College Lane
Hatfield
Herts AL10 9AB
UK

J. E. Wraith
Willink Biochemical Genetics Unit
Manchester Children's Hospital
Pendlebury
Manchester M27 4HA
UK

J. S. Wyatt
Department of Paediatrics
The Rayne Institute
University College of London
5 University Street
London WC1E 6JJ
UK

Foreword

These Proceedings of the XV Congress of Perinatal Medicine held in Glasgow 10–13th September, 1996 give an up-to-date view of the many scientific, social and ethical problems facing those who devote their working lives to the care of mothers and their infants. Congresses held every second year since 1968 have encouraged a wide range of professionals to bring their latest ideas and data for analysis and discussion. Such has been the speed of change in knowledge, understanding and practice that each of these meetings has highlighted new problems and improved methods for tackling old problems.

The opportunity was taken at the Glasgow meeting to look back 40 years at the pioneering work of Professor Ian Donald who, whilst working in Glasgow, first introduced the clinical use of ultrasound. He would have been astonished and delighted to read these Proceedings and to learn how his ideas have been developed and how technological advances have allowed us to explore the world of the developing fetus and to begin to diagnose and correct disorders identified *in utero*.

The local Organizing Committee thank all who have contributed to the conference and particularly those who have contributed to these Proceedings.

Forrester Cockburn
Congress President and President of the European Association of Perinatal Medicine 1994–96

Section I   Plenary sessions

Fetal anomalies in Europe: the EUROCAT experience

1

H. Dolk

INTRODUCTION

EUROCAT is a network of congenital malformation registers in Europe (Figure 1), covering a population of more than 400 000 births per year. The registries are population based, cover livebirths, stillbirths and terminations of pregnancy following prenatal diagnosis, use multiple sources of information to achieve more complete ascertainment and more accurate diagnostic descriptions, and extend case-finding beyond the neonatal period to register late-manifesting anomalies. A standard data set is collected on each case of congenital anomaly, and the data transmitted to a Central Registry in Brussels[1,2].

The EUROCAT network has facilitated pooling of data across registers, and also comparison of data between registers to exploit differences in health services and risk factors within Europe. This is, of course, dependent on using standard definitions and methods of data collection. Regular meetings between members of the network, as well as data validation for specific studies, form a basis for improving understanding of differences and standardization.

This paper will give some examples of the results of surveillance and research using EUROCAT data collected since 1980, including geographical differences in prevalence, the prevalence of multiply malformed children, evaluation of prenatal diagnosis of selected anomalies, and investigation of environmental risk factors.

GEOGRAPHICAL AND TEMPORAL DIFFERENCES IN PREVALENCE

Geographical differences in prevalence can give a clue to underlying genetic and/or environmental risk factors. The type of prevalence rate of interest in this context is the 'total prevalence', i.e. the number of cases found in livebirths, stillbirths and terminations of pregnancy following prenatal diagnosis, expressed as a proportion of all births. This total prevalence allows for differences in the frequency of prenatal diagnosis in different regions (see below) when assessing prevalence in relation to potential risk factors.

Figure 2 illustrates the higher average prevalence of neural tube defects in the United Kingdom and Ireland than in continental Europe. In the United Kingdom and Ireland there has been a huge decline in prevalence since the early 1960s, continuing into the 1980–92 period shown in Figure 2. In contrast, prevalence in continental Europe has remained quite stable during 1980–92. The cause of the decline in prevalence is not established, although nutritional factors can be strongly suspected since the role of periconceptional folic acid in preventing neural tube is now quite clear[3,4]. Periconceptional supplementation is estimated to halve the risk of a neural tube defect, and as European countries adopt policies to increase periconceptional intake, we should expect a further decline in total prevalence across Europe. EUROCAT registries will be crucial in describing this decline. However, recent work in some EUROCAT registries, such as Northern Netherlands and Paris[5,6], has shown that the level of awareness of women about folic acid remains low despite national policies and programs, and much work is still needed in implementing policies successfully, including consideration of fortification of foods.

3

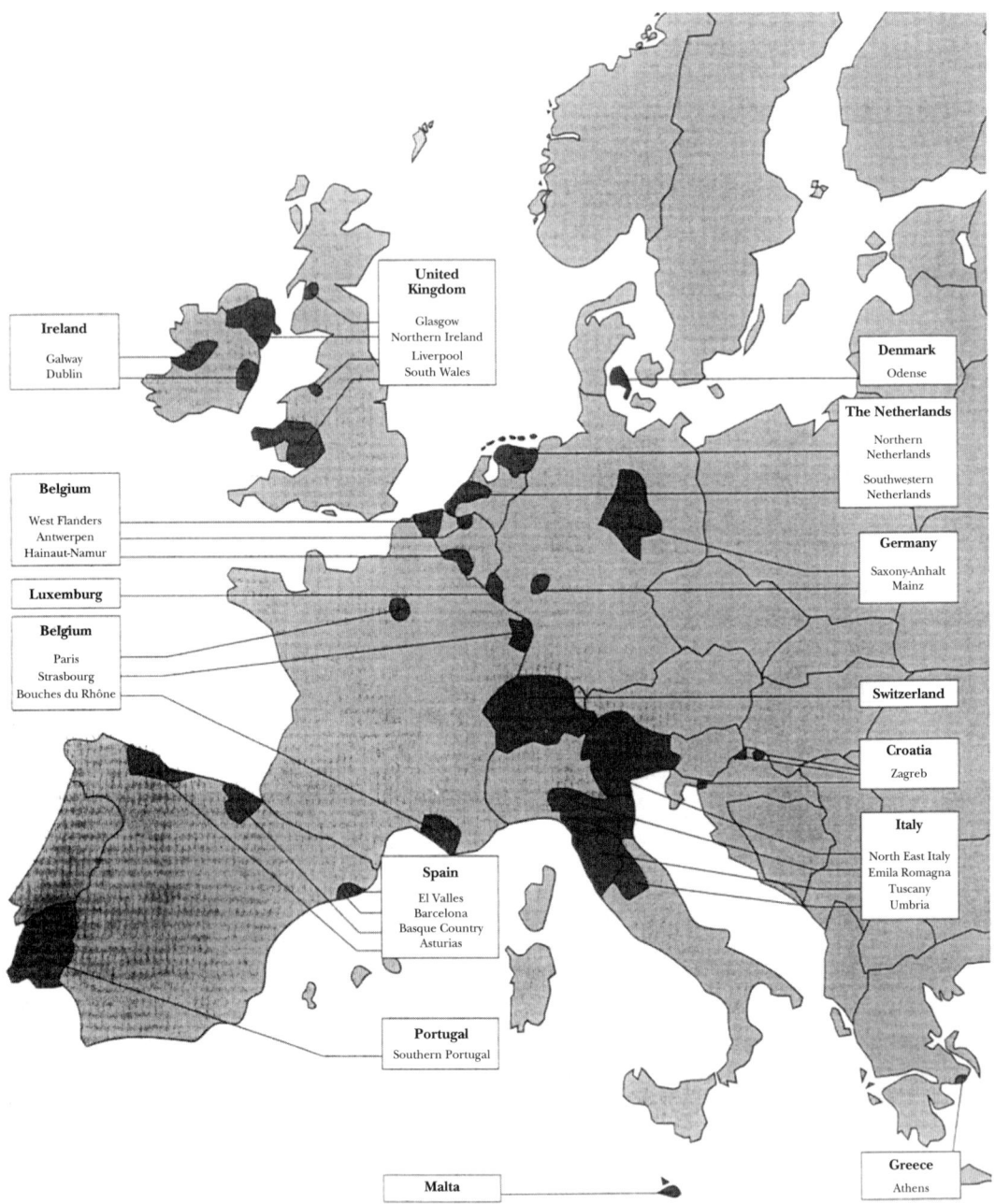

Figure 1 Map of registries participating in the EUROCAT network, showing extent of geographical area covered

The ability of registries to monitor changes in prevalence in anomalies such as neural tube defects, is dependent nowadays on the complete and accurate registration of induced abortions following prenatal diagnosis. This was more straightforward when prenatal diagnosis and termination of pregnancy were conducted in specialized centers, but more recently

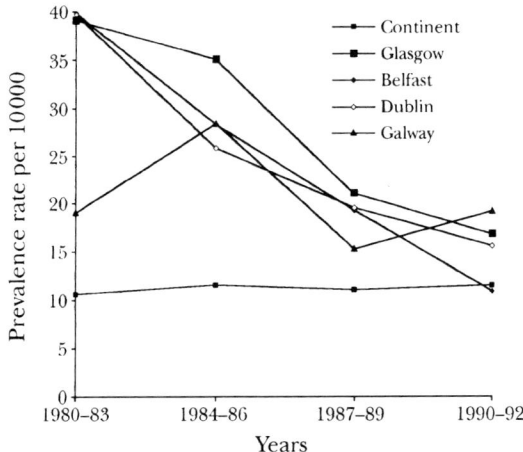

Figure 2 Total prevalence rate per 10 000 births (livebirths, stillbirths and induced abortions) of neural tube defects in four registries of United Kingdom and Ireland (Glasgow, Belfast, Dublin, Galway) and seven centers of continental Europe (Hainaut, Odense, Paris, Strasbourg, Bouches-du-Rhone, Tuscany, Northern Netherland), 1980–92

technology has enabled individual clinicians to diagnose conditions such as anencephaly without special referral, and it is now essential for all obstetricians to be aware of the need to report cases for epidemiological surveillance.

Down's syndrome also shows a wide variation in total prevalence across EUROCAT regions, from 11 to 24 per 10 000 births for 1980–92[1]. This variation can be shown to be almost entirely due to variation in the maternal-age distributions of the different populations, since older maternal age is such a strong risk factor for Down's syndrome. The proportion of older mothers (35 years and over) in the different registries varied from 5% in Hainaut, Belgium to 19% in Galway, Ireland. The proportion of births to older mothers has been increasing over time in most registries, bringing with it increases in prevalence. For example, in Paris, the proportion of older mothers nearly doubled from 11% in 1981 to 19% in 1992[1].

Facial clefts show some intriguing geographical differences[1]. Cleft lip (with or without palate) is consistently more prevalent at 15–16 per 10 000 births in the two most northern continental registries, Northern Netherlands and Odense, Denmark, compared to an average prevalence of 9 per 10 000. There are indications that prevalence decreases the more southerly the registry within continental Europe. Cleft palate, on the other hand, varies much less in prevalence around the average figure of 6.5 per 10 000, and does not show the geographical pattern of cleft lip. Both genetic and environmental differences may underly the geographical patterns, but further research is needed to elucidate this.

THE PREVALENCE OF MULTIPLY MALFORMED CHILDREN

Although it is common to look at the epidemiology of each type of congenital anomaly separately, many children are multiply malformed. Knowing more about the epidemiology of multiply malformed children can be important for treatment, for prenatal diagnosis, and for research into etiology and pathogenesis. Prospectively collected data from registries have a great advantage when analyzing multiple anomalies, since clinical series tend to be biased according to whether the baby survived, or the type of treatment needed. The best definition of a multiply malformed child depends on the purpose of the definition. For epidemiological surveillance purposes, babies with sequences of malformations such as spina bifida with club-foot and Potter sequence, are considered 'isolated' rather than 'multiply malformed', although multiple organs are affected. An analysis of data from 1986 to 1988 gave an average total prevalence of 17 per 10 000 births for multiply malformed children with two or more major anomalies, excluding syndromes, sequences and associations[7]. Figure 3 shows the proportion of cases of a range of different groups of anomalies which were associated with syndromes or were multiply malformed. For some anomalies, such as anophthalmia/microphthalmia, it is quite uncommon for the anomaly to be isolated.

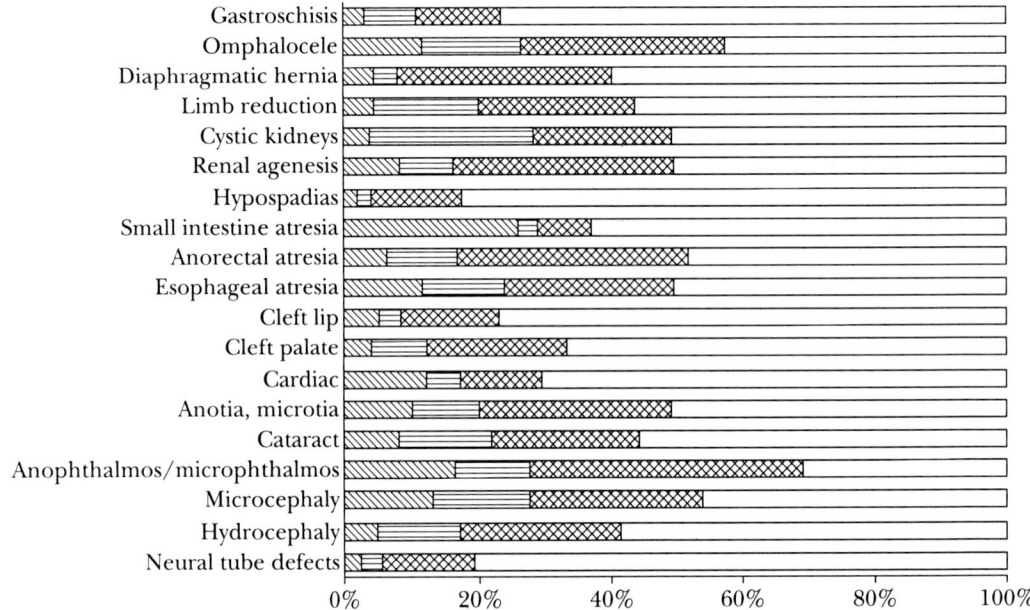

Figure 3 Proportion of cases of selected anomalies associated with syndromes and other major malformations, 1986–88, 15 EUROCAT registries. ▨ Isolated; ▧ multiply malformed; ▤ other syndromes; ▧ chromosomal syndromes

EVALUATION OF PRENATAL DIAGNOSIS

In the absence of primary prevention, it is the policy of most European countries (except Ireland and Malta) to give women the choice of prenatal diagnosis and termination of pregnancy for affected fetuses. Comparisons of the impact of prenatal screening between regions differing in the characteristics of their prenatal screening systems can be helpful in the evaluation of these systems.

In 1991–92, 13 registries were reporting terminations of pregnancy. In these registries an average of 85% of all anencephaly cases, 45% of spina bifida cases, 46% of hydrocephaly (without spina bifida), 50% of bilateral renal agenesis and 43% of omphalocele cases were terminations of pregnancy. There was marked variation between registers, not only in the total proportion of terminations, but also in the timing of prenatal diagnosis and pregnancy termination. A detailed analysis of neural tube defects[8] found that for the period 1984–86, the highest proportions of terminations for spina bifida (40–50%) were recorded in Britain and in France. However, in the two French centers with high termination rates, Paris and Strasbourg, more than one-half of terminations were performed after 28 weeks of pregnancy, whereas in the British centers the majority were performed before 20 weeks of pregnancy. Such differences may have been due to the screening method (at that time, for example, α-fetoprotein screening was only routinely offered in Britain), or to the organization of antenatal care.

Prenatal screening for Down's syndrome is tending to move from using maternal age as a sole indication, to biochemical screening for all ages. Registry data allow appreciation at a population level of the impact in terms of the proportion of terminations in each age group. Figure 4 shows the proportion of terminations among the over 35-years age-group and the under 30-years age-group in three time periods (1980–85, 1986–90, 1991–92), for two registries, Glasgow and Paris[1]. The data show that the proportion of terminations increased greatly over time in

6

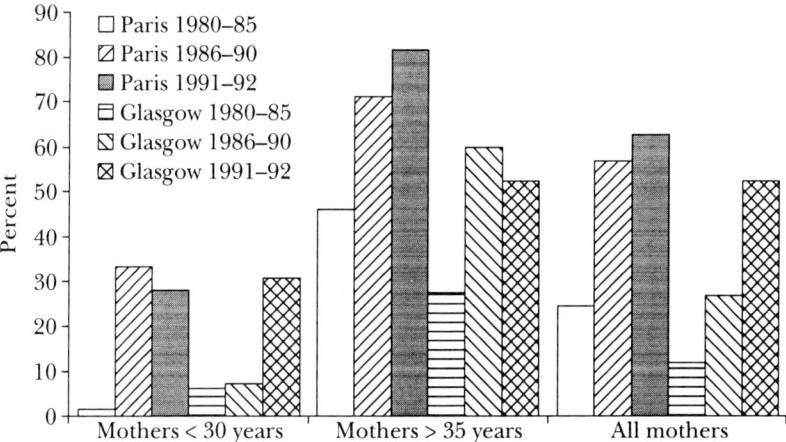

Figure 4 Terminations of pregnancy for Down's syndrome as proportion of all cases diagnosed, in Paris and Glasgow 1980–92

both centers in both age-groups. By 1991–92, the majority of cases in each of these populations were diagnosed prenatally leading to terminations of pregnancy (53% in Glasgow and 63% in Paris). Paris, over the entire 1980–92 period, had almost double the proportion of older mothers (more than 35 years) than Glasgow. Correspondingly, the proportion of all cases (including livebirths, stillbirths and terminations) of Down's syndrome with maternal age of 35 years or more as a risk factor was 56% in Paris, compared to only 34% in Glasgow. It is useful to note that as average maternal age increases, the relative gain from biochemical screening of the entire population may decrease.

Registry data are increasingly used to evaluate the population impact of prenatal screening, to compare against the published results from specialist centers. In order to improve the service at a population level, the reasons for any differences between the population impact and that recorded in specialist centers need to be investigated.

ENVIRONMENTAL RISK FACTORS

One of the major challenges for EUROCAT as a surveillance system was the Chernobyl acci-

dent[9]. Like many environmental issues today, this was a transboundary, international problem, which needed a coordinated response for evaluation. The EUROCAT response concentrated on the prevalence post-Chernobyl of Down's syndrome, and of central nervous system and eye anomalies. No significant increase was found in any registry in the immediate aftermath of Chernobyl (fetuses exposed during the first 2 months after Chernobyl), except a small cluster of four cases of neural tube defects in Odense, where less than one case was expected[10]. For those exposed during the year following Chernobyl, when exposure due to ingestion of radiocesium was rising, there was no consistent increase in prevalence across registries. There are indications, however, that the prevalence of Down's syndrome has been rising since 1988 in some areas, even after taking into account changes in the maternal age structure of the population[11]. These findings for Down's syndrome are opposite to the finding in Berlin of a cluster restricted to births in January 1987, 9 months after Chernobyl[12].

Whether after Chernobyl, or in association with local sources of pollution, it is inevitable by the statistical laws of chance that some communities will have a raised prevalence of congenital anomalies, and this 'cluster' will look as if it is associated with the environmental factor of interest. It is difficult to separate 'true' clusters (i.e. those that reflect the aggregation of a risk factor) from chance clusters, but a surveillance system has an important role in performing a priori evaluations of environmental risk factors, that is, examining health statistics in exposed and unexposed areas, rather than focusing on apparent 'clusters' without regard to the rest of the population. An example is the EUROHAZCON study, involving some of the EUROCAT registers, which is examining the risk of congenital malformation among residents near hazardous waste landfill sites[13].

On the other hand, where clusters are reported or identified during surveillance activities, investigation is important from a public health point of view, despite the possibility that the cluster is a chance occurrence, and despite the often frustrating lack of information and knowledge about the types of exposures that might underly such a cluster. Examples of recent concerns in the UK have been alleged clusters of anophthalmia, and a cluster of limb defects. The EUROCAT network is currently organizing workshops to create guidelines for good practice in investigating clusters of congenital anomalies, and member registries are already active in the response to clusters, whether by providing baseline information for comparison of rates, or by examining a suspected exposure on a more widespread basis[14], or by investigating the cluster itself.

Other environmental risk factors tend to be described according to individual exposure, rather than geographical aggregation. These include drugs and occupational exposures. A large occupational case–control study has been conducted by the collaborative effort of six EUROCAT registries. The results have particularly highlighted the risks of solvent exposure[15], which was found to be associated with an excess 42% risk of all malformations combined, and

was more specifically associated with facial clefts, omphalocele, central nervous system defects, and intestinal atresias.

It has been frequently noted that teratogenic effects of drugs tend to be picked up either by an alert clinician, or, if the relative risk is low, by studies such as case–control studies, but not by routine surveillance. For a new drug to lead to a detectable increase in frequency of a malformation in the population (that is detectable over the 'noise' of changes in diagnosis, definition and ascertainment), a large proportion of the population must be exposed and/or the drug must carry a high relative risk, and/or the drug must lead to one of the outcomes chosen for surveillance, and not a specific and rare anomaly which is lumped into a group with other more frequent anomalies[16]. One of the methods to get round some of these problems is to carry out routine surveillance which looks for associations between routinely recorded drug exposures and specific types of anomaly[17]. Using malformed controls, specific hypotheses can be tested, such as the possible association between ovulation induction and neural tube defects[18]. Surveillance systems can be used for rapid response to help evaluate newly suspected teratogens in scientific or public health terms, such as has been the case with methylene blue, chorionic villus sampling and topical retinoids[19–21].

ACKNOWLEDGEMENTS

The EUROCAT network was established as a concerted action of the BIOMED program of DGXII (Directorate General for Science, Research and Development) of the European Commission, and since 1991 has been funded by DGV, the Directorate for Employment, Industrial Relations and Social Affairs (Health and Safety Directorate).

References

1. EUROCAT Working Group (1995). *EUROCAT Report 6. Surveillance of Congenital Anomalies in Europe 1980–92.* Institute of Hygiene and Epidemiology, Brussels
2. Dolk, H., Goyens, S. and Lechat, M. F. (eds.) (1991). *EUROCAT Registry Descriptions 1979–90.* Report EUR 13615 EN, *Commission of the European Communities*
3. MRC Vitamin Study Research Group (1991). Prevention of neural tube defects: results of the MRC Vitamin Study. *Lancet*, **338**, 131–7
4. Czeizel, A. E. and Dudas, I. (1992). Prevention of first occurrence of neural tube defects by periconceptional vitamin supplementation. *N. Engl. J. Med.*, **327**, 1832–5
5. De Jong van den Berg, L. T. W., Cornel, M., Tymstra, T. and Buitendijk, S. E. (1995). Folate prophylaxis in pregnancy. *Lancet*, **346**, 1227–8
6. de Vigan, C., Raoult, B., Vodovar, V. and Goujard, J. (1996). Prevention de l'anencéphalie et du spina bifida par l'acide folique: situation en région parisienne. *JBEH*, **15**, 69–71
7. EUROCAT Working Group (1991). *EUROCAT Report 4. Surveillance of Congenital Anomalies 1980–1988.* Department of Epidemiology, Catholic University of Louvain
8. EUROCAT Working Group (1991). Prevalence of neural tube defects in 20 regions of Europe and the impact of prenatal diagnosis, 1980–86. *J. Epidemiol. Comm. Health*, **45**, 52–8
9. Dolk, H. and Lechat, M. F. (1993). Health surveillance in Europe: lessons from EUROCAT and Chernobyl. *Int. J. Epidemiol.*, **22**, 363–8
10. EUROCAT Working Group (1988). Preliminary evaluation of the impact of the Chernobyl radiological contamination on the frequency of central nervous system malformations in 18 regions of Europe. *Paediatr. Perinat. Epidemiol.*, **2**, 253–64
11. Longfield, L. (1996). *EUROCAT Registries: Identifying Trends in Down Syndrome Prevalence Rates, 1980–1992.* MSc dissertation, London School of Hygiene and Tropical Medicine
12. Sperling, K., Pelz, J., Wegner, R.-D. *et al.* (1994). Significant increase in trisomy 21 in Berlin nine months after the Chernobyl reactor accident: temporal correlation or causal relation? *Br. Med. J.*, **309**, 158–62
13. Vrijheid, M. and a EUROHAZCON Working Group (1996). Risk of congenital malformation in relation to residence near hazardous waste landfill sites in Europe. *Epidemiology*, July, abstr.
14. Bianchi, F., Calabro, A., Calzolari, E. *et al.* (1994). Clusters of anophthalmia – no link with Benomyl in Italy. *Br. Med. J.*, **308**, 205
15. Cordier, S., Bergeret, A., Ha, M. C. *et al.* (1996). Exposition professionelle aux solvants pendant la grossesse et risque de malformations congenitales. *Arch. Public Health*, **53**, 31, abstr.
16. Khoury, M. J. and Holtzman, N. A. (1987). On the ability of birth defects monitoring to detect new teratogens. *Am. J. Epidemiol.*, **126**, 136–43
17. Cornel, M. C., Erickson, J. D., Khoury, M. J., James, L. M. and Liu, Y. (1996). Population-based birth-defect and risk-factor surveillance: data from the Northern Netherlands. *Int. J. Risk Safety Med.*, **8**, 197–209
18. Cornel, M. C., Ten Kate, L. P., Dukes, M. N. G. *et al.* (1989). Ovulation induction and neural tube defects. *Lancet*, **1**, 1386 (letter)
19. EUROCAT (1991). Holoprosencephaly and exposure to topical retinoids. EUROCAT Newsletter, January
20. EUROCAT (1991). An association between methylene blue, and atresia of the ileum and jejunum. EUROCAT Newsletter, February
21. EUROCAT (1992). Chorionic villus sampling and limb reduction. EUROCAT Newsletter, March

Animal models for endoscopic fetal surgery and early human spin-off

2

J. A. Deprest, M. Miserez, V. Evrard, H. Flageole, N. A. Papadopulos, I. Dumitrascu, K. Vandenberghe, T. E. Lerut and F. Luks

INTRODUCTION

Today, the widespread use of high-resolution ultrasound allows for a more accurate and earlier diagnosis of congenital anomalies. Some of these are amenable to surgical correction, the vast majority being best managed after birth. In a limited number of conditions, however, *in utero* surgery may save the life of the fetus. This can be by correction of the malformation, arresting the progression of the disease, or temporarily treating some of the immediately life-threatening effects of the condition, leaving more definitive treatment for after birth. An international consensus, endorsed by the International Fetal Medicine and Surgery Society, has been reached on the criteria and indications for fetal surgery (Table 1)[1]. Currently only a few conditions meet these criteria. The list may change as prenatal diagnosis, medical technology and pathophysiological insight improves.

Bilateral lower urinary tract obstruction

This sporadic condition affects 1 : 5000–1 : 8000 babies. It leads to hydronephrosis, renal dysplasia and pulmonary hypoplasia, resulting in high fetal and perinatal loss. The diagnosis of lower urinary tract obstruction (LUTO) can

easily be made by ultrasound. At that time, fetal renal function can be assessed by ultrasound criteria for renal dysplasia, by analysis of fetal urine (electrolytes, β-2-microglobulin and urine osmolarity) obtained by serial bladder punctures, and urine output and clearance studies. Antenatal therapy consists of a vesico- or bilateral uretero-amniotic shunt. This has been achieved as effectively by fetoscopic or ultrasound-guided placement of a 'double pigtail' vesical stent, or *in utero* surgical vesicostomy. The goal is not to ablate the posterior urethral valves – usually the primary cause – but to restore urinary flow, to decrease compression and maintain renal function and allow normal pulmonary development. Percutaneous vesico-amniotic shunting is associated with a 5% procedure-related loss, and an overall 48% survival rate. Particularly male fetuses with posterior urethral valves are more likely to benefit from such a procedure (74% survival rate vs. 45% for controls[2]).

Congenital diaphragmatic hernia

Congenital diaphragmatic hernia (CDH) affects 1 : 5000 live-born babies, and is associated

Table 1 Criteria for fetal surgery

Accurate diagnosis and staging possible, with exclusion of associated anomalies
Natural history of the disease is documented, and prognosis established
No current postnatal therapy
In utero surgery has been proven feasible, reversing the deleterious effects of the condition in animal models
Interventions are done in specialized multidisciplinary fetal treatment centers within strict protocols, and after informing the mother and obtaining full consent

with a neonatal mortality of over 60%. The diaphragmatic defect does not challenge the fetus directly, but the associated pulmonary hypoplasia and persistent fetal circulation may be fatal to the neonate. The hypoplasia is due to *in utero* compression of the developing lungs by herniated abdominal viscera. It has been demonstrated that pulmonary hypoplasia can be reversed by *in utero* anatomical repair of the defect[3].

Congenital cystic adenomatoid malformation of the lung

Congenital cystic adenomatoid malformation of the lung (CCAM) is a space-occupying lesion that, if large enough, impairs venous return and leads to hydrops fetalis and/or causes pulmonary hypoplasia. Operative resection during gestation has been done successfully. In other fetuses, ultrasound-guided drainage of cystic parts of the lesion may decrease the compressive effects of the tumor and alleviate the fetal condition.

Sacrococcygeal teratoma

Sacrococcygeal teratoma (SCT) is the most common congenital tumor, and some lead to high output cardiac failure in the fetus, due to the shunting effect of large arteriovenous fistulae in the tumor. This condition may also cause maternal symptoms: some mothers develop a so-called pre-eclamptic 'mirror syndrome' including pulmonary edema, hypertension, and proteinuria. *In utero* resection may be of benefit to the fetus and the mother in selected cases, particularly when the diagnosis is made prior to viability. However, the vast majority are treated after birth[4].

FETAL SURGERY: OPEN APPROACH AND OPERATIVE FETOSCOPY

So far, fetal surgical interventions have only been performed in a few centers around the world[4,5]. Procedures are done under general endotracheal maternal anesthesia, providing also fetal anesthesia. Halogenated anesthetic gases are myorelaxants and suppress uterine contractility. The uterus is exposed by a large laparotomy and opened with a special stapling technique. The fetus is partially exteriorized or exposed without exteriorization, monitored and the actual surgery is done. Postoperative tocolysis includes ritodrine, magnesium sulphate, indomethacin or nitric oxide (NO). Delivery by Cesarean section is mandatory. However, the extreme invasiveness of the currently available 'open' approach has been a major drawback for antenatal surgery. All mothers experienced pre-term uterine contractions, leading to fetal loss by preterm labor in a substantial number of cases. Fetal mortality remains high, mainly due to the inability to control preterm labor, rather than to technical restrictions of operating on such frail patients. In the survivors, the surgery could prevent or slow down organ failure. Of the six patients with LUTO, pulmonary hypoplasia could be avoided in four. For CDH patients, more than half of the fetuses died perioperatively. All six survivors in the San Franciso experience were born prematurely and experienced some degree of respiratory distress, which was fatal in two[6]. The most gratifying experience has been with CCAM: five of seven operated fetuses survived until birth, without pulmonary hypoplasia[7].

The current expansion of video-endoscopic surgery, together with years of experience with fetoscopy, has paved the way for the concept of endoscopic fetal surgery[8]. The fetus, after all, is the type of patient who might benefit most from a minimally invasive approach. Key-hole access may overcome the main problem of open fetal surgery, by avoiding preterm labor triggered by a large uterine incision, or by cooling and dehydration of the fetus due to its exposure. This pathway is currently being explored in animal models, such as the fetal lamb and the non-human primate. Today, spin-off from that research and technology has materialized in procedures on the placenta and the membranes, such as fetoscopic cord ligation and neodymium:yttrium-aluminium-garnet (Nd:YAG) laser coagulation of chorionic vessels in twin–twin transfusion syndrome in a substantial number of cases. Incidentally, chorangioma, teratoma and LUTO have been named as an indication for operative fetoscopy, underlining how endoscopic modifications may offer new hope to fetal surgery.

The fetal lamb model for endoscopic fetal surgery

The ovine model has been widely used for fetal physiology and surgical experimentation. In order to study the feasibility of an endoscopic surgical approach, we developed a model in the pregnant ewe. Endoscopic access to the uterine cavity requires a small diameter, leak-proof, atraumatic cannula. Ultra-short soft-tipped balloon cannulas were therefore designed, which also prevent separation of the amniotic membranes during surgery[9]. In contrast to adult endoscopy, working space is not created by CO_2 because it has detrimental effects on the fetus[10]. Therefore, amnio-infusion with Hartmann solution at body temperature is used, to avoid fetal hypothermia, dehydration and acidosis. This medium has been shown to be safe[11–13], as long as amniodistention is done at amniotic pressure below 20 mmHg[14]. In such conditions we were able to work for up to 3 h without immediate fetal side-effects[15]. The potential for direct influence of the mode of entry or the actual surgery on vital fetal parameters has prompted the need for fetal surveillance devices. An adapted intra-amniotic temperature probe, a special pulse oximetry probe to be placed around a fetal limb, and an amniotic pressure transducer were used. Another safety aspect was that we could exclude fetal retinal injury due to bright light exposure[16]. Instrumentation adapted to the fetal size and the distention medium, which can conduct electrosurgical current, was developed. Small diameter instruments are preferred, which can maneuver around the fetus avoiding fetal trauma. A special bipolar coagulation and cutting device, or laser fibers, are used instead of conventional monopolar surgical instruments. The endoscopes used initially were 2.3–4.5 mm rod lens telescopes, but today small 0.5–2 mm fiber endoscopes are available (Karl Storz Endoskope, Tuttlingen, Germany) are used.

We also demonstrated the feasibility of fetoscopy-guided fetal endoscopy in an animal model[9]. With a 3 mm steerable endoscope, and subsequently with the 1.2 mm fiberoscope, we could access the fetal foregut *in vivo*. This technique may be an interesting research tool for gastrointestinal and pulmonary pathophysiology studies. One of the most tempting applications is fetal tracheoscopy-guided temporary tracheal obstruction.

Experimental endoscopic surgical procedures in animal models

Using the above described set-up, we and others have tried to demonstrate the feasibility of intrauterine surgical procedures in the second trimester fetal lamb (85–100 days; term = 145 days). One of the first procedures ever reported was the feasibility of intrauterine endoscopic suturing in a cleft-lip model[17]. We performed a formal surgical trial of the endoscopic creation of a lower urinary tract obstruction in early and late second trimester[15]. This procedure included dissection and ligation of delicate structures such as the urachus in the umbilical cord and the penile and abdominal urethra. Fetal survival rates of the endoscopic procedure were higher than after a similar open procedure[18]. A comparable setting has also been used to place a transabdominal stent into the fetal bladder, which could salvage renal function in cases of urinary tract obstruction[19].

The bulk of research today focuses on the treatment of congenital diaphragmatic hernia. Because of the poor outcome of anatomic *in utero* repair, another therapeutic approach is needed. An interesting alternative pathway would be the creation of a tracheal obstruction, leading to impressive lung growth and pulmonary hyperplasia, and a parallel growth of the vasculature. The pulmonary expansion gradually reduces the fetal viscera, particularly the liver, into the abdominal cavity. This pulmonary growth, in theory, should avoid the most critical neonatal problem and a formal hernia repair can be delayed until the condition of the neonate is sufficiently stable[20].

Many teams are now exploring this new approach, including the fetoscopic modification of such a procedure. In our center we have been using the fetal tracheoscopy technique to place a detachable balloon by complete endoscopic access, serving as an endotracheal 'plug'[21]. The tracheal obstruction results in reactive pulmonary hyperplasia, as demonstrated by morphometry and DNA analysis[22]. Others have also been working on tracheal obstruction techniques, using clips or endotracheal stents[23,24]. However, permanent tracheal obstruction in sheep seems to be associated with poor pulmonary maturation. An essential component for adequate respiratory function is surfactant, which reduces surface tension at the alveolar–capillary interface. *In utero* tracheal obstruction causes pulmonary growth, but decreases the number of type II pneumocytes[25,26]. Despite this, *in utero* 'unplugging' may solve this problem. We demonstrated that lambs that were obstructed for at least 2 weeks, and unplugged for at least 3 weeks prior to birth, had normal size lungs., with normal type II pneumocyte counts, suggesting normal maturation[27].

This observation may have significant implications in terms of the technique used for tracheal obstruction. The balloon obstruction device has many advantages, not only because it can be positioned completely endoscopically, but also because it can be punctured under ultrasound guidance when reversal of the obstruction is desired. However, many more questions remain, such as the potential side-effects to the fetal trachea, neonatal pulmonary function, vascularization and compliance.

Non-human primate model

One of the most significant problems of open fetal surgery is the occurrence of postoperative uterine activity, requiring massive doses of tocolytics, sometimes with significant maternal side-effects, thus limiting the widespread use of open fetal surgery[28]. The ovine model is very resistant to postoperative preterm contractions. Non-human primate models are much better in this respect. To test the hypothesis that endoscopic access to the uterine activity is associated with less uterine activity than after hysterotomy, we studied the myometrial activity in mid-trimester Rhesus monkeys (*Macaca mulatta*). A typical triple cannulation of the uterine cavity was made and the cannula left in position for 60 min. No significant postoperative premature contractions could be demonstrated, sharply in contrast to the uterine irritability following hysterotomy[29,30]. This observation has meanwhile been confirmed in humans, from the widespread clinical experience with operative fetoscopy on the cord and placenta.

Early human experience in typical indications for fetal surgery

There have been a few case reports of the successful use of endoscopy for typical indications for *in utero* surgery on the fetus. The first endoscopic vesicostomy was made in 1992 by MacMahon and colleagues[31]. At 17.5 weeks they could realize a functional bladder drainage, using a 3 mm endoscope. It closed by 33 weeks. The baby was born with a prune belly, but had normal renal function. Quintero and associates more recently suggested performing *in utero* cystoscopy to diagnose and treat LUTO. A thin flexible endoscope was passed through the lumen of a needle to observe the fetal bladder and ureters. He also ablated posterior urethral valves in a 24-week-old fetus, restoring urethral patency, but the fetus later died[32]. Whether fetal cystoscopy will contribute to a better selection of unborn patients amenable for *in utero* correction, or to guide procedures, remains to be proven.

In a recent report, Nd : YAG laser coagulation was used to treat a hydropic fetus with CCAM at 21 and 23 weeks. The tumor, however, was not completely destroyed[33]. Similarly, a laser was used by Hecher and Hackelöer[34] to reduce the flow within a SCT of a mid-trimester fetus. The procedure had to be repeated twice. The procedures described in these reports do not necessarily mimic the typical open surgical procedures. The laser vesicostomy more nearly approaches the open procedure, but the coagulation of urethral valves, lung tumor, or arteriovenous fistulae are significantly different. However, they all aim to reverse the deleterious *in utero* effects of the congenital anomalies. Therefore they merit further investigation, experimentation and perhaps application in well-selected cases.

The most challenging indication remains CDH. Endoscopy may in the future make the biggest contribution for this indication. *In utero* tracheal obstruction has already been attempted through open access. Harrison and colleagues treated eight fetuses that could not benefit from *in utero* anatomical repair[35]. He managed fetuses of 24–28 weeks, who had, together with other viscera, their liver herniating in the thorax. Liver herniation is known to be a poor prognostic factor, and actually precludes anatomical repair, as the reduction of the liver acutely impairs venous return. The fetuses did undergo tracheal obstruction either by a polymeric plug, or by clips. In four out of eight this led to the desired pulmonary response. Six were live-born, but only three survived the immediate neonatal period. Unhappily, one baby died of unrelated causes, and another baby developed a hydrocephalus, leaving only one survivor. Although at first glance these are not impressive results, one has to remember that this series included the worst subgroup of CDH patients (with herniated liver). Many of the technical problems quoted in the paper have been or will

be overcome. It also seems reasonable to expect that this procedure will be feasible by endoscopic approach, which may lead to better results. Further, endoscopy may be used to achieve other obstruction techniques, which are currently being explored in all their aspects in the animal laboratory.

CONCLUSION

The development of animal models for fetal surgery is a necessary step in the development of fetal endoscopic surgery. Models are currently being used to explore the new horizons of fetal surgery. The instruments and expertise developed have helped to improve human fetoscopic procedures on the cord and placenta, and, more recently, novel procedures on fetuses with surgical conditions.

ACKNOWLEDGEMENTS

The current research team is deeply indebted to Ivan Laermans and Rosita Kinart, biotechnicians at the Center for Surgical Technologies, for excellent care of the animals. We further acknowledge Gerard Barki and Mrs Storz-Reling from Karl Storz Endoskope, and David Russell and Piet Wuyckens from Cook for kindly providing and helping us with current and new instrumentation. This research was supported, in part, by the Belgian Council for Scientific Research, N.F.W.O. Grant no. 3.0122.94 and 3.0191.96 and by the Research Council of the KU Leuven.

References

1. Harrison, M. R. (1991). Professional considerations in fetal treatment. In Harrison, M. R., Golbus, M. S. and Filly, R. A. (eds.) *The Unborn Patient*, pp. 8–13. (Philadelphia: W. B. Saunders)

2. Nakayama, D. K., Harrison, M. R. and Delorimier, A. A. (1986). Prognosis of posterior urethral valves present at birth. *J. Pediatr. Surg.*, **21**, 43

3. Harrison, M. R., Adzick, N. S. and Flake, A. W. (1994). Congenital diaphragmatic hernia: an unsolved problem. *J. Am. Med. Assoc.*, **271**, 382–4

4. Harrison, M. R. and Adzick, N. S. (1991). The fetus as a patient. Surgical considerations. *Ann. Surg.*, **213**, 279–91

5. Bargy, F. and Sapin, E. (1992). La chirurgie foetale: pour quoi faire? *Pédiatrie*, **47**, 347–50

6. Harrison, M. R., Adzick, N. S., Flake, A. W. *et al.* (1993). Correction of diaphragmatic hernia *in utero*. VI. Hard-earned lessons. *J. Pediatr. Surg.,* **28**, 1411–18

7. Adzick, N. S., Harrison, M. R., Flake, A. W. *et al.* (1993). Fetal surgery for cystic adenomatoid malformation of the lung. *J. Pediatr. Surg.,* **28**, 806–812

8. Rodeck, C. H. (1980). Fetoscopy guided by real-time ultrasound for pure fetal blood samples, fetal skin samples and examination of the fetus *in utero. Br. J. Obstet. Gynaecol.,* **87**, 449–56

9. Luks, F. I., Deprest, J. A., Vandenberghe, K. *et al.* (1994). Fetoscopy-guided fetal endoscopy in a sheep model. *J. Am. Coll. Surg.,* **178**, 609–12

10. Luks, F. I., Deprest, J. A., Marcus, M. *et al.* (1994). Carbon dioxide pneumamnios causes acidosis in the fetal lamb. *Fetal Diagn. Ther.,* **9**, 101–4

11. Fisk, N. M., Giussani, D. A., Parkes, M. J. *et al.* (1991). Amnioinfusion increases amniotic pressure in pregnant sheep but does not alter fetal acid base status. *Am. J. Obstet. Gynecol.,* **165**, 1459–63

12. Fisk, N. M., Ronderos-Dumit, D., Soliani, A. *et al.* (1991). Diagnostic and therapeutic transabdominal aminoinfusion in oligohydramnios. *Obstet. Gynecol.,* **78**, 270–8

13. Evrard, V., Deprest, J., Luks, F., Peers, K., Van Ballaer, P., Lerut, T. and Vandenberghe, K. (1997). Amnio-infusion with Hartmann's solution: a safe distension medium for endoscopic fetal surgery in the ovine model. *Fetal Diagn. Ther.,* in press

14. Skarsgard, E. D., Bealer, J. F., Meuli, M., Adzick, N. S. and Harrison, M. R. (1995). Fetal endoscopic surgery: the relationship between insufflation pressure and the fetoplacental circulation. *J. Pediatr. Surg.,* **30**, 1165–8

15. Deprest, J. A., Luks, F. J., Peers, K. H. E. *et al.* (1995). Intrauterine endoscopic creation of urinary tract obstruction in the fetal lamb: a model for fetal surgery. *Am. J. Obstet. Gynecol.,* **172**, 1422–6

16. Deprest, J. A., Luks, F. J., Peers, K. H. *et al.* (1995). Intra-uterine exposure to video-endoscopic light in the fetal lamb. *Am. J. Obstet. Gynecol.,* **172**, 427 (Abstr.)

17. Jennings, R. W., Adzick, N. S., Longaker, M. T. *et al.* (1992). New techniques in fetal surgery. *J. Pediatr. Surg.,* **27**, 1329–33

18. Bussières, L., Wieckowski, J., Révillon, Y., Chourrout, Y., Sachs, C. and Laborde, K. (1993). Creation of experimental urethral obstruction *in utero:* evaluation of fetal renal function. *Eur. J. Pediatr. Surg.,* **3**, 161–5

19. Estes, J. M., MacGillivary, T. E., Hedrick, M. H. *et al.* (1992). Fetoscopic surgery for the treatment of congenital anomalies. *J. Pediatr. Surg.,* **27**, 950–4

20. DiFiore, J. W., Fauz, D. O., Slavin, R. *et al.* (1994). Experimental fetal tracheal ligation reverses the structural and physiological effects of pulmonary hypoplasia in CDH. *J. Pediatr. Surg.,* **29**, 248–57

21. Deprest, J. A., Evrard, V. A., Ban Ballaer, P. P., Verbeken, E., Vandenberghe, K., Lerut, T. E. and Flageole, H. (1997). Tracheoscopic endoluminal plugging using an inflatable device in the fetal lamb model. *Eur. J. Obstet. Gynaecol. Reprod. Biol.,* in press

22. Flageole, H., Evrard, V. A., Vandenberghe, K. *et al.* (1997). Tracheoscopic tracheal occlusion in the ovine model: possible application in congenital diaphragmatic hernia. *J. Pediatr. Surg.,* in press

23. Skarsgard, F. D., Meuli, M., VanderWall, K. J. *et al.* (1996). Fetal endoscopic tracheal occlusion (Fetendo-PLUG) for congenital diaphragmatic hernia. *J. Pediatr. Surg.,* **31**, 1335–8

24. Luks, F. I., Gilchrist, B. F., Jackson, B. T. and Piasecki, G. J. (1995). Endoscopic tracheal obstruction with an expanding device in a fetal lamb model: preliminary considerations. *Fetal Diagn. Ther.,* **11**, 67–71

25. Benachi, A., Bourbon, J., Delezoide, A. L. *et al.* (1996). La technique PLUG dans le traitement des hernies de coupole diaphragmatique: bénéfique ou délétère? *Méd. Foct. Echo. Gynécol.,* **27**, 25–9

26. O'Toole, S. J., Karamnaoukian, H. L., Williams, D. L. *et al.* (1996). *In utero* lung distension decreases surfactant protein gene expression. *Am. J. Resp. Crit. Care Med.,* **153**, A641

27. Flageole, H., Evrard, V. A., Piedboeuf, J. M. *et al.* (1997). The plug-unplug sequence: an important step to achieve type II pneumocyte maturation in the fetal lamb model. To be presented at the American Pediatric Surgery Association, Naples (FI), May. Submitted to *J. Pediatr. Surg.,* in press

28. Adzick, N. S. and Harrison, M. R. (1994). Fetal surgical therapy. *Lancet,* **343**, 897–902

29. Nakayama, D. K., Harrison, M. R., Seron-Ferre, M. and Villa, R. L. (1984). Fetal surgery in the primate II. Uterine electromyographic response to operative procedures and pharmacologic agents. *J. Pediatr. Surg.,* **19**, 333–9

30. van der Wildt, B., Luks, F. I., Steegers, E. A. P., Deprest, J. and Peers, K. H. (1995). Absence of electrical uterine activity after endoscopic access for fetal surgery in the Rhesus Monkey. *Eur. J. Obstet. Gynecol. Reprod. Biol.,* **58**, 213–14

31. MacMahon, R. A., Renou, P. M. M., Shekelton, P. A. and Paterson, P. J. (1992). *In utero* cystostomy. *Lancet*, **340**, 234

32. Quintero, R. A., Hume, R., Smith, C. *et al.* (1995). Percutaneous fetal cystoscopy and endoscopic fulguration of posterior urethral valves. *Am. J. Obstet. Gynecol.*, **172**, 206

33. Fortunato, S. J., Lombardi, S. J., Daniell, J. F. *et al.* (1997). Intra-uterine laser ablation of a fetal CCAM: with hydrops. *Am. J. Obstet. Gynecol.*, **176**, S84 (Abstr.)

34. Hecher, K. and Hackelöer, B.-J. (1996). Intra-uterine endoscopic laser surgery for fetal sacrococcygeal teratoma. *Lancet*, **347**, 470

35. Harrison, M. R., Adzick, N. S., Flake, A. W. *et al.* (1996). Correction of congenital diaphragmatic hernia *in utero*. VIII: Response of the hypoplastic lung to tracheal occlusion. *J. Pediatr. Surg.*, **31**, 1339–48

Immunological aspects of implantation 3

Y. W. Loke

INTRODUCTION

An important event in implantation is invasion of the uterine decidua by large numbers of placental trophoblast cells. These trophoblast cells fulfill a very important role which is to modify the walls of the decidual spiral arteries, converting them from muscular vessels into flaccid sac-like structures no longer responsive to vasoactive stimuli. This vascular transformation is essential to allow an adequate blood supply to be delivered to the rapidly growing fetoplacental unit. Failure of this process will result in a variety of pathological clinical syndromes such as infertility, miscarriage, intrauterine growth retardation (IUGR) and pre-eclamptic toxemia (PET), depending on the severity and stage of gestation when it occurs. The recent epidemiological observations that growth-retarded babies suffer from a higher incidence of diabetes and heart disease in later life suggest that inadequate development of certain organ systems in intrauterine life can also have long-term consequences. Thus, it would be important to elucidate how trophoblast migration into decidua is controlled. At present, this is not known. Because these trophoblast cells are fetally-derived and therefore foreign to the mother, it is expected that there may be some immunological recognition by the mother that could influence the migration. For this reason, reproductive immunologists are very interested in the type of immune response which may be generated locally in the uterus against trophoblast. Intriguingly, evidence to date has revealed that this uterine immune response is not the same as that encountered in classical transplantation immunology[1]. There are fundamental differences occurring in both the trophoblast and the uterus. On the trophoblast side, it is now established that the HLA antigens expressed by trophoblast are not the same as those expressed by other somatic cells. On the uterine side, the mucosa of this organ is populated by cells of the innate immune system, such as natural killer (NK) cells, rather than T and B lymphocytes characteristic of the specific acquired immune response. Thus, the immunological interaction between trophoblast and the uterus appears to be unique.

TROPHOBLAST EXPRESSION OF HLA CLASS I ANTIGENS

The genes potentially most important in initiating a maternal immune response to trophoblast are those of the major histocompatibility complex (MHC), which in humans are known as human leukocyte antigens (HLA). It is now generally accepted that extravillous trophoblast (EVT), the population that migrates into decidua during implantation, expresses the non-classical HLA-G. There is evidence for the presence of both HLA-G mRNA[2,3] and protein[4,5] in these cells. Although low levels of HLA-G message have been detected in a variety of cell types besides trophoblast, such as fetal eye, fetal thymus[6], fetal liver[7], circulating T and B cells[8] and even adult skin biopsies[9], a recent study with an HLA-G-specific antibody has localized the protein only in EVT[5]. Thus, it seems that expression of the HLA-G antigen is restricted to this trophoblast population. The HLA-G protein exists in several isoforms probably resulting from differential splicing[10]. In addition, soluble as well as membrane forms have been observed[11].

17

The function of HLA-G is unknown. It is relatively non-polymorphic at the genetic and protein level. Although a number of sequence variations in the HLA-G gene which could result in amino-acid substitutions have been reported in different individuals[12], only one of these variations is actually at a functional residue of the peptide binding groove[13]. Therefore, unlike the classical class I genes, polymorphism of HLA-G does not appear to be selected for peptide-binding diversity which implies that it has probably not evolved for classical T-cell interaction. Furthermore, the finding that HLA-G antigen is not expressed in the fetal thymus where T-cell education takes place further supports the conclusion that HLA-G is not involved in influencing the T-cell repertoire. We believe that HLA-G expressed by EVT functions as a target molecule for decidual natural killer (NK) cells rather than T cells[14,15]. However, the HLA-G molecule is capable of binding endogenous nonapeptides in the same way as classical class I molecules[16]. The peptide may merely enhance the stability of the class I molecule at the cell surface, but the possibility that it can also interact with T cells should not be entirely dismissed.

The potential role of HLA class I antigens in trophoblast-decidual NK interaction is further complicated by the finding that EVT appears to express another class I molecule besides HLA-G[17]. The identity of this molecule has been much debated, but the accumulative evidence indicates that it is probably HLA-C[18]. For a classical class I antigen, HLA-C is rather unusual and differs from HLA-A and -B in having a relatively low surface expression and being less polymorphic. Because of these characteristics, the importance of HLA-C in interacting with T cells has been questioned. Again, as for HLA-G, we believe that HLA-C expressed by EVT is recognized by decidual NK cells[1].

DECIDUAL NATURAL KILLER CELLS

The most abundant lymphoid cells in decidua are NK cells which comprise about 70% of the total population with macrophages making up 20% and T lymphocytes 10%[19]. There are insig-nificant numbers of B lymphocytes, and granulocytes are absent. The majority of the NK cells have prominent cytoplasmic granules which have led to their being called large granular lymphocytes (LGLs). The number of these NK cells is low in the proliferative stage of the menstrual cycle, gradually increases during the mid-luteal phase and reaches a peak in the late secretory phase. They will show signs of apoptosis a few days before menstruation. However, if pregnancy occurs, their number increases during the early stages of pregnancy, particularly in the decidua basalis, and then declines in the second trimester. Immunohistological studies have demonstrated these NK cells to be in close proximity to the invading trophoblast cells at the implantation site. This temporal and spatial association between decidual NK cells and EVT suggests a functional interaction between these two cell types.

Phenotypic analysis has revealed major differences between decidual NK cells and NK cells from peripheral blood, such as the expression of the NK cell marker, CD56 and the FcγRIII, CD16. In blood, 90% of the NK cells are $CD56^{dim}$ $CD16^{bright}$ and only 10% are $CD56^{bright}$ and $CD16^{dim}$. In contrast, in the uterus the majority of NK cells are $CD56^{bright}$ $CD16^-$. In addition, CD57, another marker for adult NK cells, is also not expressed by decidual NK cells. It would seem, therefore, that decidual NK cells probably represent a subpopulation of the NK-cell family which is restricted to the uterus.

The ontogeny of decidual NK cells is unclear. Two possible differentiation pathways can be proposed[1]. Decidual NK cells could have arisen from a common NK cell progenitor as those in blood, but have subsequently undergone tissue-specific differentiation under the influence of some uterine signal resulting in a unique phenotype. Alternatively, decidual NK cells may represent a distinct population which has split off early in its differentiation pathway from that in blood to settle in the uterus.

The variation in number of NK cells over the menstrual cycle and in pregnancy suggests their recruitment/maintenance is likely to be under hormonal control, but the identity of the stimulus is not known. Decidual NK cells do not express estrogen, progesterone or prolactin receptors. They do express the intermediate affinity p75 and the high affinity p55 interleukin (IL)-2R[20], and they have been observed to proliferate in the presence of IL-2 *in vitro*[21]. However, IL-2 has not been localized in decidua *in vivo*[1], and also IL-2 transforms decidual NK cells into powerful lymphokine-activated killer (LAK) cells which are capable of killing trophoblast cells *in vitro*[22], so this cytokine is unlikely to have a physiological role to play. The search is now on for a cytokine which can induce proliferation in decidual NK cells without transforming them into LAK cells *in vitro*, and which is demonstrable in uterine tissues *in vivo*.

TROPHOBLAST–DECIDUAL NK CELL INTERACTION

Although we have proposed that trophoblast invasion of the uterus during the process of implantation is controlled by decidual NK cells interacting with trophoblast HLA-G/HLA-C, elucidation of the exact mechanism of this interaction has proved elusive. This is because, compared to T cells, little is known about NK-cell biology, NK-cell target molecules, the NK-cell receptors and the outcome of any interaction between NK cells and target cells.

However, it is now generally accepted that NK cells preferentially kill target cells which have low or absent HLA class I antigen expression. This observation had led to the formulation of the 'missing self' hypothesis, which postulated that NK cells eliminated cells lacking class I molecules, in contrast to T cells which kill cells bearing foreign class I antigens. Thus the presence of class I molecules on target cells prevents NK-mediated lysis[23]. The situation has since become more complex as it is now apparent that NK cells can discriminate between different class I alleles, although they do not detect fine polymorphic differences like T cells. Instead, NK cells appear to recognize a public, perhaps primordial, polymorphism in class I molecules. A family of human NK receptors

which do recognise HLA class I antigens has recently been identified, the p58 (NKAT) family of receptors for Cw3/Cw4 and related alleles[24]. These are now designated killer inhibitory receptors (KIR). Each NK cell can express several different receptors, both KIR which recognize class I molecules, and other receptors of different molecular structure which possibly use target ligands such as oligosaccharides. It seems that this is the way receptor diversity is generated in NK cells rather than by somatic recombination of a single receptor as used by T and B cells. Expression of different combinations of these receptors on each NK cell will determine its repertoire[25]. Furthermore, the NK repertoire in blood NK cells varies between different individuals with the intriguing observation that KIR which have specificity for non-self class I molecules may occur[24]. These recent findings raise the fascinating possibility that maternal allorecognition of the fetus does occur, but it is mediated in a completely novel manner by NK cells rather than a classical allograft reaction mediated by T cells.

In the context of interaction with trophoblast, the expression of HLA-G/HLA-C by trophoblast could influence their susceptibility to decidual NK cell lysis. Exposure of human trophoblast cells to exogenous interferon (IFN)-γ, a cytokine which upregulates class I expression, has been observed to protect trophoblast cells against lysis by IL-2-stimulated decidual NK cells[26]. Similarly, HLA-G transfected into class I-deficient cell lines was found to provide some protection from lysis by freshly isolated decidual NK effectors compared to the parental cell line[27].

The additional possibility that class I signals transmitted to decidual NK cells can affect not only cytotoxicity but also influence other NK-cell function such as cytokine production would need to be explored. Decidual NK cells are known to produce a variety of cytokines and trophoblast expresses appropriate receptors for many of these cytokines. Thus a potential cytokine network may be in place at the implantation site by which decidual NK cells influence trophoblast behavior.

CONCLUSION

From this brief review, it can be seen that the immunological relationship between the implanting placenta and the maternal uterus is not governed by the laws of classical transplantation immunology. Instead, it seems to involve a more primitive defense system whose mechanism of 'self' and non-self' recognition, and the resultant reactions invoked, are more akin to those observed between unrelated invertebrates than between vertebrate allograft and host. This observation has completely altered our conceptual view of the immunology of reproduction.

ACKNOWLEDGEMENTS

Our research is supported by the Medical Research Council, Special Program of Research, Development and Research Training in Human Reproduction, World Health Organization, WellBeing (formerly Birthright), and the Wellcome Trust.

References

1. Loke, Y. W. and King, A. (1995). *Human Implantation: Cell Biology and Immunology*, (Cambridge: Cambridge University Press)
2. Yelavarthi, K. K., Fishback, J. L. and Hunt, J. S. (1991). Analysis of HLA-G mRNA in human placental and extraplacental membrane cells by *in situ* hybridization. *J. Immunol.*, **146**, 2847–54
3. Chumbley, G., King, A., Holmes, N. and Loke, Y. W. (1993). *In situ* hybridisation and Northern blot demonstration of HLA-G mRNA in human trophoblast populations by locus-specific oligonucleotide. *Hum. Immunol.*, **37**, 17–22
4. Kovats, S., Main, E. K., Librach, C., Stubblebine, M., Fisher, S. J. and DeMars, R. (1990). A class I antigen, HLA-G, expressed in human trophoblasts. *Science*, **248**, 220–3
5. Chumbley, G., King, A., Gardner, L., Howlett, S., Holmes, N. and Loke, Y. W. (1994). Generation of an antibody to HLA-G in transgenic mice and demonstration of the tissue reactivity of this antibody. *J. Reprod. Immunol.*, **27**, 173–86
6. Shukla, H., Swaroop, A., Srivastava, R. and Weissman, S. M. (1990). The mRNA of a human class I gene HLA G/HLA 6.0 exhibits a restricted pattern of expression. *Nucleic Acids Res.*, **18**, 2189
7. Houlihan, J. M., Biro, P. A., Fergar-Payne, A., Simpson, K. L. and Holmes, C. H. (1992). Evidence for the expression of non-HLA-A, -B, -C class I genes in the human fetal liver. *J. Immunol.*, **149**, 668–75
8. Kirszenbaum, M., Moreau, P., Gluckman, E., Dausset, J. and Carosella, E. (1994). An alternatively spliced form of HLA-G mRNA in human trophoblasts and evidence for the presence of HLA-G transcripts in adult lymphocytes. *Proc. Natl. Acad. Sci. USA*, **91**, 4209–13
9. Ulbrecht, M., Rehberger, B., Strobel, I., Messer, G., Kind, P., Degitz, K., Bieber, T. and Weiss, E. H. (1994). HLA-G: expression in human keratinocytes *in vitro* and in human skin *in vivo*. *Eur. J. Immunol.*, **24**, 176–80
10. Ishitani, A. and Geraghty, D. E. (1992). Alternative splicing of HLA-G transcripts yields proteins with primary structures resembling both class I and class II antigens. *Proc. Natl. Acad. Sci. USA*, **89**, 1–5
11. Fujii, T., Ishitani, A. and Geraghty, D. E. (1994). A soluble form of the HLA-G antigen is encoded by a messenger ribonucleic acid containing intron 4. *J. Immunol.*, **153**, 5516–24
12. van der Ven, K. and Ober, C. (1994). HLA-G polymorphisms in African Americans. *J. Immunol.*, **153**, 5628–33
13. Parham, P. (1995). Antigen presentation by class I major histocompatibility complex molecules: a context for thinking about HLA-G. *Am. J. Reprod. Immunol.*, **34**, 10–19
14. King, A. and Loke, Y. W. (1991). On the nature and function of human uterine granular lymphocytes. *Immunol. Today*, **12**, 432–5
15. Loke, Y. W. and King, A. (1991). Recent developments in the human maternal–fetal immune interaction. *Curr. Opin. Immunol.*, **3**, 762–6
16. Diehl, M., Münz, C., Keilholz, W., Stevanovic, S., Loke, Y. W., Holmes, N. and Rammensee, H.-G. (1996). Non-classical HLA-G molecules are classical peptide presenters. *Curr. Biol.*, **6**, 305–14
17. Grabowska, A., Carter, N. and Loke, Y. W. (1990). Human trophoblast cells in culture express an unusual major histocompatibility complex class I-like antigen. *Am. J. Reprod. Immunol.*, **23**, 10–18

18. King, A., Boocock, C., Sharkey, A., Gardner, L. and Loke, Y. W. (1996). Evidence for the expression of HLA-C class I mRNA and protein by human first trimester trophoblast. *J. Immunol.*, **156**, 2068–76

19. King, A., Wellings, V., Gardner, L. and Loke, Y. W. (1989). Immunocytochemical characterisation of the unusual large granular lymphocytes in human endometrium throughout the menstrual cycle. *Hum. Immunol.*, **24**, 195–205

20. King, A., Wheeler, R., Carter, N. P., Francis, D. P. and Loke, Y. W. (1992). The response of human decidual leukocytes to IL-2. *Cell. Immunol.*, **140**, 409–21

21. Nishikawa, K., Saito, S., Morii, T., Hamada, K., Ako, H., Narita, N., Ichijo, M., Kurahayashi, M. and Sugamura, K. (1991). Accumulation of CD16⁻ CD56⁺ natural killer cells with high affinity interleukin 2 receptors in human early pregnancy decidua. *Int. Immunol.*, **3**, 743–50

22. King, A. and Loke, Y. W. (1990). Human trophoblast and JEG choriocarcinoma cells are sensitive to lysis by IL-2 stimulated decidual NK cells. *Cell. Immunol.*, **129**, 435–48

23. Ljunggren, H. -G. and Kärre, K. (1990). In search of the 'missing self': MHC molecules and NK cell recognition. *Immunol. Today*, **11**, 237–44

24. Gumperz, J. E. and Parham, P. (1995). The enigma of the natural killer cell. *Nature*, **378**, 245–8

25. Yokoyama, W. M. (1995). Natural killer cell receptors specific for major histocompatability complex class I molecules. *Proc. Natl. Acad. Sci. USA*, **92**, 3081–5

26. King, A. and Loke, Y. W. (1993). Effect of IFN-γ and IFN-α on killing of human trophoblast by decidual LAK cells. *J. Reprod. Immunol.*, **23**, 51–62

27. Chumbley, G., King, A., Robertson, K., Holmes, N. and Loke, Y. W. (1994). Resistance of HLA-G and HLA-A2 transfectants to lysis by decidual NK cells. *Cell. Immunol.*, **155**, 312–22

Ultrasound: assessment of early human life

4

A. Kurjak

INTRODUCTION

Not so long ago, ultrasound in early pregnancy was performed only to detect an ongoing early pregnancy and to prove positive heart action. The introduction of transvaginal sonography has enabled detailed studies of early embryonic development. Adding color Doppler facilities to transvaginal ultrasound, a new diagnostic technique has been developed. This new method has enabled investigation of the functional state of an early embryo and has given new insights into the physiology of early gestation.

PLACENTAL AND EMBRYONIC CIRCULATION

By color Doppler technique, uteroplacental vessels can easily be visualized[1-5]. Pulsed Doppler waveform profiles for uterine arteries are characteristic, comprising a high peak-systolic component with a characteristic notch at the descending slope of the systole and very low end-diastolic flow. Doppler sonograms of the arcuate and radial arteries are very similar – moderate peak-systolic and end-diastolic components of blood flow are seen. A difference is seen in peripheral vascular impedance which is lower in radial than in arcuate arteries. Pulsed Doppler waveform signals obtained from the spiral arteries show low impedance to blood flow and a characteristic spiky outline. This type of waveform is indicative of high turbulence and a tortuous vessel with an irregular wall, which are the features of the spiral arteries. During pregnancy, impedance to blood flow decreases from the main uterine artery to its branches and with advanced gestational age. At the same time,

an increase of blood flow velocity is noticed (Figure 1)[1-5].

The umbilical artery can be located by transvaginal color Doppler sonography even at 6 weeks' gestation[2,3]. By the end of the 10th gestational week there is no end-diastolic component of blood flow. Between the 10th and 14th week, diastolic velocities begin to emerge, but these are incomplete and inconsistently present. There are no significant changes in umbilical artery blood flow until the 12th gestational week, when a significant decrease of vascular impedance is noticed. The anatomical changes in the villous vasculature area, which are characterized by the progressive increment of the number of the villi and the surface area occupied by the fetal vessels, must have a key role in

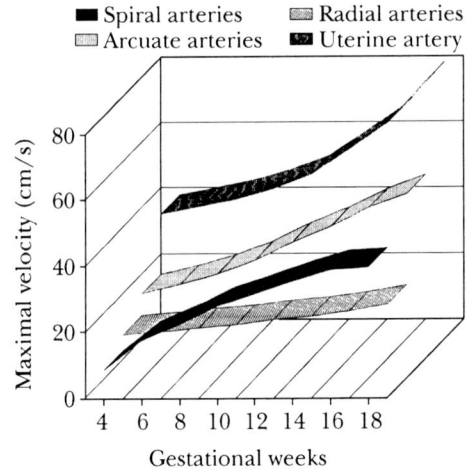

Figure 1 Peak-systolic velocity values in uteroplacental vessels

the gradual fall of blood flow impedance in the umbilical circulation.

Fetal vessels usually analyzed for assessment of fetal well-being are the aorta, carotid arteries and middle cerebral artery. Pulsations from the fetal aorta can be identified as early as the 6th week of gestation. In the fetal aorta, as in the umbilical artery, there are no significant changes of blood flow until the end of the 12th gestational week, when a significant decline of peripheral impedance is noticed. The decrease of peripheral impedance is accompanied with increment of blood flow velocities in all investigated vessels[2,3].

EARLY CEREBRAL CIRCULATION

The intracranial circulation becomes visible as early as the 7th week of gestation[6,7]. At this time discrete pulsations of the internal carotid arteries are detectable at the base of the skull. During the 9th and 10th gestational weeks, color patterns representing blood flow can be visualized in the anterolateral quadrant of the skull base. From the 10th gestational week, arterial pulsations can be detected on transverse section, lateral to the mesencephalon and cephalic flexure.

There are few transvaginal color Doppler studies of cerebral blood flow in early pregnancy[7,8]. In our study[7], middle cerebral artery blood flow was analyzed in 106 pregnant women with gestational ages from 7 to 18 weeks. They were divided into two groups: the first group included 75 clinically normal singleton pregnancies and the second one 31 patients who were admitted to our department because of vaginal bleeding. Seventeen of these complicated pregnancies ended in spontaneous abortion.

A characteristic waveform profile, i.e. a systolic component with absent end-diastolic frequencies, was observed from the 7th to the 11th gestational weeks. The end-diastolic component of the blood flow was inconsistently seen from the 11th to the 13th gestational week, earlier than has been found in other fetal vessels. From the 13th gestational week onwards, end-diastolic flow within the middle cerebral artery was consistently observed. A significant decrease of pulsatility index (PI) was observed in both groups of women and it was present 2 weeks earlier than has been noted in other parts of the fetal circulation. However, there were no significant differences in PI values between normal pregnancies and pregnancies complicated by vaginal bleeding regardless of pregnancy outcomes. Our data are in accordance with the results of the groups of Wladimiroff[9] and Van Zalen-Sprock[8], which also suggest a low vascular impedance in the fetal brain, not dependent on the changes in vascular resistance of the fetal trunk or uteroplacental circulation. In fact, cerebral vessels are a separate hemodynamic system that is independent of the other parts of the fetal circulation from the beginning of the pregnancy. Due to this mechanism, the fetal brain is probably well protected from hypoxia even in early pregnancy. Recently, more sophisticated equipment has enabled us to detect continuous diastolic flow in the middle cerebral artery of embryos between 9 and 10 weeks of gestation.

The fetal choroid plexus plays a large role in brain development. It is proportionally larger than that of an adult human being and fills more of the space of the ventricles. The choroid plexus and arachnoid membrane act together as barriers between the blood and cerebrospinal fluid. In effect, the choroid plexus is like a 'kidney' for the brain[10].

Studies evaluating the choroid plexus blood flow are limited. Our study[11] comprised 103 patients with normal pregnancies between 9 and 16 weeks' gestation. Color flow imaging was used to identify vessels in the cranium and within the choroid plexus. Pulsed Doppler signals were obtained from an internal carotid–middle cerebral artery and from choroid plexus vessels. A major cerebral vessel could be seen at 9 weeks' gestation. Choroid plexus vessels were clearly visualized at 10 weeks and 3 days of gestation. Subtle color and pulsed Doppler signals could be obtained at the inner edge of the lateral ventricle choroid plexus. The pulsed

Doppler waveform profile of choroid plexus blood vessels was characteristic. The systolic component of blood flow within a cardiac cycle was not pronounced, while the slope from the systolic peak until the end of the cycle was very gradual. The end-diastolic component could not be obtained before 12 gestational weeks. Visualization rates range from 35 to 75% for plexus vessels, and 65–100% for cerebral vessels (Figure 2). Visualization of the cerebral vessels improves with each gestational week. Choroid plexus vessels are most easily seen at 13 weeks, and then the visualization rate declines. Visual-

ization of the choroid plexus vessels increases and decreases as the gland develops and shrinks.

A steady decline in resistance and probable increment in flow is visible in cerebral and choroid plexus vessels with advanced gestational age (Figure 3). Our results showed significant flow velocity differences between the large cerebral vessels and small, choroidal vessels.

SUBCHORIONIC HEMATOMA

Subchorionic hematoma is defined sonographically as an echo-free area located between the

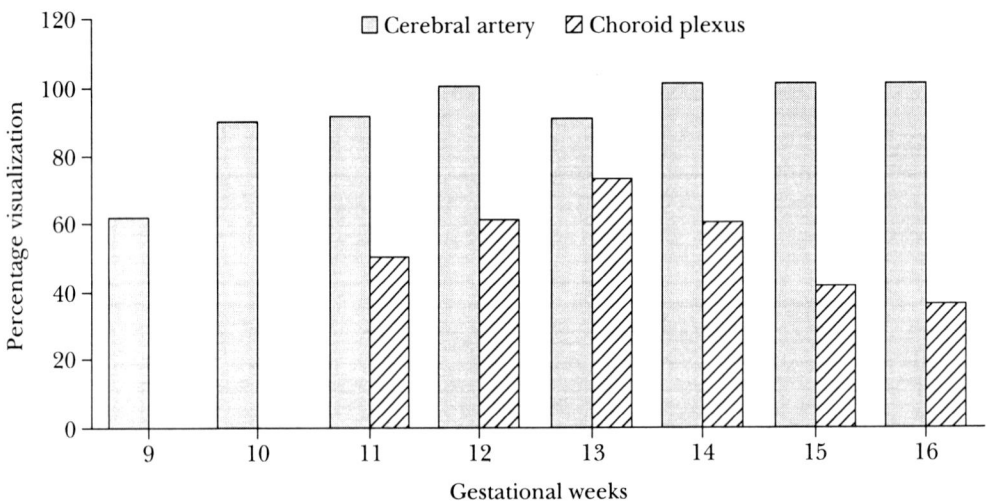

Figure 2   Visualization rate of intracranial vessels with advancing gestational age

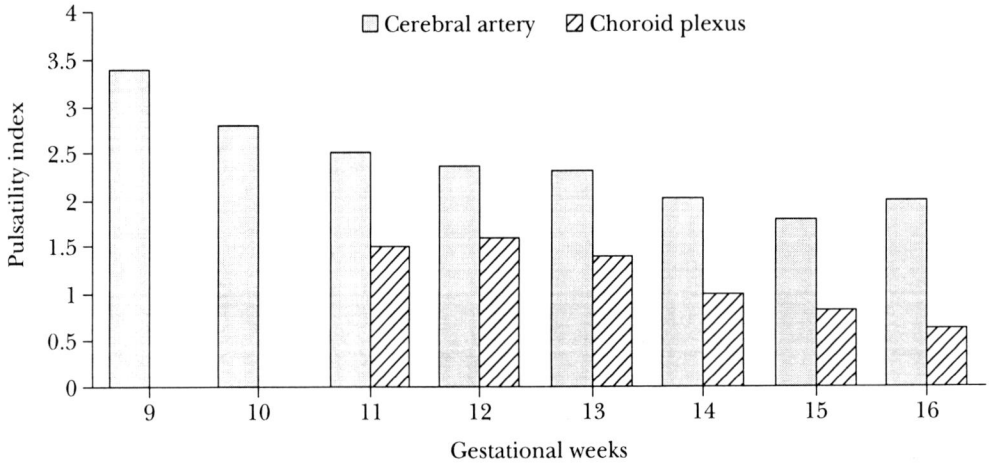

Figure 3   Pulsatility index values of intracranial arteries with advancing gestational age

membranes and the uterine wall. Physiologically, this represents a separation of the chorionic plate from the underlying decidua. The precise cause of subchorionic hematoma is unknown. Postulated associated factors include autoimmune reactions[12], coumarin drugs, or coagulation factor deficiency[13]. Color flow is necessary to confirm this observation because, occasionally, the echo-free black and white image turns out to be a highly vascularized placental site. The purpose of our recent study[14] was to evaluate the correlation between the volume of the hematoma and blood flow parameters, to estimate the frequency of spontaneous abortions and preterm deliveries in a group with subchorionic hematomata and normal pregnancies and to correlate the hematoma site with pregnancy outcome. The study comprised 59 women with vaginal bleeding, closed cervix and ultrasound findings of a living embryo and subchorionic hematoma. The gestational ages ranged from 6 to 14 weeks. More spontaneous abortions occurred in women with subchorionic hematoma, while there was no significant difference in the number of preterm deliveries. There was a positive correlation between hematoma volume and RI, and a negative correlation between hematoma volume and peak systolic velocity, probably as a consequence of mechanical compression of the spiral arteries caused by the hematoma. When pregnancy continued, these indices returned to normal values. The hematoma size did not affect pregnancy outcome, but the site did. There was no significant difference in the number of spontaneous abortions between the patients with small hematomas and those with large ones. Most hematomas associated with abortion were found in the corpus or fundus of the uterus, but not in the supracervical area. Since in most cases this is the region of the placental site, it suggests a possible disruption of placental function.

Transvaginal color and pulsed Doppler have the potential to detect patients with altered spiral artery blood flow who are at increased risk for spontaneous abortion. Furthermore, serial examinations may have a prognostic significance since they offer a direct insight into the pathophysiology of a perigestational hemorrhage. In the presence of a hematoma, the resistance is increased and blood flow is decreased. With continuation of the pregnancy and reabsorption of the hematoma, the impedance to blood flow returns to normal values.

Improvement of blood flow is predictive for normal pregnancy outcome, while decreased spiral artery blood flow indicates risk of loss during the first and second trimesters. Since no increased risk for preterm delivery was found in patients with subchorionic hematomata, it is expected that the elevated impedance to blood flow is a transitory consequence of a compression to the arterial walls by hemorrhage itself. These observations seem to be helpful in the clinical management of patients with vaginal bleeding in early pregnancy.

GESTATIONAL TROPHOBLASTIC DISEASE

Recently, transvaginal color Doppler has been reported as a useful diagnostic tool in the evaluation of gestational trophoblastic disease (GTD)[15,16]. Gestational trophoblastic disease is usually associated with increased vascular supply to the placental tissue. Therefore, color Doppler may be useful in the diagnosis of the myometrial invasion in patients with invasive mole or choriocarcinoma. It seems that presence of increased blood supply within the myometrial portion can be used in diagnosis of early invasion even before it becomes visible on B-mode.

In invasive mole and choriocarcinoma, trophoblastic invasion into myometrial tissue can be recognized as prominent color coded zones in the myometrium[15]. These zones correspond to dilated spiral arteries and newly formed vessels feeding the tumor. Since choriocarcinoma is a malignant tumor, it probably produces its own vessels, contributing to the neovascularization. All of these vessels are characterized by a high-velocity and low-impedance blood flow pattern. In patients with GTD, impedance to blood flow in uteroplacental vessels is significantly lower than in normal pregnancy[16–20]. The highest impedance is obtained in patients with complete mole, whilst the lowest values occur in choriocarcinoma. Table 1 presents peripheral impedance values in the uteroplacental vessels of patients with different types of GTD.

Transvaginal color Doppler is important in the monitoring of patients with GTD during chemotherapy[21,22]. Results showed negative correlation between β-human chorionic gonadotropin (β-hCG) titre and vascular indices in patients with GTD receiving chemotherapy. At the same time color coded spots representing newly formed vessels disappeared. Color Doppler can also be helpful in the differentiation of pathological conditions such as postabortal uterus and other endometrial pathology from GTD[23].

INTERVILLOUS BLOOD FLOW

According to the embryological textbooks, as soon as the blastocyst has implanted, maternal blood enters the future intervillous space bringing the nutrients and oxygen to the rapidly growing embryo. This classic concept has been spread by Hustin and Schaaps who performed perfusion experiments using transvaginal sonography, intervillous hysteroscopy and examination of chorionic villous sampling material[24]. Using all of these techniques, they were unable to demonstrate a true intervillous blood flow during the first 12 weeks. They suggested that during this period the tips of the spiral arteries are obstructed by intravascular trophoblastic plugs and the intervillous space is bathed by a clear fluid, possibly made of filtered plasma and uterine gland secretions. This hypothesis has been supported by the study of perfused hysterectomy specimens showing that, during the first 3 months of gestation, the embryo is totally separated from the maternal circulation by a trophoblastic shell[25]. Recent Doppler studies supported Hustin's theory that intervillous circulation normally becomes established much later in pregnancy than was previously thought[26].

Only in cases of abnormal early pregnancy has the presence of intervillous blood flow been proved before 12 weeks of pregnancy. Jauniaux and colleagues[27] found increased blood flow in the intervillous space in 16 of 23 (70%) complicated pregnancies.

However, most of these early color Doppler studies have used less sensitive equipment and have failed to demonstrate continuous blood flow in the intervillous space in the first 12 weeks. Our group used a new-generation Doppler unit to visualize color signals and obtain velocity waveforms from arterial and venous vessels of the intervillous space in normal early pregnancy.

The study group consisted of 34 patients, between 7 and 12 weeks' gestation, referred to our department because of vaginal bleeding and/or abdominal pain. The diagnosis of missed abortion (22 cases) and anembryonic pregnancy (12 cases) was made by transvaginal sonography with color Doppler imaging. The control group comprised 60 patients with normal intrauterine pregnancy whose gestational ages ranged from 6 to 12 weeks from the last menstrual period. The study was performed using Aloka SSD 2000 equipment (Aloka, Tokyo, Japan) with a transvaginal 5-MHz probe for imaging and 6-MHz pulsed Doppler system for blood flow analysis. Color Doppler was used to visualize blood flow in the uterine artery and its branches (arcuate, radial and spiral arteries) and in the intervillous space (arterial and venous flow). The resistance index (RI) and PI were calculated for arterial signals, while peak systolic velocity measurements were performed for veins of the intervillous space.

Table 1 Mean resistance index values in uteroplacental blood vessels in molar pregnancy

	Uterine artery	Arcuate artery	Radial artery	Spiral artery	Tumor vessels
Normal pregnancy	0.82	0.68	0.52	0.48	—
Hydatidiform mole	0.75	0.62	0.47	0.39	—
Invasive mole and choriocarcinoma	0.66	—	—	—	0.30

Pulsed Doppler signals obtained from intervillous arteries showed low impedance values and a characteristic spiky outline. This type of waveform profile is indicative of a high turbulence and a tortuous vessel with an irregular wall, similar to those obtained from spiral arteries. However, both RI and PI values obtained from the intervillous space were characterized by significantly lower values when compared to the spiral arteries. A continuous intervillous flow was another pattern easily detectable by highly sensitive equipment. These Doppler signals were marked by low velocity up to the 10th week of gestation. With advancing gestation the venous type of signal became stronger and randomly dispersed throughout the placenta. The blood flow velocity obtained from these vessels increased significantly from the 10th gestational week. Conversely, arterial blood flow signals did not demonstrate any difference in terms of blood flow impedance and velocity with advancing gestational age.

Our study, if supported by others, could change the suggested concept of separation of the maternal and embryonic circulation in the first trimester. The fact that we are able to demonstrate continuous circulation in the intervillous spaces in all normal pregnancies may influence our future understanding of early pregnancy physiology.

References

1. Kurjak, A., Zudenigo, D., Funduk-Kurjak, B., Shalan, H., Predanic, M. and Sosic, A. (1993). Transvaginal color Doppler in the assessment of the uteroplacental circulation in normal early pregnancy. *J. Perinat. Med.*, **21**, 25–34

2. Kurjak, A., Zudenigo, D. and Kupesic, S. (1994). Early pregnancy hemodynamics assessed by transvaginal color Doppler. In Kurjak, A. and Chervenak, F. (eds.) *The Fetus as a Patient*, pp. 435–54. (Carnforth: Parthenon Publishing)

3. Kurjak, A., Zudenigo, D., Predanic, M. and Kupesic, S. (1994). Recent advances in the Doppler study of early fetomaternal circulation. *J. Perinat. Med.*, **22**, 419–39

4. Kurjak, A., Kupesic-Urek, S., Predanic, M. and Salihagic, A. (1992). Transvaginal color Doppler assessment of the uteroplacental circulation in normal and abnormal early pregnancy. *Early Hum. Dev.*, **29**, 385–9

5. Jurkovic, D., Jauniaux, E., Kurjak, A., Hustin, J., Campbell, S. and Nicolaides, K. H. (1991). Transvaginal color Doppler assessment of uteroplacental circulation in early pregnancy. *Obstet. Gynecol.*, **77**, 365–9

6. Kurjak, A., Predanic, M. and Predanic, A. (1993). Fetal intracranial circulation. In Kurjak, A. (ed.) *An Atlas of Transvaginal Color Doppler*, pp. 71–83. (Carnforth: Parthenon Publishing)

7. Kurjak, A., Predanic, M., Kupesic-Urek, S., Funduk-Kurjak, B., Demarin, V. and Salihagic, A. (1992). Transvaginal color Doppler study of middle cerebral artery blood flow in early normal and abnormal pregnancy. *Ultrasound Obstet. Gynecol.*, **2**, 424–8

8. Van Zalen-Sprock, M. M., Van Vugt, J. M. G., Colenbrander, G. J. and Geijn, H. P. (1994). First-trimester uteroplacental and fetal blood flow velocity waveforms in normally developing fetuses: a longitudinal study. *Ultrasound Obstet. Gynecol.*, **4**, 284–8

9. Wladimiroff, J. W., Huisman, T. W. A. and Stewart, R. A. (1992). Intracerebral, aortic and umbilical artery flow velocity waveforms in the late first-trimester fetus. *Am. J. Obstet. Gynecol.*, **166**, 46–9

10. Spector, J. and Johanson, C. E. (1989). The mammalian choroid plexus. *Sci. Am.*, **6**, 48–53

11. Kurjak, A., Schulman, H., Predanic, A., Predanic, M., Kupesic, S. and Zalud, I. (1994). Fetal choroid plexus vascularization assessed by color and pulsed Doppler. *J. Ultrasound Med.*, **13**, 841–4

12. Baxi, L. and Pearlstone, M. (1991). Subchorionic hematomas and the presence of auto-antibodies. *Am. J. Obstet. Gynecol.*, **165**, 1423–6

13. Guy, G., Baxi, L. and Chao, C. (1992). An unusual complication in a patient with factor IX deficiency. *Obstet. Gynecol.*, **80**, 502–4

14. Kurjak, A., Schulman, H., Zudenigo, D., Kupesic, S., Kos, M. and Goldenberg, M. (1996). Subchorionic hematomas in early pregnancy: clinical outcome and blood flow patterns. *J. Maternal-Fetal Med.*, **5**, 41–4

15. Kurjak, A., Zalud, I., Salihagic, A., Crvenkovic, G. and Matijevic, R. (1991). Transvaginal color

Doppler in the assessment of abnormal early pregnancy. *J. Perinat. Med.*, **19**, 155–65

16. Kurjak, A., Zalud, I., Predanic, M. and Kupesic, S. (1994). Transvaginal color and pulsed Doppler study of uterine blood flow in the first and early second trimester of pregnancy: normal vs. abnormal. *J. Ultrasound Med.*, **13**, 43–7

17. Jaffe, R. (1993). Investigation of abnormal first trimester gestations by color Doppler imaging. *J. Clin. Ultrasound*, **21**, 521–6

18. Long, M. G., Boultbee, J. E., Begent, R. H., Hanson, M. E. and Bagshave, K. D. (1990). Preliminary Doppler studies on the uterine artery and myometrium in trophoblastic tumors requiring chemotherapy. *Br. J. Obstet. Gynaecol.*, **97**, 686–9

19. Taylor, K. J. W., Schwartz, R. E. and Kohorn, E. I. (1987). Gestational trophoblastic neoplasia: diagnosis with Doppler US. *Radiology*, **165**, 683–7

20. Carter, J., Fowler, J., Carlson, J., Saltzman, A., Byers, L., Carson, L. and Twiggs, L. B. (1993). Transvaginal color flow Doppler sonography in the assessment of gestational trophoblastic disease. *J. Ultrasound Med.*, **12**, 595–9

21. Zanetta, G., Lissoni, A., Colombo, M., Marzola, M., Cappellini, A. and Mangioni, C. (1996). Detection of abnormal intrauterine vascularization by color Doppler imaging: a possible additional aid for the follow up of patients with gestational trophoblastic tumors. *Ultrasound Obstet. Gynecol.*, **7**, 32–7

22. Hsieh, F. J., Wu, C. C., Chen, C. A., Chen, T. M., Hsieh, C. Y. and Chen, H. Y. (1994). Correlation of uterine hemodynamics with chemotherapy response in gestational trophoblastic tumors. *Obstet. Gynecol.*, **83**(6), 1021–5

23. Achiron, R., Goldenberg, M., Lipitz, S. and Mashiach, S. (1993). Transvaginal duplex Doppler ultrasonography in bleeding patients suspected of having residual trophoblastic tissue. *Obstet. Gynecol.*, **81**, 507–11

24. Hustin, J. and Schaaps, J. P. (1987). Echographic and anatomic studies of the maternotrophoblastic border during the first trimester of pregnancy. *Am. J. Obstet. Gynecol.*, **157**, 162–8

25. Hustin, J., Schaaps, J. P. and Lambotte, K. H. (1991). Anatomical studies of the utero-placental circulation in early pregnancy. *Obstet. Gynaecol.*, **77**, 365–9

26. Jauniaux, E., Jurkovic, D., Campbell, S., Kurjak, A. and Hustin, J. (1991). Investigation of placental circulations by color Doppler ultrasound. *Am. J. Obstet. Gynecol.*, **164**, 486–8

27. Jauniaux, E., Jurkovic, D. and Campbell, S. (1994). Doppler of the uteroplacental circulation in normal and complicated early pregnancies. X. *International Congress: The Fetus as a Patient*, Brijuni, *Abstracts*, p.42

Intrauterine growth

J. S. Robinson, J. A. Owens, I. C. McMillen, J. J. Erwich and P. C. Owens

INTRODUCTION

Intrauterine growth of the fetus and its placenta are most often characterized and described in terms of weight or length at birth and in animals at different stages of pregnancy. These measures provide an integration or summary of the many intrinsic and extrinsic factors that, directly or indirectly, influence growth during pregnancy. More accurately, true growth can only be described as a change in any of these measures with time. Mostly, although not exclusively, this has been achieved by serial ultrasound scanning at intervals throughout pregnancy. The deviations from the norm that are more commonly observed clinically are intrauterine growth restriction rather than acceleration of fetal growth, although this may be changing with the increase in the incidence of large or macrosomic babies in affluent societies.

Normal fetal growth is defined as that which is neither significantly restricted nor promoted by extrinsic factors. However, this definition requires refinement, since the maternal environment can be regarded as a component of either the extrinsic or the intrinsic environment of the conceptus. We have chosen to refer to the maternal environment as part of the extrinsic environment, despite clear recognition that successful pregnancy requires an intimate relationship between the mother and the conceptus, which includes an interchange of signals between any combination of the fetus, placenta and the mother. Cytokines, hormones, growth factors and substrates for metabolism all contribute to this exchange[1-3]. These interactions begin even before pregnancy as there is increasing evidence that factors including cytokines in semen prepare the endometrium for pregnancy.

Recently, epidemiological studies have demonstrated that different birth phenotypes, reflecting variable fetal growth, are associated with common adult diseases including hypertension, ischemic heart disease, diabetes mellitus and chronic obstructive airways disease[4]. There are also intriguing suggestions that different birth phenotypes, variations in infant growth, or maternal or fetal disorders during pregnancy affect the incidence of tumors or psychiatric disorders[5-7]. In addition, there are well described associations between antenatal factors such as intrauterine growth restriction, antepartum hemorrhage and malformation with cerebral palsy[8].

In this brief review, we shall concentrate on factors operating before or in early pregnancy that set the trajectory of growth, and those that subsequently restrict or accelerate growth. We shall also outline the evidence that these may alter or program physiological control systems in ways that could set the conditions for later emergence of adult-onset diseases.

BIRTH WEIGHT

Low birth weight is the birth of a human baby with a birth weight of less than 2500 g. More recently introduced terms include very low birth weight (< 1500 g) and extremely low birth weight (< 1000 g). Macrosomia is commonly defined as a birth weight of more than or equal to 4000 g. The incidence of low birth weight ranges from less than 5% in developed to more than 40% in less developed communities around the world[9,10]. Conversely, the incidence of macrosomia is more common in developed societies. Although it has been reported that the incidence of low birth weight has fallen in one developed society[11] (Institute of Medicine, 1990), there is a disturbing increase within one sector of that community, which has been attributed to poverty and increased substance abuse[12].

Over the last 10–20 years, there has been a steady increase in the percentage of babies with macrosomia in Canada and in the United Kingdom[13]. In the latter, the increase in the incidence of macrosomic babies began in England before it emerged in Scotland. In contrast, during the same period, there has been no change in the incidence of macrosomic babies in South Australia, a small community with a higher incidence of macrosomic babies than the United Kingdom[14]. These reports have not included detailed analysis of the factors that may have contributed to these changes in incidence. Factors which need to be considered, however, include an increase in maternal size, weight-for-height, nutrition before and during pregnancy, and the use of drugs such as tobacco[11].

SETTING THE TRAJECTORY OF GROWTH OF THE FETUS

Setting the trajectory of growth of the embryo/fetus involves the sum of several processes in early pregnancy, including genetic or epigenetic phenomena that may determine the growth rate of the embryo and fetus. The epigenetic or genetic drive to growth may be regulated in early pregnancy by the maternal hormonal, cytokine, growth factor or nutrient environment. Variation in the expression of imprinted genes is another potential route by which early events may determine the growth rate of the fetus. Normally, the sum of these events determines the rate of growth for the remainder of pregnancy. Paternal size has only a small influence on fetal size at birth[15], and presumably this is determined through the fetal genome, although seminal factors and the mito-

chondrial genome from sperm may also have to be considered.

It is well known that maternal size is a major factor that determines the size of the fetus. The effect of maternal size on growth of the fetus was first demonstrated by the classic experiments in Shetland and Shire horses of Walton and Hammond[16]. Similar observations have been made in a number of species, and, to remove the effects of the fetal genome, by embryo transfer experiments. These experiments showed that the maternal environment sets the trajectory of growth of the fetus so that its size at birth is less than, or exceeds, the normal growth of the fetus in its natural mother. A more extreme example of the latter occurs with advanced reproductive technologies in domestic animals where *in vitro* culture of the embryo, and, hence initial development in the absence of maternal influences, results in a significant proportion of excessively grown fetuses. This occurs to the extent that it has inhibited use of these technologies to rapidly increase selected strains of animals[17].

In vitro culture of ovine, caprine or bovine embryos in simple media supplemented with serum can increase size at birth to an extreme degree. In sheep, a birth weight of 11 kg has been observed and the mean birth weight is increased for embryos cultured for 1 to 5 days compared to control embryos that have been transferred from their natural to recipient mothers. The increase in size at birth is due therefore to acceleration of growth of the embryo/fetus and also due to a small increase in the length of gestation. As in other species, the maturational changes of the reproductive tract in preparation for pregnancy are accelerated by exogenous progesterone that substantially raises the maternal concentrations. This perturbation also accelerates the early development of the embryo and increases the allocation of cells to the trophectoderm in the blastocyst. In sheep, exogenous progesterone increases fetal and placental growth throughout pregnancy[18].

In contrast to these domestic animals, *in vitro* culture of murine or human embryos for shorter periods of time may inhibit embryonic and fetal growth[19,20]. This process may be linked in advanced human reproductive programs to an increased incidence of preterm births. It could also account for an increased incidence of miscarriage and antepartum hemorrhage through altered implantation and invasion of the trophoblast. Mismatch in the stages of development of the embryo and the endometrium has also been implicated in these phenomena in women with unexplained infertility[21].

Walker and his colleagues[17] have speculated that the potential mechanisms which could account for the altered rate of growth of the embryo and fetus include cytoplasmic factors, maternal–embryo signalling and imprinted genes. In their experiments, fragmentation of the cytoplasm of the blastomeres occurred and is caused by a serum component of the culture media. The cytoplasmic factors potentially responsible include inherited factors essential for early development and those that influence processes including transcription and methylation. Alternatively, removal of the embryo necessarily disrupts maternal–embryo signalling by factors including steroids (e.g. estrogens) or cytokines. They also suggested that the embryo manipulation could alter imprinting of genes such as those encoding insulin-like growth factor-II (IGF-II), the IGF type 2 receptor, H19 and Mash 2. The more recently identified genes, *Hxt* which may regulate allocation of cells to the trophectoderm in the embryo and its decidual counterpart and *Het* which may limit trophoblast formation and its invasion are also potential candidates for early alteration of embryonic and hence fetal development[22]. The role of these candidate genes as targets for epigenetic phenomena remains to be investigated.

The rate of fetal growth is lower in animals in first pregnancy and in those carrying litters or multiple pregnancies. Intriguingly, the lower birth weight in first pregnancy may be overcome in overfed pigs by exogenous progesterone administered in early pregnancy[23]. Similarly, the lower setting of the trajectory of fetal growth and subsequent constraint of fetal growth can be overcome in rodents by selecting mice with high

concentrations of IGF-I or, in rats, by exogenous IGF-I given from the beginning of pregnancy[24], but not when exogenous IGF-I is only given late in the second half of pregnancy[25].

Although birth weight is lower in multiple pregnancy in women, early investigations suggest that this is due to a decline in the rate of fetal growth, mainly in the third trimester[26]. This may account for the better perinatal survival at lower birth weights in twins and triplets than in singletons[27].

Late in pregnancy, the supply of nutrients or oxygen may alter growth rate and accelerate or restrict growth of the fetus. Thus the early setting of the genetic or epigenetic drive to growth of the fetus is subsequently modulated by the maternal or placental environment, principally through the supply of oxygen and nutrients to the fetus. The latter will also interact with the fetal endocrine environment and autonomic nervous system to modulate the distribution of cardiac output and further determine the relative growth of different organs or tissues within the fetus and the placenta.

INTRAUTERINE GROWTH RESTRICTION

During the last 10 years, there has been a remarkable increase in our knowledge of the metabolic and endocrine state of the growth restricted fetus, due to the widespread use of fetal blood sampling by cordocentesis. In the absence of infection, or genetic and chromosomal causes of growth restriction, a high proportion of the growth restricted fetuses are hypoxemic and may also be polycythemic with increased numbers of erythroblasts in the circulation. High concentrations of erythropoietin have been found in fetal fluids indicating that the fetus attempts to compensate for the hypoxemia. Hypoglycemia, increased concentration of lactate, lower concentrations of amino acids and low pH in fetal blood are correlated with the degree of hypoxemia[28]. Generally, these findings are analogous to those reported earlier in experimental intrauterine growth restriction in which placental growth and/or function has been limited by excision of placental attachment sties, ligation of a uterine or an umbilical artery, and embolization of the maternal or fetal placental circulations[1,29].

The cascade of events by which fetal growth is restricted experimentally in sheep following restricted placental growth has been characterized after prepregnancy excision of endometrial caruncles (carunclectomy). Perhaps the earliest compensatory process begins before attachment of the embryo to the remaining caruncles. At day 12–14 of the estrous cycle there are high concentrations of progesterone in the blood of the ewe after excision of caruncles. When the animal becomes pregnant, this may enhance elongation of the embryo to reach normally unused caruncles close to the utero-tubal junction or those close to the uterine cervix. By day 70, the diameter of the placentomes is significantly larger in the carunclectomized animals. Up to 90 days of pregnancy, the surface area for exchange (the feto-maternal syncytium and the trophoblast) is maintained despite a lower placental weight. No further increase in the placental surface area for exchange occurs with increasing gestational age. However, even at 90 days, maternal utero-placental blood flow is reduced. It is hardly surprising that fetal hypoxemia and hypoglycemia become evident between 90 and 120 days, as the fetus continues to grow, and the ratio of fetal weight to placental weight increases (term approximately 145–150 days).

There is a redistribution of nutrients and oxygen in the growth restricted fetuses and placentas by 120 days[29]. The fetus continues to consume oxygen and glucose at the same rate per unit mass as in controls, probably by adjusting its rate of growth to supply. To achieve this, increased extraction of oxygen (and glucose) occurs across the umbilical circulation and this may partly account for the reduction of oxygen and glucose consumption per unit mass of placenta. However, the placenta continues its output of lactate and consumes amino acids from both the maternal and fetal circulations[1,29]. The latter can only be maintained by breakdown of fetal protein. A similar process

may be inferred clinically in humans when a shrinking abdominal circumference is observed by ultrasound.

In addition to the chronic reductions in supply of substrates for the growth restricted fetus, acute-on-chronic episodes of hypoxia are evident with fetal or uterine activity, presumably due to increasing consumption or reductions in supply during these events. Decelerations of the fetal heart rate with large rises in blood pressure occur intermittently over prolonged periods. It is interesting to speculate that these acute episodes alter the setting of control mechanisms of the cardiovascular system. Such episodes may be the initiating factor in the subsequent development of high blood pressure in individuals or experimental animals, followed to adult life[30].

The combination of acute episodes and chronic reduction of supply of oxygen and glucose are likely to be responsible for endocrine changes that are common to experimental and human fetal growth restriction. These endocrine changes include reductions in the abundance of anabolic or growth promoting hormones and factors in fetal blood, including thyroid hormones, insulin, IGF-I and members of the growth hormone family. The concentrations of catabolic hormones in the blood of the growth restricted fetus are also increased (e.g. noradrenaline, adrenaline and cortisol)[1].

Four potential mechanisms could account for the increase in concentrations of noradrenaline in the growth restricted fetus. There could be increased secretion from normal numbers of noradrenaline-secreting autonomic neurones or increased secretion from the adrenal medulla driven by the hypoxemia. Alternatively, increased autonomic innervation could result from the prolonged hypoxemia and, in turn, lead to higher noradrenaline concentrations. If this hyperinnervation persists postnatally, it may, in an analogous way to the spontaneously hypertensive rat, reset the control mechanisms of blood pressure through to adult life. Finally, the placenta is a significant site of clearance of catecholamines and part of the increased concentrations may be due to decreased clearance by a smaller placenta (Simonetta and co-workers, submitted).

The plasma concentration of cortisol in the growth restricted fetus is also increased and this may enhance maturation. Although the abundance of adrenocorticotropic hormone (ACTH) immunoreactivity in fetal plasma is unchanged in fetal growth restriction, the ratio of $ACTH_{1-39}$ to larger precursor molecules is increased and this could account for enhanced adrenal growth and increased concentrations of glucocorticoids. Central resetting is also observed since pro-opiomelanocortin (POMC) mRNA is reduced in the growth restricted animals compared to controls at 140 days of gestation[31].

Experimental fetal growth restriction has allowed us to test or suggest strategies for treatment to overcome the restricted placental growth and supply to the fetus (Table 1). Maternal hyperoxia increases fetal arterial oxygen tension and the apparent margin of safety in supply of oxygen since the delivery of oxygen is increased, but this is not accompanied by an increase in oxygen consumption by the fetus or the placenta. Disturbingly, when the hyperoxia ceases, oxygen delivery to the fetus is significantly reduced relative to the control period before the hyperoxia. It should be noted here that a similar effect may occur in women carrying a growth restricted fetus when hyperoxia is stopped[32]. Small studies and randomized trials have suggested that this is a potentially useful form of therapy that requires further evaluation[33,34].

Infusion of glucose or other nutrients into the mother to increase the maternal–fetal concentration gradient may increase the supply of glucose in the fetus and this can have devastating effects, leading to increasing acidosis and rapid fetal death within a few hours.

More recently, we have tested the effects of a 10-day infusion of IGF-I to increase fetal concentrations about three-fold to achieve concentrations towards the high end of the normal physiological range[35]. In addition to stimulating growth of many, although not all, organs within the fetus, IGF-I increased vascularization of the fetal vessels within the villi of the placenta (Table 2). This increased vascularization is accompanied by a larger fall in vascular resistance determined from flow velocity waveforms obtained using Doppler ultrasound.

MATERNAL UNDER-NUTRITION

In women, maternal under-nutrition may be the commonest cause of fetal growth restriction.

Table 1 Potential strategies for treatment of intrauterine growth restriction: supplementation of the mother or the fetus

Maternal hyperoxia

Substrates
  glucose
  amino acids
  fructose, galactose, maltose, fats

Growth factors
  epidermal growth factor
  insulin-like growth factor-I
  insulin-like growth factor-II
  other growth factors, e.g. vasculo-endothelial
    growth factor (VEGF)

Increase maternal uterine blood flow
  vasodilators, e.g. nitric oxide
  growth factors

Table 2 Effects of intrafetal infusion of insulin-like growth factor-I (IGF-I) in sheep

Effects in the fetus
Organs responsive to IGF-I
  body length
  liver
  kidneys
  heart
  spleen
  parotid glands
  pituitary
  adrenal glands

Organs unresponsive to IGF-I
  gastrointestinal tract
  skeletal muscle
  appendicular skeletal bone length

Effects in the placenta
Increased fetal vascularity
Decreased connective tissue in villi
Reduced vascular resistance

Effects in the mother
Increased metabolic efficiency

Protein-energy malnutrition is common in many communities, mainly in the developing world. In affluent societies, anorexia and bulimia are associated with moderate to severe fetal growth restriction. Recently, there has been a disturbing finding that eating disorders are reported by 32.4% of women giving birth to a small-for-dates baby at term. The incidence of eating disorders was only 2.3% of all women giving birth at term[36]. There is an urgent need to extend these studies and also replicate the study of Godfrey and associates[37] of maternal diet throughout pregnancy in different communities. The composition of the diet may adversely affect fetal growth. For example, high intake of carbohydrate in early pregnancy reduces fetal and placental growth, as does a low intake of protein (from meat and dairy products) in late pregnancy[37].

The Dutch Winter Hunger of 1944–45 demonstrated that exposure to famine in late pregnancy reduced birth weight. Birth weight was not reduced when women were exposed to the famine in early pregnancy. The long-term follow-up of the children born before, during and after the famine has shown that men exposed as fetuses to famine in pregnancy and early infancy and whose birth weights were reduced, have a higher incidence of obesity than those born before or after the famine[38]. Conversely, famine exposure in early pregnancy reduced the subsequent incidence of obesity. The weight of women in middle age, who were exposed to the famine as fetuses in late pregnancy, is reduced compared to those born before or after the famine. Women whose mothers were exposed to the famine when they were fetuses in the first half of pregnancy did not themselves have lower birth weight, but their children had a high incidence of being small-for-dates at birth[39].

Transgenerational effects on the growth of the fetus have been elegantly demonstrated in rats which were exposed to moderate undernutrition for 10–12 generations. This undernutrition reduced body weight by ~40% and altered body proportions. Pregnancy outcome was adversely affected and the small malnourished rats had a high incidence of small and stillborn pups. Re-feeding the animals in pregnancy had a remarkable effect on fetal growth as it was restored to normal in the first generation. Perinatal mortality was high and perinatal damage to the mother and fetus occurred. The final adult size of surviving pups was larger than average for the control colony. It took three generations for final adult size and perinatal outcome to become similar to the control colony[40]. We and others[41] have begun to explore the effects of moderate under-nutrition at different stages of pregnancy on fetal and placental growth and metabolism. There is an interaction between nutrient stores and nutrition in early pregnancy which may increase placental weight[42] without increasing the surface area for exchange[43]. This early under-nutrition may alter glucose-insulin relationships or IGF binding proteins in the fetus in late pregnancy.

Selective reduction in protein intake in rats alters fetal and placental growth. Diets containing a range of protein content (6–18%; controls 18%) were offered to the rats in a calorically balanced diet[44]. A reduction in dietary protein to 9% increases the ratio of placental weight to fetal weight. The pulmonary tissues from these pups at birth have increased activity of angiotensin converting enzyme which is responsible for converting angiotensin-I to the active vasoconstrictor, angiotensin-II. The offspring were reared to adult life and their blood pressure was inversely related to the concentration of protein in the maternal diet. Maternal anemia in human pregnancy is also associated with an increase in placental weight to fetal weight ratio and, in other studies[4], this alteration in the placental weight to fetal weight ratio is associated with increased blood pressure in adult life. It has also been suggested that this anemia is a marker of a more generalized nutritional deficit. Crowe and co-workers[45] induced maternal anemia and this reduced placental weight and fetal weight. Soon after birth, the blood pressure of the pups from the anemic mothers was lower than that of controls. However, by 3 months of age, this had reversed and the pups from the anemic mothers had significantly higher blood pressure[45].

Our preliminary observations in guinea-pigs suggest that moderate under-nutrition, beginning about 1 month before pregnancy, substantially increases the ratio of the cells of the inner cell mass to the cells of the outer cell mass, without reducing the total numbers of the cells in the blastocyst (Jan Jaap Erwich, unpublished observation). Moderate under-nutrition from before and throughout pregnancy reduces birth weight, placental weight, and ponderal index, but increases brain weight and fat relative to body weight, and the ratio of placental weight to fetal weight in this species[46]. The consequences of chronic maternal under-nutrition in the guinea-pig for adult body composition and lipid and carbohydrate metabolism in the offspring are as yet unknown.

CONCLUDING REMARKS

Alan Lucas[47] described programming as a physiological setting by an early stimulus or insult during a sensitive or critical period of development. He also noted that the consequences can be immediate or delayed. Studies of intrauterine growth have readily demonstrated the immediate effects of restricted or accelerated growth of the embryo or of the fetus. The effects of intrauterine growth restriction on risk of fetal distress or death and long-term effects on intellectual development and cerebral palsy have been well described. The more recent epidemiological observations, that common adult diseases may have their origin in fetal life or in the perinatal period, have provided a new stimulus to investigate the regulation of fetal growth, and the long-term consequences of this stage of development. There is new evidence that perturbation of fetal and infant growth has long-term consequences for the adult in experimental animals. It is now essential to determine the mechanisms determining this relationship. Only then will it be possible to define strategies for intervention that may improve both perinatal survival and long-term outcome.

ACKNOWLEDGEMENTS

The authors gratefully acknowledge financial support from the National Health and Medical Research Council, the National Heart Foundation, the Women's and Children's Foundation and The University of Adelaide. We thank Glenys King for preparation of the manuscript and Linda Mundy and Frank Carbone for expert assistance. We also acknowledge K. Kind, A. Sohlstrom, G. Simonetta, I. Phillips, F. Lok and K. Hartwich for their major contributions to completion of these studies. Professor Robinson gratefully thanks the British Association of Perinatal Medicine for providing the opportunity to give the Overseas Founder's Lecture at the European Perinatal Association Congress which formed the basis of this manuscript.

References

1. Owens, J. A. (1991). Endocrine and substrate control of fetal growth: placental and maternal influences and insulin-like growth factors. *Reprod. Fertil. Dev.*, **3**, 501–17
2. Robertson, S. A., Seamark, R F., Guilbert, L. J. and Wegmann, T. G. (1994). The role of cytokines in gestation. *Crit. Rev. Immunol.*, **14**, 239–92
3. Robinson, J. S. and Owens, J. A. (1996). Control of fetal growth. In Hillier, S. G., Kitchener, H. C. and Neilson, J. P. *Scientific Essentials of Reproductive Medicine*, pp. 329–41. (London: W. B. Saunders)
4. Barker, D. J. P. (1994). *Mothers, Babies and Diseases in Later Life.* (London: British Medical Journal Publishing Group)
5. Barker, D. J. P., Winter, P. D., Osmond, C., Phillips, D. I. W. and Sultan, H. Y. (1995). Weight gain in infancy and cancer of the ovary. *Lancet*, **345**, 1087–8
6. Brown, A. S., Susser, E. S., Lin, S. P., Neugebauer, R. and Gorman, J. M. (1995). Increased

risk of affective disorders in males after second trimester exposure to the Dutch Hunger Winter of 1944–45. *Br. J. Psychiatry*, **166**, 601–6

7. Ekbom, A., Hsieh, C.-C., Lipworth, L., Wolk, A., Ponten, J., Adami, H.-O. and Trichopoulos, D. (1996). Perinatal characteristics in relation to incidence of and mortality from prostate cancer. *Br. Med. J.*, **313**, 337–41

8. Palmer, L., Blair, E., Petterson, B. and Burton, P. (1995). Antenatal antecedents of moderate and severe cerebral palsy. *Pediatr. Perinat. Epidemiol.*, **9**, 171–84

9. Vilar, J. and Belizan, J. M. (1982). The relative contribution of prematurity and fetal growth retardation to low birth weight in developing and developed societies. *Am. J. Obstet. Gynecol.*, **142**, 793–8

10. Ebrahim, G. J. (1984). Care of the newborn. *Br. Med. J.*, **289**, 899–901

11. Institute of Medicine (1990). *Nutrition during Pregnancy*. (Washington: National Academy Press)

12. Joyce, T. (1990). The dramatic increase in the rate of low birthweight in New York City: an aggregate time-series analysis. *Am. J. Public Health*, **80**, 682–4

13. Power, C. (1994). National trends in birth weight: implications for future adult disease. *Br. Med. J.*, **308**, 1270–1

14. Moore, V. M., Miller, A. G., Boulton, T. J. C., Cockington, R. A., Hamilton Craig, I., Magarey, A. M. and Robinson, J. S. (1996). Placental weight, birth measurements, and blood pressure at age 8 years. *Arch. Dis. Child.*, **74**, 538–41

15. Wilcox, M. A., Newton, C. S. and Johnson, I. R. (1995). Paternal influences on birthweight. *Acta Obstet. Gynecol. Scand.*, **74**, 15–18

16. Walton, A. and Hammond, J. (1938). The maternal effects on growth and conformation in Shire horse-Shetland pony crosses. Proceedings of the Royal Society Series B, **125**, 311–35

17. Walker, S., Hartwich, K. and Seamark, R. F. (1996). The production of unusually large offspring following embryo manipulation: concepts and challenges. *Theriogenology*, **45**, 111–20

18. Kleemann, D. O., Walker, S. K. and Seamark, R. F. (1994). Enhanced fetal growth in sheep administered progesterone during the first three days of pregnancy. *J. Reprod. Fertil.*, **102**, 411–17

19. Bowman, P. and McLaren, A. (1970). Viability and growth of mouse embryos after *in vitro* culture and fusion. *J. Embryol. Exp. Morphol.*, **23**, 693–704

20. Wang, J. X., Clark, A. M., Kirby, C. A., Phillipson, G., Petrucco, O., Anderson, G. and Matthews, C. D. (1994). The outcome of singleton pregnancies following *in vitro* fertilization/gamete intra-Fallopian transfer. *Hum. Reprod.*, **9**, 141–6

21. Klentzeris, L. D., Li, T. C., Dockery, P. and Cooke, I. D. (1992). Endometrial biopsy as a predictive factor in pregnancy rate in women with unexplained infertility. *Eur. J. Obstet. Gynecol. Reprod. Biol.*, **49**, 119–24

22. Cross, J. C., Flannery, M. L., Blanar, M. S., Steingrimsson, E., Jenkins, N. A., Copeland, N. G., Rutter, W. J. and Werb, Z. (1995). *Hxt* encodes a basic helix-loop-helix transcription factor that regulates trophoblast cell development. *Development*, **121**, 2513–23

23. Parr, R. A., Miles, M. A., Cash, M. P. and Waters, J. M. (1994). Timing of progesterone supplement and embryo survival in overfed gilts. Presented at the *Australian Society for Reproductive Biology*, p. 78. Brisbane, September

24. Gluckman, P. D., Morel, P. C. H., Ambler, B. H., Breier, H. T. and McCutcheon, S. N. (1992). Elevating maternal insulin-like growth factor-1 in mice and rats alters the pattern of fetal growth by removing maternal constraint. *J. Endocrinol.*, **134**, R1–3

25. O'Callaghan, S. P., Katsman, A. I., Lang, R. J., Owens, J. A., Owens, P. C. and Robinson, J. S. (1994). IGF-I treatment of pregnant rats in late gestation does not prevent fetal growth retardation following unilateral uterine artery ligation. *Placenta*, **15**, A51

26. McKcown, T. and Record, R. G. (1953). The influence of placental size on foetal growth in man, with special reference to multiple pregnancy. *J. Endocrinol.*, **9**, 418–26

27. Buekens, P. and Wilcox, A. (1993). Why do small twins have a lower mortality rate than small singletons? *Am. J. Obstet. Gynecol.*, **168**, 937–41

28. Economides, D. L. and Nicolaides, K. H. (1990). Metabolic findings in small-for-gestational-age fetuses. *Contemp. Rev. Obstet. Gynaecol.*, **2**, 75–9

29. Owens, J. A., Owens, P. C. and Robinson, J. S. (1989). Experimental fetal growth retardation: metabolic and endocrine aspects. In Gluckman, P. D., Nathanilcsz, P. W. and Johnson, B. M. (eds.) *Fetal and Neonatal Physiology*, pp. 257–80. (Ithaca, New York: Perinatology Press)

30. Folkow, B. (1978). Cardiovascular structural adaption; its role in the initiation and maintenance of primary hypertension. *Clin. Sci. Mol. Med.*, **55**, 3–22s

31. Phillips, I. D., Simonetta, G., Owens, J. A., Robinson, J. S., Clarke, I. J. and McMillen, I. C. (1996). Placental restriction alters the functional development of the pituitary-adrenal axis in the sheep during late gestation. *Ped. Res.*, **40**, 1–6

32. Bekedam, D. J., Mulder, E. J. H., Snijders, R. J. M. and Visser, G. H. A. (1991). The effects of maternal hyperoxia on fetal breathing movements, body movements and heart rate variation in growth retarded fetuses. *Early Hum. Dev.*, **27**, 223–32

33. Battaglia, C., Artini, P. G., Dambrogio, G., Galli, P. A., Segre, A. and Genazzani, A. R. (1992). Maternal hyperoxygenation in the treatment of intrauterine growth retardation. *Am. J. Obstet. Gynecol.*, **167**, 430–5

34. Nicolaides, K. H., Campbell, S., Bradley, R. J., Bilardo, C. M., Soothill, P. W. and Gibb, D. (1987). Maternal oxygen therapy for intrauterine growth retardation. *Lancet*, **1**, 942–5

35. Lok, F., Owens, J. A., Mundy, L., Robinson, J. S. and Owens, P. C. (1996). Insulin-like growth factor 1 promotes growth selectively in fetal sheep in late gestation. *Am. J. Physiol.*, **270**, (*Reg. Integr. Comp. Physiol.*, **39**), R1148–55

36. Abraham, S. and Conti, J. (1996). Disordered eating and obstetric outcome. Presented at the *RACOG Scientific Meeting*, Fiji, Abstr. 43

37. Godfrey, K., Robinson, S., Barker, D. J. P., Osmond, C. and Cox, V. (1996). Maternal nutrition in early and late pregnancy in relation to placental and fetal growth. *Br. Med. J.*, **312**, 410–14

38. Ravelli, G.-P., Stein, Z. A. and Susser, M. W. (1976). Obesity in young men after famine exposure *in utero* and early infancy. *N. Engl. J. Med.*, **295**, 249–53

39. Lumey, L. H. (1992). Decreased birthweights in infants after maternal *in utero* exposure to the Dutch famine of 1944–1945. *Paediatr. Perinat. Epidemiol.*, **6**, 240–53

40. Stewart, R. J. C., Sheppard, H., Preece, R. and Waterlow, J. C. (1980). The effect of rehabilitation at different stages of development of rats marginally malnourished for ten to twelve generations. *Br. J. Nutr.*, **43**, 403–11

41. Harding, J. E. and Johnston, B. M. (1995). Nutrition and fetal growth. *Reprod. Fertil. Dev.*, **7**, 539–47

42. McCrabb, G. J., Hosking, B. J. and Egan, A. R. (1992). Changes in the maternal body and fetoplacental growth following various lengths of feed restriction during mid-pregnancy in sheep. *Aust. J. Agric. Res.*, **43**, 1429–40

43. De Barro, T. M., Owens, J. A., Earl, C. R. and Robinson, J. S. (1992). Nutrition during early/mid pregnancy interacts with mating weight to affect placental weight in sheep. Presented at the *Australian Society for Reproductive Biology*. Adelaide, September

44. Langley, S. C. and Jackson, A. A. (1994). Increased systolic blood pressure in adult rats induced by fetal exposure to maternal low protein diets. *Clin. Sci.*, **86**, 217–22

45. Crowe, C., Dandekar, P., Fox, M., Dhinga, K., Bennet, L. and Hanson, M. A. (1995). The effect of anaemia on heart, placenta and body weight, and blood pressure in fetal and neonatal rats. *J. Physiol.*, **488**, 515–19

46. Katsman, A., Sohlstrom, A., Roberts, C., Erwich, J. J., Kind, K. and Owens, J. A. (1996). Fetal and placental growth in early and late pregnancy in guinea pigs subjected to moderate undernutrition. Presented at the *14th Meeting of Australian Perinatal Society*, Adelaide, A47

47. Lucas, A. (1991). Programming by early nutrition in man. In Bock, G. R. and Whelan, J. (eds.) *The Childhood Environment and Adult Disease*, Ciba Found. Symp. 156, pp. 38–50. (Chichester, England: John Wiley and Sons)

Maternal nutrition, fetal growth and development

6

T. K. A. B. Eskes

IMPORTANCE OF NORMAL GROWTH AND FUNCTION OF THE PLACENTA

The three major processes which determine fetal growth and development are genetic, metabolic and nutritional[1]. These processes rarely act separately because the fetus develops in concert with the placenta. In particular, widening of the maternal placental arteries (spiral arteries) is a prerequisite for normal pregnancy. During pregnancy two trophoblast invasion waves occur into the decidual and myometrial segments of spiral arteries, respectively. These trophoblast waves, occurring in the first and the second trimester, 'absorb' the endothelial lining of the spiral artery and also replace the original muscular wall with amorphous fibrinoid material[2]. It seems that the spiral arteries are liberated from the neurovascular control mechanisms, allowing an extensive dilatation and steady supply of large volumes of maternal blood to the placenta.

Occlusion or atherosis of spiral arteries can lead to placental infarction, a small-for-gestational-age infant or placental abruption.

ROLE OF HOMOCYSTEINE

Three major studies have been published indicating that homocysteine may play an important role in the pathogenesis of coronary heart disease[3], extracranial carotid artery disease[4] and venous thrombosis[5]. Homocysteine is a sulfur-containing amino-acid and lies at a metabolic branch point from which it may be trans-sulfurated to cystathionine or remethylated to form methionine. The trans-sulfuration requires the vitamin B_6-dependent cystathionine synthase.

The remethylation requires 5,10-methylene-tetrahydrofolate reductase (MTHFR) and methionine synthase (MS), which are folate- and vitamin B_{12}-dependent, respectively. The methylation serves one carbon metabolism (methyl donorship) and is essential for DNA synthesis, DNA methylation and for transfer RNA (tRNA).

The mechanisms by which elevated homocysteine concentrations promote atherosclerosis are thought to be: direct damage to the endothelium; stimulation of smooth muscle cell proliferation; enhanced low-density lipoprotein (LDL) peroxidation; impairment of the production of endothelium-derived relaxing factor, affecting the expression of thrombomodulin; and the activation of protein C.

Tsai and colleagues[6] examined the effect of homocysteine on the growth of vascular smooth muscle cells and endothelial cells. Homocysteine caused an increase in DNA synthesis in rat aortic smooth muscle cells. In contrast, homocysteine caused a dose-dependent decrease in DNA synthesis in human umbilical vein endothelial cells.

The growth-promoting effect of homocysteine on vascular smooth muscle cells, together with its inhibitory effect on endothelial cell growth, represents an important mechanism to explain homocysteine-induced atherosclerosis. It also remains to be seen what the influence of homocysteine is on the endothelial cells of spiral arteries which are invaded twice by trophoblast during pregnancy.

HYPERHOMOCYSTEINEMIA

Goddijn-Wessel and co-workers[7] demonstrated that hyperhomocysteinemia is associated with placental abruption/infarction/fetal growth retardation. In 84 women with placental abruption or infarction (study group) and 46 controls, homocysteine metabolism was investigated in the non-pregnant state by a standardized oral methionine loading test. Hyperhomocysteinemia was diagnosed in 31% of patients and 9% in controls. The median concentration of the vitamins serum folate, serum vitamin B_{12} and whole blood pyridoxal-5'-phosphate were significantly lower in women in the study group as compared to controls. It remains to be seen what the role of homocysteine is at the level of the spiral arteries because of the presence or lack of trophoblast invasion and endothelium destruction in these arteries[8].

MUTATION OF THE METHYLENE-TETRAHYDROFOLATE REDUCTASE GENE

The thermolabile enzyme, 5,10-methylene-tetrahydrofolate reductase (MTHFR), is of much interest for embryology as well as endothelial cell function. Deficiency of this enzyme has been reported as a risk factor for vascular disease[3] and also for neural tube defects[9]. The gene mutation was reported to be localized on the first chromosome[10].

In our own study of women with placental infarcts/fetal growth retardation and/or placental abruption, this mutation was found in 15% of cases and in 4% of controls (van der Molen, personal communication).

FOLIC ACID AND HOMOCYSTEINE EXPORT

Van der Molen and associates[11] studied homocysteine export from human umbilical vein endothelial cells (HUVECS) by measuring total homocysteine (tHcy) concentrations in the culture medium under standard culture conditions. Folic acid supplementation added to the culture medium lowered the tHcy export in a dose-dependent manner. Methyltetrahydrofolate (MeTHF) and folinic acid were, in this respect, about ten times more effective than folic acid. Additions to the culture medium of the other vitamins involved in homocysteine metabolism, such as vitamins B_{12} and vitamin B_6, did not have any effect on homocysteine export. There is therefore a susceptible dependency of homocysteine metabolism on folic acid in endothelial cells.

LOW SERUM FOLATE CONCENTRATIONS AND RISK OF PRETERM DELIVERY AND LOW BIRTH WEIGHT

Scholl and colleagues[12] examined the influence of folate intake from the diet and supplements by 28 weeks of gestation and third trimester circulating concentrations of serum folate on the outcome of pregnancy in women from Camden, New Jersey. Mean daily folate intake by week 28 included both dietary and supplemental folate obtained prospectively in 832 women. Circulating concentrations of serum folate as well as serum vitamin B_{12} were assayed at 28 weeks of gestation (± 2 weeks) by radioimmunoassay. The outcomes of interest included preterm delivery (< 37 weeks) and infants with low birth weight (< 2500 g). Mean folate intake was significantly correlated with circulating concentrations of serum folate ($\tau = 0.17$, $p < 0.001$). Women with a low mean daily folate intake ($240\mu g/day$) had an approximately two-fold greater risk of preterm delivery and infant low birth weight after maternal characteristics, energy intake and other correlated nutrients were controlled for. Lower concentrations of serum folate at week 28 were also associated with a greater risk of preterm delivery and low birth weight. The eventual effect of folic acid supplementation has to be tested clinically in a randomized study.

CONCLUSION

In conclusion, we can state that hyperhomocysteinemia (tHcy) is an independent risk factor for vascular disease. Hyperhomocysteinemia is also present in women who experienced fetal placental abruption and/or growth retardation with placental infarcts. The spiral arteries going to the placenta also seem to be a target. Homocysteine lies at a branch point for trans-sulfuration or remethylation. The remethylation requires 5,10-methylenetetrahydrofolate reductase and methionine synthase as enzymes and folate and vitamin B_{12} as cofactors. A mutation has been described of 5,10-methylene-tetrahydrofolate reductase which opens the possibility of discovering a gene mutation in ± 15% of these patients. Folate therapy can overcome this defective gene activity. Randomized clinical studies have yet to demonstrate the value of such prevention therapy.

ACKNOWLEDGEMENTS

The research program described here was carried out within the Institute for the Prevention of Birth Defects of the University Department of Obstetrics and Gynecology in co-operation with the Departments of Anthropogenetics, Clinical Epidemiology, Internal Medicine, Laboratory of Endocrinology and Reproduction, Pediatrics and Toxicology. The following grants are gratefully acknowledged: CDI Charity Foundation, Foundation of Primary Prevention of Birth Defects, the Dutch Prevention Foundation, the Dutch Heart Foundation, the Princess Beatrix Foundation, the Ter Meulen Foundation and the Foundation of the Catholic University.

References

1. Longo, L. D. (1984). Intrauterine growth retardation. A 'mosaic' hypothesis of pathophysiology. *Semin. Perinatol.*, **8**, 62–72
2. Pijnenburg, R. (1996). The placental bed. *Hypertension Preg.*, **15**, 7–23
3. Kang, S. S., Wong, P. W. K., Susmand, A., Sora, J., Norusis, M. and Ruggie, N. (1991). Thermolabile methylenetetrahydrofolate reductase: an inherited risk factor for coronary artery disease. *Am. J. Hum. Genet.*, **48**, 536–45
4. Selhub, J., Jacques, P. F., Bostom, A. G., D'Agostino, R. B., Wilson, P. W. F., Belanger, A. J., O'Leary D. H., Wolf, P. A., Schaefer, E. J. and Rosenberg, I. H. (1995). Association between plasma homocysteine concentrations and extracranial carotid-artery stenosis. *N. Engl. J. Med.*, **332**, 286–91
5. den Heijer, M., Blom, H. J., Gerrits, W. B. J., Rosendaal, F. R., Haak, H. L., Wijermans, P. W. and Bos, G. M. J. (1995). Is hyperhomocysteinaemia a risk factor for recurrent venous thrombosis? *Lancet*, **345**, 882–5
6. Tsai, J. C., Perrela, M. A., Yoshizumi, M., Hsieh, Ch. M., Haber, E., Schelget, R. and Lee, Mu-En. (1994). Promotion of vascular smooth muscle cell growth by homocysteine: a link to atherosclerosis. *Proc. Natl. Acad. Sci. USA*, **91**, 6369–73
7. Goddijn-Wessel, T. A. W., Wouters, M. G. A. J., van der Molen, E. F., Steegers-Theunissen, R. P. M., Blom, H. J., Boers, G. H. J. and Eskes, T. K. A. B. (1996). Hyperhomocysteinemia: a risk factor for placental abruption or infarction. *Eur. J. Obstet. Gynecol. Reprod. Biol.*, **66**, 23–9
8. Domisse, J. and Tiltman, A. J. (1992). Placental bed biopsies in placental abruption. *Br. J. Obstet. Gynaecol.*, **99**, 651–4
9. van der Put, N. M. J., Steegers-Theunissen, R. P. M., Frosst, P., Trijbels, F. J. M., Eskes, T. K. A. B., van den Heuvel, L. P., Mariman, E. C. M., den Heijer, M., Rozen, R. and Blom, H. J. (1995). Mutated methylenetetrahydrofolate reductase as a risk factor for spina bifida. *Lancet*, **346**, 1070–1
10. Frosst, P., Blom, H. J., Milos, R., Goyette, P., Sheppard, C. A., Matthews, R. G., Boers, G. H. J., den Heijer, M., Kluijtmans, L. A. J., van den Heuvel, L. P. and Rozen, R. (1995). A candidate genetic risk factor for vascular disease: a common mutation methylenetetrahydrofolate reductase. *Nature Genet.*, **10**, 111–13
11. van der Molen, E. F., van der Heuvel, L. P. W. J., Poele-Pothof, M. T. W. B. te, Monnens, L. A. H., Eskes, T. K. A. B. and Blom, H. J. (1996). The effect of folic acid on the homocysteine metabolism in human umbilical vein endothelial cells (HUVECS). *Eur. J. Clin. Invest.*, **26**, 304–9
12. Scholl, Th. O., Hediger, M. L., Schall, J. I., Khoo, Ch. S. and Fischer, R. L. (1996). Dietary and serum folate: their influence on the outcome of pregnancy. *Am. J. Clin. Nutr.*, **63**, 520–5

The mammary–enteral axis: site of genetic conflict in early life?

7

L. T. Weaver

INTRODUCTION

It is in the interests of the growing mammal to ensure that it receives a steady supply of nutrients from conception to weaning. Pregnancy and lactation are usually viewed as a co-operative interaction between mother and offspring largely for the benefit of the latter. Before birth the fetus appears entirely reliant on the mother for all its needs for development and growth, and after birth the young of most species continue to depend on the mother's milk until weaning.

Such a view has meant that the focus of most interest in materno-offspring relations has been on the transfer of nutrients and other substances form mother to young, with little concern for the needs of the former. However, the effects of natural selection on genes expressed in the fetus may be opposed by the effects of natural selection on genes expressed in the mother. Genes in offspring will be selected to increase the transfer of nutrients to fetus and infant, and maternal genes will be selected to limit transfer in excess of some maternal optimum.

It is in the interests of the mother to ensure the survival and reproduction of her progeny, which bear half of her genes. It is likewise in the interests of the offspring (fetus and infant) to make sure that it is properly nourished and protected, by not threatening its mother's health or survival. Each is also, to some extent, in conflict with the other, but neither can afford to risk its own well-being or survival for the sake of only half of its genes.

HAIG'S HYPOTHESIS

Haig[1] has likened the womb to a battlefield where from conception to birth there is rivalry between mother and embryo. While the mother retains autonomy over the embryo, by being sole provider of nutrients until it implants in the endometrium, the fetus thereafter quickly ensures that it has a secure and lasting hold over the 'means of production', its mother.

Invasion of the uterine wall by the trophoblast, breakdown of the endometrium and remodelling of the spiral arteries ensure that the fetus achieves considerable control of its own nutrient supply. However, although the placenta is an organ under genetic control of the fetus, it is also dependent on the mother, and while it maintains a continuous supply of nutrients from mother to fetus, there is interaction between the two, which may account for some of the disorders of pregnancy and the newborn.

Haig[1] has identified three areas where he believes that the struggle between the rival interests of maternal and fetal genes can be detected. The corpus luteum, by secreting progesterone, prevents menstruation and helps to prepare the endometrium for implantation. By the 7th day of pregnancy the trophoblast secretes chorionic gonadotropin (hCG) which has the effect of further stimulating progesterone secretion in the mother, thereby ensuring that the pregnancy is maintained and the position of the fetus is made more secure. Continued secretion of hCG by the placenta is a means by which the fetus 'exerts its control' over the mother.

The embryo requires a continuous supply of glucose. To maintain fetal energy needs the placenta secretes placental lactogen (hPL), which in the mother counteracts the effects of insulin, thereby causing her blood glucose levels to rise. Placental lactogen acts on maternal prolactin receptors to increase maternal resistance to insulin, and by secreting hPL the fetus maintains a high circulating blood glucose for longer periods after meals.

Fetal nutritional needs are supplied by the mother's systemic (uteroplacental) circulation which, after trophoblast invasion of the endometrium, is maintained at mean arterial pressure. Secretion by the fetus of substances that increase maternal blood pressure will therefore benefit the embryo, by increasing blood flow through the uteroplacental circulation, potentiating the transfer of nutrients and other substances from mother to fetus.

Because of the anatomical arrangement whereby the placental membranes are bathed by maternal blood into which the trophoblast can secrete bioactive substances, the fetus has an 'advantage' which it can use to manipulate maternal physiology to promote the maintenance and continuation of pregnancy. However, all these actions of the placenta, while aimed at benefiting the fetus, may have adverse effects on the mother. The rising concentrations of hCG in the mother may lead to morning sickness, those of hPL to maternal diabetes, and increased secretion of vasoactive substances by the placenta may lead to hypertension and pre-eclamptic toxemia (PET).

Mossman[2] has defined the placenta as any intimate apposition or fusion of maternal and fetal membranes for the purpose of transferring nutrients from mother to young. Such a definition can be extended, with little stretch of the imagination, to describe the 'breast and gut' or 'mammary–enteral axis' which are in essence two membranes separated by milk.

After birth, the mother continues to be the primary source of nutrition: her milk is the sole and sufficient source of nutrients for the suckling infant. Synthesized in the mammary gland and utilized at the intestinal mucosa, milk is a packaged means of transferring nutrients from mother to neonate. In this respect the breast-fed infant can be regarded as an 'extragestate fetus' until weaning. However, her mammary glands are also the source of many bioactive substances that modulate the function of the digestive system and metabolism of the neonate.

In this paper I shall discuss the relationship that exists between mother and infant through the mammary–enteral axis, and to what extent this is comparable to the placenta, which conjoins mother and fetus before birth. In doing so I shall explore the strategies that other mammals have evolved to feed their young, from birds and reptiles which produce relatively fully-formed young from eggs, to ungulates which do the same entirely *in utero*. I base my argument largely on mammals because they are, quintessentially, breast-feeders: indeed, this class of living things has been defined by this unique characteristic.

ALTRICIAL AND PRECOCIAL YOUNG

Broadly speaking, mammals have adopted one of two strategies for feeding their young: either investing most in the process of nutrient transfer in the fetal rather than the suckling period, with the production of precocial young; or the opposite, of investing in feeding the offspring on milk after birth, with the production of altricial young. These two strategies have profoundly different implications for the relationship between mother and young, which are manifest in litter size, degree of maturation of the offspring at birth, and adult feeding habits. They also have implications for the dynamics of the genetic conflict between them.

In both precocial and altricial young, milk feeding follows a period of placental nutrient transfer *in utero*. The process of supplying nutrients to the embryo as it grows to nutritional independence is equivalent to the single phase of growth and development of ancestral and modern reptiles in the egg (Figure 1).

The earliest mammals were probably small insectivore–carnivores descended from reptilian ancestors in the Triassic period around 230

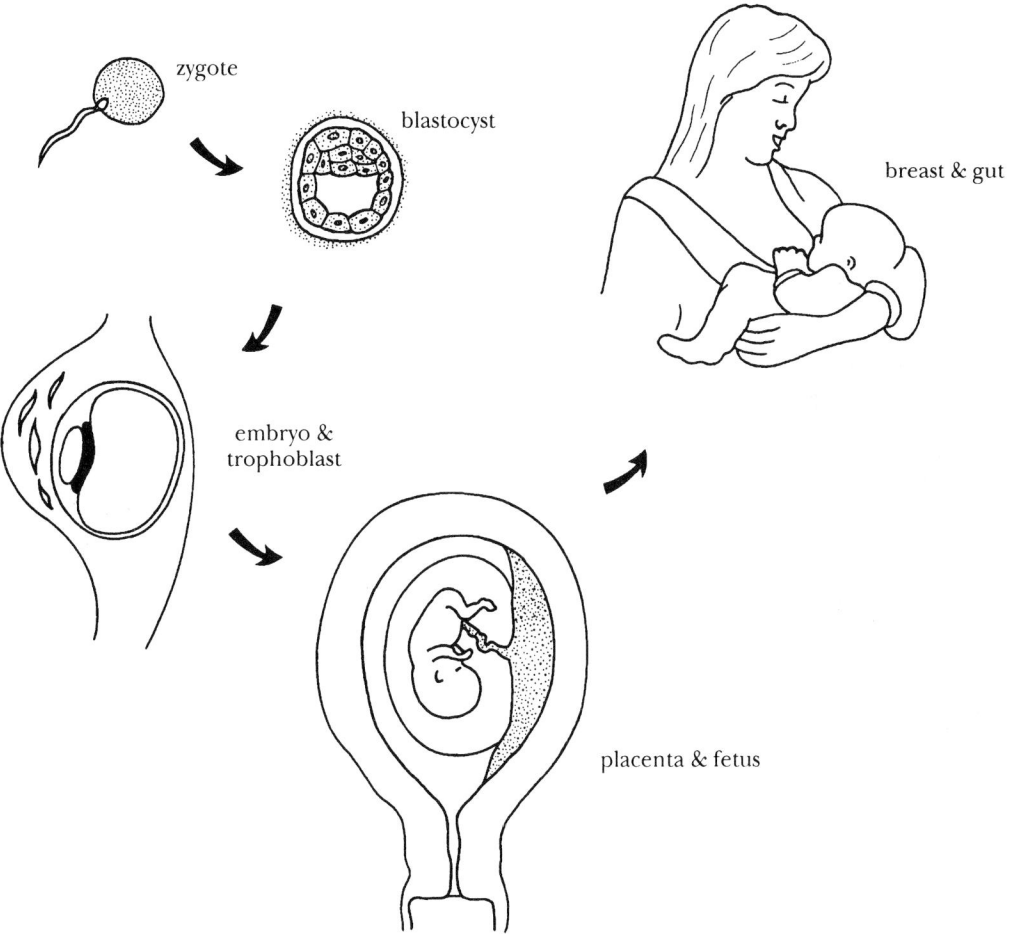

zygote

blastocyst

breast & gut

embryo & trophoblast

placenta & fetus

Figure 1 Stages in the development of the embryo. The transition from intrauterine to extrauterine life, at birth, involves a major change in the pathway of nutrients from mother to young. See text for fuller discussion

million years ago. Therapsids and proto-mammals may have laid one or two large-yolked eggs on land, from which precocial young, capable of foraging and feeding themselves soon after hatching, emerged. Another lineage of therapsids may have laid a larger clutch of smaller eggs with little yolk from which relatively altricial young hatched. Their mothers evolved a means of nourishing their offspring on the secretions of modified sebaceous glands, and a primitive form of lactation developed which sustained the young until nutritional independence.

Oviparity gave way to viviparity. The egg in which the oviparous embryo develops contains

all the necessary nutrients for growth and maturation, while the fetus *in utero* is supplied with these by the mother via the placenta before birth, and in milk after birth. The evolution of the mammary gland (and in marsupials of the pouch) freed the mother from being bound to a nest of helpless infants. Placental mammals evolved two broad patterns of reproduction, producing either precocial or altricial young.

Precocial young are born after a relatively long gestation and are comparatively mature at birth. The greater proportion of their development is undergone *in utero*, supported by the placenta, and the neonate requires a relatively short period of suckling. Accretion of essential nutrients takes place largely prenatally and early weaning and nutritional independence occur.

Altricial young are born after a relatively short gestation and are comparatively immature at birth. Placentation is brief, and growth, differentiation and development of organ systems, including the gastrointestinal tract, occur postnatally and the neonate enjoys a relatively long period of suckling. During lactation, milk is not only a vehicle for the transfer of nutrients from mother to young, but is also the principal means by which many bioactive substances are provided to the growing neonate[3].

The evolution, around 40 million years ago, of large mammals which produced a single precocial offspring after a long gestation represents the appearance, for a second time on earth, of the birth of well-developed young, but utilizing a radically different feeding strategy in early life. For them the trophoblast allows viviparity, with fetal development *in utero, ex ovo*.

However, although some precocial animals (such as the guinea pig) have reduced the suckling period to a minimum, no mammal appears to have abandoned it completely and returned to the strategy of reptiles and birds (and probably dinosaurs) of producing fully-formed progeny which are reared from birth on a non-milk diet. Perhaps milk feeding has persisted so that the mother can retain 'control' of her infant: when all the functions of the placenta, other than provision of nutrients, are taken over by the infant after birth, food supply remains the single and most fundamental function that the mother can continue to offer and control, and upon which ultimately all the others depend.

PLACENTA, BREAST AND GUT

The embryo implants in the uterine wall on around the 7th day after ovulation and is initially nourished by secretions from the endometrial glands, which contain a mixture of glycogen, protein, lipid[4] and many bioactive peptides[5]. The trophoblast then invades the endometrium and remodels the spiral arteries into low-resistance vessels that are unable to constrict. Placental villi become bathed in maternal blood.

This invasion has three consequences. First, the fetus gains direct access to the mother's arterial blood. Therefore the mother cannot reduce the nutrient content of blood reaching the placenta (and hence fetus) without reducing the nutrient supply to her own tissues. Second, the volume of blood reaching the placenta becomes largely independent of control by the local maternal vasculature. Third, the placenta is able to release hormones and other substances directly into the maternal circulation.

The consequences of these changes are to permit bidirectional transfer of substances between mother and fetus which can be both an advantage and a disadvantage to each during pregnancy. Placental secretion of hCG, hPL and other substances may promote fetal survival and well-being by manipulating maternal physiology to the benefit of the fetus and at the expense of the mother. For precocial young, a well-developed placenta with secretory properties which permit suspension of estrus and prolongation of gestation is particularly advantageous in helping the fetus to establish 'control' over the mother.

After birth, continuity of nutrient transfer is re-established via breast and gut. Milk synthesized in the former is utilized in the latter. While the mammary gland is the source of nutrients, the infant regulates the amount and frequency of milk that it receives. The human infant (born at term) is relatively autonomous in many respects, having left behind most of the other (non-nutritional) functions of the placenta at birth. Respiration becomes a task for the infant's cardiopulmonary system, excretion the function of the renal system, and thermoregulation the responsibility of the infant's metabolism of brown fat. The (remaining) nutritional function of the placenta, to serve as a means of transfer of food from mother to young, is taken over by the maternal mammary glands and the infant's digestive system (mammary–enteral axis).

Very altricial young, such as those of marsupials, plainly require from the mother more than simply nutrients. Milk is rich in protein, and after a very short period of placentation, the newborn kangaroo (joey) becomes 'fused' to the mother's teat from which passes a continuous stream of nutrients and non-nutritional substances, akin to that via the umbilical cord of eutherian mammals *in utero*. On the other hand, very precocial young have little need for either nutrients or non-nutrients in milk, having acquired them before birth.

Trivers[6] has argued that the postnatal conflict between mother and offspring is mediated primarily by 'behavioral' acts, in contrast to prenatal conflict which is mediated primarily by 'chemical' acts. However, milk may be important in this struggle not only because it is a source of nutrition to the young, but also a means of delivering non-nutritional substances to the infant. It is possible that by modulating the physiology of the newborn, milk-borne chemicals play a critical role in the struggle between mother and offspring. I suggest that, in addition to experimental evidence supporting a role for these bioactive substances in gastrointestinal maturation and nutritional adaptation, the relative maturity of the young at birth is a factor against which to judge their importance – what might be called a 'utility hypothesis' in the 'genetic conflict' between mother and young, or what advantage are they to each other?

MILK

Milk is a complex mixture of chemicals and cells. The former may be divided broadly into electrolytes (which maintain fluid homeostasis of the newborn), nutrients (energy, nitrogen, vitamins and minerals needed for growth, activity, tissue maintenance, etc.), and non-nutritional factors (which regulate cell, tissue and organ function). These non-nutritional factors include bioactive substances ranging in chemical composition from proteins and polypeptides to oligosaccharides, glycoproteins, nucleotides, sphingolipids, etc., which serve a variety of biological functions[7].

However, it is not possible to distinguish precisely between nutrients and non-nutritional substances. Some may serve more than one function, and during evolution they may have been selected for another purpose. They may be synergistically interactive and their function in the gastrointestinal tract will be determined by the balance between proteases and anti-proteases[8], and by the presence or absence of mechanisms for their uptake, processing and transfer[9]. A division of the constituents of milk into nutrients and non-nutrients does not take account of the dual (sometimes multiple) functions of many of the chemicals as they pass from mother to infant. Immunoglobulin A (IgA) for instance, while providing protection against antigens at mucosal surfaces, may also be a source of nitrogen to the newborn[10].

These dual functions of IgA illustrate an important point in the interpretation of mammalian milk composition. Most analyses of milk report the protein, fat and carbohydrate (or energy) contents, without distinguishing between nutritional and non-nutritional components. It has been estimated that up to one-third of the protein of human milk is non-nutritional, comprising immunoglobulins and other protective proteins, hormones, growth factors, digestive enzymes, etc.

Failure to distinguish between the nutritional and non-nutritional components of milks raises questions about the validity of attempts to find biological relationships between the energy and protein contents of milks and the growth rate and nutritional needs of the infant. A general feature of milk composition is that energy and protein contents are negatively correlated with maternal body weight, and positively correlated with infant weight and growth rate.

Allometric studies of lactation generally make use of the crude macronutrient composition of milks when seeking relationships between maternal and infant morphology and physiology. However, it is likely that the non-nutritional functions of a component of the protein (and probably the lipid and carbohydrate) in milk play a part in regulating these processes, rather than in providing fuel or nitrogen alone, and should be excluded from equations. The milk of altricial mammals typically has a high protein and fat content, and low carbohydrate content, while that of precocial species has the opposite; a low protein and fat and high carbohydrate content. Bearing in mind that bioactive substances are mostly polypeptides, it is possible that the presence or absence of a particular bioactive factor (or 'nutrient') could be critical in determining the rate of neonatal growth or synthesis of a particular tissue.

If this is so, allometric analysis must distinguish between altricial and precocial newborn, not because the latter have longer gestational periods and produce bigger babies (relative to maternal weight)[11], but because bioactive substances in milk are likely to be less important to the neonate, and more of the milk protein used exclusively for nutritional needs. In precocial species there is a negative correlation between milk protein concentration and neonatal weight, while in altricial species the correlation is positive.

EXTRACELLULAR AND INTRACELLULAR DIGESTION

When seeking the biological significance of bioactive substances in milks to the health, growth and development of the young, the function and relative development of the digestive system, in particular the way in which it handles proteins, must also be known. To be effective in the neonatal gastrointestinal tract, or to be absorbed and act systemically, any ingested bioactive substance must escape degradation by gastric acid and intestinal proteases[8].

In most mammals, during the period of mucosal differentiation, the apical region of the small intestinal epithelium exhibits a vesicular-tubular system adapted for the intact transfer of large molecules from the lumen into the cell[9]. The significance of this apical tubular system (ATS) to the young animal depends on the time

that it is present in the course of gut ontogeny: in altricial offspring it is active during suckling and plays an essential role in the uptake and processing of milk-borne bioactive substances. In most precocial mammals it is expressed prenatally and 'intestinal closure' occurs well before birth.

Because the gastrointestinal tract of precocial offspring is more mature and extracellular digestion predominates over intracellular digestion, bioactive substances in milk that do not resist digestion in the neonatal gut are unlikely to be of physiological importance to the newborn. Conversely, with a gastrointestinal tract that retains a system for the recognition, differential uptake and transfer of non-nutritional macromolecules, altricial newborn mammals are likely to make considerable use of bioactive substances in milk.

In altricially-born mammals the role played by the breast and gut in transferring chemicals from mother to young between birth and weaning is comparable to that undertaken by the placenta during the equivalent period in precocially-born mammals. Study of the placental barrier may offer a means by which to understand the processes of postnatal transfer of bioactive substances, and an understanding of placental transfer mechanisms can provide insight into their biological significance to the newborn infant. Indeed, both the endometrium and placenta are rich in trophic factors, and most of the growth factors and bioactive peptides found there are also present in milk.

Peaker and Neville[12] have formulated postulates that must be satisfied if non-nutritional substances in milk can be truly regarded as playing an important role in the physiology of the infant. An effect in the offspring must be obtained in response to exposure to the substance in the milk; this effect must be abolished by removal of that substance from milk and restored when it is returned; the substance must be shown to be present and active in milk; and it must retain its biological activity in the offspring to the site where it is postulated to act, or be activated by partial digestion within the gut.

BIOACTIVE SUBSTANCES IN MILK AND GENETIC CONFLICT BETWEEN MOTHER AND NEONATE

Protective factors

The protective substances in milk which help to defend the infant from infection, particularly that of the gastrointestinal tract, range from immunoglobulins and other bioactive proteins such as lactoferrin and lysozyme which neutralize antigens and interfere with bacterial metabolism and integrity, to oligosaccharides, nucleotides and trophic factors that may be involved in cell repair, immunomodulation and the maintenance of epithelial integrity.

This wide range of defensive factors has probably arisen during evolution because the principal interface between the newborn and its environment is the gastrointestinal mucosa. This is exposed to an ever-changing battery of micro-organisms and food proteins, which are constantly altering their antigenicity and pathogenicity in an attempt to secure a niche where they can propagate their genes.

The large variety of substances that milk contains and the different ways in which they contribute to the defense of the epithelium of the newborn infant against microbial and food-borne antigens, reflect the importance of this interface between organism and environment in the constant battle for survival of both it and the micro-organisms that inhabit and pass through it.

Mucosal barrier function and systemic immune defense systems are relatively naive in the human newborn. Immunoglobulin G (IgG) is transferred from mother to fetus via the placenta, but the infant does not possess a full complement of mucosal antibodies to protect it from the huge variety of antigens it will encounter throughout life. There is a particular advantage to the infant in ensuring that immunoglobulins are transferred to it intact from the mother before and after birth. Unlike growth factors or hormones, which have a fixed structure and uniform function, immunoglobulins vary almost infinitely.

Secretory immunoglobulin A (sIgA) provides protection against micro-organisms to which both the mother and infant are exposed. Via the enteromammary circulation[13], antigens recognized by M cells of maternal intestinal Peyer's patches generate primed plasma cells which migrate by the lymphoid system from her gut to her breast, providing a means of protecting the infant against the wide range of antigens to which the mother's gut has been exposed (Figure 2).

Hamilton[14] has argued that exposure of the organism to microbial antigens is a major force for genetic variation, and might even be the principal explanation for the persistence of sexual reproduction. Because the gastrointestinal mucosa is the surface of the organism which endures the most relentless and varied exposure to foreign antigens, it must have broad and adaptable defense mechanisms. The mucosal-associated lymphoid system (MALT) is an essential arm of the immune system, and for the newborn infant milk is the source of factors that afford both passive protection and help to stimulate active defenses[15].

If lactation originated form a modification of sebaceous secretions that initially served to protect the newborn from infection, it might be expected that selection of this function persisted, even when the process took on a greater nutritional importance. Altricial newborn, in remaining highly dependent on the mother for a long period, require from her much more than nutrients alone, and the high protein contents of their milks probably reflect the large amount of bioactive material in them.

Milk is rich in anti-inflammatory agents (antioxidants, growth factors, prostaglandins, lysozyme) and it appears to protect without evoking an inflammatory response. By being the principal means of controlling inflammation in the newborn (whose own defense mechanisms are immature) and of providing passive protection against antigens to which the mother has been exposed, the mother ensures the dependence of her offspring, at the same time as helping in its defense against infection. Immunoprotective and immunomodulatory substances in milk are

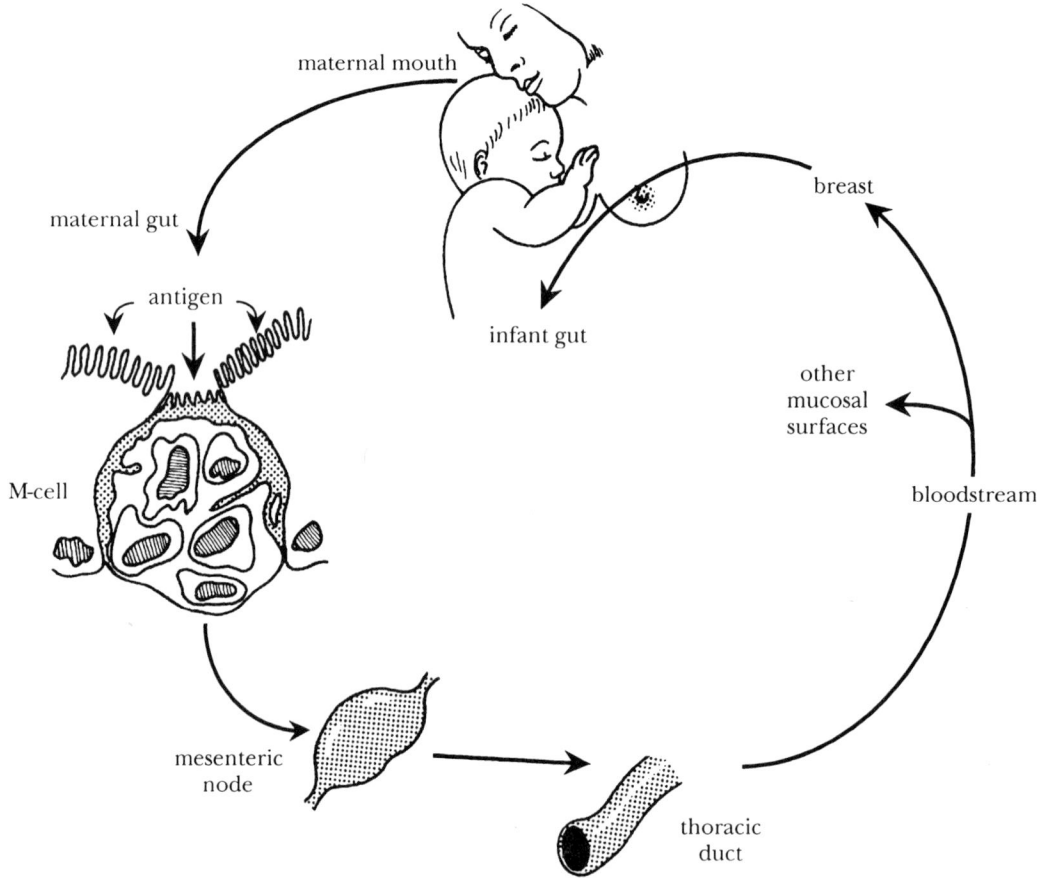

Figure 2 Enteromammary circulation. See text for explanation

therefore an example of a system that benefits the infant and leads to its continued reliance on the mother.

Trophic factors

Milk is also rich in non-nutritional polypeptides that are potentially trophic to the infant. Among these, the actions of epidermal growth factor (EGF) have been well characterized. Epidermal growth factor has trophic, mitogenic, cytoprotective and antisecretory actions: it exerts its trophic effects on epithelia where it can accelerate maturation of cell function and stimulate cell proliferation; it modulates gastric acidity by inhibiting the secretion of hydrochloric acid by parietal cells; and it modulates prostaglandin synthesis through effects on cyclo-oxygenase and lipo-oxygenase. These four biological actions are particularly relevant during the perinatal period of adaptation from intrauterine to extrauterine nutrition, when there is initiation of enteral feeding with exposure of the mucosa to 'foreign' antigens, acceleration of epithelial turnover and gastric acid secretion.

Because of its potentially critical role in early life, it is likely that there has been conservation of EGF in mammalian milks and selection of processes in the newborn that rely on its action. Epidermal growth factor is present in murine milk, and when given intraperitoneally to pregnant mice it accelerates maturation of brush border enzymes[16]. It also stimulates DNA and protein synthesis when applied topically to organ cultures of fetal rat small intestine[17]. Postnatally, EGF is trophic to the small intestine of the adult rat when administered systemically, but when given orogastrically it is trophic only when co-administered with a protease inhibitor or with a competitive substrate such as casein[18].

The gastrointestinal tract of the rat is capable of taking up EGF prenatally and postnatally[19,20], whence it may pass intact to the circulation and reach the liver and peripheral tissues. Epidermal growth factor resists degradation in the gastrointestinal tract. It is also secreted by ulcer-associated cells, suggesting that it has a function in mediating cellular repair. In infants with damage to the small intestinal mucosa from necrotizing enterocolitis and microvillus atrophy, systemically-delivered EGF leads to enterocyte proliferation and repair[21,22].

As a biologically active polypeptide, EGF may play a critical role in genetic conflicts in early life. Milk contains EGF and there are receptors for it on infant cells. Peaker and Neville's postulates[12] have been satisfied in some rodents, in which the milk-borne growth factor appears to act as a 'messenger' sent from mother to offspring. Evidence suggests that EGF is most useful to altricial young and to human infants born preterm or with damage to the gastrointestinal mucosa. The effects of deprivation of milk-borne bioactive substances on the welfare and survival of the newborn are demonstrated forcefully in the preterm baby, which, if not fed on human milk, is at ten times greater risk of necrotizing enterocolitis than if it is[23].

Milk provides EGF in far greater concentrations than endogenous production by the neonate, flooding its gut with bioactive substances at every feed. As the infant grows and becomes increasingly independent, its endogenous production increases and its requirements decrease. To be effective, protease activity must be low in the neonatal gut, or protease inhibitors or antagonists must be provided simultaneously in milk. By providing abundant quantities in association with factors that potentiate their action in the neonatal gut, protective and trophic factors in milk may be part of a system that makes the infant dependent on the mother, and a means by which she exerts her control over her offspring. This may be especially so in the altricial newborn, in which the gastrointestinal tract is not fully differentiated, and immature in its defense and barrier functions.

CONCLUSIONS

Haig[1] and Trivers[6] have explored the selective pressures acting on parents and offspring before and after birth, and pointed out that there is an overlap of self interest between each but not an identity of self interest. The infant is far from independent of the mother at birth, but as lactation progresses parental investment in the young decreases, culminating in a break in this interdependence at weaning, when behavioral acts of conflict may reach their peak.

Selective pressures act on the mammary gland, challenging it to secrete substances that improve the chances of infant survival and reproductive fitness. Selective pressures also act on the young to maximize the advantages it takes of the milk, and thereby its chances of survival to reproductive age. Counterbalancing these are selective pressures acting to conserve the mother's energies and to promote independence of the offspring as early as possible. The conflict between mother and young is expressed in the former as a decision to what extent to commit precious resources to (invest in) its young, and in the latter to what degree to remain dependent on the mother, in particular rely on her milk. Within the two extremes, from producing extremely precocial young through considerable investment in the embryo *in utero*, to producing extremely altricial offspring which depend on prolonged milk feeding, the genetic conflicts between mammalian mothers and their offspring are played out.

The choice between producing precocial or altricial offspring involves a switch from devoting care to the young while in the womb, where two-way interaction between mother and fetus of the kind outlined by Haig[1] can occur, to devotion of a greater proportion of maternal care to the process of suckling after birth, when the infant makes rising demands on the mother at the same time as growing increasingly independent.

This decision between short gestation and long lactation (altricial young) or long gestation and short lactation (precocial young) involves a trade-off not only in the energetics of food supply, but also in systems of defense against infection and of epithelial repair and function. The embryo may be protected from infection in the womb, but once born requires protection against a multitude of micro-organisms. The greatest selection pressures on the infant are on its defense mechanisms against infection of the gastrointestinal tract and systems for the maintenance of epithelial function and integrity, where exposure to potentially pathogenic micro-organisms is most relentless.

A price that must be paid by the mother of altrical young is that she must supply more than simply nutrients after birth. She must ensure that her offspring receives all the other factors that enable it to survive outside the womb and to undergo considerable development and maturation from the immature state in which it is born. The mother of precocial young accomplishes this well before birth, and this challenge to the mother is greatest for marsupials which spend a large proportion of their 'fetal' life in a pouch fused to a teat by which milk is supplied continuously.

In transferring non-nutritional substances to her suckling young, the mother, particularly that of altricial offspring, is also in a position to manipulate its physiology in ways that may be not only to its advantage, but also to hers. In producing altricial young whose gastrointestinal tracts and metabolisms are immature, the mother can take responsibility for making up for deficiencies in digestive function by secreting compensatory substances in her milk. By limiting the duration of gestation she also avoids the danger of the fetus trying to regulate her physiology by secreting substances into her circulation.

For altricial young, which remain dependent on the mother for a considerable period of time, the wide array of bioactive substances that must be transferred in milk afford opportunities for conflict between each. While the fetus appears to take advantage of its facility to secrete substances into the maternal circulation prenatally, after birth it makes demands on the mother's milk by sucking; the more it sucks the more it gets. To counter this demand, milk secretion is regulated in the mammary gland, but the mother also floods the infant's gastrointestinal tract with non-nutritional substances every time it feeds.

Among these proteins are casomorphins (α, β and κ) which have opioid effects. Their actions on the gastrointestinal tract are to slow down transit rate, to inhibit gastric acid and cholecystokinin secretion, and to potentiate somatostatin secretion, all actions that limit nutrient uptake. In addition, human milk contains benzodiazepine-like substances which modulate the activity of γ-aminobutyric acid (GABA), a major inhibitory neurotransmitter in the central nervous system. If GABA receptors in the infant are a target of maternal sedatives in milk, then the mother has a potent way of 'controlling' her infant and delivering to it other bioactive substances that modulate its physiology.

The genetic conflict hypothesis predicts that there is an advantage to both mother and infant in her expending energy on producing milk that contains a wide variety of protective and trophic factors. Numerous genes have been selected in the newborn to account for the defense and barrier functions of its gastrointestinal secretions, epithelium and immune system.

Numerous genes have also been selected in the mother to account for the extraordinarily complex and diverse array of substances that she secretes in her milk to protect her infant. Their number and diversity reflect the equal number and diversity of mechanisms that microorganisms adopt to colonize, invade and infect their host. The newborn infant is particularly vulnerable, and such maternal adaptations involve not just the immune system, but also the secretion in milk of proteins, oligosaccharides, glycoproteins, polypeptides, etc., which have specific and definable effects on microorganisms, compromising their survival in the gastrointestinal tract. In the infant, genes will be selected that make optimum use of the milk it receives. Thus nutrients and non-nutrients will be well utilized and the gastrointestinal tract will have unique mechanisms, such as antiproteases, specific receptors and specialized pathways for the uptake of intact bioactive substances.

If the hypothesis proposed here is to be tested, we need to know much more about the non-nutritional composition of the milk of mammals. Oftedal[24] has drawn attention to the paucity of data on the macronutrient content of mammalian milks, and pointed out that the most reliable measures come from samples obtained at peak lactation. However, to test the present hypothesis we need to have information on the changing nutrient and non-nutrient composition of milk during the immediate neonatal period from many mammals, spanning the full range of those born in an extreme altricial state (such as marsupials) to precocial newborn (such as the lamb or guinea pig). We also need to know more about the protein requirements for growth of altricial neonates: what proportion of nitrogen is used for this purpose and what represents non-nutritional protein; and the site and mechanisms of action

and uptake of bioactive substances in the neonatal gastrointestinal tract[25].

The mammary–enteral axis that all mammals have conserved, is much more than a conduit for the passage of nutrients from mother to young: it is a vital part of the means by which the mother maximizes the likelihood of the survival to reproduction of her offspring (and thereby perpetuation of half of her genes) and of the means by which the young makes maximal use of maternal provisions, employing bioactive substances secreted in milk to optimize adaptation to extrauterine life. The advantage of breast feeding may be marginal for the human neonate which appears capable of being reared on adapted cow's milk, but for many other mammals, particularly those that are suckled for a significant period, lactation is a time of genetic conflict between mother and offspring, and the milk she secretes contains not just food, but also ammunition for the struggle between them.

ACKNOWLEDGEMENT

I am grateful to Jean Hyslop for preparing the figures.

References

1. Haig, D. (1993). Genetic conflicts in human pregnancy. *Q. Rev. Biol.*, **68**, 495–532
2. Mossman, H. W. (1937). Comparative morphogenesis of the fetal membranes and accessory uterine structures. *Contrib. Embryol.*, **158**, 133–247
3. Weaver, L. T. (1993). Egg, placenta, breast and gut: comparative strategies for feeding the young. *Endocr. Regul.*, **27**, 95–104
4. Boyd, J. D. (1959). Glycogen in early human implantation sites. *Endocrinology*, **6**, 26–34
5. Fay, T. N. and Grudzinskas, J. G. (1991). Human endometrial peptides: a review of their potential role in implantation and placentation. *Hum. Reprod.*, **6**, 1311–26
6. Trivers, R. L. (1974). Parent–offspring conflict. *Am. Zool.*, **14**, 249–64
7. Koldovsky, O. and Thornburg, W. (1988). Hormones in milk. *J. Pediatr. Gastroenterol. Nutr.*, **6**, 172–96
8. Britton, J. R. and Koldovsky, O. (1989). Development of luminal protein digestion: implications for biologically active dietary polypeptides. *J. Pediatr. Gastroenterol. Nutr.*, **9**, 144–62
9. Weaver, L. T. and Walker, W. A. (1989). Uptake of macromolecules in the neonate. In Lebenthal, E. (ed.) *Human Gastrointestinal Development*, pp. 731–48. (New York: Raven Press)
10. Prentice, A., Ewing, G., Roberts, S. B., Lucas, A., MacCarthy, A., Jarjou, L. M. and Whitehead, R. G. (1987). The nutritional role of breast milk IgA and lactoferrin. *Acta Paediatr. Scand.*, **76**, 592–8

11. Martin, R. D. (1984). Suckling effects and adaptive strategies in mammalian lactation. *Symp. Zool. Soc. London*, **51**, 87–117

12. Peaker, M. and Neville, M. C. (1991). Hormones in milk: chemical signals to the offspring. *J. Endocrinol.*, **131**, 1–3

13. Kleinman, R. E. and Walker, W. A. (1979). The enteromammary immune system. *Dig. Dis. Sci.*, **24**, 876–82

14. Hamilton, W. D. (1964). The genetical evolution of social behaviour. *J. Theoret. Biol.*, **7**, 1–52

15. Kraehenbuhl, J.-P. and Neutra, M. R. (1992). Molecular and cellular basis of immune protection of mucosal surfaces. *Physiol. Rev.*, **72**, 853–79

16. Calvert, R., Beaulieu, J.-F. and Menard, D. (1982). Epidermal growth factor accelerates maturation of fetal mouse intestinal mucosa *in utero*. *Experientia*, **38**, 1096–7

17. Conteas, C. N., De Morrow, J. M. and Majumdar, A. P. N. (1986). Effect of epidermal growth factor on growth and maturation of fetal and neonatal rat intestine in organ culture. *Experientia*, **42**, 950–2

18. Playford, R. J., Woodman, A. Z., Clark, P., Watanapa, P., Vesey, D., Deprez, P. H., Williamson, R. C. N. and Calam, J. (1993). Effect of luminal growth factor preservation on intestinal growth. *Lancet*, **341**, 844–8

19. Weaver, L. T., Gonnella, P. A. and Israel, E. J. (1990). Uptake and transport of epidermal growth factor by the small intestinal epithelium of the fetal rat. *Gastroenterology*, **98**, 828–37

20. Gonnella, P. A., Siminoski, K., Murphy, R. A. and Neutra, M. R. (1987). Transepithelial transport of epidermal growth factor by absorptive cells of suckling rat ileum. *J. Clin. Invest.*, **80**, 22–32

21. Walker-Smith, J. A., Phillips, A. D., Walford, N., Gregory, H., Fitzgerald, J. D., MacCullagh, K. and Wright, N. A. (1985). Intravenous EGF-urogastrone increases small intestinal cell proliferation in congenital microvillous atrophy. *Lancet*, **2**, 1239–40

22. Sullivan, P. B., Brueton, M. J., Tabara, Z., Goodlad, R. A., Lee, C. T. and Wright, N. A. (1991). EGF in necrotising enterocolitis. *Lancet*, **338**, 53–4

23. Lucas, A. and Cole, T. J. (1990). Breast milk and neonatal necrotising colitis. *Lancet*, **336**, 1519–23

24. Oftedal, O. T. (1984). Milk composition, milk yield, and energy output at peak lactation: a comparative review. *Symp. Zool. Soc. London*, **51**, 33–85

25. Weaver, L. T. (1992). Breast and gut: the relationship between lactating mammary function and neonatal gastrointestinal function. *Proc. Nutr. Soc.*, **51**, 155–63

The minds of our children

F. Cockburn

INTRODUCTION

'And a woman who held a babe against her breast said,
"Speak to us of children."
And he said:
"Your children are not your children.
They are the sons and daughters
of Life's longing for itself.
They come through you but not from you,
and though they are with you
yet they belong not to you.
You may give them your love but not your thoughts,
for they have their own thoughts.
You may house their bodies but not their souls,
for their souls dwell in the house of tomorrow,
which you cannot visit, not even in your dreams.
You may strive to be like them, but seek not to
make them like you.
For life goes not backwards nor tarries
with yesterday.
You are the bows from which your children as living
arrows are sent forth."'

Kahlil Gibran, *The Prophet*[1]

If asked where your mind is you would have little difficulty in locating it somewhere inside your head. In earlier times you might have been persuaded that your 'self' or mind lay in your heart, liver or diaphragm, for the function and structures of the brain and nervous system were not known.

Even with newer brain scanning techniques such as positron emission tomography (PET) and functional magnetic resonance imaging, together with centuries of philosophical debate and psychological experimentation and observation, we find it difficult to define what constitutes the mind. Everyone has a mind. We

identify our 'self'. Every individual has a unique identity of mind which has been developed from before birth and throughout our lives. We can change our minds at any age sometimes for rational and at other times for irrational reasons.

However, the basis of our mindful thinking processes has been determined largely in our formative years. Children of 5 years certainly have minds of their own. Ask any parent. Most mothers are aware that even their infants (Latin – *infans*: English – not speaking) have minds of their own. Although words and language may not be necessary for the development of the mind they are essential for its description or definition.

WHAT IS THE MIND?

One definition from *Chambers Twentieth Century Dictionary* is 'that which thinks, knows, feels and wills'. Other words and phrases used to describe attributes of the mind include: memory, thought, judgement, opinion, reason, purpose, inclination, attention, consciousness, wits, intellect, sanity, right senses, personality, identity, self and soul.

It is the ability of the human to undertake abstract thought and to develop ideas which differentiates man from other animals. The mind of man is his most important attribute.

Aristotle gave much thought to the origin of the mind and of reason. He did not deny that humans have innate reason, i.e. they were born with reason. On the contrary, he thought that reason is man's most distinguishing characteristic but our reason or mind is completely empty until we have sensed something. So man has no innate 'ideas'. They are learned. Most of this learning takes place within the first year or two of life.

THE ANATOMY OF THE MIND

No textbook or CD-ROM of anatomy can show you the anatomy of the mind. Neither can they demonstrate the memory which is a major component of the mind. Scientific studies of memory have revealed that there are different forms of memory. Short-term memory is the system we use to hold on to small amounts of information for brief periods. This we use to remember speech long enough to gain meaning for conversation and to do mental arithmetic. Some attributes of the mind use short-term memory but most lie within the domain of long-term memory.

There are three major categories of long-term memory. Memories of events (episodic memory), acquisition and use of general knowledge (semantic memory) and acquisition and use of motor and cognitive skills (procedural memory) appear to be represented and stored within the brain using different neural mechanisms. Episodic memory is 'housed' in the hippocampus, parts of the thalamus and in connecting neuronal pathways[2].

Lasting traces of a series of visual images, sensations or emotions must be translated from their origins, e.g. light, color, pain, endocrine hormone release, to a network of neuronal synapses where electrochemical energy allows the integration, interpretation and storage of the signals for later recall. A fuller understanding of these processes will be reached during the next millennium.

THE EMBRYONIC AND FETAL BRAIN

The period of human development from 20 to 60 days post-conception has been termed arbitrarily embryogenesis because it is during this phase that most organs are formed and their relationships established. However, development of the brain and nervous system of the human continues throughout embryonic and fetal life and into the first year or two of postnatal life[3–6]. Fundamental developmental processes during embryonic and fetal growth of the brain include: regional differences in molecular composition controlled by regional gene expression, cell replication and programmed cell death, induction and intercellular communication, cell migration, movement of contiguous cell populations (folds, fusions, merges and separations), mechanical effects, and circulatory and metabolic homeostasis. Maternal infections, malnutrition, physical insults, and metabolic disorders such as diabetes mellitus, phenylketonuria and maternal ingestion of teratogens such as alcohol, increase the risk of congenital anomalies of the brain by affecting these processes.

There are three main types of genes, based on the function of the gene products. Mutations of *housekeeping* genes, which code for polypeptides present in the cytoplasm of every cell, are probably lethal in early gestation. *Structural* (tissue-specific) gene mutations cause defects in specific cells. *Regulatory* genes (master genes) code for polypeptides that are active in cell nuclei, modifying the array of transcribed genes from the totipotent cells of the 2–8-cell embryo to the specialized cell populations of later embryonic development. Proliferation and differentiation of cells during embryogenesis is largely controlled by growth and transcription factors. Transcription factors controlled by regulatory genes are responsible for a cascade of temporally and spatially organized events that cause the formation of, for example, the neural tube and corpus callosum. Neurotrophins and neurotrophin receptors affect not only neuronal survival, but also affect proliferation, differentiation, phenotypic expression and recovery after injury[7]. Abnormal transcription regulation can therefore cause profound errors of nervous system embryogenesis. Mitochondrial DNA mutations can also predispose to congenital anomalies and dysfunction of the brain[8].

Neuronal development starts in embryonic life and by 22 weeks' gestation most neurones have formed and have migrated from their area of origin, in the subependymal regions, to the cortical surface where they will form grey matter. During the second half of pregnancy the cells develop complex arborizations and after birth there is a very rapid increase in the numbers of synaptosomes in these neurones. At birth the term infant brain weighs about 350 g or 10% of the total body weight.

THE HUMAN INFANT BRAIN

There is a peak of glial cell division during the first 6 months of postnatal life and neuroglial cells envelop neuronal axons to create myelin sheaths particularly during the first 18 months of life[9]. During the first year brain weight increases threefold from about 350 to 1100 g. Throughout the first year of life the increase in infant brain weight parallels that of total body weight gain and remains at 10% of total body weight. Table 1 shows infant brain growth and cerebral cortex composition during the first year of life. It can be seen that 47% of the increase in brain weight during the first year takes place in the cortex and that the bulk of the dry weight of cortex is lipid, predominantly phospholipid. Sixty percent of the total energy intake of the infant during the first year is used by the brain largely to construct neuronal membrane and deposit myelin. Fat from human milk and from infant formulae is not simply a source of hydrocarbon for energy production but is comprised of a series of complex lipid structures necessary for the creation of cell membrane.

THE COMPOSITION OF NEURONAL MEMBRANES

Animal membranes, whether at the cell surface or forming part of an intracellular organelle such as a mitochondrion or peroxisome, are predominantly phosphoglycerols and unesterified cholesterol. In neuronal membranes there are in addition to these, sphingomyelins (phosphosphingolipids) and cerebrosides (glycosphingolipids). Singer and Nicolson proposed the 'fluid mosaic model' of membrane structure in which phospholipid is present as a bimolecular sheet with fatty acids held in the interior of the bilayer and with polar phospholipid head groups on the internal and external faces of the membrane[10]. Lipid bilayers provide flexible and adaptable structures into which are inserted proteins and glycoproteins such as enzymes, receptors and transmembrane transporter proteins. The major membrane phospholipids contain two fatty acids and a substituted (amino) alcohol attached to a glycerol phosphate backbone which is hydrophilic. The alcohol head group and the attached fatty acids have major effects on the functions of the membrane[11]. Phosphatidylcholine (PC), phosphatidylethanolamine (PE), phosphatidylserine (PS) and phosphatidylinositol (PI) are the major components of neuronal membranes. PC confers structural stability to the neuronal membrane[12] while the carboxyl group of PS functions as an ion exchange site[13]. Incorporation of peptides and proteins responsible for enzymatic activity and neurotransmission in phospholipid membranes, are not only dependent upon genetic control but also on the distribution of PS and PE and their fatty acid moieties in the membrane[12–14]. Incorporation

Table 1 Infant brain growth and composition during the first year of life. Each increase in weight is expressed as a percentage of the weight of the previous item in the table

	Percentage	*Weight* (g)
Increase in brain weight	—	750
Increase as cortex	47	350
Increase as cortex (dry weight)	35	125
Increase as lipid	60	75
Increase as phospholipid	65	50
Increase as docosahexaenoic acid	8	4

of proteins and peptides into the PS- and PE-rich areas of membrane is critically dependent upon the chain length, degree of unsaturation and hence configuration of the two fatty acids attached to each PS and PE moiety[15]. Polyunsaturated docosahexaenoic acid (DHA) of these moieties preferentially crosslinks with proteins and the degree of unsaturation conveyed by these molecules can mediate the activities of membrane bound enzymes[16,17]. Very high concentrations of DHA attached to PS and PE at the inner aspect of the phospholipid bilayer, is necessary for the promotion of the rapid and repeated complex biochemical activities which allow neurotransmission to take place at the neuronal synaptosomes. This is particularly important in the retina to allow the rapid conversion of light energy into electrical impulses in the retinal photoreceptors[18,19].

Whereas protein synthesis will cease if essential amino acid supplies are absent, incorporation of fatty acids into membrane phospholipids in the absence of long-chain polyunsaturated fatty acids (LCPUFA) proceeds with the substitution of fatty acids of similar chain length and desaturation, but none the less with the result that there are significant changes in membrane properties. Control mechanisms responsible for the distribution of different phospholipids and their fatty acids are at present unknown. Insertion of substitute LCPUFA may render the membrane metabolically unstable and more permeable to water (and electrolytes)[20].

We have recently demonstrated that the phosphatidylethanolamine and phosphatidylserine fatty acid composition in the neurones of cerebral cortex in formula-fed infants, is significantly depleted in docosahexaenoic acid when compared with the concentrations found in breast-fed infants[21,22]. Where there is dietary deficiency of LCPUFA of the n-3 series which includes DHA, n-6 fatty acids substitute for them. In formula-fed preterm infants deficient in n-3 and in n-6 LCPUFA, the n-9 fatty acids Mead and dihomo-Mead acids are substituted[21]. Arachidonic acid (AA) is a major active n-6 fatty acid and docosapentaenoic acid (DPA) is the fatty acid which is preferentially substituted for DHA. Animal studies have also shown that in n-3

fatty-acid deficiency states there is selective substitution of DHA in neuronal phospholipid membrane by DPA[23-25].

The preferential replacement of DHA in the phospholipid membrane by DPA can be seen to affect both phosphatidylethanolamine and phosphatidylserine from cerebral cortex (Figure 1). Synthesis of both DHA and DPA from the parent essential fatty acids, α-linolenic and linoleic respectively, are dependent upon a series of elongases and desaturases some of which may not function in early infancy[26].

Recent studies from our Department have shown that the cerebral white matter of artificially fed infants also contains relatively less DHA and a relative excess of AA. Measurements of concentrations of the major fatty acids of myelin, nervonic and lignoceric acid,

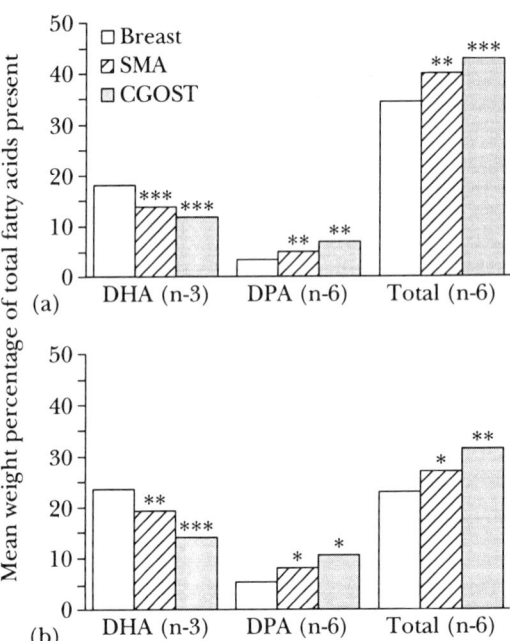

Figure 1 The mean weight percentage of total fatty acids present in (a) phosphatidylethanolamine and (b) phosphatidylserine of cerebral cortex from breast- and artificially fed infants during the first year of life. The SMA formula contained relatively greater concentrations of the essential fatty acid precursor of DHA, namely α-linolenic acid, than either Cow and Gate or Ostermilk (CGOST) formulae in each case. DHA (n-3), docosahexaenoic acid; DPA (n-6), docosapentaenoic acid; ***significant difference by Student's *t*-test, $p < 0.001$; **$p < 0.01$; *$p < 0.05$

showed that in artificially fed infants there was significant delay in the appearance of these very long chain fatty acids in the brain white matter[27]. Nervonic acid is undetectable in artificial formulae whereas in mature human milk nervonic acid contributes up to 0.32% of the total fatty acids. This dietary supply probably enables the earlier incorporation of nervonic acid into the cerebrosides of breast-fed infants. Delay in the appearance of these fatty acids in the white matter may indicate delayed myelination in artificially fed infants and this could have long-term adverse consequences.

ADVERSE EFFECTS OF ALTERED NEURONAL PHOSPHOLIPID COMPOSITION

There is now a balance of evidence which shows that human milk conveys significant advantage to preterm and term infants' visual and cognitive functions when compared with those of infants fed standard infant formulae[28,29]. Preterm infants fed human milk have higher developmental status at 18 months and a higher intelligence quotient in later childhood than those fed infant formulae[30,31]. There are also significantly altered electro-retinographic patterns with delayed rod photoreceptor maturation in preterm infants fed standard formulae compared to those who are breast fed. Visuocortical functions are better in breast-fed infants or in infants fed formula supplemented with DHA[32]. It has been shown that term infants' visual responses at 5 months after birth correlate with erythrocyte DHA concentrations[33]. Term infants fed breast milk have also been shown to have better stereo-acuity and better matching ability at 3 years of age than do formula-fed children[34].

Preterm infants fed breast milk or DHA-supplemented formulae perform significantly better than standard formula-fed infants on the Bayley mental scales[35–37]. Evidence for improved intellectual function in term infants who have been breast fed in comparison to those fed formula with inadequate DHA content is building up. Although most publications show that breast-fed infants have a higher mean IQ than

artificially fed infants there is often difficulty in interpretation due to social and educational factors. Another factor to be considered in comparisons between the visual function and intellectual function of breast-fed infants and those fed formulae without added DHA and AA, are the relative concentrations of these polyunsaturated fatty acids and also the relatively low concentrations of DHA found in human milk in some women with inadequate dietary intake of n-3 fatty acids[38].

SENSORY INPUT AND THE DEVELOPMENT OF THE HUMAN INFANT BRAIN AND MIND

The developing human infant brain requires visual, aural and emotional stimuli as well as good nutrition to properly develop the brain pathways which subserve and integrate normal brain development and function. For example, failure to stimulate the eye results in a failure of development of the occipital neurones subserving the functions of that eye[39]. Sensory input to the normal term human infant is largely dependent upon the mother's physical, intellectual and emotional state and on the family- and social support she receives. Psychological research into affect development suggests both that there is a particular developmental period that is most important in the development of emotional regulation[40], and that the age at which the infant is capable of regulating emotional expression may differ for each of the discrete emotions[41]. The mother, or other primary care-giver, by providing well-modulated stimulation, facilitates the growth of connections between cortical limbic and subcortical limbic structures that neurobiologically mediate self-regulatory functions[42]. Interactions between mother and infant, particularly in response to stressful transactions during the first 2 years of life are instrumental in determining the final structural maturation of an adaptive cortical system that can self-regulate emotional states. Schore[42] argues that early relational experiences directly influence the emergence of a frontolimbic system in the right hemisphere that can adaptively auto-regulate both positive and negative effect in response to changes in the socio-emotional environment. He further argues that failure of the mother and infant to develop this type of affect regulation and cortical and subcortical limbic structures, can result in the developmental psychopathology that underlies various forms of later psychiatric disorder. There is experimental evidence to show an increased risk of insecure attachments if day care, as typically provided in Western society, begins in the first year and is extensive in duration[43]. There is an increasing number of reports demonstrating that extensive non-maternal and non-paternal care in the first 2 years of life is a risk factor for the increased development of insecure patterns of attachment and elevated levels of aggression[44-49].

In addition to lack of good parenting within the first 2 years there are other exogenous influences which can pollute the developing minds of children. Adverse factors include irresponsible and thoughtless production of media material that can distort behavioral and social values. Just as abuse of alcohol and drugs can affect the physical structure and the fetal brain *in utero* these same toxins can distort the functioning of the mother and father's behavior towards the child, and thus distort the values of the child. Abuse of religious ideas can similarly create distortions within the naïve mind of the child. Various religions which may be defined as repositories in the minds of men which encompass their hopes, fears and aspirations, can have a very beneficial effect on codes of behavior and social interaction. Most religions have learned group behaviors with roles governing social activities which are beneficial, although each religion has its own code of ethics. Abuse of religious training can cause deviant development of the mind. Similarly, abuse of politics can result in racialism and nationalism to a degree which distorts the behaviors of the naïve mind. Other social pressures, particularly over-population and war situations, can create permanent scars within the minds of children.

Factors which can counteract these environmental pollutants include responsible parenthood, good education, good legislation and a balance between population size and natural resources.

CONCLUSION

Mammals probably first appeared on earth about 250 million years ago and placental mammals in the last 100 million years. The first hominids appeared between 4 and 5 million years ago and the early genus *Homo* around 2.5 million years ago. Modern man (*Homo sapiens sapiens*), characterized by a large and complicated brain, has during the last 40 thousand years evolved the complex society we know today. During this last 10 thousand years man has learned to cultivate plants and to farm animals and fish for food consumption. After the agricultural revolution came the industrial revolution and with it, during this past century, the practice of using modified bovine milks and synthetic plant-based milks to feed newborn human infants. The evolutionary processes which allowed man to develop considerable intellectual achievements have taken many thousands of years. During this last 100 years there has been a move from natural human mammalian feeding processes and a disruption of the normal maternal/infant involvement during the first 2 years of life throughout many countries of the world. A strong commercial drive to displace natural feeding of the human infant, together with altered family and work patterns has resulted in very low levels of breastfeeding in 'developed' countries. Although the World Health Organization (WHO) has made strenuous efforts to redress the imbalance created by these pressures, there is still a great need to alert the population to the needs both nutritional and emotional of the young human infant during the first years of life. It is important that the best formulae possible are developed and to this end some manufacturers are now adding DHA to infant formulae. However, it is essential that women are encouraged to feed their own infants and thus provide the best nutrient and also the best opportunity for optimal learning interactions between mother and infant. The brains and minds of our children are our most precious resource.

ACKNOWLEDGEMENTS

I gratefully acknowledge the work of my colleagues Dr J. Farquharson, Miss E. C. Jamieson, Dr K. Abbasi, Dr W. J. A. Patrick, Dr A. G. Howatson, Mrs N. Caine and Dr R. W. Logan, and my secretary Mrs Myra Fergusson and Miss J. Hyslop, medical artist, for their help in the preparation of the text.

References

1. Gibran, K. (1926). Speak to us of children. *The Prophet*, 1996 reprint, p. 20. (London: William Heinemann)
2. Lathe, R. and Morris, R. G. (1994). Analysing brain function and dysfunction in transgenic animals. *Neuropathol. Appl. Neurobiol.*, **20** (4), 350–8
3. Kostovic, I. (1990). Zentral nervensystem. In Hinrichsen, K. V. (ed.) *Human Embryologie*, pp. 381–448. (Berlin: Springer-Verlag)
4. Kostovic, I. (1990). Structural and histochemical reorganisation of the human prefrontal cortex during perinatal and postnatal life. *The Prefrontal Cortex. Prog. Brain Res.*, 85, pp. 223–40
5. Goldman-Rakic, P. S. (1992). Neuronal development and plasticity of association cortex in primates. *Neurosci. Res. Prog. Bull.*, **20**, 520–32
6. Kostovic, A., Judas, M., Petanjek, Z. and Simic, G. (1995). Ontogenesis of goal-directed behavior: anatomo-functional considerations. *Int. J. Psychophysiol.*, **19**, 85–102
7. Kalcheim, C. (1996). The role of neutrophins in development of neural-crest cells that become sensory ganglia. *Philos. Trans. Biol. Sci.*, **351**, 375–81
8. Brown, G. K. (1992). Pyruvate dehydrogenase Elα deficiency. *J. Inher. Metab. Dis.*, **15**, 625–33
9. Dobbing, J. (1981). The later development of the brain and its vulnerability. In Davis, J. A. and Dobbing, J. (eds.) *Scientific Foundations of Paediatrics*, 2nd edn., pp. 744–59. (London: William Heinemann)
10. Singer, S. J. and Nicolson, G. L. (1972). The fluid mosaic model of the structure of cell membranes. *Science*, **175**, 720–31
11. Stubbs, C. D. and Smith, A. D. (1984). The modification of membrane polyunsaturated fatty acid composition in relation to membrane fluidity and function. *Biochim. Biophys. Acta*, **779**, 89–137
12. Cullis, P. R. and De Krui, J. F. F. B. (1979). Lipid polymorphism and the functional roles of lipids in biological membranes. *Biochim. Biophys. Acta*, **559**, 399–420
13. Cook, A. M. Low, E. and Ishijimi, M. (1972). Effect of phosphatidylserine decarboxylase on neuronal excitation. *Nature (London) New Biol.*, **239** (92), 150–1
14. Fenske, D. B., Jarrell, H. C., Guo, Y. and Hui, S. W. (1990). Effect of unsaturated phosphatidylethanolamine on the chain order profile of bilayers at the onset of the hexagonal phase transition. ^{2}H–NMR study. *Biochemistry*, **29**, 11122–9
15. Salem, Jr, N., Kim, H. Y. and Yergey, J. A. (1986). Docosahexaenoic acid: membrane function and metabolism. In Simopoulos, A. P. *et al.* (eds.) *Health Effects of Polyunsaturated Fatty Acids in Seafoods*, pp. 263–317. (London: Academic Press Inc.)
16. Orlacchio, A., Maffei, E., Binaglia, L. and Porcellati, G. (1981). The effect of membrane phospholipid acyl-chain composition on the activity of brain beta-n-acetyl-D-glucosaminidase. *Biochem. J.*, **195**, 383–8
17. Tanaka, R. (1969). Comparison of lipid effects on K$^+$–magnesium Mg^{2+} activated p-nitrophenylphosphatase and sodium Na$^+$–K$^+$–Mg^{2+} activated adenosine tryphosphatase of membrane. *J. Neurol. Chem.*, **16**, 1301–7
18. Weidmann, T., Pates, R., Beach, J. *et al.* (1986). Lipid–protein interactions mediate the photochemical function of rhodopsin. *Biochem.*, **27**, 64–9
19. Wood, J. (1990). Essential fatty acids and their metabolites in signal transduction. *Biochem. Soc. Trans.*, **18**, 755–86
20. Stubbs, C. D. and Smith, A. D. (1990). Essential fatty acids in membrane: physical properties and function. *Biochem. Soc. Trans.*, **18**(5), 779–81
21. Farquharson, J., Cockburn, F., Patrick, W. J. A., Jamieson, E. C. and Logan, R. W. (1992). Infant cerebral cortex phospholipid fatty acid composition and diet. *Lancet*, **340**, 810–13
22. Farquharson, J., Jamieson, E. C., Abbasi, K. A., Patrick, W. J. A., Logan, R. W. and Cockburn, F. (1995). Effect of diet on the fatty acid composition of the major phospholipids of

infant cerebral cortex. *Arch. Dis. Child.*, **72**, 198–203

23. Bourre, J. M., Pascal, G., Durand, G., Masson, M., Dumont, O. and Piciotti, M. (1984). Alterations in the fatty acid composition of rat brain cells (neurones, astrocytes and oligodendrocytes) and of subcellular fractions (myelin and synaptosomes) induced by a diet devoid of n-3 fatty acids. *J. Neurochem.*, **43**, 342–8

24. Galli, C., Trzechiak, H. I. and Paoletti, R. (1971). Effects of dietary fatty acids on the fatty acid composition of brain ethanolamine phosphoglyceride: reciprocal replacement of n-6 and n-3 polyunsaturated fatty acids. *Biochim. Biophys. Acta*, **248**, 449–54

25. Mohrhauer, H. and Hollman, R. T. (1963). Alterations of the fatty acid composition of brain lipids by varying levels of dietary essential fatty acids. *J. Neurochem.*, **10**, 523–30

26. Farquharson, J., Jamieson, E. C., Logan, R. W., Patrick, W. J. A., Howatson, A. G. and Cockburn, F. (1995). Age- and dietary-related distributions of hepatic arachidonic and docosahexaenoic acid in early infancy. *Pediatr. Res.*, **38**, 361–5

27. Farquharson, J., Jamieson, E. C., Logan, R. W., Patrick, W. J. A., Howatson, A. G. and Cockburn, F. (1996). Docosahexaenoic and nervonic acids in term and preterm infant cerebral white matter. *Prenat. Neonat. Med.*, **1**, 1–7

28. Gibson, R. A. and Makrides, M. (1996). Early fatty acid supply and mental development. In Boulton, J., Larou, Z. and Rey, J. (eds.) *Long-term Consequences of Early Feeding.* Nestle Nutrition Workshop Series, Vol. 36, pp. 19–33. (Philadelphia: Lippencott-Raven)

29. Standing Committee on Nutrition of the British Paediatric Association (1994). Is breastfeeding beneficial in the UK? *Arch. Dis. Child.*, **71**, 376–80

30. Lucas, A., Morley, R. Cole, T. J. *et al.* (1990). Early diet in preterm babies and developmental status at 18 months. *Lancet*, **1**, 1477–81

31. Lucas, A., Morley, R., Cole, T. J., Lister, G. and Leeson-Payne, C. (1992). Breast milk and subsequent intelligence quotient in children born preterm. *Lancet*, **339**, 261–4

32. Uauy, R., Birche, D. and Perano, P. (1992). Visual and brain function measurements in studies of n-3 fatty acid requirements of infants. *J. Pediatr.*, **120**, S168–80

33. Makrides, M., Simmer, A., Goggin, M. and Gibson, R. A. (1993). Erythrocyte docosahexaenoic acid correlates with the visual response of healthy term infants. *Pediatr. Res.*, **33**, 424–7

34. Birche, D., Hoffman, D., Hale, L., Everett, M. and Uauy, R. (1993). Breastfeeding and optimal visual development. *J. Pediatr. Ophthalmol. Strabismus*, **30**, 33–8

35. Carlson, S. E., Werkman, S. H., Peeples, J. M. and Wilson, W. M. (1994). Long chain fatty acids and early visual and cognitive development of preterm infants. *Eur. J. Clin. Nutr.*, **48**, S27–30

36. Carlson, S. E. and Werkman, S. H. (1996). A randomised trial of visual attention in preterm infants fed DHA until 2 months. *Lipids*, **31**, 85–90

37. Werkman, S. H. and Carlson, S. E. (1996). A randomised trial of visual attention in preterm infants fed DHA until 9 months. *Lipids*, **31**, 91–7

38. Neuringer, M., Reisbick, S. and Janowsky, J. (1994). The role of n-3 fatty acids in visual and cognitive development: current evidence and methods of assessment. *J. Pediatr.*, **125**, S39–47

39. Hubel, D. H. (1978). *Effects of Deprivation on the Visual Cortex of Cat and Monkey*, Vol. 72, pp. 1–51. (New York: Harvey-Lect)

40. Gottman, J. M. and Fainsilber-Katz, L. (1989). Effects of marital discord on young children's peer interaction and health. *Dev. Psychol.*, **25**, 371–81

41. Buechler, S. and Izard, C. E. (1983). On the emergence, functions and regulation of some emotion expressions in infancy. In Plutchik, R. and Kellerman, H. (eds.) *Emotion. Theory, Research and Experience*, Vol. 3, pp. 292–313. (New York: Academic Press)

42. Shore, A. N. (1994). Affect regulation and the origin of the self. (Hillsdale, NJ: Lawrence Erlbaum Associates)

43. Bretherton, I. (1992). The origins of attachment theory: John Bowlby and Mary Ainsworth. *Dev. Psychol.*, **28**, 759–75

44. Belsky, J. and Rovine, M. J. (1988). Non-maternal care in the first year of life and security of the infant–parent attachment. *Child Dev.*, **59**, 157–67

45. Belsky, J. and Braungart, J. M. (1991). Are insecure-avoidant infants with extensive day-care experience less stressed by and more independent in the strange situation? *Child Dev.*, **62**, 657–71

46. Barglow, P., Vaughn, B. and Molitor, N. (1987). Effects of maternal absence due to employment on the quality of infant-attachment in a low-risk sample. *Child Dev.*, **58**, 945–54

47. Haskins, R. (1985). Public school aggression among children with varying day-care experience. *Child Dev.*, **56**, 689–703

48. Lamb, M. E., Sternberg, K. J. and Ketterlinus, R. (1992). Child care in the United States. In Lamb, M. E., Sternberg, K., Hwang, C. P. and Brobeg, A. G. (eds.) *Child Care in Context*, pp. 207–22. (Hillsdale, NJ: Lawrence Erlbaum Associates)

49. Scarr, S. and Eisenberg, M. (1993). Child care research: issues, perspectives and results. *Ann. Rev. Psychol.*, **44**, 613–44

Section II Symposia

Delivery of the very-low-birth weight infant

9

P. J. Steer

Delivery of the very-low-birth weight infant can be considered under three main headings.

WHEN TO DELIVER THE VERY-LOW-BIRTH WEIGHT INFANT

This is not as simple a decision as might be thought. There are situations when delivery is necessary for the safety of the baby or mother – for example with fulminating pre-eclampsia, placental abruption or fetal growth restriction. In a recent study of babies of between 500 and 800 g birth weight[1], such indications accounted for 12% of 111 cases. In the remainder, however, the birth was not planned – 35% preterm pre-labor rupture of membranes, 28% idiopathic preterm labor and 25% preterm labor associated with multiple pregnancy. This latter in particular complicates the decision from a logistic point of view – the facilities available always need to be considered.

In addition, the diagnosis of preterm labor is often difficult. The meta-analysis of 16 trials of betamimetics in preterm labor showed that in the control groups with no treatment, 35% of women with apparently definite preterm labor delivered at term[2].

Tocolysis is often suggested as a means of preventing the delivery of the very-low-birth weight infant. The delivery rate with threatened preterm labor can be reduced from 37 to 24% within 48 h, but even when it can be used, there is no overall effect on the proportion of babies delivering at term, or on perinatal death[2]. In fact, tocolysis is only appropriate for about 20% of women in preterm labor[3]; in the rest it is contraindicated because of ruptured membranes (less effective and a risk of infection),

medical complications indicating delivery, or advanced cervical dilatation (≥ 3 cm). Some tocolytics are now obsolete because of unacceptable side-effects (ethyl alcohol, isoxuprine hydrochloride) but even those in general use have many problems (Table 1). New tocolytics have been proposed, such as calcium antagonists (e.g. nifedipine)[4,5], oxytocin antagonists (such as atosiban)[6] and nitric oxide donors such as glyceryltrinitrate[7]. However, their efficacy and safety have yet to be shown. The effect of antibiotics is as yet unclear and must await the completion of the Oracle trial, co-ordinated from Leicester, UK by Professor D. Taylor and colleagues.

Table 1 Risks of tocolysis

β-*Agonists*
Fluid overload/pulmonary edema
Myocardial ischemia
Hyperglycemia
Hypokalemia
Death

Indomethacin
Maternal
  Peptic ulceration
  Gastro-intestinal bleeding
  Thrombocytopenia
  Allergic reactions
Fetal/neonatal
  Pulmonary hypertension secondary to closure
    of the ductus
  Necrotising enterocolitis
  Intraventricular hemorrhage

Magnesium sulfate
Adult respiratory distress syndrome
Respiratory depression
Cardiac arrest
Low therapeutic ratio

There are many specific contraindications to tocolysis; a selection are shown in Table 2.

WHERE TO DELIVER THE VERY-LOW-BIRTH WEIGHT INFANT

Ideally, all very-low-birth weight infants should be delivered in a tertiary referral center. However, risk assessment will select only a small proportion of preterm infants for special surveillance[8] and many women will present in labor at sites where intensive care for the infant is not readily available. '*In utero* transfer' is often cited as the solution, but many mothers and babies can be put at risk by transfer. In one study of 190 *in utero* transfers in the Liverpool region, 66 women (35%) had co-existing diseases and post-delivery had considerable morbidity, 17 (9%) needed prolonged intensive care, 32 (17%) were being treated with antihypertensives and/or anticonvulsants, some intravenously, and 32 (17%) were being treated with tocolytics[9]. There is the risk of hemorrhage, unrecognized fetal hypoxia, and even delivery while in transit. Mothers may have less confidence in their new birth attendants, there may be change and confusion in the management strategy, and the new and unfamiliar environment can be frightening to the family. Mothers may even die if there is a delay in delivery while a unit with a free cot(s) is identified[10].

HOW TO DELIVER THE VERY-LOW-BIRTH WEIGHT INFANT

Keirse[11], in his meta-analysis of the mode of delivery of the very-low-birth weight infant, has stated that 'the data are not sufficient to justify a policy of elective Caesarean delivery of the small baby'. The hazards of Cesarean section in this setting are increased; the lower segment is poorly formed and the procedure is often technically difficult. There is an increased risk of hemorrhage and infection. In general, if the

Table 2 Contraindications to tocolysis

Fetal death
Fetal distress
Lethal fetal abnormality
Chorioamnionitis – PPROM?
Antepartum hemorrhage
Maternal disease (cardiac, thyroid, diabetic)
Delivery indicated (severe pre-eclampsia)

PPROM prelabor preterm rupture of membranes

presentation is cephalic, Cesarean section is usually done for the same indications as for a term baby. For example, the presence of an abnormal fetal heart rate pattern increases the risk of neonatal respiratory distress syndrome[12], and the longer the pattern is abnormal, the higher the risk of cere' al palsy[13]. If the presentation is by the breech, the literature is very sparse, and has recently been reviewed by Penn and colleagues[14]. The data suggest that Cesarean is slightly safer for the baby, but carries substantial maternal morbidity. At present, the issue is so finely balanced that parental choice should be taken into account. If the pregnancy is multiple, it has become 'the norm' to perform a Cesarean section, despite the evidence which fails to support this approach[15–17].

Finally, there was for a while a trend to advocate the use of classical Cesarean sections between 23 and 30 weeks, when the lower segment is poorly formed, in the belief that this would be less traumatic for the baby. However, data from Edinburgh[18] and St. Mary's in London (L. Stacey and P. Steer, unpublished data) reviewed 38 Cesareans at less than 30 weeks gestation, and found that all 21 babies born by the lower segment incision survived, whereas nine of 17 born by the classical incision died. There was no evidence that the classical incision made the delivery easier, and in two cases in the St. Mary's series, the mothers went on to rupture their classical scars antenatally in their next pregnancies, in one case with the loss of the baby at 32 weeks' gestation.

References

1. Iannucci, T., Tomich, P. and Gianopoulos, J. (1996). Etiology and outcome of extremely low-birth weight infants. *Am. J. Obstet. Gynecol.*, **174**, 1896–1902

2. Keirse, M. (1995). Betamimetics in preterm labour. In Keirse, M., Renfrew, M., Neilson, J. and Crowther, C. (eds.) *The Cochrane Pregnancy and Childbirth Database.* (Oxford: Update Software, c/o BBC Publications)

3. Tucker, J., Goldenberg, R., Davis, R., Copper, R., Winkler, C. and Hauth, J. (1991). Etiologies of preterm birth in an indigent population: is prevention a logical expectation? *Obstet. Gynecol.*, **77**, 343–7

4. Kuperminc, M., Lessing, J. B., Yaron, Y. and Peyser, M. R. (1993). Nifedipine versus ritodrine for suppression of preterm labour. *Br. J. Obstet. Gynaecol.*, **100**, 1090–4

5. Glock, J. L. and Morales, W. J. (1993). Efficacy and safety of nifedipine verses magnesium sulfate in the management of preterm labor: a randomized study. *Am. J. Obstet. Gynecol.*, **169**, 960–4

6. Goodwin, T. M., Paul, R., Silver, H., Spellacy, W., Parsons, M., Chez, R. *et al.* (1994). The effect of the oxytocin antagonist atosiban on preterm uterine activity in the human. *Am. J. Obstet. Gynecol.*, **170**, 474–8

7. Lees, C., Campbell, S., Jauniaux, E., Brown, R., Ramsay, B., Gibb, D. *et al.* (1994). Arrest of preterm labour and prolongation of gestation with glyceryl trinitrate, a nitric oxide donor. *Lancet*, **343**, 1325–6

8. Mercer, B., Goldenberg, R., Das, A., Moawad, A., Iams, J., Meis, P. *et al.* (1996). The preterm prediction study: a clinical risk assessment system. *Am. J. Obstet. Gynecol.*, **174**, 1885–95

9. Ryan, T. and Kidd, G. (1989). Maternal morbidity associated with *in utero* transfer. *Br. Med. J.*, **299**, 1383–5

10. Levene, M. I., Wild, J. and Steer, P. J. (1992). Higher multiple births and the modern management of infertility in Britain. *Br. J. Obstet. Gynaecol.*, **99**, 607–13

11. Keirse, M. (1995). Elective versus selective caesarean delivery of the small baby. In Keirse, M., Renfrew, M., Neilson, J. and Crowther, C. (eds.) *Pregnancy and Childbirth Module, the Cochrane Database of Systematic Reviews.* (Oxford: Update Software)

12. Hobel, C. J., Hyvarinen, M. A. and Oh, W. (1972). Abnormal fetal heart rate patterns and fetal acid-base balance in low birth weight infants in relation to the respiratory distress syndrome. *Obstet. Gynecol.*, **39**, 83–8

13. Shy, K. K., Luthy, D. A., Bennett, F. C., Whitfield, M., Larson, E. B., Van Belle, G. *et al.* (1990). Effects of electronic fetal monitoring, as compared with periodic auscultation, on the neurologic development of premature infants. *N. Eng. J. Med.*, **322**, 588–93

14. Penn, Z. J., Steer, P. J. and Grant, A. (1996). A multicentre randomised controlled trial comparing elective and selective caesarean section for the delivery of the preterm breech infant. *Br. J. Obstet. Gynaecol.*, **103**, 684–9

15. Davison, J., Easterling, T. R., Jackson, J. C. and Benedetti, T. J. (1992). Breech extraction of low-birth-weight second twins: can cesarean section be justified? *Am. J. Obstet. Gynecol.*, **166**, 497–502

16. Dommergues, M., Mahieu-Caputo, D., Mandelbrot, L., Huon, C., Moriette, G. and Dumez, Y. (1995). Delivery of uncomplicated triplet pregnancies: is the vaginal route safer? *Am. J. Obstet. Gynecol.*, **172**, 513–17

17. Wildschut, H., Roosmalen, J., Leeuwen, E. and Keirse, M. (1995). Planned abdominal birth compared with planned vaginal birth in triplet pregnancies. *Br. J. Obstet. Gynaecol.*, **102**, 292–6

18. Haddad, N. and Irvine, D. (1988). Classical versus lower segment caesarean section in very preterm deliveries. *Lancet*, **1**, 762

Postnatal management of the very-low-birth weight infant

10

O. Linderkamp

INTRODUCTION

Most very-low-birth weight (VLBW) infants are healthy at birth, although premature infants more often suffer from malformation and intrauterine growth retardation than full-term infants. However, due to their immaturity, VLBW infants need special support, and often intensive care, since they are not ready to adjust to extrauterine life. Stewart and Hope[1] have shown that in 90% of VLBW infants with periventricular leukomalacia, this complication results from postnatal events. The major goals of the management of the VLBW infant are:

(1) Survival;

(2) Normal maturation and growth;

(3) Prevention of damage by intensive care techniques; and

(4) Prevention of psychosocial problems.

This chapter focuses on the three topics that are major research areas of the Neonatology Division in Heidelberg.

PREVENTION AND TREATMENT OF HYPOTENSION AND ISCHEMIC ORGAN DAMAGE

Arterial blood pressure increases with birth weigh and postnatal age[2]. The circulation of the healthy VLBW infant is characterized in high blood flow dynamics in spite of low arterial driving pressure. Thus, the resistance to blood flow (exerted by the vessel geometry and viscosity of blood) is extremely low in VLBW infants[3]. These peculiar flow conditions , which appear to work very well *in utero*, make the VLBW infant extremely vulnerable to any circulatory disturbance.

Low arterial blood pressure in VLBW infants is common during the first hours after birth. In most VLBW infants, arterial blood pressure increases spontaneously within 6 h of birth, thereby suggesting that in hypotensive, but otherwise stable infants, an expectant approach may be adequate[4]. However, an expectant approach to hypotension in VLBW infants may lead to cerebral leukomalacia and hemorrhage[5,6] since impaired autoregulation in these infants causes a parallel fall of blood pressure and cerebral blood flow[7-9]. Low arterial blood pressure in many VLBW infants shortly after birth may explain why blood flow velocity in the cerebral arteries of preterm infants at 28 weeks of gestational age decreases by about 50% during the first 2 h after birth when compared with fetuses of the same gestational age[10]. Moreover, hypotension and low blood volume at birth predispose the VLBW infant to increased risks of severe respiratory distress syndrome and bronchopulmonary dysplasia[11].

Hypotension in VLBW infants may be due to hypovolemia, heart failure, systemic vasodilatation or impaired venous return to the heart. Several studies have shown that the arterial blood pressure in hypotensive preterm infants increases in response to blood volume expansion[6-9]. On the other hand, studies on the relationship between blood volume and arterial blood pressure yielded conflicting results. In VLBW infants of 2–8 h postnatal age, a poor relationship existed between blood volume and systolic blood pressure[12]. In a study of 95 VLBW infants, we showed that during the first 2 h after birth, 58% of VLBW infants with systolic blood pressures below 35 mmHg had a low blood volume (< 70 ml/kg) and responded to volume expansion with a marked rise in systolic blood pressure, whereas VLBW infants with normal or high blood volume (> 70 ml/kg) did not respond to volume expansion (Linderkamp and colleagues, unpublished data). This may explain why other authors observed a more pronounced increase in arterial blood pressure with dopamine treatment when compared to volume expansion[13,14].

Systemic vasodilatation may occur as a result of treatment with morphine, diazepam, muscle relaxants or vasodilators. Since generalized vasodilatation increases the vascular capacity, usually volume expansion will compensate for the vasodilatation. Impaired venous return to the heart often occurs during mechanical ventilation due to increased intrathoracic pressure. Minimization of the alveolar and intrathoracic pressure may be achieved with high frequency oscillatory ventilation. We have recently shown that cardiac output and blood flow velocity in cerebral and intestinal arteries may markedly improve with high frequency oscillatory ventilation[15].

Placental transfusion provides the neonate with both volume expansion and red blood cells. In the 1960s, several reports suggested that placental transfusion of preterm infants may decrease their risk of respiratory distress syndrome[11]. Recently, two randomized controlled studies have been performed on the effects of delayed cord-clamping in vaginally born VLBW infants[16,17]. These studies showed a marked increase in the hematocrit value after delayed cord clamping and no effect of the mode of cord clamping on the incidence of cerebral hemorrhage. Moreover, Kinmond and colleagues[17] reported decreased red cell transfusion requirements and decreased oxygen dependence in the infants with delayed cord clamping. We are currently investigating the effects of delayed cord clamping in VLBW infants born by Cesarean section. Our preliminary results show that a sufficient placental transfusion can be achieved

if the VLBW infant is kept 40 cm below the placenta and the cord is clamped after 30 s.

Gill and Weindling[14] performed a randomized controlled trial to compare the effects of plasma vs. dopamine in the hypotensive VLBW infant. Plasma up to 40 ml/kg was successful in 45%, whereas dopamine up to $10 \, \mu g \, min^{-1} \, kg^{-1}$ succeeded in 89% of the hypotensive infants. These data agree with our results that approximately 50% of hypotensive VLBW infants suffer from hypovolemia and therefore benefit from volume expansion.

Based on these results, we suggest the following approach in VLBW infants with low blood pressure during the first hours after birth:

(1) Abnormalities frequently associated with hypotension (e.g. acidosis, hypoxemia, sepsis) are treated;

(2) If no signs of cardiac failure are evident, infants are given 10 ml/kg of a volume expander (e.g. serum) over 30–60 min;

(3) If the arterial blood pressure tends to increase, but remains low, the serum infusion is repeated;

(4) If there is no or little response to volume expansion, treatment with catecholamines or dexamethasone is initiated; and

(5) Additional circulatory measurements (e.g. echocardiography) may be helpful to distinguish hypovolemia from cardiac failure.

PREVENTION AND TREATMENT OF RETINOPATHY OF PREMATURITY

Retinopathy of prematurity (ROP) appears to develop in two phases[18,19]. Early vasoconstriction damage to endothelial cells and obliteration of retinal microvessels develop in response to high oxygen pressure or other factors (e.g. intensive light, radicals). Vasoproliferation follows, perhaps in response to an angiogenic factor released by the hypoxic retina.

In a prospective study on 2392 premature infants born in the Rhine-Neckar region between 1984 and 1995, multivariate analysis yielded the following significant risk factors for ROP[20]:

(1) Low birth weight;

(2) Low gestational age;

(3) Total volume of transfused red cells;

(4) Mechanical ventilation > 7 days; and

(5) Postnatal transport.

Preventive measures include strict monitoring if arterial oxygen (O_2) and carbon dioxide (CO_2) pressures and arterial blood pressure, and avoidance of postnatal transport, intense illumination and iron overload (transfusions). We have shown in a randomized controlled study that prolonged covering of the eyes of VLBW infants for prevention of retinal illumination does not decrease the incidence of ROP[21]. This may be explained by cyclical illumination in our preterm ward. Reduced daylight is present during the day, whereas at night light is reduced to almost complete darkness. Since increased oxygen supply may stop retinal vasoproliferation, we try to achieve regression of vasoproliferation by keeping the arterial oxygen saturation (SaO_2, measured by pulse oxymetry) continuously high if ROP stage II or III has developed. At stage II we keep SaO_2 between 93 and 96% and at stage III (extraretinal proliferation) between 95 and 99%.

Retinopathy of prematurity stage III + (threshold retinopathy) requires treatment for prevention of retinal detachment. Seiberth and co-workers[22] yielded better results with diode-laser coagulation when compared to cryopexia for treatment of severe ROP. After cryopexia, in nine out of 39 infants (23%) both eyes became blind, whereas after diode-laser coagulation only one eye in 25 infants (2% of all eyes) became blind.

GENTLE INDIVIDUALIZED CARE FOR THE VLBW INFANT

Preterm infants are usually exposed to the technical environment of a neonatal intensive care unit (NICU) which provides a lot of life-saving methods, but often fails to consider the individual needs of the infants and their parents. Several groups have performed intervention programs on preterm infants and their parents to minimize the adverse effects of hospitalization. Most programs aimed to compensate for the intensive hospital care of preterm infants that was assumed to be necessary for their survival[23,24].

At the present time, the impact of psychological and social support on the wellbeing of preterm infants and their parents is becoming an issue of major interest for neonatologists[25,26]. Several neonatologists have published successful programs which try to eliminate as much intensive care as possible and to introduce as much psychological and social support as possible. Wung (unpublished observations, cited by Avery and associates (1987). *Pediatrics*, **79**, 26–30) from the United States was the first to suggest the restriction of mechanical ventilation to those who really need it (Table 1). Jacobsen and associates[27] and Faxelius and co-workers[28], from Scandinavia, managed to decrease the number of infants receiving mechanical ventilation to less than 50% by applying early continuous positive airway pressure (CPAP). Marcovich[29] from Austria recently reported that

Table 1 Indications for mechanical ventilation of very low-birth weight infants

	Conventional	Wung (New York)	Marcovich[29] (Vienna)
Arterial SaO_2 ($FiO_2 > 60\%$)	< 88%	< 88%	< 88%
Arterial PcO_2 (mmHg)	> 50	> 65	> 90
pH	< 7.25	< 7.15	< 7.10
Severe respiratory distress	yes	yes	no
Apneas in the first days	few	several	numerous

FiO_2, fraction of inspired oxygen

in her unit only 20% out of 42 VLBW infants required mechanical ventilation. Marcovich suggests restriction of all means of intensive care such as blood sampling, transcutaneous blood gas monitoring, and insertion of venous and arterial lines. On the other hand, she encourages skin contact (including Kangaroo care) between infants and parents, and also between infants and staff.

Als and co-workers[30] have recently shown that individualized developmental care decreases the time of mechanical ventilation and hospital treatment, and reduces the risk for cerebral hemorrhage and adverse neurological outcome. Mechanical ventilation may impair cerebral perfusion, thereby increasing the risk for cerebral ischemia and hemorrhage[31]. Moreover, mechanically ventilated infants are at high risk of developing severe pulmonary damage and bronchopulmonary dysplasia. Mechanical ventilation is extremely stressful and sometimes painful for the infants and it separates them from their parents. Thus, modern neonatal intensive care should minimize intensive care, but maximize psychosocial support. Provision of gentle and individualized care for preterm infants includes:

(1) Restriction of artificial ventilation and other means of intensive care to the infants who really need them;

(2) Eliminating as much as possible any activity that produces distress for the infants and their parents;

(3) Shaping the environment within the intensive care unit so that it is the least disruptive and the most comforting to the infant and the parents; and

(4) Allowing as much skin-to-skin contact of infants and their parents as possible (including Kangaroo care).

Prenatal counselling of the parents by neonatologists and other staff facilitates the decision making by parents for perinatal interventions and improves the postnatal communication and wellbeing of parents in the NICU. Intervention before birth may prolong pregnancy in mothers with early contractions[32]. Early visits of the mothers to their infants are facilitated by the localization of the NICU in the delivery unit. For nurses, physicians and other staff, psychological and medical care are of equal importance. The NICU and other neonatal units provide all the necessary intensive care techniques, including recent new developments (e.g. oscillatory ventilation), but also a kind and home-like environment. The wards are quiet, auditory stimulation is provided by the parents and by cassette recorders and not by technical devices. Reduced daylight is present during the day, whereas at night light is reduced to almost complete darkness. Reduced light levels relieve the infants of stress and appear to decrease the risk of retinopathy[21].

Early skin-to-skin contact (including Kangaroo care) between parents and infants is encouraged. Several studies have shown that Kangaroo care is safe even for VLBW infants with body weights below 1000 g[33–36]. It increases the confidence of the parents and appears to improve regular breathing and heart rate in some preterm infants. A self-help group has special parents' rooms in the neonatal wards where parents regularly meet with 'veteran' parents and staff members. Moreover, the self-help group provides continuous support for families with preterm infants and other high-risk neonates. Mothers are encouraged to provide breast milk for their infants[37] and to participate in nursing procedures as early as possible.

Mechanical ventilation is the most important single factor for long-term problems resulting from intensive care in preterm infants[20,31]. On

Table 2 Details of preterm infants born in the Perinatal Center of Heidelberg[38]

		1991	1992	1993
Number of infants	< 1000 g	28	30	26
	1000–1500 g	61	47	52
Mechanically	< 1000 g	86	80	62
ventilated (%)	1000–1500 g	38	32	21
Mortality (%)	< 1000 g	18	20	12
	1000–1500 g	8	4	4

the other hand, many preterm infants cannot survive without mechanical ventilation and the delayed commencement of mechanical ventilation can result in hypoxia and brain damage. It is, therefore, extremely important to start mechanical ventilation at the right time, but to avoid mechanical ventilation in the infants who do not really need it. Only experts in neonatology are capable of making the proper decisions on the treatment required for tiny preterm infants.

By using the indications for mechanical ventilation introduced by Wung (Table 1), we managed to decrease both the percentage of mechanically ventilated preterm infants and their mortality between 1991 and 1993 (Table 2). In 1993, only 35% of the infants with birth weight below 1500 g were intubated and mechanically ventilated. This agrees with results reported by other neonatal centers using similar approaches[27,28] (Wung, unpublished observations).

References

1. Stewart, A. and Hope, P. (1988). Outcome of very low birthweight or very preterm infants with special consideration of perinatal events. In Kubli, F., Patel, N., Schmidt, W. and Linderkamp, O. (eds.) *Perinatal Events and Brain Damage in Surviving Children*, pp. 258–64. (Heidelberg: Springer)

2. Versmold, H. T., Kitterman, J. A., Phibbs, R. H., Gregory, G. A. and Tooley, W. H. (1981). Aortic blood pressure during the first 12 hours of life in infants with birth weight 610 to 4,220 grams. *Pediatrics*, **67**, 607–13

3. Linderkamp, O. (1996). Pathological flow properties of blood in the fetus and neonate. *Clin. Hemorheol.*, **16**, 105–16

4. Moscoso, P., Goldberg, R. N., Jamieson, J. and Bancalari, E. (1983). Spontaneous elevation in arterial blood pressure during the first hours of life in the very-low-birth-weight infant. *J. Pediatr.*, **103**, 114–17

5. Miall Allen, V. M., De Vries, L. S. and Whitelaw, A. G. L. (1987). Mean arterial blood pressure and neonatal cerebral lesions. *Arch. Dis. Child.*, **62**, 1068–9

6. Bada, H. S., Korones, S. B., Perry, E. H., Arheart, K. L., Ray, J. D., Pourcyrous, M., Magill, H. L., Runyan, W., Somes, G. W., Clark, F. C. and Tullis, K. V. (1990). Mean arterial blood pressure changes in premature infants and those at risk for intraventricular hemorrhage. *J. Pediatr.*, **117**, 607–14

7. Greisen, G., Pryds, O., Rosén, I. and Lou, H. (1988). Poor reversibility of EEG abnormaility in hypotensive, preterm neonates. *Acta Paediatr. Scand.*, **77**, 785–90

8. Jorch, G. and Jorch, N. (1989). Failure of autoregulation of cerebral blood flow in neonates studied by pulsed Doppler ultrasound of the internal carotid artery. *Eur. J. Pediatr.*, **146**, 468–72

9. Kempley, S. T. and Gamsu, H. R. (1993). Arterial blood pressure and blood flow velocity in major cerebral and visceral arteries. II. Effects of colloid infusuion. *Early Hum. Dev.*, **35**, 24–30

10. Kurmanavichius, J., Karrer, G., Hebisch, G., Huch, R. and Huch, A. (1991). Fetal and preterm newborn cerebral blood flow velocity. *Early Hum. Dev.*, **26**, 113–20

11. Linderkamp, O. (1982). Placental transfusion: determinants and effects. *Clin. Perinatol.*, **9**, 559–92

12. Bauer, K., Linderkamp, O. and Versmold, H. T. (1993). Systolic blood pressure and blood volume in preterm infants. *Arch. Dis. Child.*, **69**, 521–2

13. Rennie, J. M. (1989). Cerebral blood flow velocity variability after cardiovascular support in premature babies. *Arch. Dis. Child.*, **64**, 897–901

14. Gill, L. B., Weindling, L. M. L. (1994). Randomized controlled trial to compare plasma protein fraction and dopamine in the hypotensive very low birthweight infant. *Pediatr. Res.*, **35**, 273

15. Nelle, M., Zilow, E. P. and Linderkamp, O. (1995). Circulatory performance in neonates on high-frequency oscillation. *Int. Care Med.*, in press

16. Hofmeyr, G. J., Gobetz, L., Bex, P. J., Van der Griendt, M., Nikodem, C., Skapinker, R. and Delahunt, T. (1993). Periventricular/intraventricular hemorrhage following early and delayed umbilical cord clamping. A randomized controlled trials. *Online J. Curr. Clin. Trials Doc.*, **110**

17. Kinmond, S., Aitchison, T. C., Holland, B. M., Jones, J. G., Turner, T. L. and Wardrop, C. A. (1993). Umbilical cord clamping and

preterm infants: a randomised trial. *Br. Med. J.*, **306**, 172–5

18. Avery, G. B. and Glass, P. (1988). Retinopathy of prematurity: what causes it? *Clin. Perinatol.*, **15**, 917–28

19. Phelps, D. L. (1988). Reduced severity of oxygen-induced retinopathy in kittens recovered in 28% oxygen. *Pediatr. Res.*, **24**, 106–9

20. Seiberth, V., Linderkamp, O., Freiwald, R. Knorz, M. C. and Liesenhoff, H. (1997). Risk factors in retinopathy of prematurity. A multivariate statistical analysis. *Grafe's Arch. Ophtalmol.*, in press

21. Seiberth, V., Linderkamp, O., Knorz, M. C. and Liesenhoff, H. (1994). A controlled clinical trial of light and retinopathy of prematurity. *Am. J. Opthalmol.*, **118**, 492–5

22. Seiberth, V., Linderkamp, O., Knorz, M. C. and Liesenhoff, H. (1995). Diode laser photocoagulation for 3 + retinopathy of prematurity. *Graef's Arch. Clin. Exp. Ophtalmol.*, **233**, 489–93

23. Hall, W. G. and Oppenheim, R. W. (1987). Developmental psychobiology: prenatal, perinatal and early postnatal aspects of behavioral development. *Annu. Rev. Psychol.*, **38**, 91–128

24. Affleck, G., Tennen, H. and Rowe, J. (1991). Infants in Crisis. *How Parents Cope with Newborn Intensive Care and its Aftermath.* (New York, Berlin, Heidelberg: Springer)

25. Freud, W. E. (1988). Prenatal attachment, the perinatal continuum and the psychological side of neonatal intensive care. In Fedor-Freyberg, P. G. and Vogel, M. L. V. (eds.) *Prenatal and Perinatal Psychology and Medicine*, pp. 217–34. (Carnforth, Lancashire, UK: Parthenon Press)

26. Minde, K. (1986). Bonding and attachment: its relevance for the present-day clinician. *Dev. Med. Child. Neurol.*, **28**, 803–6

27. Jacobsen, T., Gronvall, J., Peterson, S. and Anderson, E. (1993). "Minitouch" treatment of very low-birth-weight infants. *Acta Paediatr. Scand.*, **82**, 934–8

28. Faxelius, G., Katz-Salamon, L. M. and Lagercrantz, H. (1994). Scandinavian VLBW infants in the Stockholm County. *Early Hum. Dev.*, **39**, 139–40

29. Marcovich, M. (1995). Vom sanften Umgang mit Frühgenborenen. Neue Wege in der Neonatologie. *Int. J. Prenat. Perinat. Psychol. Med.*, **7**, 57–71

30. Als, H., Lawhon, G., Duffy, F. H., McAnulty, G. B., Gibes-Grossman, R. and Blickman, J. G. (1994). Individualized developmental care for the the very-low-birth-weight preterm infant. Medical and neurofunctional effects. *J. Am. Med. Assoc.*, **272**, 853–8

31. Bozynski, M. E. A., Nelson, M. N., Matalon, T. A. S., O'Donnel, K. J., Naughton, P. M., Vasan, U., Meier, W. A. and Ploughman, L. (1987). Prolonged mechanical ventilation and intracranial hemorrhage: impact on developmental progress through 18 months in infants weighing less than 1,200 grams. *Pediatrics*, **79**, 670–6

32. Sontheimer, D., Gassen, M., Feltner-Heller, H., Stober, B., Bastert, G. and Linderkamp, O. (1995). Prevention of prematurity in women with premature labour. *Int. J. Prenat. Perinat. Psychol. Med.*, **7**, 31–8

33. Anderson, G. C. (1991). Current knowledge about skin-to-skin (kangaroo) care for preterm infants. *J. Perinatol.*, **91**, 216–26

34. Bauer, J., Sontheimer, D., Fischer, C. B. and Linderkamp, O. (1996). Metabolic rate and energy balance in very low birthweight infants during Kangaroo holding by their mothers and fathers. *J. Pediatr.*, **129**, 608–11

35. Sontheimer, D., Fischer, C. B., Scheffer, F., Kaempf, D. and Linderkamp, O. (1995). Pitfalls in respiratory monitoring during Kangaroo care. *Arch. Dis. Child.*, **72**, F115–17

36. Whitelaw, A., Heisterkamp, G., Sleath, K., Acolet, D. and Richards, M. (1988). Skin to skin contact for very low birthweight infants and their mothers. *Arch. Dis. Child.*, **63**, 1377–81

37. Morley, R. and Lucas, A. (1993). Early diet and outcome in prematurely born children. *Clin. Nutr.*, **12** (Suppl. 1), S6–11

38. Linderkamp, O. (1995). Minimization of intensive care for tiny preterm infants. In Bitzer, J. and Stauber, M. (eds.) *Psychosomatic Obstetrics and Gynaecology*, pp. 243–7. (Bologna, Italy: Monduzzi Editore, International Proceeding Division)

Nutrition of the very-low-birth weight infant

11

P. J. J. Sauer, M. Saenz de Pipaon Marcos and M. G. A. Baartmans

'You cannot feed a baby with mathematics, you must feed a baby with brains'.

Abraham Yacoup, one century ago.

The optimal nutrition of the very-low-birth weight (VLBW) infant remains a topic of continuous debate, despite extensive research over the last three decades. In this chapter we would like to discuss some of the recent results obtained by different investigators and, based on this review, give guidelines on how to feed the VLBW infant.

HOW MUCH TO FEED

The majority of studies done so far, at least in human infants, have focused on the question of the optimal intake of calories and protein. These studies have mainly been conducted in relatively healthy, growing, appropriate for gestational age (AGA) preterm infants. Important studies regarding the optimal intake of energy and protein have been conducted by Kashyap and colleagues[1,2]. They compared the effect of three formulae, differing in energy and protein content, on gain in weight, length, head circumference and body composition. They compared formulae providing 120 kcal and 2.4 g protein $kg^{-1} day^{-1}$, 120 kcal and 3.5 g protein $kg^{-1} day^{-1}$ and 148 kcal and 3.5 g protein $kg^{-1} day^{-1}$, respectively. The higher protein intake resulted in greater rates of weight gain, length gain, and gain in head circumference. Increasing the energy intake to 148 kcal $kg^{-1} day^{-1}$ further increased the rate of weight gain, but mainly as a result of fat accretion. These results are in line with many other studies (for review, see reference 3). It is clear that growth can be stimulated by increasing protein and energy intake. However, protein intakes greater than 3.5–4 g $kg^{-1} day^{-1}$ are unlikely to be utilized completely for anabolism and hence will be catabolized, resulting in the metabolic effects characteristic of excessive protein intake. Increasing the energy intake to values above 120–130 kcal $kg^{-1} day^{-1}$ mainly results in increases in fat deposition. The energy balance of a growing AGA preterm infant receiving approximately 130 kcal $kg^{-1} day^{-1}$ is given in Figure 1.

The needs of the sick preterm infant as well as the small for gestational age (SGA) infant are largely unknown. There are indications that infants born SGA have a higher need of energy and possibly also of proteins than their AGA counterparts[4,5]. In an (unpublished) study comparing the growth of AGA and SGA infants receiving either 100 or 120 kcal $kg^{-1} day^{-1}$, we observed a lower weight gain in the SGA infants at 120 kcal $kg^{-1} day^{-1}$ compared to their AGA counterparts, while the SGA almost ceased

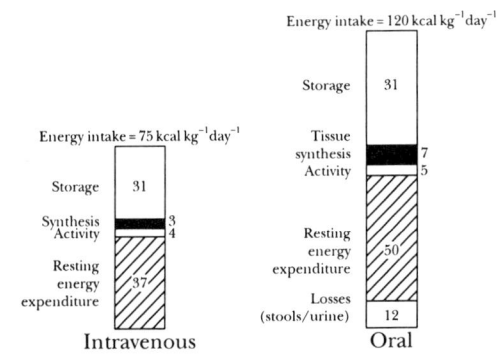

Figure 1 Estimated energy balance in orally fed preterm neonates. Reproduced from reference 3 with kind permission from Springer-Verlag

growing at intakes of 100 kcal kg^{-1} day^{-1}, in contrast to the AGA infants. Using stable isotopes to measure protein turnover, we also collected evidence that 3.5 g kg^{-1} day^{-1} protein is a lower limit for SGA infants. The optimal energy and protein intake for infants with diseases, like bronchopulmonary dysplasia (BPD), is largely unknown. Weight gain is often unsatisfactory in BPD infants. This could be due to either a reduced tolerance of oral feeding, a lower absorption or a higher energy expenditure. A number of studies have evaluated the energy expenditure of BPD infants and found it to be elevated[6,7]. However, these studies, which used indirect calorimetry as well as stable isotopes, may have had methodological flaws[8]. Therefore, the results of these studies should be interpreted with caution. More studies on these topics are needed, but it is very likely that both SGA infants and infants with BPD do need extra energy and protein.

We have studied the optimal composition and structural position of different fatty acids. The absorption of medium chain fatty (MCT) acids is better than that of long chain fatty (LCT) acids. The absorption of long chain fatty acids is dependent on their position on the glycerol molecule. There seems to be no advantage in adding MCT to formulae[9]. A formula in which the saturated long chain fatty acids are on the sn-2 position of glycerol and the unsaturated fatty acids on the 1 and 3 positions seems optimal, improving both the fatty acid and calcium absorption[10].

ESSENTIALITY OF AMINO ACIDS

Traditionally, amino acids are divided into essential and non-essential amino acids. Essential amino acids are defined as amino acids in which the carbon skeleton cannot be synthesized by the human body. Twenty amino acids are known to be incorporated into body proteins. In the classical studies that distinguished essential from non-essential amino acids, one amino acid was deleted from the diet and growth or protein balance was used to define the essentiality. Based on these studies, nine amino acids were classified as essential (Table 1).

More recent studies, however, have indicated that a number of amino acids might be partially indispensable for preterm and term infants, although they are not indispensable for adults. Jackson and colleagues[11] were the first to study the conditional essentiality of an amino acid in infants using stable isotopes. After the administration of [^{15}N]glycine, ^{15}N is lost in urinary urea. However, in human milk-fed LBW infants, no or minimal loss of ^{15}N-urinary urea was found. Jackson speculated that all the glycine was incorporated into protein and therefore not lost in urine. We observed the same phenomenon in both VLBW-SGA infants fed formula and in VLBW infants not receiving any dietary protein on day 4 of life[12]. All these results indicate that glycine might be conditionally indispensable for VLBW infants.

Recent studies have also shown that other amino acids might be indispensable for VLBW infants. We observed in VLBW infants a linear relationship between plasma cysteine levels and rate of protein synthesis on day 1 of life[13]. Infants fed a total parenteral nutrition (TPN) solution without cysteine have low plasma cysteine levels. This is attributed to a low activity of hepatic cystathionase, a key enzyme in the transulfuration pathway. Miller and co-workers[14] studied the essentiality of amino acids by

Table 1 Classification of amino acids and taurine as indispensable, conditionally indispensable, or dispensable for low-birth weight infants. Reproduced from reference 16 with kind permission from Kluwer Academic Publishers

Dispensable	Indispensable	Conditionally indispensable*
Alanine	Histidine	Arginine
Asparagine	Isoleucine	Cysteine
Aspartate	Leucine	Glutamine
Glutamate	Lysine	Glycine
Serine	Methionine	Proline
	Phenylalanine	Taurine†
	Threonine	Tyrosine
	Tryptophan	
	Valine	

*Insufficient evidence for the classification of these amino acids as either dispensable or indispensable for the growth and development of low-birth weight infants; †taurine is not synthesized into protein

infusing ^{13}C-labelled glucose as precursor of the carbon skeleton of amino acids. They found almost no enrichment in plasma cysteine and tyrosine, again showing a potential essentiality of these amino acids. Recently they observed no enrichment in plasma amino acids but an enrichment in apo-B lipoprotein[15]. This can be explained by a limited synthesis of these amino acids, which are then immediately incorporated into newly synthesized protein and not released into plasma.

Pencharz and associates[16] have done extensive studies to determine the essentiality of amino acids in newborn pigs and in human adults. They infused different amounts of individual amino acids and looked at protein synthesis, nitrogen retention and the oxidation of the infused amino acid. For tyrosine they could, for instance, show that a low intake results in a low nitrogen retention and a low oxidation rate of tyrosine. Increasing the intake of tyrosine caused an increased nitrogen retention as well as increase in tyrosine oxidation. The level of intake at which protein synthesis or nitrogen retention reaches a maximal plateau and oxidation of the amino acid starts to increase, might be the optimal level of intake.

Human milk contains rather low amounts of, for instance, cysteine, tyrosine and glycine. The exact requirements of these amino acids in the preterm infant are yet to be established. More studies are needed to better define the amino acid requirements of these infants. It is not unreasonable, however, to speculate that a number of TPN solutions and also human milk and preterm infant formulae might be too low in individual amino acids.

Glutamine

Glutamine is a preferential fuel for rapidly dividing cells such as enterocytes, lymphocytes and macrophages. Traditionally, glutamine was thought to be non-essential and was not included in parenteral feeding because of its relative instability in solution. Nowadays it is possible to keep glutamine stable in nutrient solution[17].

During catabolic illness, the plasma concentration of glutamine decreases and recent studies have demonstrated that glutamine may be a conditionally essential amino acid during this period[18]. Glutamine appears to be beneficial when depletion is severe and/or when intestinal mucosa is damaged by insults such as starvation, chemotherapy or radiation therapy[19]. There have been no extensive studies in preterm infants. Lacey and colleagues[20] studied 44 extremely low-birth weight infants (ELBW) who received glutamine in their parenteral nutrition and concluded that glutamine is safe for use in ELBW premature infants, and the most beneficial effect was seen in the cohort less than 800 g ($n = 24$). To confirm these observations larger multicenter trials are needed.

WHAT TO FEED

The optimal nutrition for the VLBW infant should satisfy its nutritional and other needs while preventing unwanted side-effects. Estimated needs for a number of nutrients are given in Table 2. Human milk, including the milk of the mother delivering preterm, does not contain sufficient amounts of energy and protein, especially approximately 3 weeks after delivery. It is of interest to note that a higher protein and energy content of preterm human milk is found during the first 2–3 weeks of life, a period when only part of the total intake is given orally. Human milk is considered to have many advantages over formula feeding. We will discuss below a few of the potential beneficial effects of human milk. Potential advantages of human milk are:

(1) Reduced incidence of infections;

(2) Reduced incidence of necrotizing enterocolitis;

(3) Presence of nucleotides;

(4) Presence of growth factors;

(5) Presence of cholesterol;

(6) Presence of polyunsaturated fatty acids (PUFA);

Table 2 Calculated nutrient intakes from preterm human milk during the 1st, 2nd and 4th weeks of lactation and mature donor human milk compared with estimated nutritional needs of low-birth weight infants

Component (unit kg^{-1} day^{-1})	Preterm milk			Mature milk	Estimated nutrient needs
	Week 1	Week 2	Week 4		
Energy (kJ)*	504	504	504	504	504
Fluid volume (ml)	180	180	180	190	150
Protein (g)	3.9	3.4	2.8	2.4	3.5
Sodium (mEq)	4.0	2.7	1.8	2.0	3.5
Calcium (mg)	53	46	42	47	160–200
Phosphorus (mg)	25	27	23	26	80–100

*1 kJ = 0.239 kcal

(7) Prevention of allergy; and

(8) Improvement of cognitive and psychomotor development.

Human milk and infections

Many aspects of the human immune system are incompletely developed at birth and this immaturity is most profound in the preterm infant. Both the cellular and humoral defence mechanisms are immature. The transfer of antibodies that usually takes place during the last trimester of pregnancy, has not been possible. Human milk contains a number of defence agents like lactoferrin, lysozyme and secretory immunoglobulin A (IgA). Moreover, it contains cells like macrophages. Feeding human milk also has an effect on the bacterial flora in the gut, favoring the growth of bifidobacteria and a number of Gram-negative bacteria. Theoretically, therefore, human milk has advantages regarding the incidence of infections in newborn infants. However, surprisingly few studies have been done in preterm infants. Studies comparing the incidence of infections in VLBW infants receiving human milk with that of infants receiving formula are lacking. Two studies showed that supplemental feeding of expressed human milk reduced the incidence of infections in VLBW infants. However, one study was done in India[21] and the other in the 1960s[22]. These studies, therefore, have a limited relevance to modern neonatal intensive care units (NICUs). More clinical research should be carried out to ascertain whether human milk has indeed a protective effect against infections in VLBW infants.

Incidence of necrotizing enterocolitis

Many studies have investigated the relationship between type of feeding and necrotizing enterocolitis (NEC) and, in particular, the potential preventive effect of human milk. Some studies showed a protective effect of human milk[23], while others found no difference in incidence of NEC between human milk- and formula-fed infants[24]. NEC is most likely a disease caused by a multitude of factors and it will therefore be difficult to pinpoint one factor as being either causative or protective. One of the most cited studies on the protective effect of human milk against NEC has been published by Lucas and Cole[23]. In their paper they showed a significantly lower incidence of NEC in the human milk-fed group than in the formula-fed group. A careful look at this paper, however, gives a slightly different impression. The incidence of NEC was not different between groups born at a gestational age of less than 30 weeks. Significance was reached by a surprisingly high incidence of NEC in formula-fed infants born at more than 31 weeks' gestation, especially in the group born at 34–36 weeks. Necrotizing enterocolitis is, these days, in most modern NICUs, mainly a problem of infants below 30 weeks' gestation. It is unclear whether human milk has a protective effect in these infants. Finally, it is interesting to note that NEC has almost disappeared for more than 10 years in our unit[25]. One possible explanation might be our feeding policy of not starting oral feedings before day 7 of life in VLBW infants.

Nucleotides

Nucleotides consist of a nitrogenous base, a pentose sugar and one or more phosphate groups. The nitrogenous base is either a purine or a pyrimidine whose atoms are primarily derived from amino acids[26]. Cellular nucleotides may be found in millimolar concentrations. Nucleotides participate in a wide variety of biochemical processes. They serve as the ubiquitous high-energy source adenosine triphosphate (ATP), as monomeric precursors of nucleic acids, as physiological mediators, as components of coenzymes and as activated intermediates. Nucleotides can be endogenously synthesized but this synthesis rate might be limited in preterm infants, making these compounds 'conditionally essential'. Several studies, both in humans and animals, have investigated the potential beneficial effects of adding nucleotides to the diet[27]. Results are summarized in Table 3. The effects, as found in humans, are rather limited and of short duration. More studies are therefore needed to distinguish the exact role of nucleotides in the feeding of VLBW infants.

Growth factors

Growth factors can be defined as low molecular weight proteins (mostly in the range 3000–70 000) that initiate growth responses in target cells through binding to highly specific cell-surface receptors, an interaction that is followed by internalization of the entire complex into the cell. This interaction leads to an increase in both cell size and number, through a stimulation of various anabolic cellular pathways including nutrient uptake, transport, DNA synthesis, RNA synthesis and protein synthesis, together with a co-ordinated inhibition of catabolic pathways, such as protein degradation[28].

Human milk contains an impressive number of growth factors and the list of known growth factors has expanded considerably in recent years (Table 4). There is almost no solid published evidence of a physiological role of milk growth factors in the neonate. However, indirect evidence for a putative role includes the following: the concentration of some of the factors is higher in milk and colostrum than in maternal serum (epidermal growth factor (EGF) and insulin). It has been shown that EGF is absorbed intact following oral administration and may, therefore, produce biological effects on non-gastrointestinal targets in the neonate. The third observation is that the growth factor concentration in milk is high enough to evoke a growth stimulus using cultured cells[29].

In the 1970s and 1980s, researchers demonstrated, in animal studies, that milk is a potent stimulator of growth both *in vivo* and *in vitro*[30–32]. Klagsbrun[33] provided the first *in vitro* evidence that human milk contains mitogenic factors and Ichiba and co-workers[34] showed the growth promoting activity of human milk on (human) fetal intestinal cell lines.

Epidermal growth factor is found in higher concentrations in pre- than in postpartum

Table 3 Reported effects of dietary nucleotides in humans and in animals (from reference 27)

	Human	Animal
Promotion of small intestinal growth		+
Increased small intestinal disaccharidase activity		+/–
Intestinal hyperemia		+
Protection against diarrheal disease	+	+
Effects upon stool flora	+	
Enhanced cellular immunity	+	+/–
Enhanced humoral immunity		+
Effects upon hepatic composition		+
Increased blood levels of long-chain polyunsaturated fatty acids	+/–	+/–
Effects upon serum lipoproteins	+/–	

Table 4 Gastrointestinal (GI) trophic factors. Reproduced from reference 17 with kind permission from W. B. Saunders Company

For the GI tract	GI secretion	Factors affecting GI motility
Nutrients, especially iron, zinc, vitamin B_{12}, vitamin A, folate, arginine, glutamine	secretin gastrin gastric inhibitory peptide pancreatic polypeptide vasoactive intestinal peptide neurotensin	motilin enteroglucagon vasoactive intestinal peptide neurotensin enteroglucagon cholecystokinin
Hormones and peptides Epidermal growth factor Transforming growth factor Insulin-like growth factor Insulin Growth hormone Glucocorticoids Somatostatin Bombesin Intestinal peptide YY		
Others Polyamines Nucleotides		

mammary secretions, suggesting that it may act as a local regulator of prepartum mammary gland development. Limited degradation of EGF in the gastric milieu of the suckling rat and preterm infant suggests that milk-borne EGF may retain bioactivity in the newborn gastrointestinal tract. In rodents, milk-borne EGF is involved in the regulation of the timing of eyelid opening and tooth eruption, and in intestinal, hepatic, pancreatic and lung development. Data on the effect of EGF on the developing human gastrointestinal tract are limited primarily to *in vitro* studies[17,35].

Milk insulin-like growth factor-1 (IGF-1) is derived primarily from maternal serum. Also IGF-binding proteins are reported in milk. Bioactivity of IGFs is retained in the gastrointestinal tract and studies in calves, septic rats and dexamethasone-treated rats suggest the important role of IGF-1 in the gastrointestinal tract[36,37]. Orally administered bovine whye growth factor extract (WGFE) containing IGFs, EGF, platelet-derived growth factor (PDGF), transforming growth factor-β (TGF-β), as well as uncharacterized growth factor activity, was effective in reducing intestinal damage caused by injection in adult rats of a high dose of the chemotherapy drug, methotrexate. Insulin-like growth factor-1

(oral or systemic) was ineffective in this setting. This last study outlined the fact that growth stimulation is most effective when growth factors are administered in a combined form[38].

Cholesterol

Human milk contains ample amounts of cholesterol (10–15 mg/100 ml)[39], while the level in formulae is rather low. Different studies, mainly in baboons, have studied the effect of breast vs. formula feeding in early life on cholesterol metabolism in later life. The results of these studies are partly summarized in Figure 2.

Feeding baboons in early life with human milk with cholesterol results in lower serum cholesterol, high-density lipoprotein-1 (HDL_1) and HDL_2 cholesterol concentrations and bile acid production rates in later life, and in higher low-density lipoprotein (LDL) receptor messenger RNA (mRNA) concentrations[40]. It is likely that there is an imprinting of cholesterol metabolism in early life that has a sustained effect until adulthood. A rather conflicting study from the same group of authors, however, showed that baboons fed formula in early life were more able to tolerate a cholesterol challenge in later life than human milk-fed

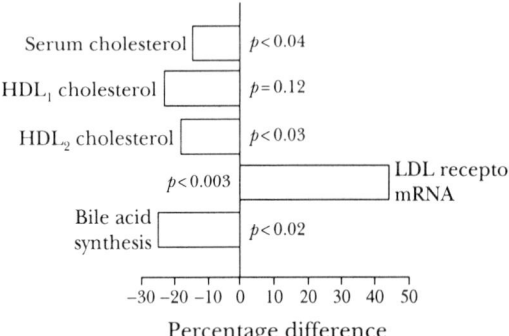

Figure 2 Long-term effects of breast vs. formula feeding on cholesterol metabolism (from reference 41). HDL, high-density lipoprotein; DL, low-density lipoprotein

baboons[41]. Under conditions of normal feeding in adulthood, baboons fed human milk in infancy might be better off, but during high-cholesterol challenges formula-fed animals might have advantages.

A recent study in human infants, using stable isotopes to quantitate cholesterol synthesis, showed a lower cholesterol synthesis rate in human milk-fed infants compared to formula-fed counterparts[42]. Endogenous cholesterol synthesis might be down regulated in human milk-fed infants. It is unknown whether this phenomenon causes the above mentioned 'imprinting'. Fall and associates[43] compared serum cholesterol in 50–60-year-old adults fed either human milk or formula in infancy. Those adults who were breastfed but weaned before the age of 1 year or who received both breast and bottle feeding showed lower cholesterol levels compared to adults exclusively breastfed for more than 1 year or exclusively formula-fed. We should realize immediately, however, that the fat composition of the formula given to these individuals (high in milk fat) is not at all comparable to that of the modern formulae. The question of whether cholesterol should be added to the feeding of the VLBW infant remains unanswered. More studies are needed. At the same time we should realize that cholesterol is an important component for brain growth and therefore important for the preterm infant.

Polyunsaturated fatty acids

It has been known for some time that there are two families of fatty acids that are essential for human health: n-3 and n-6 essential fatty acids. The parent compounds of these fatty acids are α-linolenic acid (C18-3n3) and linoleic acid (C18-2n6), respectively. From these parent compounds important fatty acids like arachidonic acid (AA) (C20-4n6) and docohexaenoic acid (DHA) (C22-6n3) are formed via chain elongation and desaturation. Arachidonic acid is an important precursor for prostanoids, while DHA is an important component of cell membranes in the retina and the brain. Human milk contains PUFAs, while older formulae for both preterm and term infants are devoid of these compounds. Several studies showed decreasing plasma and tissue levels of AA and DHA in preterm infants fed a formula devoid of PUFAs[44,45]. It was therefore speculated that PUFAs are semi-essential for preterm infants. Recently we showed that, in contrast to what was previously thought, preterm infants are able to synthesize AA and DHA[46]. An explanation for these findings might be that the need for AA and DHA is so high in the preterm infant that, despite endogenous production, plasma levels decrease when no additional dietary PUFAs are given.

Many studies have recently focused on the potential beneficial effects of adding PUFAs to the feeding[47]. Uauy[44] was the first to observe improved visual acuity in infants fed a DHA-supplemented formula. A number of studies have subsequently been done, so far, however, without completely convincing evidence of the beneficial effect of adding PUFA to the feeding of the preterm infant. A summary of a number of recent studies is given in Table 5. More studies and in particular studies with much larger numbers of infants, are needed to answer the question of whether PUFAs are essential for preterm infants.

Allergy

Many studies have investigated the relationship between human milk, formula and allergy.

Table 5 Positive effects of adding docosahexaenoic acid (DHA) to formulae containing α-linolenic acid (experimental) compared with α-linolenic acid alone (control): randomized trials in preterm infants. Reproduced from reference 47 with kind permission from Kluwer Academic Publishers

Retinal physiology	enhanced at 36 weeks PMA unchanges at 57 weeks PMA
Visual acuity	higher at 48 and/or 57 weeks PMA unchanged at 69, 79 and 92 weeks PMA
Look duration	shorter look duration at 69, 79 and 92 weeks PMA (the only ages studied) shorter look duration at 92 weeks PMA (the only age studied) in a second trial
Bayley MDI	higher 12-month scores in infants discharged from hospital and fed a nutrient-enriched (preterm) formula until 48 weeks PMA (both control and experimental groups had normal biochemical indices of vitamin A, zinc and protein status by 48 weeks PMA) no effect on 12-month Bayley MDI in infants discharged from the hospital on term formula (both control and experimental groups had evidence of marginal vitamin A, zinc and protein status at 48 weeks PMA)

PMA = post-menstrual age; Bayley MDI = mental developmental index

Almost all studies have been done in term infants. The results of the different studies are somewhat conflicting. The general message, however, seems to be that breastfeeding is protective against allergy in cases where there is a genetic predisposition of the infant to allergy. Studies on this issue in preterm infants are lacking.

Cognitive and psychomotor development

The effect of early feeding on the development of VLBW infants has been extensively studied by Lucas and co-workers[48]. They have followed a large cohort of infants fed either human milk (expressed vs. banked) or formula (preterm vs. term formula). By analyzing their results in varying ways, a number of observations have been made. In one study the authors showed a significantly higher psychomotor development index (PDI) and mental developmental index (MDI) at 18 months in infants fed the preterm formula (higher protein and energy content) compared to those fed the term formula[48]. In other studies they found that infants fed banked human milk had higher PDI scores at 18 months than those fed term formula, and had developmental scores similar to infants fed the preterm formula[49]. As banked human milk contains significantly lower amounts of protein and energy than the preterm formula, while the development was comparable, the authors suggested that other factors in human milk may have a favorable effect on neurodevelopment in preterm infants. In a recent study Lucas and colleagues[49] showed higher IQ scores at 8 years of age in VLBW infants fed human milk vs. formula in infancy. In this paper the authors, however, do not describe the composition of the formula given to the infants. It is unclear whether these infants were fed a preterm or a term formula. Another very important confounding variable in all studies of this group is the very marked difference in social class between the infants of mothers giving breastfeeding and the formula-fed counterparts, the social class of the breast-feeders being much higher. It is very well known, especially in preterm infants, that there is a relationship between outcome and social class. Although the authors commented that they corrected statistically for this difference, the magnitude of the difference in social class makes the other results unconvincing. A final issue that should be considered in evaluating the results of Lucas and associates is the rather variable period that the test-feeding was given in infancy, ranging from 2 weeks to approximately 2 months. The feeding after discharge was also not controlled. Therefore more studies are needed to really answer the question if breastfeeding in itself improves the cognitive and psychomotor development in VLBW infants.

WHEN TO FEED

There is a wide variety in timing of initiation of enteral feedings in VLBW infants between different NICUs. Some units start on the first day of life, other units wait until the infant is 'stable', others only start after weaning from the ventilator, while in our unit it is practice to start enteral feeding after 7 days. Potential advantages of starting early feeding are stimulation of gut growth and maturation, stimulation of gut hormones and attainment of early total enteral feeding (with less need for TPN). The latter might result in an earlier regain of birth weight and better postnatal growth. A potential negative effect of early administration of enteral feeding is a supposed higher incidence of NEC. This prompted us to delay the introduction of enteral feeding to day 7 of life with a concomitant virtually complete disappearance of NEC[21].

Studies in animals have shown a reduction in gut mass, mucosal weight, protein and DNA content in animals fed intravenously compared with those receiving the same solution orally[50]. A reduction in the levels of sucrase, maltase and lactase was also observed. These results were observed after withholding oral feeding for 1 week in rats. It is difficult, however, to translate these results immediately to humans as the rate of growth in rats is quite different from that of humans. Heird and colleagues[51] showed in dogs that feeding colostrum for 24 h resulted in a significant increase in DNA, protein and protein/DNA ratio of the ileum and jejunum over the values found directly after birth. No increase, however, was observed in the formula-fed animals.

Oral feeding induces the maturation of the gastrointestinal tract and especially alters the permeability for large molecules. Different studies, both in humans and animals, have shown that gut permeability decreases with the introduction of feeding, both in humans and animals[52,53]. Gut closure, however, is especially observed when human milk is given and is less

obvious during the first days of life in cases where formula is administered. Administration of enteral feeding also promotes the motility of the intestine. Large volumes of undiluted feeding, however, might impair gastric emptying[54].

Despite the theoretical advantages of starting some feeding and especially breastfeeding at a low volume early in life, surprisingly few studies have investigated the beneficial effects in humans. In many studies, published from the USA, starting feeding at day 5 of life was considered early feeding and starting at day 19–21 was regarded as late feeding (for review see reference 55). One recent paper studied the effect of starting a low volume hypocaloric feeding (either diluted formula or breast milk) within 24 h after birth or after resolution of the initial disease[56]. In the early feeding group the time to reach full oral feeding was shorter (10 ± 3 vs. 13 ± 4 days) while weight gain above birth weight at day 30 was higher (223 ± 125 vs 95 ± 161 g kg^{-1} day^{-1}). No other differences were observed. Despite the theoretical advantages of early 'minimal' enteral feeding in sick VLBW infants, more studies are needed to prove its real value.

HOW TO FEED

Feeding can be given either continuously or as a bolus every 1–3 h. Continuous feeding might result in better tolerance of feeding and a better absorption while intermittent feeding might result in higher and more variable levels of gut hormones. A recent study showed no differences between infants fed intermittently and those fed continuously in tolerance or absorption of formula feeding[57]. Gain in weight, length and head circumference was also not different between groups. The choice between intermittent or continuous feeding therefore remains individual and can be tailored to the individual infant.

CONCLUSION

Despite an enormous number of studies done over the last decades on the optimal nutrition of very low-birth weight infants, many unanswered questions remain as to how much to feed, what to feed, when to feed and how to feed these infants. Nevertheless, the following scheme to feed a preterm infant with a birth weight less than 1500 g seems reasonable.

Suggested nutritional management of VLBW infants

First 5–7 days of life

'Minimal enteral feeding' approximately 20 ml kg^{-1} day^{-1} breast milk (if available). Parenteral nutrition with 2.5 g kg^{-1} day^{-1} protein and 2.5 g kg^{-1} day^{-1} lipids.

After 5–7 days

Increase enteral feeding with 20 ml kg^{-1} day^{-1}. Use 'fortified' human milk or preterm formula. Gradual decrease of TPN.

How long to give an enriched formula to a VLBW infant?

It is practice in most hospitals to give an enriched feeding of either breastmilk or a preterm formula until discharge from hospital. In cases where there are no complications, infants are discharged usually with a weight between 2 and 2.5 kg. The growth rate of an infant is high until a weight of approximately 3.5 kg or the term age. The needs regarding protein, energy, calcium and sodium for instance are still high at this early discharge. Therefore enriched feeding, with either the supplemented breastmilk or the preterm formula, should be continued at least until the term age or a weight of 3.2 kg.

The results of the continuation of preterm formula for a period of 6–9 months have been published recently. Both studies showed a higher linear growth and weight gain in infants receiving the enriched formula[58,59]. It also improved bone calcification. More studies are needed to see if an enriched formula also improved psychomotor development.

References

1. Kashyap, S., Forsyth, M., Zucker, C., Ramakrishnan, R., Dell, R. B. and Heird, W. C. (1986). Effects of varying protein and energy intakes on growth and metabolic response in low birth weight infants. *J. Pediatr.*, **108**, 955–63
2. Kashyap, S., Schulze, K. F., Forsyth, M., Zucker, C., Dell, R. B., Ramakrishnan, R. and Heird, W. C. (1988). Growth, nutrient retention, and metabolic response in low birth weight infants fed varying intakes of protein and energy. *J. Pediatr.*, **113**, 713–21
3. Sauer, P. J. J. (1991). Neonatal energy metabolism. In Cowett, R. M. (ed.) *Principles of Perinatal-neonatal Metabolism*, pp. 583–608. (New York, Berlin and Heidelberg: Springer-Verlag)
4. Davies, P. S. W., Clough, H., Bishop, N. J., Lucas, A., Cole, J. J. and Cole, T. J. (1996). Total energy expenditure in small for gestational age infants. *Arch. Dis. Child. Fetal Neonatal Ed.*, **74**, F208–10
5. Picaud, J. C., Putet, G., Rigo, J., Salle, B. L. and Senterre, J. (1994). Metabolic and energy balance in small- and appropriate-for-gestational-age, very low-birth-weight infants. *Acta Paediatr. Suppl.*, **405**, 54–9
6. Kurzner, S. I., Garg, M., Bautista, D. B., Sargent, C. W., Bowman, C. M. and Keens, T. G. (1988). Growth failure in bronchopulmonary dysplasia: elevated metabolic rates and pulmonary mechanics. *J. Pediatr.*, **112**, 73–80
7. Yeh, T. F., McClenan, D. A., Ajayi, O. A. and Pildes, R. S. (1989). Metabolic rate and energy balance in infants with bronchopulmonary dysplasia. *J. Pediatr.*, **114**, 448–51
8. Kalhan, S. C. and Denne, S. C. (1990). Energy consumption in infants with bronchopulmonary dysplasia. *J. Pediatr.*, **116**, 662–4
9. Sulkers, E. J., Van Goudoever, J. B., Luenisse, C., Wattimena, J. L. D. and Sauer, P. J. J. (1992). Comparison of two preterm formulas with or without addition of medium-chain triglycerides (MCTs). 1. Effects on nitrogen and fat balance and body composition changes. *J. Pediatr. Gastroenterol. Nutr.*, **15**, 34–41
10. Carnielli, V. P., Luijendijk, I. H. T., Van Goudoever, J. B., Sulkers, E. J., Boerlage, A. A.,

Degenhart, H. J. and Sauer, P. J. J. (1995). Feeding premature newborn infants palmitic acid in amounts and stereoisomeric position similar to that of human milk: effects on fat and mineral balance. *Am. J. Clin. Nutr.,* **61**, 1037–42

11. Jackson, A. A., Shaw, J. C. L., Barber, A. and Golden, M. H. N. (1981). Nitrogen metabolism in preterm infants fed human donor breast milk: the possible essentiality of glycine. *Pediatr. Res.,* **15**, 1454–61

12. Van Lingen, R. A., Van Goudoever, J. B., Luijendijk, I. H. T., Wattimena, J. L. D. and Sauer, P. J. J. (1992). Effects of early amino acid administration during total parenteral nutrition on protein metabolism in pre-term infants. *Clin. Sci. (Colch.),* **82**, 199–203

13. Van Goudoever, J. B., Colen, T., Wattimena, J. L. D., Huijmans, J. G. M., Carnielli, V. P. and Sauer, P. J. J. (1995). Immediate commencement of amino acid supplementation in preterm infants: effect on serum amino acid concentrations and protein kinetics on the first day of life. *J. Pediatr.,* **127**, 458–65

14. Miller, R. G., Jahoor, F. and Jaksic, T. (1995). Decreased cysteine and proline synthesis in premature neonates fed intravenous glucose. *Program Issue APS-SPR Ped. Res.,* **37**, 314A (abstr.)

15. Keshen, T. H., Jahoor, F. and Jaksic, T. (1996). Intracellular compartmentation of cysteine in premature neonates. *Program Issue APS-SPR Ped. Res.,* **39**, 313A (abstr.)

16. Pencharz, P. B., House, J. D., Wykes, L. J. and Ball, R. O. (1996). What are the essential amino acids for the preterm and term infant? In Bindels, J. G., Goedhart, A. C. and Visser, H. K. A. (eds.) *Recent Developments in Infant Nutrition,* pp. 278–96. (Dordrecht, Boston and London: Kluwer Academic Publishers)

17. Carver, J. D. and Barness, L. A. (1996). Trophic factors for the gastrointestinal tract. *Clin. Perinatol.,* **23**, 265–85

18. Souba, W. W. (1991). Glutamine: a key substrate for the splanchnic bed. *Annu. Rev. Nutr.,* **11**, 285–308

19. Van Der Hulst, R. R. W. J., Van Kreel, B. K., Von Meyenfeldt, M. F., Brummer, R. J. M., Arends, J. W., Deutz, N. E. P. and Soeters, P. B. (1993). Glutamine and the preservation of gut integrity. *Lancet,* **341**, 1363–5

20. Lacey, J. M., Crouch, J. B., Benfell, K., Ringer, S. A., Kristann Wilmore, C., Maguire, D. and Wilmore, D. W. (1996). The effects of glutamine-supplemented parenteral nutrition in premature infants. *J. Parent. Enteral. Nutr.,* **20**, 74–80

21. Narayanan, I., Prakash, K., Bala, S., Verma, R. K. and Gujral, V. V. (1980). Partial supplementation with expressed breast-milk for prevention of infection in low-birth-weight infants. *Lancet,* **2**, 561–3

22. Winberg, J. and Wessner, G. (1971). Does breast milk protect against septicaemia in the newborn? *Lancet,* **1**, 1091–4

23. Lucas, A. and Cole, T. J. (1990). Breast milk and neonatal necrotising enterocolitis. *Lancet,* **336**, 1519–23

24. Kliegman, R. M., Pittard, W. B. and Fanaroff, A. A. (1979). Necrotizing enterocolitis in neonates fed human milk. *J. Pediatr.,* **95**, 450–3

25. Spritzer, R., Koolen, A. M. P., Baerts, W., Fetter, W. P. F., Lafeber, H. N. and Sauer, P. J. J. (1988). A prolonged decline in the incidence of necrotizing enterocolitis after the introduction of a cautious feeding regimen. *Acta Paediatr. Scand.,* **77**, 909–11

26. Leach, J. L., Baxter, J. H., Molitor, B. E., Ramstack, M. B. and Masor, M. L. (1995). Total potentially available nucleotides of human milk by stage of lactation. *Am. J. Clin. Nutr.,* **61**, 1224–30

27. Carver, J. D. and Walker, W. A. (1995). The role of nucleotides in human nutrition. *Nutr. Biochem.,* **6**, 58–72

28. James, R. and Bradshaw, R. A. (1984). Polypeptide growth factors. *Annu. Rev. Biochem.,* **53**, 259–92

29. Ballard, F. J., Nield, M. K., Francis, G. L., Dahlenburg, G. W. and Wallace, J. C. (1982). The relationship between the insulin content and inhibitory effects of bovine colostrum on protein breakdown in cultured cells. *J. Cell Physiol.,* **110**, 249–54

30. Stoddart, R. W. and Widdowson, E. M. (1976). Changes in the organs of pigs in response to feeding for the first 24 h after birth. 3. Fluorescence histochemistry of the carbohydrates of the intestine. *Biol. Neonate,* **29**, 18–27

31. Simmen, F. A., Cera, K. R. and Mahan, D. C. (1990). Stimulation by colostrum or mature milk of gastrointestinal tissue development in newborn pigs. *J. Anim. Sci.,* **68**, 3596–603

32. Burrin, D. G., Shulman, R. J., Reeds, P. J., Davis, T. A. and Gravitt, K. R. (1992). Porcine colostrum and milk stimulate visceral organ and skeletal muscle protein synthesis in neonatal piglets. *J. Nutr.,* **122**, 1205–13

33. Klagsbrun, M. (1978). Human milk stimulates DNA synthesis and cellular proliferation in cultured fibroblasts. *Proc. Natl. Acad. Sci. USA,* **75**, 5057–61

34. Ichiba, H., Kusuda, S., Itagane, Y., Fujita, K. and Issiki, G. (1992). Measurement of growth promoting activity in human milk using a fetal small intestinal cell line. *Biol. Neonate,* **61**, 47–53

35. Donovan, S. M. and Odle, J. (1994). Growth factors in milk as mediators of infant development. *Annu. Rev. Nutr.,* **14**, 147–67

36. Baumrucker, C. R. and Blum, J. W. (1993). Secretion of insulin-like growth factors in milk and their effect on the neonate. *Livestock Prod. Sci.*, **17**, 825–8

37. Read, L. C., Tomas, F. M., Howarth, G. S., Martin, A. A., Edson, K. J., Gillespie, C. M., Owens, P. C. and Ballard, F. J. (1992). Insulin-like growth factor-I and its N-terminal modified analogues induce marked gut growth in dexamethasone-treated rats. *J. Endocrinol.*, **133**, 421–31

38. Read, L. C., Steeb, C. B., Lamb, J. and Howarth, G. (1996). Effects of orally administered milk growth factor on gut growth and repair. *Proceedings of 5th International Symposium on Hormones and Bioculture Substances in Milk*, Smolenice, Slowakia Republic, p. 22

39. Bitman, J., Wood, D. L., Mehta, N. R., Hamosh, P. and Hamosh, M. (1986). Comparison of the cholesteryl ester composition of human milk from preterm and term mothers. *J. Pediatr. Gastroenterol. Nutr.*, **5**, 780–6

40. Mott, G. E., Jackson, E. M., De Lallo, L., Lewis, D. S. and McMahan, C. A. (1995). Differences in cholesterol metabolism in juvenile baboons are programmed by breast- versus formula-feeding. *J. Lipid Res.*, **36**, 299–307

41. Mott, G. E., Jackson, E. M., McMahan, C. A. and McGill Jr, H. C. (1990). Cholesterol metabolism in adult baboons is influenced by infant diet. *J. Nutr.*, **120**, 243–51

42. Hachey, D. L., Pond, W. G. and Wong, W. W. (1996). Is dietary cholesterol beneficial to the infant? In Bindels, J. G., Goedhart, A. C. and Visser, H. K. A. (eds.) *Recent Developments in Infant Nutrition*, pp. 251–9. (Dordrecht, Boston and London: Kluwer Academic Publishers)

43. Fall, C. H. D., Barker, D. J. P., Osmond, C., Winter, P. D., Clark, P. M. S. and Hales, C. N. (1992). Relation of infant feeding to adult serum cholesterol concentration and death from ischaemic heart disease. *Br. Med. J.*, **304**, 801–5

44. Uauy, R. D., Birch, D. G., Birch, E. E., Tyson, J. E. and Hoffman, D. R. (1990). Effect of dietary omega-3 fatty acids on retinal function of very-low-birth-weight neonates. *Pediatr. Res.*, **28**, 485–92

45. Carnielli, V. P., Pederzini, F., Vittorangeli, R., Luijendijk, I. H. T., Boomaars, W. E. M., Pedrotti, D. and Sauer, P. J. J. (1996). Plasma and red blood cell fatty acid of very low birth weight infants fed exclusively with expressed preterm human milk. *Pediatr. Res.*, **39**, 671–9

46. Carnielli, V. P., Wattimena, D. J. L., Luijendijk, I. T. H., Boerlage, A., Degenhart, H. J. and Sauer, P. J. J. (1996). The very low birth weight premature infant is capable of synthesizing arachidonic and docosahexaenoic acids from linoleic and linolenic acids. *Pediatr. Res.*, **40**, 169–74

47. Carlson, S. (1996). LCPUFA and functional development of preterm and term infants. In Bindels, J. G., Goedhart, A. C. and Visser, H. K. A. (eds.) *Recent Developments in Infant Nutrition*, pp. 218–24. (Dordrecht, Boston and London: Kluwer Academic Publishers)

48. Lucas, A., Morley, R., Cole, T. J., Gore, S. M., Lucas, P. J., Crowle, P., Pearse, R., Boon, A. J. and Powell, R. (1990). Early diet in preterm babies and developmental status at 18 months. *Lancet*, **335**, 1477–81

49. Lucas, A., Morley, R., Cole, T. J., Lister, G. and Leeson-Payne, C. (1992). Breast milk and subsequent intelligence quotient in children born preterm. *Lancet*, **339**, 261–4

50. Levine, G. M., Deren, J. J., Steiger, E. and Zinno, R. (1974). Role of oral intake in maintenance of gut mass and disacchardie activity. *Gastroenterology*, **67**, 975–82

51. Heird, W. C., Schwarz, S. M. and Hansen, I. H. (1984). Colostrum-induced enteric mucosal growth in beagle puppies. *Pediatr. Res.*, **18**, 512–15

52. Beach, R. C., Menzies, I. S., Clayden, G. S. and Scopes, J. W. (1982). Gastrointestinal permeability changes in the preterm neonate. *Arch. Dis. Child.*, **57**, 141–5

53. Weaver, L. T., Laker, M. F., Nelson, R. and Lucas, A. (1987). Milk feeding and changes in intestinal permeability and morphology in the newborn. *J. Pediatr. Gastroenterol. Nutr.*, **6**, 351–8

54. Berseth, C. L. (1996). Gastrointestinal motility in the neonate. *Clin. Perinatol.*, **23**, 179–90

55. Gross, S. J. and Slagle, T. A. (1993). Feeding the low birth weight infant. *Clin. Perinatol.*, **20**, 193–209

56. Troche, B., Harvey-Wilkes, K., Engle, W. D., Nielsen, H. C., Frantz III, I. D., Mitchell, M. L. and Hermos, R. J. (1995). Early minimal feedings promote growth in critically ill premature infants. *Biol. Neonate*, **67**, 172–81

57. Silvestre, M. A. A., Morbach, C. A., Brans, Y. W. and Shankaran, S. (1996). A prospective randomized trial comparing continuous versus intermittent feeding methods in very low birth weight neonates. *J. Pediatr.*, **128**, 748–52

58. Lucas, A., Bishop, N. J., King, F. J. and Cole, T. J. (1992). Randomised trial of nutrition for preterm infants after discharge. *Arch. Dis. Child.*, **67**, 324–7

59. Cooke, R. J., Griffin, I., Wells, J., Smith, J., Robinson, S. and Leighton, M. (1996). Feeding preterm infants after hospital discharge. 1. Effect of type of formula on nutrient intake and growth. *Program Issue APS-SPR Ped. Res.*, **39**, 307A (abstr.)

Nursing of the very-low-birth weight infant: the search for clinical strategies

12

B. Persson

BACKGROUND

All newborn infants are vulnerable and their future health and well-being depend on the amount and quality of care provided. Protection, warmth, nutrition, love and attention are the principal requirements.

Childhood morbidity in developed countries has changed during this century especially over the past decades. Iatrogenic, social, emotional and chronic problems have largely replaced acute infections as the principal causes of child morbidity. The term 'new morbidity' has been coined to describe this change, under which a range of problems can be grouped – behavior disorders, suboptimal nutrition, child abuse and neglect and special needs[1]. New medical technology has had a strong impact on one such area: the handling of low-birth weight infants and the long-term, high technology care after preterm delivery. The high technology environment of the neonatal intensive care units is quite different from the intrauterine milieu. It is conceivable that the imposed stay in such an environment, even in the absence of major medical complications, could have an impact on the future development and behavior of the neonate, either directly or through the experience of the parents and their subsequent parenting skills and expectations[2].

The focus on medical issues in neonatology has changed from infection and temperature-control in the 1970s, to technological advances concerning laboratory tests, ventilation and monitoring in the 1990s. The disadvantages with the explosion of diagnostic and therapeutic technology have sometimes been a lack of harmony between the biological, psychological and social circumstances necessary for an infant's future health and quality of life.

In a long-term prospective, controlled study in Sweden, 20 extremely-low-birth weight (< 1000 g) infants with birth weights between 500 and 900 g and gestational ages between 24 and 30 weeks were compared with 20 4-year-old full-term infants for growth, health, development and quality of life. The results disclosed few neurological impairments. However, there were developmental inconsistencies and a high incidence of behavioral problems. The behavioral symptom interview showed an increased rate of hyperactivity and difficulties in concentrating[3].

Taking these kinds of results as a background, there has been a shift in emphasis from survival only, to improvement of the future quality of life for this group of babies.

NURSERY ENVIRONMENTAL RISKS

The advantages of caring for sick infants 'outside' of hospitals were already being reported at the beginning of this century[4]. American studies in the 1940s showed that babies in institutions for the abandoned, whilst continuing to receive the same kind of daily care, had been lacking a loving caregiver. Even with adequate food, hydration and warmth these babies suffered from numerous infections, underwent growth and mental retardation and experienced severe emotional disturbances. This led to the theory that, for optimal survival, babies need loving care as well as warmth, food and liquid[5].

The birth of a premature infant and its first weeks of life are well known to be a time of stress and crisis for parents, involving feelings of either guilt, or failure due to the inability to carry the pregnancy to term, or of uncertainty about the infant's health status and fears of parenting the infant. This had already been described in 1960 by Kaplan and Mason[6]. In these early beginnings of neonatal care, surroundings were kept very sterile, with masks, gowns and gloves for everyone. This was necessary, because most babies that died, did so due to infection. Parents did not touch their baby until discharge. Preterm children born prior to the 1970s were also more likely to be neglected or even physically abused than children born at term[7]. The importance of the first few days after birth for infant–mother attachment was reported by Klaus and Kennell[8]. In addition to medical complications, these studies led to an increasing area of concern regarding iatrogenic effects occurring during the separation of mother and infant. These authors reported in 1976: 'Although we have only begun to understand the complex process of the attachment of parents to their newborn infant, those responsible for the care of mothers and infants should re-evaluate hospital procedures that interfere with early, sustained mother–infant contact'[9]. Many studies were carried out in the late 1970s to evaluate these new findings. In Sweden, for example, a group of mothers had skin-to-skin contact with their infants for 15 min after delivery. When they were compared with mothers who had been cared for according to regular hospital routines, it was revealed that the group of extra-skin-to-skin-contact mothers breast-fed for an average of 2 months longer[10].

EXPLORING NEW SOLUTIONS

Between the 1970s and early 1980s many suggestions for new solutions and innovations towards providing a better understanding of the environmental impact on the infant and the family were generated. Some theorists reasoned that the boring environment provided *lack of stimulation*. Some investigators hypothesized

that the neonatal environment was a *source of sensory deprivation* and various types of stimulation, i.e. auditory, kinesthetic, tactile, vestibular/proprioceptive and visual, were offered[11]. Programs with rocking chairs, waterbeds to simulate intrauterine movement and experiments with sounds of mother's voice and taped music were started. Nurses encouraged parents to hold, talk to and play with their baby and toys and teddy-bears were placed inside the incubators. Most of these studies revealed certain kinds of benefits to the stimulated infant in, for example, weight gain and improved function on developmental assessments.

In addition, the impacts of other changes in the infant's environment or care have been investigated; for example, on *Maternal education* as part of the discharge planning[12], and on the use of *non-nutritive sucking*, sucking of a pacifier in connection with tube-feeding to enhance the rate of weight gain[13]. A Swedish study showed that the sucking of a pacifier before, during and after tube feeding appeared to induce increased vagal nerve activity, reducing tube-feeding time, and decreasing somatostatin release, thereby facilitating tube-feeding and digestion[14].

REDUCTION OF HANDLING AND POSITIONING

Noise pollution

The Academy of Pediatrics in 1974[15] and Long and associates in 1986[16] addressed the effects of noise pollution, caused by both staff and equipment, on the neonate, and cited hypoxemia as an outcome. A frequently quoted study reported that preterm infants were constantly interrupted in their rest, as often as 132 times per day[17]. They had fewer and shorter periods of quiet sleep than term infants and rest periods of only 4.6–19.2 min between handlings. Gorski in 1983[18], and with colleagues[19] in several later studies, also raised concerns about the intensive care environment in relation to optimal development: 'Stimulation or social interaction, if poorly timed, could ultimately stress a vulnerable infant as much as medical procedures'.

Skin-to-skin care

In Bogota, Colombia, an alternative neonatal care arose out of severe economic limitations and problems with nosocomial and cross-infections. Infants, placed in a skin-to-skin position with their mothers, survived, in spite of their impoverished home environments[20]. This care, the 'kangaroo method' (K-method) was introduced by two pediatricians, Edgar Ray and Hector Martinez, of Bogota, Colombia. It is based on a deep respect for natural processes and for the mothers and infants own capability. The K-method in a modified form, i.e. skin-to-skin contact, and with the infant placed on the mother's chest dressed only in a diaper, was introduced in several neonatal units in western countries during the 1980s[21]. Studies reported that the position provided opportunities for closeness and mutual stimulation between the mother and the premature infant[22], longer breast-feeding and less crying[23]. The skin temperature was well maintained through skin-to-skin contact, even with infants as small as 1000 g, in a warm room with a hat and a blanket. Apneas were not precipitated and oxygenation was well maintained. Far from compromising respiration in infants with chronic lung disease, skin-to-skin contact was associated with an overall improvement in their oxygenation[24].

Developmental care

The 1980s were marked by an intensification of the belief that stimulation can be stressful to premature infants and that the nursery environment is sometimes overstimulating. Several studies proposed that, before stimulation programs were initiated, the infant's environment needed to have noxious stimuli removed and that the stimulation should be individualized to the infant.

Heidelise Als' synactive theory of premature infant development[25] provides a framework for individualized developmental care. This framework identifies premature infant behaviors that envelope a body language that communicates stress. They synactive theory of infant development looks at the integration of the neurological subsystems and their interaction with the environment. The philosophy is centered around stress reduction, promoting infant development and opportunities for parenting.

THE SPIRIT OF THE UNITED NATIONS CONVENTION ON THE RIGHTS OF THE CHILD

This convention, accepted in 1989, acts as a guide in all public health efforts with children[26]. The convention stresses that, because of their vulnerability, children have a right to expect special consideration and that in every situation, the needs and the voice of the child must be heard and respected. One of the most fundamental principles is stated in the formulation 'for the best interest of the child', first mentioned in the third article: 'The necessity of every medical intervention has to be scrutinized in this respect to assure that the interventions really are necessary and performed in a manner which is for the best interest of the child'[27].

CHANGE OF FOCUS

This philosophy and these aims are essentially those of a commitment in neonatal intensive care wards around the world today to create an optimal nursing care environment for preterm infants and their parents, by continuously searching for strategies to enhance their health and life quality. This background, together with my daily clinical observations, were the key for a range of clinical development projects at the neonatal ward in Helsingborg, Sweden. With the aim of working with *the family as an inseparable entity*, the following studies began. The purpose was to understand better both infants' and parents' requirements and to integrate and implement this knowledge, together with current research findings into a comprehensive care philosophy for the ward that functions as the base for developing local standard routines and criteria for continuous quality improvements.

A RETROSPECTIVE, COMPARATIVE STUDY USING THE K-METHOD AS A COMPLEMENT TO THE STANDARD INCUBATOR CARE[28]

Subjects

The sample consisted of 66 consecutive mother–infant pairs. The total sample comprised two groups of infants: 33 who received the kangaroo method of care (K-group) and 33 who received standard prematurity care (SPC-group). Mothers in both groups were encouraged to hold their infants as much as they desired, so that there was an equal distribution of mothers breast-feeding and of holding their infants. The two groups were matched for parity, gestational age and birth weight. A demographic profile was conducted.

Results

Infants in the K-group (Table 1) gained more weight per week, stayed fewer days in the incubator and were also younger when first taken out of the incubator, they had a shorter length of hospital care, and were more often breast-fed upon discharge, as compared to infants in the standard prematurity care group.

No physiological problems were found in the two groups during the study period. Mothers in the K-group were more likely to be breast-feeding upon discharge (82%) as compared to those in the SPC-group (45%). Infants in the SPC-group had significantly longer stays in the

incubator as well as in the hospital. Their weight gain was, on average, 42 g lower per week than that of the K-group. This result needs further investigation as a loss of weight for a premature baby presumably gives rise to the need for additional interventions.

The benefits derived from the mutual stimulation of skin-to-skin care were: enhanced opportunities for breast-feeding and its continued success up to the time of hospital discharge, improved infant comfort and weight gain and readiness to leave the incubator and hospital.

CAN WE CREATE A MORE OPTIMAL HOSPITAL ENVIRONMENT?[29]

Method

This paper describes an attempt at exploring a practical change, by creating a care model (Figure 1) for the ward, with the K-method as the key to creating a more optimal clinical environment for both infants and parents, and an evaluation where a group of nurses were engaged in compiling data obtained from semi-structured interviews with parents of infants below 1500 g. The results were analyzed first individually and then in the group. Then there followed an implementation and integration period of the K-method in a nursing care model, begun as a first step towards common goals and some broad, acceptable standards that can, in the future, be constantly assessed and improved in quality.

Table 1 Age when first taken out of incubator, weight gain, days in incubator and hospital, and proportion breastfed at discharge, by group status. Data are expressed as mean (SD) or number (%)

Variable	K-group (n = 33)	SPC-group (n = 33)	Statistics
Age at first time out of incubator (days)	4.36 (4.7)	8.0 (5.9)	$t = 2.80$ $p < 0.01$
Weight gain per week (g)	237.48 (96.4)	195.5 (82.9)	$t = 1.90$ $p < 0.05$
Days in incubator	20.9 (13.9)	30.5 (15.7)	$t = 2.61$ $p < 0.05$
Total days in hospital	41.6 (16.9)	49.4 (18.9)	$t = 1.76$ $p < 0.05$
Breast-fed upon discharge	27 (82)	15 (45)	$\chi^2 = 7.92$ $p < 0.005$

K, kangaroo method; SPC, standard prematurity care

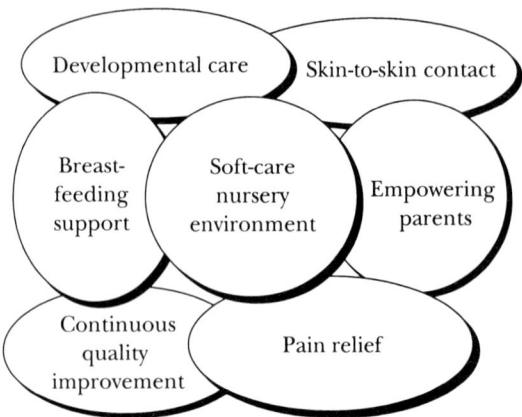

Figure 1 Neonatal nursing model – a biopsychosocial approach

Main findings

The following are some typical themes of importance to the parents as determined from the interview material:

(1) To be prepared during pregnancy for the preterm delivery;

(2) The premature delivery created feelings of disappointment and sorrow over 'the delivery one did not get';

(3) The staff – too many of them always around observing the family members;

(4) Taking part in the daily care and planning is important, not just visiting the infant;

(5) The clinical environment – creates hostile feelings which can be an obstacle for full participation;

(6) The contact with the infant demands possibilities for presence and participation;

(7) Family relationships suffered; and

(8) After discharge – much overprotecting and worries.

Conclusions

What can be done? An analysis of the care model was drawn up (Figure 1). The aforesaid studies took place at ward and group meetings and were also presented at parents' meetings in order to obtain their feed back.

THE SOFT CARE NURSERY

The model consists of the main themes from the parent interviews, combined with today's new focus in neonatal research and development. It embodies an attempt at creating an integrated nursing care model for a neonatal intensive care unit; a basic model, a philosophy and standard routine the aim of which is to develop criteria that can be constantly assessed and improved in quality.

Soft care

Much of the work in an intensive care ward is necessary and lifesaving, but perhaps medical and technical advances have made us too eager, so we forget the therapeutic value of rest and deep sleep. We must create a balance between medical procedures and good primary care, by conscientiously planning our ward routines and by training ourselves to be aware of the infants' signals of worry, stress and pain. With the help of a few rather simple care-giving practices, we can create a more secure nursery environment, which more resembles that of the uterus and which might possibly lead to a reduction in the risk of stress and relationship problems that could occur after the infant's discharge and which are a result of the intensive care and hospital environment.

The infant's right to rest, darkness, closeness, pain relief and individual care

The infant is given assistance in maintaining a flexed position, applicable also during care-giving procedures, in order to maintain its neurological balance. The incubator beds are made 'cosy' with soft towels folded and placed to form a little nest. The incubator tops are covered to protect the baby from bright lights and sounds. The light is dimmed and individual light is only used when the infant requires treatment or care.

Conversation in the nursery is kept to a minimum and with low voices. The staff are trained to continuously and systematically observe the infant for signs of stress and restlessness. Painful procedures and blood tests are co-ordinated so as to allow the infant longer periods of uninterrupted sleep. Pain relief and/or sedation should be administered when needed. As soon as the infant is stable enough to be moved, he is removed from the incubator and placed skin-to-skin on the mother's breast for warmth and mutual stimulation and to allow breast-feeding. The parents participate as much as possible in the care of their baby.

Create a care chain

Every effort should be made to establish an early contact with 'future' parents so as to inform them about the ward, e.g. parents in all prenatal classes and those women admitted to the maternity ward due to pregnancy complications. The family should be actively involved in the care as soon as possible and a small 'family area' created near the ward where siblings can play and where it is possible to take a rest and eat a meal.

All the nursing and medical plans and procedures should be formulated *with* the parents, the purpose being to involve them in the decision making. Weekly parental meetings are arranged for information, education and discussions. Discharge is done through a 'soft' approach and always with the door left open for telephone contacts, home-visits and/or outpatient visits.

Develop a care setting

In an effort to reach an understanding in our work, we must not forget the impression the physical environment has on human beings. Neonatal units are usually planned as standard intensive care units. It is therefore an important aspect of the work to try to create better surroundings for the family. It is possible to create a ward environment with both a high standard of hygiene, good practical working conditions and a warm and friendly environment for the families.

The professionals – a team with a mutual philosophy

Every child and family is assigned their own doctor and primary nurse. They are responsible for medical care, support, information and the medical and nursing procedures. The team is enlarged, as and when necessary, with, for example, the psychologist, physiotherapist or district nurse. It is important to develop a strong, multi-disciplinary co-operation, to enable the entire staff to strive after a mutual care philosophy and it is therefore also necessary, that any changes in development, quality controls and improvement programs be a joint effort.

Adapt the organization to the infant's needs

Ward staff are divided into teams to diminish the amount of people around each family. The teams follow their patients throughout the entire hospital stay, from intensive care to discharge and to outpatient visits. The team have their 'own' doctor and together they hold regular meetings at which primary nurses receive directions about the infant's individual care plan. In a ward where doctors are often highly specialized, it is important that nurses develop their skills in different fields as a complement to medical care. It could be, for example, in the field of intensive care methods, family education, breast-feeding, developmental care, quality improvement etc. The head nurse has to maintain and develop the competence of the nursing staff to enable the care philosophy to be achieved and is actively engaged in the constant evaluation of routines and methods by assessing and improving the quality.

SUMMARY AND DISCUSSION

The last decade has been marked by the more extensive development of care practices in the neonatal intensive care units as nurses and physicians have begun to realize the impact on the results. Medical and physiological issues in neonatology have been at the forefront and have often overshadowed nursing issues. Nursing has always been a model of holistic care but was rarely fully integrated into the daily clinical guidelines, the organization or scheduling by the staff. Our history is filled with examples of how advice and dogmas have been based more on belief than on real knowledge.

A good start is to observe attentively the mother–child interaction and to explore the biological, behavioral and social backgrounds to it. Because nurses are constantly at the bedside, in intimate contact with the patients and their families, their intervention in the form of implementing skin-to-skin care, developmental care and other recent solutions for preventing the environmental risks in our neonatal intensive units is almost inevitable. Indeed much research remains to be done about the assessment tools, validation of our interpretations of an infant's behavior and on the testing of the outcomes of specific interventions.

Nursing care routines must be based on a theoretical background, in the same way that the management of complicated respiratory, circulatory and metabolic disturbances of perinatal adaptation is. Ethics is another area we come face to face with every day. Basically, ethics involves doing good rather than harm to these babies and their families. They are highly vulnerable to what we do, and since we expose them to medical treatment that will profoundly affect their lives, we must also be responsible for and committed to how we do this. As we examine our own ethical initiatives in neonatal nursing so must we also listen to our families and fully participate in their empowerment. We must see ourselves as vital links between our patients and their future.

References

1. Fasting, U. (1995). The new iatrogenesis. In Lindström, B. and Spencer, N. (eds.) *Social Paediatrics*, pp. 259–70. (New York and London: Oxford University Press)
2. Lacy, J. B. and Ohlsson, A. (1993). Behavioral outcomes of environmental or care-giving hospital-based interventions for preterm infants: a critical overview. *Acta Paediatr.*, **82**, 408–15
3. Stjernquist, K. and Svenningsen, N. W. (1995). Extremely low-birth-weight infants less than 901 g: development and behaviour after 4 years of life. *Acta Paediatr.*, **84**, 500–6
4. Chapin, H. D. (1908). A plan of dealing with atrophic infants and children. *Arch. Pediatr.*, **25**, 491
5. Spitz, R. (1945). Hospitalism: an inquiry into the genesis of psychiatric conditions in early childhood. In Eissler, R. S. (ed.) *Psychoanalytic Study of the Child*, pp. 53–74. (New Haven, CT: Yale University Press)
6. Kaplan, D. N. and Mason, E. A. (1960). Maternal reactions to premature birth viewed as an emotional disorder. *Am. J. Orthopsychiatry*, **30**, 539–52
7. Minde, K. (1984). The impact of prematurity on the later behavior of children and on their families. *Clin. Perinatol.*, **11**, 227–44
8. Klaus, M. H. and Kennell, J. H. (1970). Mothers separated from their newborn infants. *Pediatr. Clin. N. Am.*, **17**, 1015–37
9. Klaus, M. H. and Kennell, J. H. (1976). *Maternal-infant bonding*, p. 240. (Saint Louis: C. V. Mosby Company)
10. Public Health (1987). Low birth weight 1975–85 and perinatal mortality. *Public Health*, **101**, 1–2
11. Field, T. (1980). Supplemental stimulation of preterm neonates. *Early Hum. Dev.*, **4**, 301–14
12. Rauh, V. A., Nurcombe, B., Achenback, T. and Howell, C. (1990). The mother-infant transaction program. *Clin. Perinatol.*, **17**, 31–45
13. Measel, C. P. and Anderson, G. C. (1979). Non-nutritive sucking during tube feeding: effect on clinical course in premature infants. *J. Obstet. Gynecol. Neonatal Nurs.*, **8**, 265–72
14. Widström, A. -M., Marchini, G., Matthiesen, A. -S., Werner, S., Winberg, J. and Uvnäs-Moberg, K. (1988). Non-nutritive sucking in tube-fed preterm infants: effects on gastric motility and gastric content of somatostatin. *J. Pediatr. Gastroenterol. Nutr.*, **7**, 517–23
15. Committee on Environmental Hazards (1974). Noise pollution: neonatal aspects. *Acad. Pediatr.*, **54**, 476–8
16. Long, J. G. (1980). Noise and hypoxemia in the intensive care nursery. *Pediatrics*, **65**, 143–5

17. Moore, T. (ed.) (1976). Disturbance and Infant's Rest. Iatrogenic Problems in Neonatal Intensive Care. In *Report of the 69th Ross Conference on Pediatric Research*, Columbus, Ohio, pp. 74–97, May

18. Gorksi, P. (1983). Direct computer recording of premature infants and nursing care: distress following two interventions. *Pediatrics*, **72**, 198–202

19. Gorski, P. A., Huntington, L. and Lewkowicz, D. J. (1990). Handling preterm infants in hospitals. *Clin. Perinatol.*, **17**, 102–12

20. Rey, E. S. and Martinez, H. G. (1983). Manejo Rational del Nino Prematuro. In *Conference Proceedings I: Curso de Medicina Fetal y Neonatal*, Bogota, Columbia, pp. 137–51 (Spanish)

21. Anderson, G. C., Marks, E. A. and Wahlberg, V. (1986). Kangaroo care for premature infants. *Am. J. Nurs.*, 807–9, July

22. Affonso, D., Wahlberg, V. and Persson, B. (1989). Exploration of mothers' reactions to the kangaroo method of prematurity care. *Neonatal Network*, **7**, 43–51

23. Whitelaw, A. (1986). Skin-to-skin contact in the care of very low birth weight babies. *Pediatrics*, **9**, 270–4

24. Acolet, D., Sleath, K. and Whitelaw, A. (1989). Oxygenation, heart rate and temperature in very low birth weight infants during skin-to-skin contact with their mothers. *Acta Paediatr. Scand.*, **78**, 189–93

25. Als, H. (1986). A synactive model of neonatal behavioral organization: Framework for the assessment of neurobehavioral development in the premature infant and for support of infant and parents in the neonatal intensive care environment. *Physical Occup. Ther. Paediatr.* **6**, 3–53

26. *UN Convention on the Rights of the Child* (1989). (New York: United Nations)

27. Lindström, B. (1995). For the best interests of the child – UN Convention on the Rights of the Child. In Lindström, B. and Spencer, N. (eds.) *Social Paediatrics*, pp. 36–44. (New York and London: Oxford University Press)

28. Wahlberg, V., Affonso, D. and Persson, B. (1992). A retrospective comparative study using the kangaroo method as a complement to the standard incubator care. *Eur. J. Public Health*, **2**, 34–7

29. Persson, B. (1995). Can we create a more optimal hospital environment? In Lindström, B. and Spencer, N. (eds.) *Social Paediatrics*, pp. 527–39. (New York and London: Oxford University Press)

Forty years of ultrasound

13

J. E. E. Fleming, I. H. Spencer and M. A. Nicolson

In 1984, I was asked by the British Medical Ultrasound Society to form a historical collection to record the development of medical ultrasound. This was an understandable request as I had worked with Professor Ian Donald for some years and had been given some historically significant items for safe keeping. However, my background is engineering, not history, and this project had little more than the status of a hobby until 2 years ago when our new Professor, Iain Cameron, suggested that the Wellcome Unit for the History of Medicine might be interested in making use of the collection. The response has been enthusiastic and exciting. Within months Malcolm Nicolson had obtained a grant from the Wellcome Trust. This enabled us to employ Ian Spencer to work as a research assistant on a study of the development of medical ultrasound in Glasgow (1954–76). All I had been able to do was to collect hardware and papers, good ways to fill a few rooms and filing cabinets and interest a few visitors; Malcolm and Ian have now breathed life into the enterprise. To date their work has included interviewing colleagues and contemporaries of Professor Donald, a study of his correspondence and the presentation of papers on issues such as 'The Role of Medical Ultrasound in the Abortion Debate in Scotland'[1], 'Clinical Ultrasound and Inter-Professional Rivalries'[2] and 'Ultrasound and the Fetal Image'[3].

This paper concentrates on the work in and around Glasgow and Scotland and, in particular, that of Ian Donald (Figure 1). His contribution was important because of his sustained and concerted efforts, and because of his unfailing enthusiasm and faith that ultrasound really would be valuable. This continued throughout all his time in Glasgow, after he had officially retired and virtually until he died in 1987. What basis did he have for this extraordinary exertion? Were those often described experiments in the Babcock and Wilcox factory really significant? Did that fabled day, the 21 July 1955, play such an important part in showing Donald the way to go? Malcolm Nicolson suggested that we re-enact the experiments. We did this on 19th July 1996 – almost 41 years on to the day.

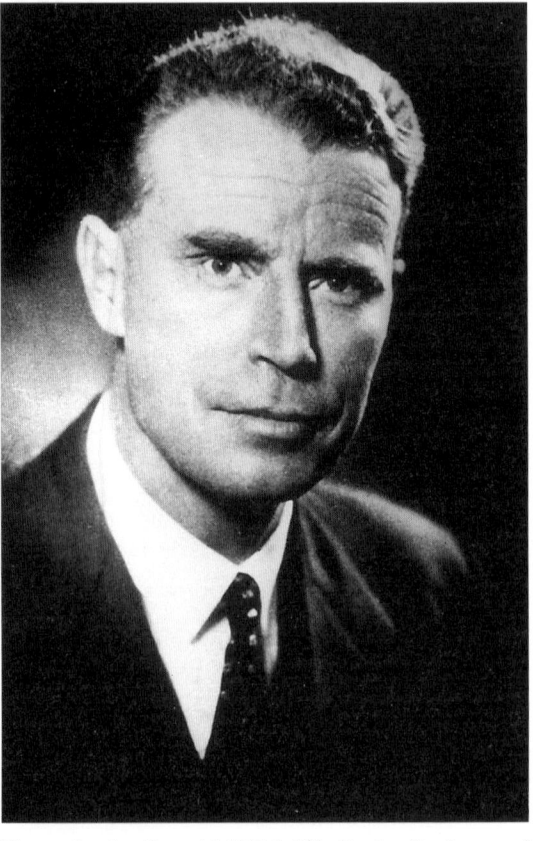

Figure 1 Ian Donald (1910–87), Regius Professor of Midwifery, University of Glasgow 1954–76

The experiments at Babcock and Wilcox are vividly described by Donald[4]. 'I shall always remember that lovely sunny afternoon of the 21 July 1955 when we took down to the factory in Renfrew two cars with their boots loaded up with recently excised fibroids, small, large and calcified, and a huge ovarian cyst. The people in the factory had also supplied an enormous lump of steak by way of a control material. Then there followed a series of fascinating experiments behind closed doors in their research department. We applied their ultrasonic probe directly to the various tissues and noted the type of echoes which appeared on their cathode ray screens. There were no facilities for photography and the factory artist was called in to sketch the results. These were beyond my wildest dreams and clearly showed the difference between a fibroid and an ovarian cyst. This may sound laughable, but to me this was fundamental and exciting. I could see boundless possibilities in the years ahead. Curiously enough nobody would accept the lump of steak at the end of the day!'. After this Ian Donald continued to experiment in the Western Infirmary in Glasgow using a Kelvin Hughes Mk2 flaw detector which he had managed to borrow. The instrument was used on patients before operation and then on the cysts and tumors after removal. Donald and his colleagues also did A-Scans of their own legs and observed the difference between their full and empty bladders.

To re-enact these experiments we borrowed a Kelvin Hughes Mk4 flaw detector as used in Babcock and Wilcox in the 1950s (Figure 2). It was fortunate that the equipment, with only a few minor repairs, still worked after more than 40 years. We invited as many people as possible who had been around at the time, and some of those who are now involved in studying the history. To avoid ethical problems we asked the Professor of Veterinary Anatomy and a veterinary ultrasound expert, Jack Boyd, for assistance. He and his staff were of immense help, providing suitable animal tissues and facilities. A video camera was used to record the trace on the flaw detector (we have never found any further mention, or evidence, of the somewhat mysterious company artist). The Medical Illustration Department, Yorkhill Hospitals Trust, supported us with their usual skill and enthusiasm. They made a video recording, and took still photos, during the whole 3 h of activity.

I had, of course, expected that it would all work but gradually I came to realize that such expectations were the result of over 30 years of immersion in ultrasound. That is not how it would have appeared to Ian Donald in 1955. With that frame of mind, seeing the difference between cystic and solid tissue, or the changes in the echoes from a full bladder (mine!) to one that was half empty (Figure 3), really was remarkable and one could begin to feel a little of the revelation that it would have been, and to understand his words about it being laughable, but fundamental and exciting. Furthermore, it has to be remembered that these traces were obtained using an instrument designed for testing steel and welds, it had not been modified in any way for medical use. Perhaps it worked, and worked so well, and gave Donald such excitement because he had asked the right question – will ultrasound distinguish between cystic and solid masses?

The experience has certainly given us a much clearer understanding of the state of ultrasound in 1955. We also more fully understand the difficulty in interpreting the A-Scan traces. There is much more to learn from a study of the recordings and from the comments of a number

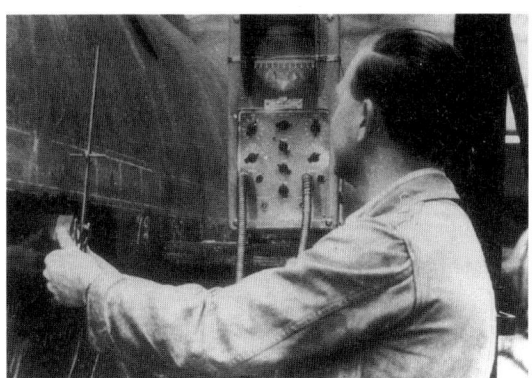

Figure 2 The late Mr J. Davis operating a Kelvin Hughes Mk4 flaw detector in the factory of Babcock and Wilcox Ltd, Renfrew, in about 1955

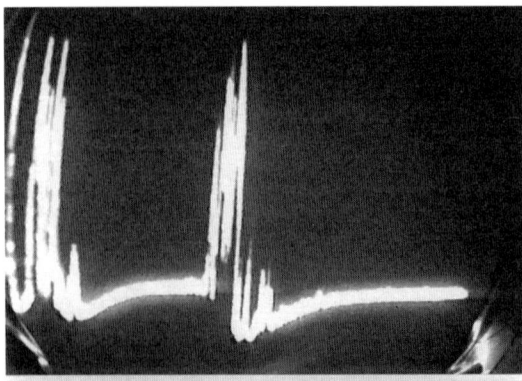

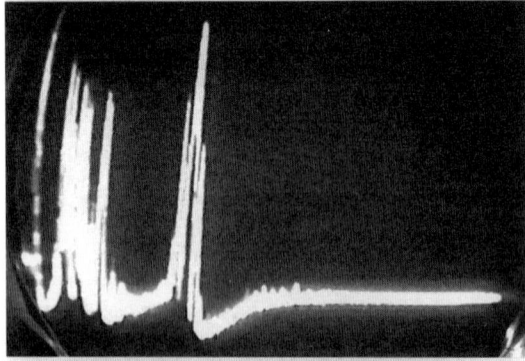

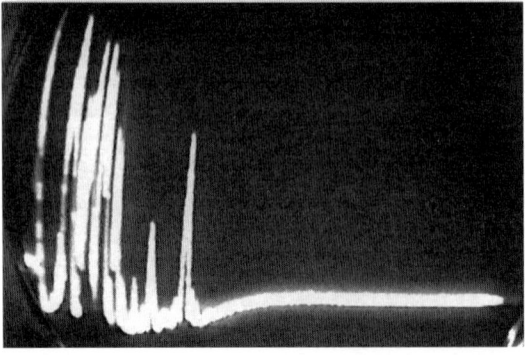

Figure 3 A-Scan traces recorded at the re-enactment of Professor Donald's early experiments from an adult male bladder. From top to bottom: full bladder; after voiding 400 ml; and after a further 300 ml

of people who were not able to be present at the re-enactment.

Donald's experiments had been possible because industrial flaw detectors were available. The credit for the first instrument goes to Firestone[5], working with the Sperry Corporation and Michigan University. He had patented his Reflectoscope and used it to examine metal components for defects and grain structure. Close on his heels were Uchida in Japan and Sproule[6] working at Kelvin Hughes Ltd in the UK, and later in Canada. Kelvin Hughes had a factory in Glasgow so here we see the beginning of a clustering of interests. By 1952, Douglass Howry[7] for one had recognized that ultrasound had a potential value in medicine; the seeds were sown and waiting to be nurtured and brought to fruition by people like Ian Donald.

Ian Donald came to Glasgow in 1954, having accepted the Regius Chair of Midwifery (now Obstetrics and Gynaecology) and was looking for a new research project[4]. Chance, or as I see it, a positive response to opportunity led to the visits to Babcock and Wilcox and later to the involvement of Tom Brown, an engineer at Kelvin Hughes. These events have been fully described elsewhere[8]. Brown's first contributions were to improve the Mk2 A-Scan unit and then to acquire a better instrument, a KH Mk4 flaw detector. About this time Ian Donald was joined by Dr John MacVicar, who later became Professor of Obstetrics and Gynaecology in Leicester. As mentioned earlier, they experimented with the A-Scan on patients prior to operation and then looked for similar traces from the cysts and tumors after removal. Using themselves as controls, they did A-Scans of their legs and showed the difference between their full and empty bladders.

Brown's next and vital contribution was to realize the limitations of A-Scan and to design and build a B-Scan machine (Figures 4 and 5). This was not the earliest two-dimensional scanner but it was the first in which the transducer was placed in direct contact with the patient. In the hands of Donald and MacVicar it was a major step forward and culminated in the publication by Donald, MacVicar and Brown of 'Investigation of abdominal masses by pulsed ultrasound'[9], a dry sounding paper but the one that Donald considered to be his most important and the first of a stream of papers on ultrasound from his department.

This success was followed by the design and construction of the unique automatic contact

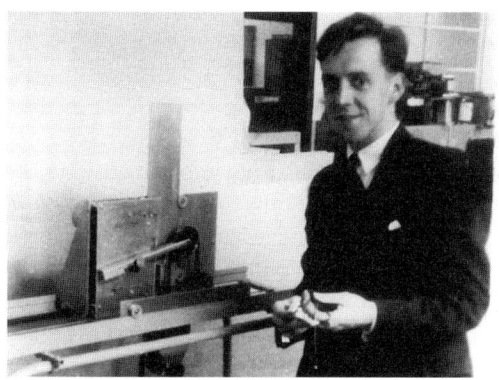

Figure 4 T. G. Brown working on the first two-dimensional contact scanner in the laboratories of Kelvin Hughes (Smiths Industries), Hillington, Glasgow in about 1956. This machine was used to produce the images in the paper by Donald, MacVicar and Brown in 1958 (reference 9)

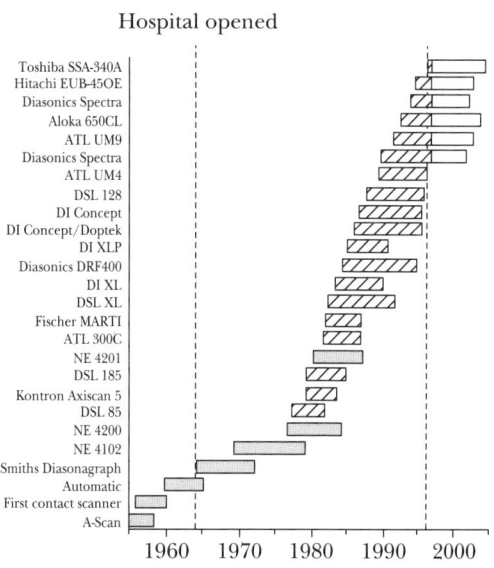

Hospital opened

Toshiba SSA-340A
Hitachi EUB-45OE
Diasonics Spectra
Aloka 650CL
ATL UM9
Diasonics Spectra
ATL UM4
DSL 128
DI Concept
DI Concept/Doptek
DI XLP
Diasonics DRF400
DI XL
DSL XL
Fischer MARTI
ATL 300C
NE 4201
DSL 185
Kontron Axiscan 5
DSL 85
NE 4200
NE 4102
Smiths Diasonagraph
Automatic
First contact scanner
A-Scan

1960   1970   1980   1990   2000

Figure 6 This chart shows the periods of use of ultrasound machines starting with the A-Scan in the Western Infirmary, Glasgow and then in the ultrasound department established by Professor Ian Donald in The Queen Mother's Hospital. Following the A-Scan there are two classes of scanner: the static, indicated by dark bars; and the real-time indicated by hatched boxes. The right hand vertical broken line marks the year 1996. The anticipated life of scanners beyond that date is indicated by extending the bars to the right without hatching. The acceptance of ultrasound and the advent of real-time is obvious from the sudden change of slope which occurred in the late 1970s

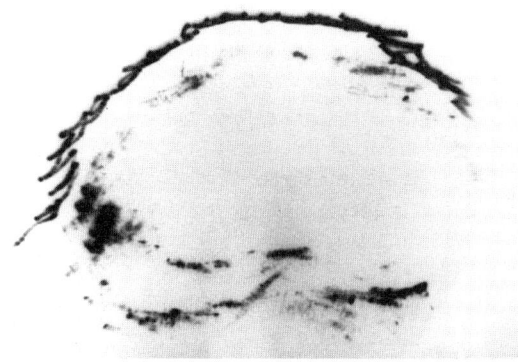

Figure 5 An image of a serous cystadenoma made in about 1957 using the machine in Figure 4

scanner. This enormous machine was in regular weekly use when I came to Glasgow in 1962. The images it produced firmly established the value of ultrasound and during its life it was used on thousands of patients until replaced by the Diasonograph, the first scanner to be produced in quantity. Twelve Diasonographs had been built when the board of Smiths Industries (Kelvin Hughes' parent company) decided to close the loss-making Glasgow factory. This seemed like the end. However, after protracted negotiations, Nuclear Enterprises Ltd, in Edinburgh, bought the interest and stock and went on to greatly improve the Diasonograph. They produced some hundreds of scanners known as NE4101, NE4102, NE4200 and a range of variants. The 'end' had just been the 'end of the beginning'.

The Diasonographs and NE machines, all static scanners, enabled Ian Donald, his colleagues and disciples in many parts of the world to show that ultrasound had great value and potential. Then in the mid-1970s, a major change occurred as can be seen from the chart (Figure 6) of machines purchased in The Queen Mother's Hospital; the large hand operated static scanners were being replaced by real-time machines.

Some precursors of the change to real-time can be found. A film made Howry and Holmes[10] shows cross-sections of the neck of a patient sitting in a tank of water while being scanned with a transducer oscillating at a few sweeps per second. Then, in 1964, the Kretztechnik company in Austria and the East German ophthalmologist, Werner Buschmann[11], built a 10-element concave array for examining the eye. Around the same time the Siemens Vidoson appeared; this remarkably simple machine was designed by Krause and Soldner[12]. Whether it was, when it first appeared, truly valued for its real-time capability is not clear. However, it was very successful and sold in large numbers. In spite of this commercial success it was not developed to any great extent. The reasons for this, which probably include technological problems and misperceptions of the market, would be interesting issues to study.

What did advance was the development of array transducers; again it was a case of concerted and dedicated effort this time by workers in Holland[13] and the team in Advanced Diagnostic Research in Arizona[14]. The aim seems to have been to use ultrasound to study the dynamics of the heart. In that context the shortcomings of the limited field of view, poor resolution, poor beam shape and gaps in the image were more acceptable. The value of real-time for looking at other parts of the body seems not to have been immediately obvious.

Now it is clear that real-time machines had great inherent advantages. They gave bright immediate images with frame-freeze and they were small machines that could be easily transported and demonstrated. Altogether these factors and the growing acceptance of ultrasound widened the market, and sales and hence the funds for research and development increased. These changes, combined with the rapid advances in electronics, resulted in the price of machines falling in real terms to about a third between 1976 and 1992, in spite of their greatly increased electronic complexity. The developments which took place overcame the shortcomings of real-time.

Running almost in parallel with the development of two-dimensional imaging has been the advance of Doppler. Ignoring Doppler's industrial antecedents, the most obvious steps have been the simple, but useful, fetal heart detector, instruments for measuring blood velocity, the development of real-time spectral analysis and the combining of B-Scan and Doppler in 'duplex' systems. Then an almost unnoticed paper in 1982 by Namekawa and co-workers[15], working at Aloka, laid the foundations of color Doppler; rapid improvement followed, leading to two-dimensional images overlaid with color to indicate blood or tissue velocity. More recently, we have seen the development of 'power' Doppler to give a display indicating tissue perfusion.

This is a brief and selective summary of the 40 or so years during which the combined efforts of medics, engineers, physicists and industrialists have developed ultrasound from the A-Scans in industry to marvellous, almost photographic, images with color depicting flow or perfusion; to provide a somewhat broader overview a list of historical landmarks is given below. Ultrasound is so widely used that some radiologists claim it now provides 40% of all medical imaging. Its use has spread to almost every medical specialty, not only gynecology and obstetrics as pioneered by Ian Donald. Ultrasound images have become a commonplace icon in newspapers and on television, indicating fetal life or representing a hospital environment, in spite of the fact that the images are built up from the echoes of high frequency sound pulses as were first seen in barely intelligible A-Scan traces.

ULTRASOUND MUSEUMS

A Kelvin Hughes Mk2 flaw detector of the type used by Ian Donald in his early experiments is in the Science Museum, London, where there are a few other ultrasound items including the Diasonograph used by Professor Stuart Campbell when working at Queen Charlotte's Hospital.

The British Medical Ultrasound Society Historical Collection was established in 1984 and a small selection of items from this collection were on display in the exhibition associated with this Congress. The Collection contains over 60 items of hardware, scanners and associated equipment, a wide range of manufacturer's literature and a substantial and increasing archive of unique documents. Many items of hardware are on display, or can be seen, in the Department of Obstetrics and Gynaecology, University of Glasgow, The Queen Mother's Hospital, Yorkhill, Glasgow, G3 8SJ. The archive material is also available for viewing and study. In the long term, the Collection will pass into the care of the Hunterian Museum, University of Glasgow, G12 8QQ. For more details please contact any of the authors of this paper.

A collection is also held by the American Institute of Ultrasound in Medicine in Washington, DC. This collection and archive are largely the result of the work of Professor Barry Goldberg, who organized a Symposium on the history of medical ultrasound in Washington in 1988.

Recently, an Ultrasound Museum has been established in Dresden by the German Society of Ultrasound in Medicine. This is intended to focus, although not exclusively, on the development of ultrasound in the German speaking countries of Central Europe[16].

DIAGNOSTIC ULTRASOUND: HISTORICAL LANDMARKS

This very brief, rather selective, set of 'landmarks' acknowledges only a few of the multitude of people who have contributed to the development of medical diagnostic ultrasound.

1842 J. C. Doppler wrote paper on the Doppler effect.

1880 J. and P. Curie discovered piezo-electric effect.

1917 P. Langevin built first piezo-electric transducers, found lethal effects on fish.

1942 K. T. Dussik made efforts to use through-transmission in neurology.

1945 F. A. Firestone developed supersonic reflectorscope (A-Scan).

1948 D. Howry started experimental work.

1949 G. D. Ludwig and F. W. Struthers worked on detection of gallstones and foreign bodies.

J. J. Wild started experimental work.

R. Uchida (Japan) built an A-Scan instrument.

D. O. Sproule (UK) developed supersonic flaw detector.

1950 J. J. Wild and D. Neal wrote first paper on detecting changes of texture in living tissue.

L. A. French, J. J. Wild and D. Neal worked on detection of cerebral tumors.

1954 K. Tanaka started using contact scanning for neurology.

Ian Donald started experimental work.

Elder and Hertz wrote first paper on echo-cardiology.

J. J. Wild and J. M. Reid worked on visualization of breast lesions.

D. Howry, J. Holmes and colleagues wrote papers on visualization of soft tissues.

H. P. Kalmus and co-workers wrote papers on acoustic flowmeter systems.

1956 T. G. Brown joined Ian Donald and improved A-Scan.

Denver group wrote paper on three-dimensional and stereo methods.

S. Satomura was studying heart with Doppler.

G. Baum, J. G. Henry and colleagues wrote papers on ophthalmic ultrasound.

T. Cieszynski developed first intra-luminal transducer.

1957 T. G. Brown built contact scanner for Ian Donald.

Baldes and associates 'Forum on ultrasonic measurement of blood velocity'.

1958 First paper from Donald, MacVicar and Brown.

1959 T. G. Brown started work on automatic contact-scanner.

Franklin, Baker and co-workers developed pulsed Doppler flowmeter.

97

1962 B. Sunden (Sweden) started using 1st B-scanner sold by Kelvin Hughes.
Kato showed that red blood cells were source of Doppler shift signals.

1963 First Kelvin Hughes (Smiths) Diasonograph manual contact scanners sold.
Denver contact scanner in use.

1964 Denver group's first publication on obstetric use of contact scanner.
Physionic Porta-Arm scanner delivered to Denver group.

1965 Buschmann showed 10-element array for the eye.
1st International Congress, Pittsburgh, 33 papers from nine countries.
SmithKline Instruments Doptone fetal heart detector on market.

1966 K. Kato described directional Doppler.
Postgraduate course on Diagnostic Ultrasound started in Denver.

1967 W. Krause and R. Soldner developed Siemens 'Vidoson' real-time scanner.
Cardiac scanning by Kikuchi and Tanaka.

1968 J. C. Somer developed electronic phased array sector scanner.
D. A. Lobdell worked on the annular array.

1969 Peronneau produced flow profiles with multigate Doppler.
Kretztechnik built vaginal transducer for A. Kratochwil (Austria).

1970 Courses on Diagnostic Ultrasound started in Glasgow.

1971 N. Bom linear array 'for moving cardiac structures'.

1972 First commercial linear array scanner from Advanced Diagnostic Research.

1973 D. L. King wrote first paper on use of linear array; referred only to cardiac use.

1974 F. E. Barber, D. W. Baker and co-workers developed Duplex echo-Doppler scanner.
Coglan and associates developed time compression spectrum analyzer.

1977 T. G. Brown (Sonicaid) Multiplanar three-dimensional scanner in production.

1982 K. Namekawa, C. Kasai and colleagues (Aloka) described color Doppler at The World Federation for Ultrasound in Medicine and Biology, 1982.
Acuson delivered first 'computed sonography' system.

1983 The performance of ultrasound systems
–96 has rapidly improved, color Doppler imaging, giving both velocity and 'power' displays has become commonplace and three-dimensional imaging is arriving on the scene. It has been estimated that ultrasound now accounts for 40% of all medical imaging.

For more details please contact the author or refer to the excellent and comprehensive bibliography compiled by White and associates[17].

ACKNOWLEDGEMENTS

We would like to thank the following: Wellcome Trust for their grant 'The development of medical ultrasound in Glasgow, 1954–1976'; Mr B. Donnelly, Axiom Ltd, Clifford Lane, Glasgow, for the loan of a Kelvin Hughes Mk4 flaw detector; Dr K. P. Hanretty for the loan of equipment to record the A-Scan trace; Medical Illustration, Yorkhill Hospitals Trust, Glasgow; Mitsui Babcock Energy Ltd; and the Department of Veterinary Anatomy, Glasgow University.

References

1. Spencer, I. H., Fleming, J. E. E. and Nicolson, M. (1996). The role of medical ultrasound in the abortion debate in Scotland. Presented at *Scottish Medical Sociology Group of the British Sociological Association*, May, Pitlochry

2. Spencer, I. H., Fleming, J. E. E. and Nicolson, M. (1996). Clinical ultrasound and inter-professional rivalries. Presented at *Society for the History of Technology Annual Meeting*, August, London

3. Nicolson, M., Spencer, I. H. and Fleming, J. E. E. (1996). Ultrasound and the construction of the fetal image. Presented at *Conference of the Medical Sociology Group of the British Sociological Association*, September, Edinburgh

4. Donald, I. (1974). Sonar – the story of an experiment. *Ultrasound Med. Biol.*, **1**, 109–17

5. Firestone, F. A. (1945). The Supersonic Reflectoscope for interior inspection. *Metal Prog.*, **48**, 505

6. Desch, C. H., Sproule, D. O. and Dawson, W. J. (1946). The detection of cracks in steel by means of supersonic waves. *J. Iron Steel Instr. London*, **153**, 319–53

7. Howry, D. H. and Bliss, W. R. (1952). Ultrasonic visualisation of soft tissue structures of the body. *J. Lab. Clin. Med.*, **40**, 579–92

8. Fleming, J. E. E. (1995). Medical ultrasound from A-Scan to real-time. In Reed, G. B., Claireaux, A. E. and Cockburn, F. (eds.) *Diseases of the Fetus and Newborn*, pp. 867–74. (London: Chapman and Hall)

9. Donald, I., MacVicar, J. and Brown, T. G. (1958). Investigation of abdominal masses by pulsed ultrasound. *Lancet*, **1**, 1188–95

10. Howry, D. H. and Holmes, J. (1954/5). *A New Diagnostic Tool.* 16-mm cine film, duration 20 min, University of Colarado. Copy in British Medical Ultrasound Society Collection

11. Buschmann, W. (1964). Ein neues Gerat die Ultraschalldiagnostik. Presented at *Symposium Internationale de Diagnostica Ultrasonica in Ophthalmologia*, Berlin, 3–5 June 1964, Augenklinik der Charite, Humboldt-Universitat zu Berlin, pp. 31–5

12. Krause, W. and Soldner, R. (1967). Ultrasonic imaging technique (B-scan) with high image rate for medical diagnosis. *Electromedica*, 35, 8–11

13. Bom, N., Lancee, C. T., Honkoop, J. and Hugenholtz, P. G. (1971). Ultrasonic viewer for cross-sectional analysis of moving cardiac structures. *Biomed. Eng.*, **6**., 500–3, 508

14. King, D. L. (1973). Real-time cross-sectional ultrasonic imaging of the heart using a linear array multi-element transducer. *J. Clin. Ultrasound*, **1**, 196–200

15. Namekawa, K., Kasai, C., Tsukamoto, M. and Koyano, A. (1982). Realtime bloodflow imaging system utilising auto-correlation techniques. In Lerski, R. A. and Morley, R. (eds.) *Proceedings of WFUMB-82*, the *Third Meeting of the World Federation for Ultrasound in Medicine and Biology*, Brighton, UK, 26–30 July, pp. 203–8. (Oxford: Pergamon Press)

16. Editorial (1996). Ultrasound Museum in Dresden, *EFSUMB Newsletter*, **10** (1), 9

17. White, D. N., Clark, G., Carson, J. and White, E. (eds.) (1982). *Ultrasound in Biomedicine: Cumulative Bibliography of the World Literature to 1978.* (Oxford: Pergamon Press)

Ultrasound screening for fetal abnormalities in the United Kingdom

14

M. J. Whittle

INTRODUCTION

Information concerning screening for fetal abnormalities in the UK by ultrasound is difficult to establish. No database exists which gives an accurate insight but a recent, currently unpublished, survey by the Royal College of Obstetricians and Gynaecologists (RCOG) and Royal College of Radiologists (RCR) suggested that about 80% of women were offered an anomaly scan at 18–20 weeks.

There has been considerable pressure both from health care purchasers and, to some extent, from patients themselves, for the professionals to justify a policy of routine, as opposed to selective scanning. However, the fact that about 95% of fetal abnormalities occur unexpectedly means that the only effective method of detection is by some form of screening policy.

Whilst it may be self-evident that the detection of the majority of fetal abnormalities can only be through screening, accurate information on detection rates using ultrasound is extremely difficult to determine from the standard literature. In fact there is only one database in the UK and that is in the Northern Region[1]. It indicates that ultrasound may be effective for conditions such as neural tube defects but not particularly good for other anomalies, particularly those involving the cardiovascular system. A further analysis of the data[2] indicated that when a termination was done on the basis on a scan, autopsy showed concordance with regard to prognosis in 99.5% of cases, although the exact diagnosis was refined in 35%. This suggests that, overall, ultrasound is better at estimating severity rather than providing absolute diagnostic accuracy. A fetal anomaly register has just been established in the West Midlands but data are not yet available and a database from Scotland is in the process of publication.

THE EFFECTIVENESS OF ULTRASOUND

In the analysis of effectiveness two issues need to be addressed, namely the ability of ultrasound to detect certain abnormalities and the consequences flowing from that detection. The detection of an anomaly by ultrasound screening may lead to either termination of the pregnancy or provide an opportunity for the planning of both intrauterine treatment and appropriate management at, and after, delivery.

Detection rates

Often individual papers do not clearly indicate how a study was undertaken, who was doing the scanning and on what standard of machine. Follow-up is variable and postdelivery ascertainment unreliable, especially for those conditions which may not be clinically obvious.

It is important to distinguish between the need to identify those conditions which carry high morbidity and are therefore a large burden for both family and State, and those conditions which are likely to be fatal. The aims are different for these two circumstances; in the former the aim is to reduce morbidity either by termination of the pregnancy or by optimizing management to minimize morbidity. The aim in the second is to reduce the need for the mother

Table 1 Average detection rates for fetal abnormalities from the ultrasound literature

System	Average detection rate (%)
Central nervous system	80
Cardiovascular system	20
Renal system	66
Anterior abdominal wall	80
Skeletal system	35
Aneuploidy	24

to go through a pregnancy certain to result in a non-viable fetus; it may also prevent inappropriate obstetric management.

Average detection rates for various conditions are shown in Table 1. These are drawn from the literature and no particular judgement has been made about whether contributing papers are good or not[3-11]. In fact, the reality of detection rates is that they are generally likely to be lower than shown. However, the Table indicates that for central nervous system defect, typically neural tube defects, detection is generally high at around 80%. Conversely, serious cardiac defects may have detection rates which at best are around 20%. Major abnormalities are relatively easy to detect, so that conditions such as anencephaly, body stalk abnormality or even severe skeletal dysplasia will be found with a high degree of probability

The detection of chromosome disorders by ultrasound remains debatable but the use of nuchal translucency described by one large study looks promising[11]. The study comprises approximately 20 000 cases, although follow-up is available on only about 2700 who underwent chorionic villus sampling (CVS) because of a positive nuchal translucency. Using these data gives a detection rate of about 80% for chromosome abnormalities but the test is undertaken between 10 and 14 weeks and at this stage in pregnancy about 50% of Down's syndrome and about 80% of Edward's syndrome fetuses will abort spontaneously. The results are interesting in that those babies with apparently normal karyotypes had a perinatal mortality rate of about 40/1000, suggesting that the presence of a nuchal translucency in the absence of

aneuploidy indicates increased pregnancy risk. Whether this test will prove cost-effective as a screen for chromosome abnormalities remains to be seen and other groups, albeit with smaller numbers, have not been able to reproduce the results.

The variables which determine detection do not only depend on the type of lesion and whether it is single or multiple, but also on such matters as the maternal size, fetal position and gestational age. Only the last of these can be controlled and the optimal time for scanning is usually set at around 18–20 weeks. Thus, cardiac abnormalities are difficult to identify at 15 weeks since a reliable four-chamber view can be difficult to achieve at that time. However, by 20 weeks a clear view of the heart will be possible in about 90% of fetuses and around 10–35% of anomalies will be seen. After 24 weeks it may be possible that half of the serious lesions will be seen. Other variables include the skill and training of the operator and the quality of the equipment. These are important issues and recent data[12] suggest that improved training and experience can influence detection rates.

Management strategies

Philosophical changes have occurred over the years with regard to the management of fetal abnormalities. Previously, the identification of an abnormal fetus was a prelude to termination of the pregnancy. These decisions were sometimes taken without due discussion and the realization that a proportion of abnormalities may in fact not be lethal and, with appropriate treatment, may have relatively low morbidity. Knowledge of the natural history of many of the disorders which can nowadays be diagnosed is often scanty but this area is rapidly expanding.

Cardiac abnormalities offer a good example. Ten years ago it was usually considered that the univentricular heart was incompatible with life. Today babies can undergo a series of procedures from which maybe 50% survive. Thus, although some couples may decide on termination in this condition as the best solution for them, this approach is not one to be automatically adopted. Some evidence exists to suggest that prior awareness that a cardiac lesion exists improves overall outcome[13].

On the other hand, the consequences of being born with spina bifida are still regarded as very severe and in spite of enormous experience, improvements have not been greatly evident. Morbidity may be reduced by elective Cesarean section, although confirmation of this observation requires larger studies and generally babies with spina bifida may survive but with considerable morbidity and requiring multiple surgical procedures. Only about 12% of babies born with myelomeningocele will have 'minimal handicap'[14].

In contrast, experience with anterior abdominal wall defects, such as gastroschisis, suggests that their prior diagnosis and delivery under optimal circumstances in a suitable high-risk unit improves outcome[15]. The morbidity of the lesion is relatively small when there is the opportunity for correct management, this only being possible in prenatally diagnosed cases.

The only firm evidence that ultrasound screening may have an impact on perinatal mortality comes from the Helsinki study[16] which indicated that the reduction noted was partly explained by 50% fewer babies being born alive with fetal abnormality because of their prior termination.

PATTERN OF SCREENING FOR FETAL ABNORMALITIES IN THE UK

These data are drawn from a RCOG/RCR survey completed in 1994 and currently unpublished. The survey involved 256 departments throughout the UK and 168 returns were received, a 65% response. About 77% of departments offered women a booking scan, which appeared to be most frequently performed at about 14 weeks, and 82% a routine scan for fetal anomaly screening usually undertaken at between 18 and 20 weeks (mean 19 weeks). Only 5% of departments undertook a routine third trimester scan.

Certain elements were examined in nearly all cases (approximately 90%), such as the biparietal diameter, ventricles, cerebellum, spine, four-chamber view, bladder and stomach. About 80% looked for diaphragm, limbs, hands/feet, femur length, cord insertion, kidneys and placental position. Around 50% looked at the orbits, lips, situs and nuchal fold and cord vessels.

However, palate, nostrils and fingers/toes were only sought in about 25%, just over 20% examined the outflow tracts and only 8% the short axis view of the heart. Only 2% used color flow.

Of those units which did not have a routine anomaly scanning policy, 90% used an alternative such as maternal serum α-fetoprotein (AFP). About a third stated that they planned to introduce a routine anomaly scanning policy within 6 months of the survey, i.e. within 1996.

THE ORGANIZATION OF SCREENING FOR FETAL ABNORMALITIES IN THE UK

The ideal screening method for fetal abnormalities would be one which was easy to administer, cheap and which had low false positive and negative rates. Clear objectives must be defined so that in general the important issues, discussed above, will be addressed, namely that screening will identify conditions that are relatively common, are of high morbidity and mortality or amenable to intrauterine or postnatal treatment.

The two highly morbid conditions are neural tube defects and Down's syndrome. In the former both biochemical screening and ultrasound seem reasonably effective, and in welltrained hands about 85% of spina bifida will be detected and virtually all anencephaly. In Down's syndrome early ultrasound (10–14 weeks) may be capable of detecting up to 80%, whilst biochemistry may detect potentially 65%. In both these circumstances it is possible that the overall performance of biochemical testing in low-risk groups may be better since the test is simpler to administer. Evidence that screening has had an impact on both these conditions is evident.

In neural tube defect, the birth prevalence of this condition has changed from 6.6/1000 births in 1964–1968 to 1.04/1000 in 1979–1989 and the pregnancy prevalence has changed from 5.63/1000 to 3.02/1000 over the same time span. Thus the overall prevalence fell by 46% but the birth prevalence fell by 82%, the latter change arising both as a result of the natural fall in the incidence of the condition and from screening for the condition[17]. It is now rare for a baby to be born with an unexpected neural tube defect[1].

The incidence of liveborn Down's syndrome babies has fallen from 1.1/1000 to 0.9/1000 between 1989 and 1993[18]. This reflects the increased number of antenatal diagnoses made over this period, which to some extent antedates the time when widespread biochemical screening became available. One might anticipate, therefore, an even more significant fall in subsequent years.

ORGANIZATION IN THE UK

Although prenatal screening may be feasible it is essential that it is accompanied by a robust support service which includes the availability of appropriate counselling and easy referral to specialist centers.

In 1982 the RCOG established a working party to investigate the possibility of setting up three subspecialty programs in the UK – fetal medicine, gynecological oncology and reproductive medicine[19]. Fetal medicine was to encompass special training in both fetal conditions and maternal disease and, in effect, Fetal Medicine Centres have now been established in all regions of the UK. They provide advice to doctors within their region, and occasionally to outside regions, with particular reference to prenatal diagnostic problems and treatment.

The funding arrangements are complex and unsatisfactory and difficulties have recently arisen as a result of the organizational changes in the National Health Service. Tertiary units may have contracts with hospitals in their region to undertake care of individual cases but the effort involved is inadequately compensated by this method. Conversely, extracontractual referrals are more representative of the work involved in a financial sense but the mechanism for collecting these funds is unreliable.

The disintegration of the regional system has meant that competition has developed between units, leading to duplication of effort and a reduction in the experience base for individual units.

CONCLUSIONS

Ultrasound offers the opportunity for the effective screening of pregnancies for fetal abnormalities. However, the technique was introduced without properly designed studies so that its efficacy remains uncertain. Nevertheless, ultrasound examination remains an important part of the obstetric examination and, in combination with biochemical methods, may provide an effective method of identifying seriously morbid conditions such as neural tube defects and Down's syndrome and fatal conditions like anencephaly. Its performance with other conditions may be less reliable but it will also identify those babies with conditions requiring postnatal treatment and so allow appropriate delivery arrangements to be made.

References

1. Northern Region Survey Steering Group (1992). Fetal abnormality; an audit of its recognition and management. *Arch. Dis. Child.*, **67**, 770–4
2. Brand, I. R., Kaminopetros, P., Cave, M., Irving, H. C. and Lilford, R. J. (1994). Specificity of antenatal ultrasound in the Yorkshire region; a prospective study of 2261 ultrasound detected anomalies. *Br. J. Obstet. Gynaecol.*, **101**, 392–7
3. Carrera, J. M., Torrents, M., Mortera, C., Cusi, V. and Munoz, A. (1995). Routine prenatal

ultrasound screening for fetal abnormalities; 22 years experience. *Ultrasound Obstet. Gynecol.*, **5**, 174–9

4. Chitty, L. S., Hunt, G. H., Moore, J. and Lobb, M. O. (1991). Effectiveness of routine ultrasonography in detecting fetal structural abnormalities in the low risk population. *Br. Med. J.*, **303**, 1165–9

5. Crane, J. P., Le Fevre, M. L., Winborn, R. C., Evans, J. K., Ewigman, B. G., Bain, R. P., Frigoletto, F. D., McNellis, D. and the RADIUS Study Group (1994). A randomised trial of prenatal ultrasonographic screening; impact on the detection, management and outcome of anomalous fetuses. *Am. J. Obstet. Gynecol.*, **171**, 392–9

6. Goncalves, L. F., Jeanty, P. and Piper, J. M. (1994). The accuracy of prenatal ultrasonography in detecting congenital anomalies. *Am. J. Obstet. Gynecol.*, **171**, 1606–12

7. Levi, S., Schaaps, J. P., De Havay, P. and Defoort, P. (1995). End-result of routine ultrasound screening for congenital anomalies: The Belgium Multicentre Study 1984–1992. *Ultrasound Obstet. Gynecol.*, **5**, 366–71

8. Luck, C. (1992). Value of routine ultrasound scanning at 19 weeks; a four year study of 8849 deliveries. *Br. Med. J.*, **304**, 1474–8

9. Rosendahl, H. and Kivinen, S. (1989). Antenatal detection of congenital malformation by routine ultrasound. *Obstet. Gynecol.*, **73**, 947–51

10. Shirley, I. M., Bottomley, F. and Robinson, V. P. (1992). Routine radiographer screening for fetal anomalies by ultrasound in an unselected low risk population. *Br. J. Radiol.*, **65**, 564–9

11. Pandya, P. P., Snijders, R. J. M., Johnson, S. P., Brizot, M. de L. and Nicolaides, K. H. (1995). Screening for fetal trisomies by maternal age and fetal nuchal translucency thickness at 10 to 14 weeks of gestation. *Br. J. Obstet. Gynaecol.*, **102**, 957–62

12. Stoll, C., Dott, B., Alembik, Y. and Roth, M. P. (1995). Evaluation of routine prenatal diagnosis by a registry of congenital anomalies. *Prenat. Diagn.*, **15**, 791–800

13. Cohen, D. M. (1992). Surgical management of congenital heart disease in the 1990s. *Am. J. Dis. Child.*, **146**, 1447–52

14. Sturgiss, S. and Robson, S. (1995). Prognosis for fetuses with antenatally detected myelomeningocoele. *Fetal Matern. Med. Rev.*, **7**, 235–49

15. Roberts, J. P. and Burge, D. M. (1990). Antenatal diagnosis of abdominal wall defects: a missed opportunity. *Arch. Dis. Child.*, **65**, 687–9

16. Saari-Kempainen, A., Karjalainen, O., Ylostalo, P. and Heinonen, O. P. (1990). Ultrasound screening and perinatal mortality; controlled trial of systematic one-stage screening in pregnancy. *Lancet*, **336**, 387–91

17. Omran, M., Stone, D. H. and McLoone, P. (1992). The Chief Scientist reports ... Pattern of decline in prevalence of anencephaly and spina bifida in a high risk area. *Health Bull.*, **50**(5), 407–13

18. Alberman, E., Mutton, D., Ide, R., Nicholson, A. and Bobrow, M. (1995). Down's syndrome births and pregnancy termination in 1989–1993. *Br. J. Obstet. Gynaecol.*, **102**, 445–7

19. Royal College of Obstetricians and Gynaecologists (1982). *Report of the RCOG Working Party on Further Specialisation within Obstetrics and Gynaecology.* (London: Royal College of Obstetricians and Gynaecologists)

Fetal behavior

15

D. James

INTRODUCTION

The normal term human fetus is a sophisticated organism from a neurological point of view[1]. The advent of ultrasound has meant that we have been able to study the neurodevelopment of the fetus, or fetal behavior. Behavior is defined as the interaction of an organism with its environment[2]. Human fetal neurobehavioral development has been studied in three ways:

(1) By passive observation of fetal activity[3];

(2) By recording the reaction of a fetus to a stimulus[4]; and

(3) By documenting fetal habituation, that is the cessation of a response to a repeated stimulus[5].

This last response represents a simple form of learned behavior and potentially is the most sophisticated method of assessment of the three.

PASSIVE BEHAVIOR

Fetal activity is detectable with ultrasound as early as 7 weeks. De Vries and colleagues[6] reported that the first movements seen in the fetus were extensions and flexions of the fetal spine visible from 7 weeks. This was followed by the onset of a wide variety of distinct types of movement over the next 6–8 weeks. Indeed, all the movements observed in term fetuses were already present by 15 weeks, provided a sufficiently long observation time was used to compensate for the low incidence of many movements (such as breathing) in early pregnancy (see Table 1). The only difference in these early movements and those seen at term

is in their greater sophistication, co-ordination and integration later in pregnancy.

As pregnancy advances a cyclicity of fetal behavior develops. The first to be recognized is a diurnal pattern which has been reported from as early as 20–22 weeks[7] through to the end of pregnancy[8].

From the end of the second trimester shorter cycles of fetal behavioral variation can be recognized. Initially, the fetus shows alternating rest–activity cycles (also called active–quiet and ultradian rhythms). Thus, for example, prior to 24 weeks, the longest period of inactivity or quiescence in the human fetus is 6 min, whereas after 32 weeks most quiet intervals are between 10 and 40 min[9]. Using this arbitrary 6-min rule, rest–activity cycles are rarely seen prior to 24 weeks but by 29 weeks they are seen in over 80% of recordings from normal fetuses[9].

This continuing development of the fetal neurological system can be seen in the

Table 1 The appearance of fetal movements in early pregnancy (adapted from reference 6)

Movement	Gestation of first appearance (week)
Any movement	7
Startle	8
Generalized movements	8
Hiccups	8
Isolated arm movements	9
Head retroflexion	9
Hand–face contact	10
Breathing	10
Jaw opening	10
Stretching	10
Head anteflexion	10
Yawn	11
Suck and swallow	12

manifestation of behavioral states by the end of pregnancy. Behavioral states are fixed and recurring associations between body movements, eye movements and heart rate in the fetus, which change within 3 min[3]. They are defined in Table 2 and their characteristics are described in Table 3. The existence of State 3F is disputed[10]. Behavioral states are present in over 80% of recordings from normal fetuses at 36 weeks[10].

There is a progressive increase in the tone of the fetus as pregnancy advances. This reflects maturation of both the central nervous system (especially the cerebellum) and the musculoskeletal system. This may be useful as a general neurological screening tool in the future.

The development of fetal heart rate (FHR) characteristics during normal pregnancy represents a combination of the effects of both local and central factors[11]. During normal pregnancy the mean baseline FHR declines significantly as gestation advances, with the mean value being approximately 155 bpm at 16 weeks and falling by approximately 1 bpm per week to reach a mean value of 130 bpm at 40 weeks[11]. Thus the normal range of the FHR at the start of the third trimester is 120–160 bpm, whereas at term it is 110–150 bpm. Most of the other features of the FHR are positively correlated with advancing gestation. Thus as pregnancy progresses there are significant rises in the proportion of fetal movements associated with FHR accelerations, the rate of rise of the accelerations and the maximum height of the accelerations[11]. There is also an initial increase in the variability of the baseline FHR over the first two trimesters. However, over the last trimester this continues to rise in periods of activity but falls again in periods

of quiescence[11]. A sinusoidal FHR pattern may reflect underlying pathology, especially severe fetal anemia or shock. However, it can also be a normal feature found in association with fetal mouthing movements[12].

The onset of both hiccups and breathing has been described at 8–10 weeks[6], corresponding to the time of development of the diaphragm. However, their developmental trends are very different, with fetal hiccups being the predominant type of diaphragmatic movement up to 26 weeks and fetal breathing being more common thereafter[13]. This suggests that the centers controlling fetal breathing are not only different but also are more complex than those that control hiccups.

STIMULATED BEHAVIOR

The most commonly studied stimulus to fetal behavior is the 'acoustic larynx'[4], which emits a broad band of frequencies resulting in both vibratory and acoustic components to the stimulus. A normal term healthy human fetus responds to such a vibroacoustic stimulus (VAS) by manifesting an increase in baseline FHR, an increase in frequency and duration of FHR accelerations, an increase in duration of body

Table 3 Characteristics of behavioral states in full-term normal human fetuses (from reference 10)

State	% Time observed	Mean duration (min)	Range (min)
1F	30.1	21.8	3–38
2F	57.5	31.6	3–94
4F	9.5	37.8	4–137

Note: no 3F was observed in this study; state was not defined for 2.9% of the observational period

Table 2 Behavioral states in full-term normal human fetuses (from reference 3)

State description	Somatic movements	Eye movements	Baseline FHR pattern
1F	Absent except for occasional startle	Absent	Low variation
2F	Present in bursts	Present	High variation
3F*	Absent	Present	High variation
4F	Present	Present	Sustained tachycardia

FHR = fetal heart rate; *the existence of State 3F is disputed (see text and reference 10)

movements but a reduction in duration of fetal breathing[4]. The earliest response has been noted at 22 weeks, but by 28 weeks all females and by 30 weeks all male fetuses appear to respond in some degree[14]. However, the appearance of fetal movement and FHR responses appear to be developmentally distinct processes.

HABITUATION

Habituation is a decrease and eventual cessation of a behavioral response that occurs after an initially novel stimulus is repeatedly presented. It is widely accepted as a basic form of learning and a normal pattern reflects an intact and fully functioning central nervous system[15]. A number of different stimuli have been used. Leader and colleagues[16] examined habituation of the fetal movement and FHR response to repeated vibroacoustic stimulation using an electric toothbrush applied to the maternal abdomen. They demonstrated that in over 50% of normal term low-risk fetuses habituation occurred after 10–20 stimuli and only 7% took more than 50 stimuli to habituate.

It appears that the fetal ability to habituate to this stimulus is related to long-term neurodevelopmental outcome. Leader and colleagues took the same cases that they had used to study habituation (above)[16] and measured their General Intelligence Quotient (GIQ) scores at 1 year postnatal age. They found that those infants who, as fetuses, took over 50 stimuli to habituate ('slow habituators') had significantly lower GIQ scores than the 'normal habituators' (less than 50 stimuli)[15].

A gestational effect has also been reported for fetal habituation, with the rate of habituation becoming significantly faster as gestational age increases. This phenomenon is thought to reflect the maturation of the neural circuitry responsible for this form of learning[17].

Finally, fetal habituation has been used to study cognition and language development. Term fetuses are able to discriminate between different sounding vowels[18], to recognize their mother's voice and to differentiate between male and female voices[19].

BIOLOGICAL INFLUENCES ON FETAL BEHAVIOR

A number of biological or physiological factors influence fetal behavior. Arguably the two most important factors are gestational age and behavioral state. There are ethnic differences[20]. There is no agreement about the influence of uterine contractions and labor on fetal behavior. Similarly, there are conflicting reports in the literature about the effects of heat and maternal exercise, although this is perhaps not surprising given the varied nature of the thermal stress and exercise used in the different studies.

PATHOLOGICAL INFLUENCES ON FETAL BEHAVIOR

Intrauterine growth retardation

Alteration of fetal behavior in growth retardation has been studied by several groups. The definitions of intrauterine growth retardation (IUGR) have varied in the different reports. Causes of growth restriction are many and include congenital abnormality and infection. The most common identifiable cause is uteroplacental insufficiency and this is the commonest cause in most of the studies of fetal behavior in association with IUGR, although many of the reports have failed to document the cause. However, the commonly agreed effects of pathological undergrowth on fetal behavior are[21]: reduced quantity and quality of fetal movements, a delay in maturation of FHR patterns and behavioral states, a progressive fall in FHR variation with chronic hypoxia, a lower incidence and shorter duration of fetal breathing, a reduced FHR and fetal movement response to VAS, and a longer time being taken to habituate, if at all.

Maternal diabetes

Behavior is altered in fetuses of diabetic mothers[22,23]. In summary, such fetuses show a delay in onset of general fetal movements in early pregnancy, but an earlier onset and greater frequency of fetal breathing movements (probably related to higher maternal glucose values) and an increased activity in late pregnancy[22,23].

Maternal drugs

Many drugs have been studied with respect to fetal behavior. Most are depressive to all forms of fetal activity with the exception of amphetamines and β-sympathomimetic agents which have been shown to be stimulatory.

Other pathologies

There is a dispute in the literature as to whether fetal infection affects behavior. Fetal abnormalities of various sorts have been reported to be associated with abnormalities of behavior – passive[24], stimulated[14] and habituation[25].

APPLICATION IN PRACTICE

The main drawbacks of fetal behavioral analysis in a research activity are that it is impractical, time-consuming, laborious and, in part, subjective[1,2]. These problems are being overcome in two stages[1]; first, by the identification and recording of fetal behavior (principally FHR and fetal movement) using Doppler ultrasound and, second, by the analysis by computer of the signals thus generated.

These methods have been applied to the study of: passive fetal behavior using FHR alone[26], fetal movements alone[27] and FHR and fetal movements in combination[1]; stimulated behavior[28]; and habituation[29].

In our own work we have studied both passive FHR and activity in fetuses detected using Doppler ultrasound and analyzed by computer 'on line'. Using this approach we have been able to confirm many of the observations in pathological pregnancies previously reported using conventional behavioral methods. Thus, for example, we have shown that fetuses with intrauterine growth retardation and abnormal umbilical artery Doppler recordings but normal biophysical profile scores have significantly reduced fetal activity at all gestations compared to normal and significantly reduced periods of high variation in the more severe/earlier onset cases presenting at 28–31 weeks. In contrast, fetuses of diabetic mothers manifest no changes in FHR variation but show increased fetal activity, which is statistically significant at 36 weeks and above. The effects of fetal abnormality on FHR and activity recorded and analyzed in this way vary with the diagnosis. Some conditions have normal FHR variation. If it is abnormal it is usually in the form of an increased duration of low FHR variation. Most of the abnormal fetuses we have studied have abnormal fetal activity (either reduced or increased).

Given the practical methodological problems of conventional fetal behavioral analysis, it is not surprising that the only clinical applications of behavior research are antenatal FHR monitoring and biophysical profile testing. Whilst both are in widespread clinical use, the results from meta-analysis of randomized trials of these two methods have failed to show any benefit from their use alone as the final arbiter of fetal well-being. However, it must be admitted that the total numbers in all those trials were small.

CONCLUSIONS

Ultrasound makes detailed study of fetal neurobehavioral development possible. Development is affected by both biological and many pathological factors (not just hypoxia). Newer technology holds out the promise of objective clinical applications. So far, most studies of fetal development have concentrated on the last trimester. In principle it is important to examine the development in early pregnancy. Yet it is uncertain how rewarding that will be since the fetus is, by definition, more immature. In the future, assessment of fetal behavior will have a place in clinical practice as an adjunct to other methods of fetal assessment for screening, diagnosis and predicting prognosis. However, those methods will have to be objective and only introduced after sufficiently large randomized, controlled trials have been assessed.

References

1. James, D., Pillai, M. and Smolenic, J. (1995). Neurobehavioural development in the human fetus. In Lecanuet, J. P., Fifer, W. P., Krasnegor, N. A. and Smotherman, W. P. (eds.) *Fetal Development – a Psychobiological Perspective*, pp. 107–28. (New Jersey: Lawrence Erlbaum Assoc. Inc.)

2. Vindla, S. and James, D. (1995). Fetal behaviour as a test of fetal wellbeing (Commentary). *Br. J. Obstet. Gynaecol.*, **102**, 597–600

3. Nijhuis, J., Prechtl, H. F. R., Martin, C. B. and Bots, R. S. G. M. (1982). Are there behavioural states in the human fetus? *Early Hum. Dev.*, **6**, 177–95

4. Gagnon, R., Hunse, C., Fellows, F., Carmichael, L. and Patrick, J. (1987). Human fetal responses to vibratory acoustic stimulation from twenty-six weeks to term. *Am. J. Obstet. Gynecol.*, **157**, 1375–81

5. Leader, L. R., Baillie, P., Martin, B. and Vermeulen, E. (1982). The assessment and significance of habituation to a repeated stimulus by the human fetus. *Early Hum. Dev.*, **7**, 211–19

6. De Vries, J. I. P., Visser, G. H. A. and Prechtl, H. F. R. (1987). The emergence of fetal behaviour: I. Qualitative aspects. *Early Hum. Dev.*, **15**, 301–22

7. De Vries, J. I. P., Visser, G. H. A., Mulder, E. J. H. and Prechtl, H. F. R. (1987). Diurnal and other variations in fetal movement and heart rate patterns at 20 to 22 weeks. *Early Hum. Dev.*, **15**, 333–48

8. Patrick, J., Campbell, K., Carmichael, L., Natale, R. and Richardson, B. (1982). Patterns of gross fetal body movements over 24 hours observation interval in the last 10 weeks of pregnancy. *Am. J. Obstet. Gynecol.*, **136**, 471–7

9. Pillai, M. and James, D. (1990). The importance of the behavioural states in biophysical assessment of the term human fetus. *Br. J. Obstet. Gynaecol.*, **97**, 1130–4

10. Pillai, M. and James, D. K. (1990). Behavioural states in normal mature human fetuses. *Arch. Dis. Child.*, **65**, 39–43

11. Pillai, M. and James, D. K. (1990). The development of fetal heart rate patterns during pregnancy. *Obstet. Gynecol.*, **76**, 812–16

12. Pillai, M. and James, D. K. (1990). Sinusoidal fetal heart rate associated with fetal mouthing. *Eur. J. Obstet. Gynecol. Reprod. Biol.*, **38**, 151–6

13. Pillai, M. and James, D. K. (1990). Hiccups and breathing in the human fetus. *Arch. Dis. Child.*, **65**, 1072–5

14. Groome, L. J., Gotleib, S. J., Neely, C. L. and Waters, M. D. (1993). Development trends in fetal habituation to vibroacoustic stimulation. *Am. J. Perinatol.*, **10**, 46–9

15. Leader, L. R. and Bennett, M. J. (1995). Fetal habituation and its clinical application. In Leven, M. I. and Lilford, R. J. (eds.) *Fetal and Neonatal Neurology and Neurosurgery*, pp. 45–60. (Edinburgh: Churchill Livingstone)

16. Leader, L. R., Baillie, P., Martin, B. and Vermenlen, E. (1982). Fetal habituation in high risk pregnancies. *Br. J. Obstet. Gynaecol.*, **89**, 441–6

17. Groome, L. J., Watson, J. E. and Dykman, R. A. (1994). Heart rate changes following habituation testing of the motor response in normal human fetuses. *Early Hum. Dev.*, **36**, 69–77

18. Hepper, P., Scott, D. and Shahidullah, S. (1992). Newborn and fetal response to maternal voice. *J. Reprod. Infant Psychol.*, **11**, 147–53

19. Lecanuet, J. P., Granier-Deferre, C., Jacquet, A. Y., Capponi, I. and Ledru, I. (1993). Prenatal discriminating of a male and female voice uttering the same sentence. *Early Dev. Parent*, **2**, 217–28

20. Johnson, M. J., Paine, L. L., Mulder, H. H., Cezar, C., Gegor, C. and Johnson, T. R. (1992). Population differences of fetal biophysical and behavioural characteristics. *Am. J. Obstet. Gynecol.*, **166**, 138–42

21. James, D. and Pillai, M. (1993). Behavioural development and intrauterine growth retardation. *Curr. Obstet. Gynaecol.*, **3**, 196–9

22. Mulder, E. J. H. and Visser, G. H. A. (1991). Growth and motor developments in fetuses of women with type-1 diabetes. I. Early growth patterns. *Early Hum. Dev.*, **25**, 91–106

23. Mulder, E. J. H. and Visser, G. H. A. (1991). Growth and motor developments in fetuses of women with type-1 diabetes. II. Emergence of specific movement patterns. *Early Hum. Dev.*, **25**, 107–15

24. Horimoto, N., Koyanagi, T., Maeda, H., Satoh, S., Takashima, T., Miniami, T. and Nakani, C. (1993). Can brain impairment be detected by *in utero* behavioural patterns? *Arch. Dis. Child.*, **69**, 3–8

25. Hepper, P. G. and Shahidullah, S. (1992). Habituation in normal and Down's syndrome fetuses. *Q. J. Exp. Psychol.*, **44B**, 305–17

26. Dawes, G. S., Redman, C. W. G. and Smith, J. H. (1985). Improvements in the registration and analysis of fetal heart rate records at the bedside. *Br. J. Obstet. Gynaecol.*, **92**, 317–25

27. Melendez, T. D., Rayburn, W. P. and Smith, C. V. (1992). Characterisation of fetal body movement recorded by the Hewlett-Packard M-1350-A fetal monitor. *Am. J. Obstet. Gynecol.*, **167**, 700–2

28. Ling, N. P. (1991). Auditory evoked response of the human fetus: simplified methodology. *J. Perinat. Med.*, **19**, 177–83

29. Groome, L. J., Mooney, M. M. and Dykman, R. A. (1994). Motor and cardiac response during habituation testing: demonstration of exaggerated cardiac reactivity in a subgroup of normal human fetuses. *Am. J. Perinatol.*, **11**, 73–9

Progress report of the study group on environmental and lifestyle influences in pregnancy and later outcome of the children

16

J. G. Koppe and R. Zetterström

HISTORY

After the 1992 Congress in Amsterdam, at the instigation of Rolf Zetterström, a meeting was organized in Amsterdam with the aim of co-ordinating studies in Europe on the influence of alcohol and drugs in pregnancy. Among the members of the group were Hans-Ludwig Spohr from Germany, Hans-Christoph Steinhausen from Switzerland, May Olofson from Denmark, and Per-Anders Rydelius, Kerstin Strömberg and Lillemor Nordberg from Sweden, all experts on the alcohol problem; Anneloes van Baar, Kees Boer, Marian van Huis, Sri Soepatmi and Boudewijn Gunning from The Netherlands and Gianluigi Conte from Italy, all experts on the drugs problem; and Sabine Koch from Germany and Arianne Dessens from The Netherlands, experts on the use of anticonvulsants. During this meeting an overview was given of the above-mentioned problems, by the different members, and we came to the conclusion that a structured follow-up program for children affected by these problems had to be developed. The presentations were published as a supplement of *Acta Paediatrica*[1].

A second meeting was organized by Rolf Zetterström and Per-Anders Rydelius in Stockholm in 1994, and in the same year during the Congress of the European Association of Perinatal Medicine (EAPM) in Helsinki it was decided to formalize our group as a study group of the EAPM, and to broaden the scope to include environment and lifestyle influences. Therefore, the influences of stress, poly-chloro-biphenyls (PCBs) and dioxins, malnutrition, smoking and irradiation were added. During the second meeting in Stockholm, the emphasis was on the alcohol problem. A series of lectures was given, including an outstanding one on the relation of alcoholism and genetic make-up. It was realized that the detection of alcohol-drinking mothers is a major problem. It was decided to formulate a proposal for a combined study under the auspices of the European Community and to approach the department of the European Community in Luxembourg, since they had a public health program.

A third meeting took place in 1995, again in Amsterdam. Sponsorship by the European Community was not forthcoming. Scientifically, however, we came to a consensus. It was agreed that a co-operative study should begin in the form of a prospective longitudinal study on small-for-gestational-age (SGA) children, because within this group babies exposed to alcohol would be found. Most of the other above-mentioned problems in pregnancy also result in intrauterine growth retardation. Rolf Zetterström formulated a protocol and this protocol was discussed and agreed upon by a steering group in Denmark in December 1995.

OVERVIEW OF THE PROBLEMS

It is in the group of SGA babies that most of the babies damaged by external environmental influences are found. This is not a group to which much attention is given. At birth these babies seldom need intensive care, especially those with a gestational age of more than 30 weeks and a birth weight of more than 1500 g. A blood sugar measurement may be performed but the cause of the growth retardation is seldom known and mostly not studied. Failure to pay attention to this group of babies in the perinatal period results in a failure to identify the problems these children may develop later in life, such as learning difficulties, behavioral problems, psychiatric disorders and even criminality. If Barker's hypothesis proves true, diabetes, lung problems and coronary disease in adulthood are also threats.

Exposures during pregnancy can be divided into three groups: voluntary exposure, involuntary exposure, and therapeutic exposure.

Voluntary exposure

This is related to lifestyle. Alcohol, smoking and drugs are among the most important damaging substances. In 30% of all pregnancies alcohol is consumed, and about 10% of these mothers are heavy drinkers who consume more than 80 g of pure alcohol each day. Although it is unknown what quantity of alcohol is damaging, an amount of 80 g each day means a high risk of growth retardation, mental retardation and craniofacial-abnormalities. Detection of these heavy-drinking mothers is difficult, since most deny it. A biochemical marker in the blood has not yet been found. Carbohydrate-deficient transferrin could be such a marker, but more studies are needed. It is possible that history-taking by computer would be more accurate as there are indications that women are more honest with a computer than with another human being. The alcohol problem will be a major concern to the study group.

Smoking in pregnancy is also a habit in 30% of pregnant mothers. In recent years there has been a decrease in smoking of 4% in Holland, but the people that do smoke consume more. The average number of cigarettes smoked per person rose to 23 a day; shag is also smoked in similar quantities, and is even worse because concentrations of nicotine are higher in this type of tobacco. In Holland the income from taxes on tobacco increased in recent years, to 3 billion guilden a year. Effects on the unborn baby are primarily intrauterine growth retardation, solutio placentae, placenta previa, bleeding in pregnancy, prolonged rupture of membranes, preterm delivery and an increased perinatal mortality. Nicotine, carbon monoxide and the heavy metal cadmium are probably causing the fetal damage. Cadmium accumulates in the placenta and causes a dysfunction resulting in growth retardation of the baby. In smoking mothers the placenta is not smaller, but is dysfunctional.

Drugs and especially hard drugs like heroin in pregnancy is one of the research lines studied at the University of Amsterdam. In the Netherlands about 20 000 people are enslaved to hard drugs. In comparison with Germany and France, Holland has a four-times lower mortality in this group thanks to our drug policy. Also in the population with AIDS only 15% is drug-addicted, compared with 40–70% in other European countries. Millions of sterile syringes and needles have been provided in Holland resulting in a prevention of AIDS in the drug-addicted group. Although heroin seems to be less harmful to the unborn child than alcohol, more long-term follow-up studies are needed in this group.

Involuntary exposure

This results from several environmental and lifestyle factors. Stress, such as in jobs where the pregnant mother has to stand many hours during the day, is known to be a cause of both growth retardation and preterm delivery. Studies are in progress to measure the effect of stress, and this factor might be of great importance in pregnancies today.

Another involuntary exposure of the baby is to PCBs and dioxins accumulated in the mother's adipose tissue during the years before conception and transferred to the baby via the yolk sac and placenta. In western industrialized countries background levels of these chemical pollutants are high, so that 10% of babies are at risk of negative effects on growth, cognitive functioning and immunity. Why these chemicals have an effect on neurodevelopment is unknown; it might be that an imbalance in thyroid hormone metabolism plays a role, but abnormalities in the neurotransmitter dopamine have been described. Besides these effects, enzymes can be easily induced in the liver by these chemicals, disrupting normal levels of hormones such as estrogens, or vitamin K. Both thrombosis and bleeding are found in animal studies, and the late hemorrhagic disease of the newborn might be caused by PCBs and dioxins[2].

Heavy metals like mercury and lead are not a great problem in our society. However, levels of lead should not exceed 100 µg/l in the maternal plasma.

Irradiation, such as that subsequent to the disaster in Chernobyl, is certainly a factor of concern. High doses (above 100 rems) can cause growth retardation, an increased risk of leukemia, congenital anomalies and cancer of the thyroid gland. However, the screens of computers and televisions seem to be safe. A dose of less than 5 rems per year is probably safe.

Malnutrition during pregnancy is also a source of problems. In general this happens under poor social circumstances, and to separate the effect of underfeeding and poor socioeconomic factors is impossible. In Holland during World War II starvation was introduced as a punishment in the months November 1944–May 1945, in a population which previously had rather good socioeconomic circumstances. After the war Clement Smith studied the effects on birth weight and found a decrease of about 300 g[3]. Later, Zena Stein and Mervin Susser did studies on the conscripts born in the starvation period. They found more obesity among the boys[4]. Studies are ongoing in both males and females born or conceived in the starvation period, at the University of Amsterdam in cooperation with Barker. An interesting finding of Susser and Linis, that in the group conceived when starvation was at its height (February–March 1945), there is a peak of schizophrenia[5].

Therapeutic exposure

That medicaments can also influence the development of the fetus is well known because of the thalidomide drama. After that finding the question arose as to the safety of anticonvulsants in pregnancy. Anticonvulsants proved to be unsafe, especially when several medicaments were used together. Cleft lip and palate, and heart defects are known to be caused by anti-epileptic medication. In a recent study, effects on the gender-identity and an increase in transsexualism have also been found on long-term follow-up of children of mothers using anticonvulsants[6].

Most of the above-mentioned environmental exogenous influences can disturb the same biochemical pathways resulting in the same abnormalities. For instance, phenobarbital and PCB 153 are both strong enzyme inducers of the same group of enzymes, and the same clinical abnormalities can be expected. Genetic background is very important to determine the ultimate effect of exogenous influences.

PROPOSED STUDY

The study group agreed to set up a project to study SGA-babies with the title: 'Small-for–gestational age infants, etiology and prognosis', a prospective longitudinal study from pregnancy and birth into infancy, childhood and adolescence. No consecutive longitudinal prospective studies on the risk of sequelae in this group have, to our knowledge, been performed. Retrospective studies done in different parts of the world all indicate a high risk of short stature, lower weight, lower IQ and neurological abnormalities[7–11]. Causes of intrauterine growth retardation include deficient fetal supply as in hypertension of pregnancy, congenital anomalies, congenital infections, multiple pregnancies and external toxic influences. It is on this last group that our study group is focusing. About 20% of SGA children belong to this group. It is important to develop strategies and interventions to prevent and/or cure the growth retardation, the abnormal neurodevelopment and behavioral problems in this so far neglected group of babies. The proposed study will be performed in different countries of Europe, since we expect that the problems are different depending on the environment. Colleagues who are interested in participating are invited to contact the co-ordinator, Janna G. Koppe.

References

1. Drug- and alcohol dependency during pregnancy, long-term effects on child development. (1994). *Acta Paediatr.*, **83**, (Suppl.), 404

2. Koppe, J. G., Pluim, E. and Olie, K. (1989). Breastmilk, PCBs, dioxins and vitamin K deficiency: discussion paper. *J. Royal Soc. Med.*, **82**, 416–20

3. Smith, C. A. (1947). Effects of wartime starvation in Holland on pregnancy and its products. *Am. J. Obstet. Gynecol.*, **53**, 599–608

4. Stein, Z A., Susser, M., Saenger, G. and Marolla, F. (1975). Famine and Human Development. The Dutch Hunger Winter of 1944–1945. (London: Oxford University Press)

5. Susser, E. S. and Lin, S. P. (1992). Schizophrenia after prenatal exposure to the Dutch Hunger Winter of 1944–1945. *Arch. Gen. Psychiatry*, **49**, 983–8

6. Dessens, A. B. (1996). Prenatal exposure to phenobarbital and diphantoin: a study on long-lasting consequences. Thesis. University of Amsterdam, September 1996

7. Paz, I., Gale, R. and Laor, A. (1995). The cognitive outcome of full-term small for gestational age infants at late adolescence. *Obstet. Gynecol.*, **85**, 452–6

8. Low, J. A. and Handley-Derry, M. H. (1992). Association of intrauterine fetal growth retardation and learning deficits at age 9 to 11 years. *Am. J. Obstet. Gynecol.*, **167**, 1499–505

9. Smedler, A. C. and Faxelius, G. (1992). Psychological development in children born with very low birthweight after severe intrauterine growth retardation: a 10-year follow-up study. *Acta Paediatr.*, **81**, 197–203

10. Hadders-Algra, M., Huiosjes, H. J. and Touwen, B. C. (1988). Preterm or small for gestational age infants. Neurological and behavioural development at the age of 6 years. *Eur. J. Pediatr.*, **147**, 460–7

11. Cnattingius, S. and Axelsson, O. (1987). Perinatal outcome for small for gestational age infants from an unselected area-based population. *Early Hum. Dev.*, **15**, 95–101

Environmental influences on the embryo and fetus: alcohol

17

H. L. Spohr

INTRODUCTION

In the Western industrialized countries, chronic alcoholism is currently one of the leading diseases afflicting the population and is, in addition to this, a serious socioeconomic burden. Chronic alcohol abuse is on the rise and affects increasingly younger sectors of the population. An estimated 20% of alcohol dependent women are of child-bearing age.

Maternal drug and alcohol abuse puts children at risk, both prenatally through possible teratogenic effects and postnatally through a compromised home environment. In the USA, national figures based on maternal hospital discharge diagnoses indicate that approximately 375 000 (11%!) of neonates are prenatally exposed to illicit drugs and/or alcohol[1].

The objective of the present paper is to reveal the relationship between chronic maternal alcohol abuse during pregnancy and *in utero* damage to the child as well as to document the long-term consequences for the affected patients.

CLINICAL PICTURE

The syndrome, which was first described by Jones and Smith[2] 23 years ago and independently identified in France[3], has been frequently diagnosed in recent years in infants and young children from every racial group throughout the Western world. Among the various possible teratogenic effects of alcohol abuse, the fetal alcohol syndrome (FAS) and fetal alcohol effects (FAE) are regarded as the most serious consequences of intrauterine alcohol exposure. Today alcohol is recognized as a leading teratogenic agent for developmental brain damage and long-lasting central nervous system (CNS) dysfunction and is, together with Down's syndrome and neural tube defects, considered to be a leading cause of congenital mental retardation.

Fetal alcohol syndrome is a birth defect but, unlike phokomelia or club foot, which are major malformations observable at birth, this syndrome has more subtle physical characteristics with a typical pattern of minor anomalies, particularly observable in the face, but often with persistent devastating psychiatric and mental consequences.

The diagnosis is made when there is confirmation of a history of maternal alcohol abuse and when examination reveals a cluster of three main characteristic criteria:

(1) Prenatal or postnatal growth retardation (height and weight below the 10th percentile when corrected for gestational age);

(2) CNS dysfunction (any neurological abnormality, hyperactivity, learning and/or memory problems, attentional deficits, developmental delay or intellectual impairment); and

(3) Characteristic craniofacial abnormalities, including at least two of the following three: microcephaly; short palpebral fissures; poorly developed philtrum, thin upper lip and flattening of the maxillary area[4].

All is to be expected in a syndrome with such individual variety of teratogenic susceptibility, not all children exposed to alcohol during pregnancy fulfil these criteria. The full-blown syndrome is the most severe form of damage occurring *in utero* as a result of chronic maternal alcohol abuse. The term 'fetal alcohol effects' (FAE) may be used when a child shows two rather than all three of the above-listed indicators, to describe mild or abortive forms of the syndrome, and is not a strict medical diagnosis but a descriptive term to describe observed effects in children that could have been caused by prenatal alcohol exposure. Patients with FAS are not necessarily more severely affected than those with FAE, but very often they may be. Children with FAE may be in need of the same intensive care as those with FAS, but it is particularly difficult for these children to get the needed help and services because they will not be recognized as suffering from intrauterine alcohol exposure and often do not have a medical diagnosis.

DIAGNOSTIC DIFFICULTIES

In spite of the fact that alcohol teratogenicity is well known among pediatricians today, most of the neonatal medical staff fail to recognize FAS and FAE in newborn infants[5,6]. The reasons for this striking underestimation of one of the major causes of congenital mental retardation are manifold.

(1) In general, FAS is estimated to occur in 0.3–1.9 per 1000 live births in Western societies[7], but drinking behavior and chronic alcoholism depend strongly on prosperity, industrialization and on religious influences, so the prevalence of the syndrome varies widely among different countries and between rural areas and big cities. Many neonatologists may not see many *in utero* alcohol damaged newborns depending on the place where they work. (In some Indian reservations in the USA, the incidence of FAS is reported to be 1 : 50 live births).

(2) Communication between obstetric and pediatric medical staff should be improved, particularly when providing care for pregnant women and newborn infants at high risk for complications due to maternal alcohol or other drug abuse[5].

(3) As a rule, the syndrome is characterized only by non-specific abnormalities at birth. There exist similarities to other disorders which can be differentiated only by experienced examination. Some birth defect syndromes which resemble FAS are Cornelia de Lange syndrome, Noonan syndrome and some rare chromosomal diseases. Intrauterine growth retardation, on the other hand, is one of the more consistent findings in FAS at birth and should be used as a possible predictor for intrauterine alcohol exposure[6].

In summary, a diagnosis of FAS/FAE should be taken into consideration in a pregnant woman with a history of taking some (2–4) alcoholic beverages per day, and delivering a small-for-date baby which may look a little bit peculiar.

LONG-TERM PERSPECTIVES OF FETAL ALCOHOL SYNDROME

In contrast to the extended research on moderate alcohol consumption during pregnancy[8,9], there is still limited knowledge about the long-term development and adolescent outcome of children diagnosed as having FAS[10].

In 1977–1979 we started a longitudinal project involving small infants and children living in the former city of West Berlin and suffering from varying degrees of FAS. Many of these

Table 1 Symptoms of juvenile fetal alcohol syndrome

Small head circumference/microcephaly
Stocky stature/growth retardation
Developmental and cognitive deficits
Psychiatric and behavioral problems
Craniofacial features:
short palpebral fissures
thin upper vermillion
prominent nasal bridge
mild midface hypoplasia
strabismus/myopia
maladjusted teeth

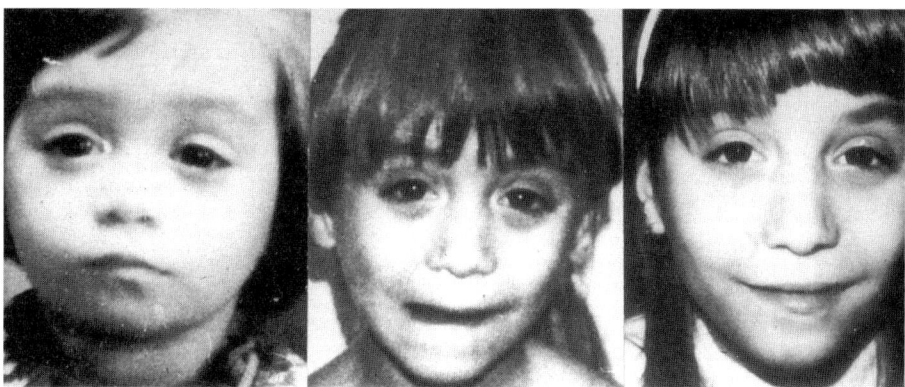

N. V. Moderate FAS at 10 months, 3 years, 10 years

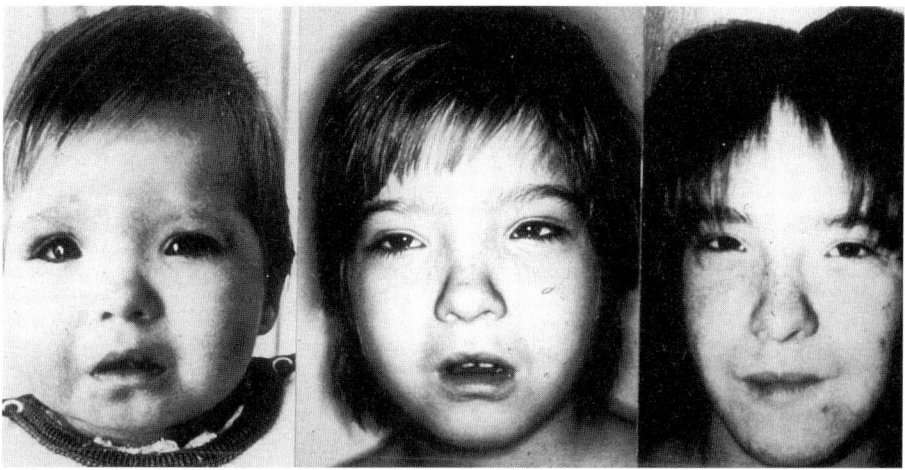

S. C. Moderate FAS at 8 months, 3 years, 15 years

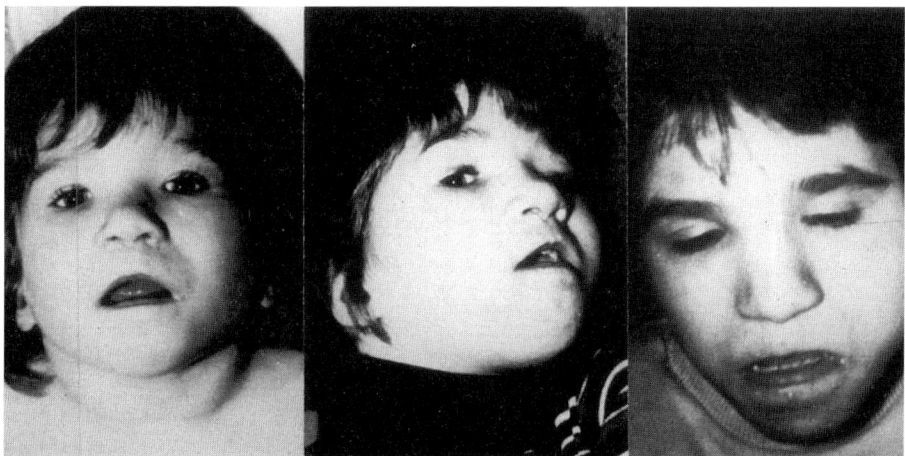

C. B. Severe FAS at 3 years, 5 years, 16 years

Figure 1   Facial symptoms in three patients with fetal alcohol syndrome (FAS) during the course of their development

patients could be followed up into adolescence and the follow-up study documented the developmental changes from FAS in childhood to adolescence[11]. Although the usual pronounced growth retardation and the craniofacial dysmorphia typical for early childhood gradually diminish in the growing patient, a characteristic dysmorphic pattern nevertheless persists. Familiarity with this pattern aids in the diagnosis of the syndrome at a later age – school age or even puberty[12]. The typical persistent or newly-acquired symptoms are summarized in Table 1 (juvenile alcohol syndrome).

The cardinal signs of juvenile FAS are growth retardation, observed in half of the examined cases, and persistent microcephaly, observed in nearly two-thirds of the patients. Being underweight, which is typical in infancy and early childhood, and only rarely amenable to therapeutic measures, is partially corrected. Weight gain is observed, especially in adolescent female patients. In many adolescent FAS patients, a particular facies is still discernible. This, however, changes in the course of time and in comparison to the typical syndrome-pattern of childhood.

As Figure 1 shows, a triad of signs persists besides the small head: short palpebral fissures, indistinct philtrum and a thin upper lip. Additionally, often only discernible in the course of development, misaligned teeth, strabismus, myopia or hypermetropia may appear.

Another symptom characteristic of the juvenile FAS patient is the persistent disturbance in juvenile mental development. The degree of the intellectual impairment remains relatively stable, although, in some cases, there is a further deterioration over the course of time. When the diagnosis was made in early childhood, 25% of our patients were classified as having a severe form, a further 25% as having a moderate form, and half of the examined children as having a mild form of FAS. The patients in the last group, especially, were given a favorable developmental prognosis with predominantly normal intellectual development. Unfortunately, 10–14 years later we have to admit that the prognosis was often too favorable. Only 30% of the patients followed up had an age-appropriate IQ and a predominantly normal social development, whereas developmental and cognitive handicaps persisted in 70% of the adolescents.

Additionally, there are a lot of noticeable psychiatric problems that unfold in a very constant pattern throughout childhood development in FAS patients[13]. This psychopathological profile can also appear with slightly lower intensity in adolescence. Among the persisting disorders are abnormal habits and stereotypies, emotional disorders, sleep disturbances and, above all, hyperkinetic disorders. Surprisingly, these psychopathological symptoms are observed in mildly as well as in severely affected patients. This psychiatric 'profile' of symptoms is to a large extent responsible for the severe psychosocial difficulties with which the adolescent juvenile FAS patients have to cope when entering adulthood.

References

1. Grant, T. M. M., Ernst, C. C. and Streissguth, A. P. (1996). Intervention with high risk mothers abusing alcohol and drugs: the Seattle advocacy model. *Am. J. Publ. Health* in press
2. Jones, K. L. and Smith, D. W. (1973). Recognition of the fetal alcohol syndrome in early infancy. *Lancet*, **2** (7836), 999–1001
3. Lemoine, P., Harousseau, H., Borteyru, J. P. and Menuet, P. J. (1968). Les enfants de parents alcooliques: anomalies observees. A propos de 127 cas. *Quest Med.*, **21**, 476–82
4. Sokol, R. J. and Clarren, S. K. (1989). Guidelines for use of terminology describing the impact of prenatal alcohol on the offspring. *Alcoholism*, **13**, 597–8
5. Little, B. B., Snell, L. M., Rosenfeld, C. R., Gilstrap, L. C. and Gant, N. F. (1990). Failure to recognize fetal alcohol syndrome in newborn infants. *Am. J. Dis. Child.*, **144**, 1142–6

6. Schöneck, U., Spohr, H. L., Willms, J. and Steinhausen, H. C. (1992). Alkoholkonsum und intrauterine Dystrophie. *Monatsschr. Kinderheilk,* **140**, 34–41

7. Abel, E. L. and Sokol, R. J. (1987). Incidence of the fetal alcohol syndrome and economic impact of FAS-related anomalies. *Drug Alcohol Depend.,* **19**, 51–70

8. Streissguth, A. P., Barr, H. M. and Sampson, P. D. (1990). Moderate prenatal alcohol exposure: effects on child IQ and learning problems at age 7 1/2 years. *Alcohol Clin. Exp. Res.,* **14**, 662–8

9. Florey, C., Taylor, D., Bolumar, F., Kaminski, M. and Olsen, J. (eds.) (1992). Maternal alcohol consumption and its relation to the outcome of pregnancy and child development at 18 months. *Int. J. Epidemiol.,* **21** (Suppl. 1)

10. Streissguth, A. P., Aase, J. M., Clarren, S. K., Randels, S. P., La Due, R. A. and Smith, D. F. (1991). Fetal alcohol syndrome in adolescents and adults. *J. Am. Med. Assoc.,* **265**, 1961–7

11. Spohr, H. L., Willms, J. and Steinhausen, H. C. (1993). Prenatal alcohol exposure and longterm developmental consequences: a 10-year follow-up of 60 children with fetal alcohol syndrome (FAS). *Lancet,* **341**, 907–10

12. Spohr, H. L., Willms, J. and Steinhausen, H. C. (1994). The fetal alcohol syndrome in adolescence. *Acta Pädiatr.,* **404**, 19–26

13. Steinhausen, H. C., Willms, J. and Spohr, H. L. (1993). The long-term psychopathological and cognitive outcome of children with fetal alcohol syndrome. *J. Am. Acad. Child Adolesc. Psychiatr.,* **32**, 990–4

Drugs of addiction

18

M. Hepburn

INTRODUCTION

Drug use is increasing in many countries throughout the world. In Britain the increase has been particularly marked among young women, so the problem of drug use during pregnancy is increasingly common, with the need to provide appropriate care an increasing challenge for maternity services. To meet this need it is essential to know local patterns and changes in patterns of drug use. It is also important to remember that, while drug use occurs throughout society and often without significant addiction problem, drug use is disproportionately associated with socioeconomic deprivation[1]. Problem drug use causes many problems and also exacerbates those due to deprivation. Drug use during pregnancy is therefore associated with poorer health for both mother and baby and also with less effective service use. It also has adverse social effects and can compromise parenting skills so services which provide care for pregnant drug-using women must be acceptable to the women and address both medical and social issues.

In Glasgow the Women's Reproductive Health Service (WRHS), based at Glasgow Royal Maternity Hospital (GRMH), provides care for women with severe social problems[2]. From a pilot clinic established in 1986, it was expanded in 1990 to provide city-wide cover. Drug use, the single most common problem, is experienced by more than half those who attend and the service has now cared for more than 900 pregnant drug-using women with more than 800 deliveries. Numbers are steadily increasing and the annual attendance rate, regularly in excess of 100, reached 150 in the year to April 1996. Drug use is managed not in isolation but in the context of other problems due to deprivation

and consequently, through a network of community clinics, the service provides multidisciplinary care which deals with all problems both medical and social[3].

In Scotland heroin is the most frequently reported drug of abuse, followed by the benzodiazepine temazepam[4]. In Glasgow, where polydrug use is common, these two drugs are frequently used together and often in combination with other substances. Amphetamine use is relatively common but cocaine use, as yet, is not, while alcohol consumption, high in Scotland as a whole, is very low among women who use illicit drugs. One major change to this pattern since the establishment of the WRHS has been that buprenorphine, commonly used in the 1980s and the most frequently encountered drug in the early days of the service, has now been replaced by heroin.

HEALTH OF THE MOTHERS

The poor nutrition commonly associated with deprivation is exacerbated by drug use. Regular weighing may be an ineffective tool in monitoring fetal growth and well-being but it is useful in monitoring the stability of an individual's drug use. Injection of drugs may cause vascular damage and result in infection both local and systemic. Venous access may therefore be difficult, while abscess formation at the injection site is common. Breast abscesses can be a particular problem due to increased use of breast veins for injection during pregnancy. Septicemia may result from infected drug injection, with endocarditis a common complication, which makes routine cardiovascular assessment at booking important. Prophylactic antibiotic cover may be required for delivery and also for procedures such as dental extraction. The latter is frequently necessary because dental decay is common and requires treatment since reduced consumption of analgesic drugs might precipitate toothache and jeopardize attempts at control of drug use. Infection with blood-borne viruses, especially human immunodeficiency virus (HIV), and hepatitis B and C, is a well publicized risk of injecting drug use, with almost half of those infected with HIV in Scotland infected by this route. However, the possibility of sexual transmission of HIV and hepatitis B and the delay between infection and seroconversion, precludes the use of screening to accurately identify all infected individuals. Thus, while all pregnant women should be offered information about blood-borne viruses with the option of screening, this is to enable them to make appropriate management choices. Effective infection control will be achieved not by screening but by the recognition that all pregnant women are at risk of blood-borne viruses and consequently the GRMH employs a policy of single-tier management with universal precautions. All women are regarded as potentially infected with HIV and other blood-borne viruses and infection control measures are adopted appropriate to the procedure, not the patient.

HEALTH OF THE BABIES

Precise fetal effects from maternal drug use will depend on the drugs used and the level and pattern of use but fall into two main categories. First, there are increased rates of perinatal mortality and morbidity attributable largely to increased rates of low birth weight and preterm delivery[5]. An increased risk of sudden infant death is also reported. All are multifactorial and, in particular, heavy use of tobacco by drug-using women makes a major contribution to low birth weight. Preterm delivery is postulated to result from increased uterine activity due to recurrent drug withdrawals as a result of erratic use. More severe withdrawals due to antenatal detoxification have been reported to cause fetal death[6]. However, in Glasgow, drug-using women have always been offered the option of antenatal detoxification and among the first 300 drug-using women delivered in the Women's Reproductive Health Service rates of preterm delivery and low birth weight were lower among those who underwent detoxification than among those who did not (Table 1). Since the two groups were self-selected and not comparable this does not suggest that detoxification is safer – and indeed does not provide any information on the relative safeties of detoxification and maintenance therapy – but it does suggest that detoxification is less hazardous to the fetus than previously reported. Nevertheless, antenatal detoxification is still widely regarded as advisable only if restricted to mid-trimester and with very slow rates of reduction, while prescription of a substitute drug with a longer half-life such as methadone is advocated both to increase stability of drug use and to reduce injecting, with its attendant risks. It has also been suggested that to effectively achieve these objectives high doses of methadone are necessary.

Maternal drug use may also lead to withdrawal symptoms in the neonate. These range in severity from mild irritability to major

Table 1 Outcome of pregnancy by antenatal management of drug use

	Perinatal deaths	Delivery < 37 weeks	Birth weight < 2.5 kg	Birth weight < 10th centile	Total deliveries
Cold turkey detoxification	0	5 (8.1%)	3 (4.8%)	5 (8.1%)	62
Methadone detoxification	0	13 (12.8%)	19 (18.6%)	16 (15.7%)	102
No detoxification	5	22 (16.2%)	26 (19.1%)	26 (19.1%)	136

cerebral irritation with convulsions. Babies of drug-using women, while hungry, are often poor feeders and if withdrawal symptoms are severe may have unacceptable weight loss. These effects are largely dose-dependent but while there is a general correlation between the severity of symptoms and the mother's level of drug use this will not necessarily apply to individual cases. An individual baby's condition therefore cannot be predicted from, nor provide an accurate measure of, the mother's level of use. It should also be remembered that methadone causes neonatal withdrawal symptoms at least as severe as those due to the opiates for which it provides a substitute. Thus, maintaining drug use at the lowest level compatible with stability – including the option of complete detoxification – provides the best protection against neonatal withdrawal symptoms. Treatment of withdrawal symptoms in the baby can be either by substitution therapy with gradual withdrawal or by symptomatic therapy. In Glasgow where polydrug use is common the latter approach is adopted. Treatment is not routinely given but where necessary phenobarbitone is prescribed as an anticonvulsant and a sedative to allow more effective feeding. Although substitute therapy is not prescribed, women are encouraged to breast feed to reduce the severity of neonatal withdrawal symptoms by provision of continued small doses of drugs in the breast milk. While in Glasgow breast feeding is culturally unacceptable among women from deprived backgrounds, this argument has persuaded some women to try it.

No service can operate in a vacuum, however, so management in the WRHS is influenced by the existence of and policies of other drug services. The WRHS was established against a background of limited substitute prescribing in the city so few women would have the option of receiving methadone postnatally. This contributed to the decision to allow women the option of antenatal detoxification and helped strengthen their resolve and consequently their success in doing so. Additionally, doses of methadone prescribed by the WRHS were relatively low and this in turn no doubt contributed

to the favorable pregnancy outcomes observed, regardless of whether or not the women underwent antenatal detoxification. Indeed, among the first 200 drug-using women delivered in the service, outcomes of pregnancy in terms of rates of preterm delivery and low birth weight (< 2.5 kg), as well as rates of admission to the Special Care Nursery, were comparable to those among women with social problems other than drug use delivered in the same period (Hepburn, unpublished data). Glasgow now has an established drug treatment network providing services, including prescription of methadone, with marked benefits in terms of reduced injecting and greater stability of drug use. Increasingly, pregnant drug-using women attending the WRHS for the first time are already receiving methadone and many are stable on doses much higher than those previously prescribed by the WRHS. Although the increased availability of postnatal methadone has lessened the pressure to undergo antenatal detoxification, most women are still keen to and do reduce their level of drug use to reduce the chance of severe withdrawal symptoms in the baby. However, care must be taken not to jeopardize stability and inevitably doses of methadone used during pregnancy are now significantly higher. Among babies born to the 199 drug-using women delivered during the 2 years 1994/95, 36.2% were admitted to the Special Care Nursery compared to a rate of 16.5% during the first 5 years of the service (Table 2). While the groups differ in some respects and outcomes of pregnancy in terms of preterm delivery and low birth weight are therefore not strictly comparable, the increased admission rate to the Special Care Nursery corresponded to an increase in the number of babies requiring treatment for withdrawal symptoms. Thus, while prescription of methadone has its undoubted benefits, it is not without its disadvantages, while treatment of the two types of neonatal problems also provides potential for conflict. This dilemma therefore reinforces that which is true of drug treatment as a whole; namely that neither maintenance therapy nor abstinence provides the ideal solution, that both should be regarded as part

Table 2 Outcome of pregnancy among drug users by year of delivery

	Perinatal deaths	Delivery < 37 weeks	Birth weight < 2.5 kg	Birth weight < 10th centile	Admission to SCN	Total deliveries
1986–90	2	19 (9.5%)	25 (12.5%)	24 (12.0%)	33 (16.5%)	200
1994–5	6	27 (13.6%)	38 (19.1%)	49 (24.6%)	72 (36.2%)	199

SCN = Special Care Nursery

of the spectrum of harm reduction, and that all drug treatment inevitably involves compromise and should therefore be tailored to individual needs and wishes.

SOCIAL OUTCOME

The WRHS was developed in close collaboration with the Social Work Department, whose management policy recognizes that adequate child care depends less on drug use *per se* than on the effect of drug use on the mother's lifestyle, a view long recognized and becoming increasingly widespread[7]. Thus, while pregnant drug-using women attending the WRHS can choose maintenance therapy or detoxification or any combination of these options, it is emphasized that reduction should not be at the expense of stability. They are reassured that the Social Work Department shares the view that stability is more important than abstinence for adequate child care. The role of the social worker is therefore supportive rather than punitive and a named social worker is allocated early in pregnancy with a remit aimed at prevention rather than crisis intervention.

Multidisciplinary meetings are held at 32 weeks' gestation at which goals are set, problems identified and management plans agreed. Involvement of the partner and/or family is also encouraged where this is likely to be supportive. Confidentiality is important and prior consent to the involvement of others must always be sought. However, this will be encouraged by the recognition that late accidental disclosure without breach of confidentiality – as for example with development of obvious neonatal withdrawal symptoms – may ultimately prove more damaging. It is vitally important to establish an effective community network to provide support both before and after delivery. This should involve medical, non-medical, statutory and voluntary services as well as family and friends. A multidisciplinary approach to the care of pregnant drug-using women will promote good pregnancy outcomes. A similar approach after delivery offers the best hope of keeping mother and baby together. At all stages success is more likely if the woman is an active and voluntary participant in the decision-making process.

References

1. Scottish Office Home and Health Department (1994). Drugs in Scotland: meeting the challenge. *Report of the Ministerial Drugs Task Force.* (Edinburgh: Her Majesty's Stationery Office)
2. Hepburn, M. (1991). Social problems. In Hall, M. H. (ed.) *Antenatal Care: Clinical Obstetrics and Gynaecology, International Practice and Research*, pp. 149–68. (London: Bailliere Tindall)
3. Hepburn, M. (1996). Drug use in pregnancy. *Druglink*, July/August, 12–14
4. Scottish Health Service Common Services Agency, Information and Statistics Division

(1993). *Scottish Drug Misuse Database Bulletin 1993.* (Edinburgh: Common Services Agency)

5. Alroomi, L., Davidson, J., Evans, T. J., Galea, P. and Howat, R. (1988). Maternal narcotic abuse and the newborn. *Arch. Dis. Child.*, **63**, 81–3

6. Vaille, C. (1985). Risks incurred by children of drug addicted women: some medical and legal aspects. *Bull. Narcotics*, **37**, 149–56

7. National Local Authority Forum on Drugs Misuse in conjunction with Standing Conference on Drug Abuse (1989). Drug using parents and their children. *2nd Report of NLAFDM/SCODA.* (London: NLAFDM/SCODA)

Hypertension in pregnancy 19

E. Halmesmäki, R. Kaaja, H. Laivuori, A. Orpana, V. Ranta and O. Ylikorkala

INTRODUCTION

The problems associated with elevated blood pressure in pregnancy are global, but maternal and fetal morbidity and mortality depend on local resources and practices, in and between different countries. Thus the severity of problems of attendance at antenatal clinic and when diagnosed vary, being most serious and leading to highest maternal and fetal morbidities and mortalities in the developing countries. This is understandable as in those countries only 50–70% of pregnant women receive some antenatal care, and the care is substandard in 20–30%[1]. However, also in developed countries like the UK, complications associated with high blood pressure during pregnancy are the third, and in the USA, the second leading cause of maternal mortality.

Elevated blood pressure in pregnancy can be either of chronic (chronic hypertension) or pregnancy-associated (pregnancy-induced hypertension) origin, or complicated by proteinuria (pre-eclampsia). There are several theories of the etiology and pathogenesis of hypertension in pregnancy, some of which are under active research in our unit. In the following paper we will give a short review of our latest studies in this field.

'FRESH MATING' THEORY AND PRE-ECLAMPSIA

Some previous data have indicated an extremely high incidence of pregnancy-induced hypertension even in multigravidae who had conceived after minimal cohabitation with a new partner[2], and, furthermore, a high frequency of pre-eclampsia in pregnancies from donor insemination[3]. A mother is exposed to paternal antigens through sperm and seminal plasma, which are highly antigenic[4,5]. This exposure may be important to prevent the maternal immunological system becoming active against fetal tissues. Therefore, we decided to study whether paternal antigens really would protect against the risk of pregnancy-induced hypertension and pre-eclampsia, and evaluated a group of 186 women who had desired pregnancy with the present partner for 2–10 years.

Forty-three of the women had a child with another partner, and four of these 43 pregnancies had been complicated by pre-eclampsia. Indications for donor insemination were a sperm count less than 1.0 million/ml in 92 men and a genetic disease in one man. The partners of these men were made pregnant by 1–3 attempts with donor sperm (insemination in 53, *in vitro* fertilization in 40). In the remaining 93 men, the sperm count was between 1.0–50 million/ml, and the partners of these men were finally made pregnant using husbands' sperm either spontaneously ($n = 26$), or by using insemination ($n = 22$) or *in vitro* fertilization ($n = 45$).

The courses of the pregnancies were carefully followed at prenatal clinics. Pre-eclampsia was defined as blood pressure exceeding 140/90 mmHg after 20 weeks of gestation, or as a significant rise in systolic (≥ 30 mmHg) or in diastolic (≥ 15 mmHg) pressure, and the presence of proteinuria (> 0.3 g/l in a 24-h specimen). Pregnancy-induced hypertension was diagnosed when blood pressure was > 140 /90 mmHg without proteinuria after the 20th gestational week, and chronic hypertension when blood pressure was $> 140/90$ mmHg already before the 20th week of pregnancy.

Altogether seven women in the donor group (7.5%) and ten women in the control group (10.8%) were hypertensive during pregnancy. Pre-eclampsia developed in two women in the donor group (2.2%) and in six women in the control group (6.5%). Two women in the donor group (2.2%) and four women in the control group (4.3%) developed pregnancy-induced hypertension. Three women in the donor group (3.2%) had chronic hypertension. Thus our data were strongly against the proposal that there would be more hypertensive complications in donor pregnancies without previous exposure to the fertilizing sperm. In contrast, women inseminated with donor sperm tended to show a reduced risk of hypertensive pregnancy complications (odds ratio 0.39) although this difference was not statistically significant (95% CI 0.12–1.28). Thus it appeared unlikely that paternal antigens affected such a maternal immunological acceptance of the fetus which might be a factor in pre-eclampsia and the etiological factor must be sought elsewhere.

PRE-ECLAMPSIA AND INSULIN RESISTANCE SYNDROME

Hyperinsulinemia and insulin resistance are typical for hypertensive individuals. Furthermore, these individuals often have elevated serum triglyceride and decreased high-density lipoprotein (HDL) cholesterol levels. The primary abnormality may be insulin resistance, causing hyperinsulinemia, hypertension, hypertriglyceridemia, and low serum HDL cholesterol. The condition is well proven in men and non-pregnant women, but analogy can be observed with pregnancy-induced hypertension as well. Pregnancy-induced hypertension is more common in women with impaired glucose tolerance[6] and is accompanied by elevated serum triglyceride levels[7].

To study metabolic disorders associated with pregnancy-induced hypertension, we analyzed serum insulin, lipids, lipoproteins, and the stable urinary metabolites of prostaglandin (PG)I_2 and thromboxane A_2 (TxA$_2$) in 31 hypertensive (blood pressure > 140/90 after 20 weeks

of pregnancy) and 21 normotensive pregnant women[8]. In eight of the hypertensive women proteinuria of > 0.5g/24 h developed as a sign of pre-eclampsia; the other 23 women developed only pregnancy-induced hypertension.

Pregnancy-induced hypertension was associated with 18% lower ($p < 0.05$) mean serum HDL$_2$ cholesterol levels and 65% higher ($p < 0.05$) mean triglyceride levels when compared with controls. Proteinuria was not associated with any greater changes in the lipid patterns. Hyperinsulinemia was significant in the women with pregnancy-induced hypertension; also the concentrations of uric acid were higher than in controls. The urinary excretion of PGI$_2$ metabolites was reduced in hypertensive patients, but no change in the excretion of TxA$_2$ metabolites was found.

Our findings in pregnancy-induced hypertensive patients resemble the key characteristics of insulin resistance syndrome[9], and even hyperuricemia has recently been associated with insulin resistance of non-pregnant subjects[10]. These findings may be associated with endothelial cell dysfunction associated with pre-eclampsia, but whether endothelial cell dysfunction is a primary abnormality or secondary – induced for example by maternal lipids as suggested by recent observations[11] – is not known. It has been shown, however, that the sera of women with pre-eclampsia is characterized by high availability of free fatty acids, and that the sera stimulate the synthesis of triglycerides by the endothelial cells[12]. These findings are supported by our results, indicating a significant abnormality in lipid patterns of patients with pregnancy-induced hypertension. Whether these changes are primary or secondary, and whether the pre-eclamptic women do have lower insulin sensitivity, remains to be studied in the future.

ENDOTHELIAL CELLS IN PRE-ECLAMPSIA AND NITRIC OXIDE PRODUCTION

As mentioned above, endothelial cell dysfunction may play a role in pre-eclampsia. For example, the production of anti-aggregatory and vasodilatory prostanoid prostacyclin is reduced in this disorder[13], and we therefore studied whether the production of another important vasodilator, nitric oxide (NO), formed from L-arginine by the calcium-dependent NO synthetase, is reduced as well[14]. Deficiency in calcium-dependent NO production may play a role in pre-eclampsia, because in experiments with rodents, constant administration of a calcium-dependent NO synthesis inhibitor produces symptoms resembling those of human pre-eclampsia[15].

In a study of 11 patients with severe pre-eclampsia and ten normotensive pregnant women, we isolated human umbilical vein endothelial cells for analysis of maximal calcium-ionophore A23187-stimulated NO production[14]. The production was measured as accumulation of nitrate and nitrite in the culture medium, and it was related to the number of viable endothelial cells. To be sure of precise estimations of the number of cells achieved from different cell cultures, we did paired comparisons between the cells achieved from pre-eclamptic and normotensive patients, and used cellular mitochondrial activity to measure the cell count[16]. The results were obtained with serial dilutions of cell cultures to achieve a standard curve from normotensive women.

We found no difference between the cell number-related NO production capacity of pre-eclamptic and normotensive pregnancies, but the total NO production of cells from pre-eclamptic patients was significantly lower than that of cells from normotensive women. This difference was caused by a larger number of viable endothelial cells from normotensive pregnancies.

Our results indicated that lower production of NO metabolites resulted from a smaller number of endothelial cells achieved from pre-eclamptic pregnancies. This cannot be regarded as contradictory to previous data of normal urinary excretion of nitrate and nitrite[17] and decreased serum nitrate levels[18] in pre-eclampsia, as there may be multiple, even exogenic, sources for both urinary and serum nitrite and nitrate[19]. Taken altogether, if impaired NO production plays a role in pre-eclampsia, it does not cause a major defect in NO production capacity of the vascular endothelial cells of the umbilical vein.

METABOLIC FUTURE OF WOMEN WHO HAVE HAD A PRE-ECLAMPTIC FIRST PREGNANCY

As stated above[8], women with pre-eclampsia and pregnancy-induced hypertension display hyperinsulinemia, hypertriglyceridemia and low HDL cholesterol levels. They seem to have a form of the insulin resistance syndrome, but not necessarily gestational diabetes. Whether these changes are only transiently associated with pregnancy has been unclear. We studied 22 women who had had a typical pre-eclamptic first pregnancy between 1976 and 1978, with normal blood pressure and no proteinuria 6 weeks after the pregnancy[20]. To study whether the hyperinsulinemia and other abnormalities in carbohydrate and lipid metabolism still persisted 17 years later, we analyzed their serum insulin, their blood glucose in a 3-h 75-g oral glucose tolerance test (OGTT), and their lipid and uric acid levels, and compared them to those of 22 control women of the same age who had had a normotensive first pregnancy between 1976 and 1978. The patients and controls were comparable as regards body mass index (BMI), but both the mean systolic and diastolic blood pressures were higher in women with prior pre-eclampsia than in the control women.

Blood baseline glucose, and glucose during the OGTT were comparable in the two groups. The insulin levels of the women with prior pre-eclampsia were significantly elevated at baseline and at 3 h. The area under the insulin curve was larger in women with prior pre-eclampsia. Total cholesterol, LDL and HDL cholesterol, triglyceride and uric acid concentrations did not differ significantly between the two groups. In women with prior pre-eclampsia the fasting insulin correlated positively with serum triglyceride and systolic and diastolic blood pressures, and the area under the insulin

127

curve correlated negatively with the HDL_2 cholesterol.

Thus, pre-eclamptic women seem to be characterized, not only during the pre-eclamptic pregnancy, but also during their later life, by hyperinsulinemia. The hyperinsulinemia in these patients may be either associated with the previous pre-eclampsia or be of inherited origin. As the relationships found in our study are typical for insulin resistance[21], the latter assumption of an inherited feature seems more likely. Although the etiology of pre-eclampsia is unknown and possibly multifactorial, one risk factor might be insulin resistance. If so, pre-eclampsia should have occurred in all subsequent pregnancies of these women as well, and, in fact, nine of 15 women had had pre-eclampsia or pregnancy-induced hypertension in future pregnancies.

In conclusion, the impact of pregnancy-induced hypertension on the future risk of hypertension in later life is significant, but the risk also seems to be increased after pre-eclampsia[22,23]. Not only high risk of hypertension, but even the risk of ischemic heart disease seems to be increased in these women in later life[24].

References

1. Engelhardt, T., Moodley, J. and Motlhabani, B. (1996). Does antenatal care in developing countries prevent eclampsia? A retrospective analysis at King Edward VIII Hopsital, Durban, South Africa. *Hypertension in Pregnancy*, **15**, 87–94

2. Robillard, P.-Y., Hulcey, T. C., Perianin, J., Janky, E., Miri, E. H. and Papiernik, E. (1994). Association of pregnancy-induced hypertension with duration of sexual cohabitation before conception. *Lancet*, **344**, 973–5

3. Need, J. A., Bell, B., Meffin, E. and Jones, W. R. (1983). Pre-eclampsia in pregnancies from donor inseminations. *J. Reprod. Immunol.*, **5**, 329–38

4. Bronson, R., Cooper, G. and Rosenfeldt, D. (1984). Sperm antibodies: their role in infertility. *Fertil. Steril.*, **42**, 171–83

5. Kajino, T., Torry, T. S., McIntyre, J. A. and Faulk, W. P. (1988). Trophoblast antigens in human seminal plasma. *Am. J. Reprod. Immunol. Microbiol.*, **17**, 91–5

6. Suhonen, L. and Teramo, K. (1993). Hypertension and preeclampsia in women with gestational glucose intolerance. *Acta Obstet. Gynecol. Scand.*, **72**, 269–72

7. Potter, M. F. and Nestel, P. J. (1979). The hyperlipidemia of pregnancy in normal and complicated pregnancies. *Am. J. Obstet. Gynecol.*, **133**, 165–70

8. Kaaja, R., Tikkanen, M. J., Viinikka, L. and Ylikorkala, O. (1995). Serum lipoproteins, insulin, and urinary prostanoid metabolites in normal and hypertensive pregnant women. *Obstet. Gynecol.*, **85**, 353–6

9. Ferrannini, E., Buzzigoli, G., Bonadonna, R., Giorico, M. A., Olegini, M. and Graziadei, L. (1987). Insulin resistance in essential hypertension. *N. Engl. J. Med.*, **317**, 350–7

10. Vuorinen-Markkola, H. and Yki-Järvinen, H. (1994). Hyperuricemia and insulin resistance. *J. Clin. Endocrinol. Metab.*, **78**, 25–9

11. Lorentzen, B., Endresen, M. J., Haug, E. and Henrikssen, T. (1991). Sera from preeclamptic women increase the content of triglycerides and reduce the release of prostacyclin in cultured endothelial cells. *Thromb. Res.*, **63**, 363–72

12. Endresen, M. J., Lorentzen, B. and Henrikssen, T. (1992). Increased lipolytic activity and high ratio of free fatty acids to albumin in sera from women with preeclampsia leads to triglyceride accumulation in cultured endothelial cells. *Am. J. Obstet. Gynecol.*, **167**, 440–7

13. Ylikorkala, O. and Viinikka, L. (1992). The role of prostaglandins in obstetric disorders. *Baillières Clin. Obstet. Gynaecol.*, **6**, 809–27

14. Orpana, A. O., Avela, K., Ranta, V., Viinikka, L. and Ylikorkala, O. (1996). The calcium-dependent nitric oxide production of human vascular endothelial cells in preeclampsia. *Am. J. Obstet. Gynecol.*, **174**, 1056–60

15. Yallampalli, C. and Garfield, R. E. (1993). Inhibition of nitric oxide synthesis in rats during pregnancy produces signs similar to those of preeclampsia. *Am. J. Obstet. Gynecol.*, **169**, 1316–20

16. Scudiero, D. A., Shoemaker, R. H., Paull, K. D., Monks, A., Tierney, S., Nofziger, T. H., Currens, M. J., Seniff, D. and Boyd, M. R. (1988).

Evaluation of a soluble tetrazolium/fomazan assay for cell growth and drug sensitivity in culture using human and other tumor cell lines. *Cancer Res.*, **48**, 4827–33

17. Cameron, I. T., van Papendorf, C. L., Palmer, R. M. J., Smith, S. K. and Moncada, S. (1993). Relationship between nitric oxide synthesis and increase in systolic blood pressure in women with hypertension in pregnancy. *Hypertension in Pregnancy*, **12**, 85–92

18. Seligman, S. G., Buyon, J. P., Clancy, R. M., Young, B. K. and Abramson, S. B. (1994). The role of nitric oxide in pathogenesis of preeclampsia. *Am. J. Obstet. Gynecol.*, **171**, 944–8

19. Benjamin, N. and Vallace, P. (1994). Plasma nitrite as a marker of nitric oxide production. *Lancet*, **344**, 960

20. Laivuori, H., Tikkanen, M. J. and Ylikorkala, O. (1996). Hyperinsulinemia 17 years after pre-eclamptic first pregnancy. *J. Clin. Endocrinol. Metab.*, **81**, 2908–11

21. DeFronzo, R. A. and Ferrannini, E. (1991). Insulin resistance: a multifaced syndrome responsible for NIDDM, obesity, hypertension, dyslipidemia, and atherosclerotic cardiovascular disease. *Diabetes Care*, **14**, 173–94

22. Adams, E. M. and MacGillivray, L. (1961). Long term effect of preeclampsia on blood pressure. *Lancet*, **2**, 1373–5

23. Sibai, B. M., El-Nazer, A. and Gonzales-Rutz, A. (1986). Severe preeclampsia-eclampsia in young primigravid women: subsequent pregnancy outcome and remote prognosis. *Am. J. Obstet. Gynecol.*, **155**, 1011–16

24. Jonsdottir, L. S., Arngrimsson, R., Geirsson, R. T., Sigvaldason, H. and Sigfusson, N. (1995). Death rates from ischemic heart disease in women with a history of hypertension in pregnancy. *Acta Obstet. Gynecol. Scand.*, **74**, 772–6

Diabetes and pregnancy

20

F. A. Van Assche

INTRODUCTION

Although substantial progress has been made in the physiopathology and management of diabetes and pregnancy, major problems remain unsolved. Furthermore, diabetes and pregnancy remains an important medical complication, with implications for mother and child in the short and long term. Gestational diabetes has not a significantly increased perinatal mortality, but fetal hyperinsulinism and macrosomia is present; the outlook for the pre-existing insulin-dependent pregnant diabetic has improved, but major complications, such as congenital malformations, sudden fetal death and the association with pre-eclampsia, need better understanding.

SCREENING FOR GESTATIONAL DIABETES

Gestational diabetes is defined as carbohydrate intolerance of variable severity with onset or first recognition during the current pregnancy[1]. Gestational diabetes occurs more frequently in older and overweight pregnant women. It is a heterogeneous disorder and affects 2–3% of pregnancies in the Western world[2,3]. The metabolic adaptation which occurs during normal pregnancy involves apparent deterioration of glucose tolerance and hyperinsulinism, but only in a minority of women are the diagnostic criteria for gestational diabetes present[4]. Insulin secretion is increased during pregnancy and there is evidence that insulin resistance exists[5,6]. The morphological basis for this hyperinsulinism during pregnancy is marked β-cell hypertrophy and hyperplasia, and hyperactivity of individual β-cells[7].

The diabetic ketoacidosis, hyperosmolar coma and vascular complications seen in type I diabetes are extremely rare in gestational diabetes. Cousins[8] found that the incidence of pre-eclampsia was increased in women with gestational diabetes. Perinatal mortality and morbidity are affected by this complication. Gestational diabetes is also a risk factor for the development of diabetes in later life. The first studies were those of O'Sullivan[9] who reported a high incidence of diabetes mellitus many years after pregnancies complicated by gestational diabetes. Further studies have confirmed these original findings[10–14].

In the past, gestational diabetes was reported to be associated with an increased perinatal mortality[15–17]. More recently it has been shown that the perinatal mortality is not different from that of the general population. However, gestational diabetic women receive more obstetric attention and there is increased perinatal mortality in undiagnosed gestational diabetes[18]. Perinatal mortality therefore remains an indication to screen for gestational diabetes. Perinatal morbidity, in particular fetal macrosomia, is also increased in gestational diabetes. Fetal macrosomia is associated with an increased number of operative deliveries and with shoulder dystocia[19,20]. There is also evidence that infants born to mothers with gestational diabetes have an increased risk of becoming diabetic in later life[21].

It therefore remains necessary to screen for gestational diabetes and if possible to perform general screening of all pregnant women[22]. However, there are a large number of glucose challenge procedures, with no agreement on the diagnostic criteria for gestational diabetes and there is not much hope of standardization in the near future[22]. Venous or capillary blood can be used, the glucose load can be oral or intravenous, and the glucose challenge can be 50, 75 or 100 g. The original Somogyi-Nelson method of glucose measurement has been changed over the years to the glucose oxidase or hexokinase method. Furthermore, there are geographical, ethnic and racial differences in the deterioration of glucose metabolism[23]. Screening for glycosuria is not a strong index of gestational diabetes, since in pregnancy glucose in the urine does not reflect hyperglycemia.

In the USA, screening of the total pregnant population is advised using a 50 g, 1 h challenge test; the American College of Obstetricians and Gynecologists advocate a glucose threshold of 140 mg per cent or 7.8 mmol/l (using venous plasma or serum and glucose oxidase or hexokinase techniques). Screening should be performed at 26–28 weeks, but retesting later in pregnancy might be reasonable for some patients such as obese and older women[22]. The use of the glucose reflectance meter may facilitate general screening in the future. However, lack of precision of the meters can be responsible for missing pregnant women who need further testing[24,25]. Other challenge tests and also random blood glucose testing have been used but have not shown any advantage over the 50 g challenge test[22]. The measurement of glycosylated hemoglobin and glycosylated proteins has inadequate sensitivity and specificity for screening[26,27].

The standard method for the diagnosis of gestational diabetes still remains the 100 g oral glucose challenge, although the World Health Organization has recommended a 75 g load (as in the non-pregnant population). The interpretation of the test goes back to the original study of O'Sullivan and Mahan[28]. Carpenter and Coustan[29], using venous plasma and the glucose oxidase or hexokinase techniques, converted the O'Sullivan and Mahan[28] criteria as shown in Table 1.

These criteria are close to the data of the European collaborative study where a glucose load of 75 g was used, but the blood sampling varied in the different centers[30]. It must be stressed that international comparisons of the prevalence of diabetes during pregnancy are difficult because of the different methods and cut-off points for diagnosis. Furthermore, there are major ethnic variations[31].

Gestational diabetes remains a risk factor for mother and child. It is therefore necessary to screen for this disorder during pregnancy. Universal screening with a 50 g, 1 h glucose challenge is recommended. The final diagnosis is made with a 100 g oral glucose tolerance test. This clearly means that women with risk factors (severe obesity, a history of diabetes in the family, a personal birth weight of more than 4500 g, pre-eclampsia, polyhydramnios, fetal macrosomia, perinatal death, congenital anomalies) need a 100 g oral glucose tolerance test.

PREPREGNANCY CARE

There is growing evidence that tight control of diabetes before pregnancy improves fetal and maternal outcome. Education and management may prevent congenital malformations and early pregnancy loss and can also improve the maternal condition[32]. Many studies have shown that congenital malformations are more numerous in infants of type I diabetic mothers[33–38] and these are becoming the leading cause of perinatal morbidity and mortality in such infants. Kucera[39] reviewed the world literature between 1930 and 1964: the incidence of congenital malformations in diabetic pregnancies was 4.8% compared with 1.65% in normal pregnancies. Anomalies of the central nervous system, heart, skeleton, gastrointestinal

Table 1 Criteria used by Carpenter and Coustan[29], converted from those of O'Sullivan and Mahan[28], for diagnosis of gestational diabetes

	Blood level of glucose
Fasting	95 mg%; 5.3 mmol/l
1 h	180 mg%; 10.0 mmol/l
2 h	155 mg%; 8.7 mmol/l
3 h	140 mg%; 7.8 mmol/l

tract and genitourinary tract are predominant. Poor metabolic control and the severity of diabetes is correlated with the high incidence of congenital anomalies[34,40]. An association is also found with a high level of glycosylated hemoglobin in the first trimester of pregnancy[41]. Furthermore, optimal treatment with insulin in the critical periods of organogenesis reduces the rate of fetal malformations in the rat[42,43].

The first study in human pregnancy showing a reduction of congenital malformations by intensive diabetic management prior to conception was from Karlsburg, Germany[44]. The incidence of congenital malformations was 0.8% in the pregnancies of women given intensive treatment prior to conception and 7.8% in those pregnancies where intensive treatment started at 8 weeks. Studies in Europe and the USA confirmed these positive findings[45–47]. Strict metabolic control early in pregnancy reduces the number of congenital malformations at birth but does not prevent the excess frequency at conception, as is the case with tight glycemia control prior to conception[38].

The relationship between poor diabetic control before conception or early in pregnancy and an increased rate of spontaneous abortion is not so clear. Miodovnik and colleagues[49] concluded that control of blood sugar is crucial around conception and in the early weeks of pregnancy to reduce the risk of an early abortion. Abortions after 10 weeks are probably due to congenital malformations. Studies in diabetic rats have shown delayed morphological development of blastocysts even in the preimplantation period and also more degenerate embryos[50].

It therefore seems necessary for each diabetic woman planning a pregnancy to undergo preconceptual counselling. The existence of hypertension, vasculopathy, proliferative retinopathy and neuropathy must be determined. Proliferative retinopathy should be treated by laser coagulation. The woman and her partner should be told that, in the case of severe diabetes, certainly in association with hypertension, life-threatening complications for her-

self and the fetus do exist and, exceptionally, she should be advised not to become pregnant.

The most important goal of preconceptual care is to motivate intensive self-management in order to obtain normoglycemia. The woman must be instructed on self-monitoring her blood glucose and must learn about diet, physical activity and an efficient insulin regimen. Only when constant normoglycemia is achieved can the future of the conceptus and maternal health be assured.

The key points of preconceptual counselling are clearly described by J. Steel, who was one of the first to indicate the importance of this approach[51]. After 20 years of experience in Scotland, it appears necessary that, for all diabetic women of reproductive age, health care providers should regard this visit as a preconception visit.

MEDICAL APPROACH TO THE PREGNANT DIABETIC WOMAN

Normoglycemia from the preconceptual period until the time of delivery must be achieved in pregnant women with pre-existing diabetes. In order to reach these goals, intensive education of the diabetic woman is necessary. The skills, knowledge and experience of doctors and non-medical advisers are also important. During their reproductive years, diabetic women must be treated by a diabetologist with clinical and research interests in diabetic pregnancy. Of even more importance, a multidisciplinary approach is necessary, including the general practitioner, nurse, dietician, physician, obstetrician and neonatologist. In most centers care is performed in a combined obstetric– diabetic antenatal clinic.

Self-monitoring of capillary blood glucose must be taught before conception and continued throughout pregnancy. There is no evidence that any special insulin regimen is better than others[52]. Frequent daily use of short- and medium-acting insulin and pen injectors or pumps delivering insulin subcutaneously are accepted alternatives. Optimal blood glucose levels are 4.0 mmol/l (80 mg per cent) preprandial and 6.0 mmol/l (120 mg per cent) postprandial. Since hypoglycemia can occur in the first trimester, it is advisable to use the same dose of insulin as that used before conception. With further progression of pregnancy, the dose of insulin will increase. There is universal agreement that the measurement of glycosylated hemoglobin is the gold standard for the evaluation of good diabetic control. Levels below 7.5% should be achieved[52]. During labor and delivery, blood glucose is controlled by an intravenous infusion of dextrose and insulin.

Gestational diabetes can be treated by diet alone or by diet and insulin therapy. It is usual to start with dietary control. When blood sugar levels remain high or when fasting blood glucose is elevated, insulin should be given and adjusted in order to maintain normoglycemia. One insulin injection daily in the morning will control hyperglycemia. A review of current practice shows that only 15% of women with gestational diabetes require insulin[53].

Weiss and co-workers[54] have suggested intensive management of the fetus in gestational diabetes by measuring insulin in the amniotic fluid. In the case of fetal hyperinsulinism, treatment with increasing doses of insulin is advised. The intention of controlling fetal hyperinsulinism is to prevent macrosomia and neonatal complications. However, intensive treatment with insulin has reduced the rate of macrosomia[55]. Experimental and epidemiological data indicate that long-term complications can be prevented by correct insulin therapy during gestational diabetes[56].

There are no clear data available concerning the use of active agents in delaying digestion or absorption of nutrients. The use of oral hypoglycemic agents is a matter of controversy, and is mostly regarded as being contra-indicated in Western medicine.

OBSTETRIC APPROACH TO THE PREGNANT DIABETIC WOMAN

Perinatal mortality in the pregnancies of women with pre-existing diabetes has been reduced over the last few decades. Congenital malforma-

tions and unexpected stillbirths remain the leading causes of death. Intrauterine deaths can still occur in type I diabetic pregnancies with poor control and in women with complications such as polyhydramnios, pre-eclampsia, macrosomia and intrauterine growth retardation[57]. The most important obstetric management therefore includes the detection of congenital anomalies, fetal surveillance and the prevention or early detection of complications of pregnancy. Congenital malformations can be detected by ultrasound examinations between 16 and 20 weeks of pregnancy. Pedersen and Mølsted-Pedersen[58] have shown that fetuses with early growth retardation have a higher incidence of congenital malformations. Ultrasound is also the most suitable method for the evaluation of fetal growth. Increased thoracic diameter and increased abdominal circumference are markers for macrosomia[59]. However, the exact prediction of fetal weight remains difficult[60]. In diabetic vasculopathy, asymmetric growth retardation can be detected during the second half of pregnancy[61]. Biophysical methods, such as fetal heart heart rate monitoring and the biophysical profile are superior to the older fetoplacental function tests for fetal surveillance, certainly during the third trimester. It is our experience that abnormalities of these tests are more ominous for the fetus of a diabetic woman than for the fetus of a woman with other complications of pregnancy.

Maternal complications are still frequently seen in diabetes and pregnancy[8]. Hypertension during pregnancy and pre-eclampsia are increased in gestational diabetes and in the pregnant woman with pre-existing diabetes. Garner and associates[62] found an incidence of pre-eclampsia of 9.9% in diabetic pregnancies compared with 4.3% in non-diabetic women. Van Assche and colleagues[63] found an increased production of thromboxane between 28 and 32 weeks of pregnancy in diabetic women without clinical vascular complications at the time of testing. The highest levels were found in those women who subsequently developed pre-eclampsia. It was concluded that increased thromboxane generation could be related to the occurrence of pre-eclampsia and the use of antiplatelet therapy to prevent pre-eclampsia warrants further investigation. However, pre-eclampsia will keep its secrets and prevention of the disease will be difficult. When polyhydramnios is found, fetal anomalies must be excluded and re-evaluation of strict diabetic control is advisable[8]. Polyhydramnios can be caused by excessive fetal urine production secondary to hyperglycemia. Premature rupture of the membranes, preterm labor, cord prolapse and abruptio placentae are known risk factors. Preterm labor can lead to the birth of a premature baby. On the other hand, the use of β-agonists and corticosteroids can result in maternal hyperglycemia, hyperinsulinemia, hypocalcemia, ketoacidosis, pulmonary edema and angina[64]. When these drugs are used, intensive diabetic monitoring is mandatory. Magnesium sulfate and calcium channel blockers may be worthwhile alternatives[65]. Urinary tract infections are not more common in diabetic pregnancies but pyelonephritis increases the risk of perinatal morbidity[66].

In older studies it was recommended that type I diabetic women should be delivered between 35 and 36 weeks of pregnancy in order to avoid the high number of intrauterine deaths. In the last decade it has been suggested that diabetic pregnancies under tight control and without complications should be allowed to continue to term. Under these circumstances, an amniocentesis to determine fetal maturity seems unnecessary. For cervical ripening and induction of labor, local prostaglandin E_2 administration is of substantial benefit. Close supervision of the progress of labor and continuous electronic fetal monitoring are mandatory. The incidence of Cesarean section varies between 17 and 83%[60]. Failed induction, macrosomia causing obstructed labor and fetal distress are the main reasons for abdominal delivery[8]. Coustan and co-workers[67] have shown that, with close supervision, the Cesarean section rate can be reduced without increased perinatal risk. However, in the presence of a macrosomic fetus, Cesarean section is advisable in order to avoid shoulder dystocia. Indeed, the physique of the

infant, with broad shoulders and a short neck, may predispose to the dangerous complication of shoulder dystocia.

The obstetric management of the mother with gestational diabetes is mainly concentrated upon the detection of fetal macrosomia. Maresh and Beard[68] suggest that, in the absence of any obstetric complication, spontaneous labor can be awaited. However, in more severe gestational diabetes, certainly in the case of macrosomia, management similar to that of the pregestational diabetic is recommended[69]. Congenital malformations and early fetal loss are probably not increased in gestational diabetes.

THE EFFECT OF MATERNAL DIABETES ON THE FETUS AND OFFSPRING

Alterations in the intrauterine environment affect fetal growth and development. In diabetic pregnancies not complicated by vasculopathy, fetal hyperinsulinism and macrosomia are mostly present. However, when vasculopathy and nephropathy are associated, intrauterine growth restriction and hypoinsulinism are common findings. Both conditions may have long-term consequences. At the present time, human and experimental data in the rat are available.

The advantage of research in the rat is that a better exploration of the underlying mechanisms is possible. Offspring of rats which were hyperglycemic throughout the last week of gestation, appear at adulthood as normal healthy animals with a normal body weight, normal basal glucose and insulin levels and a morphologically normal endocrine pancreas[70,71]. When stressed, however, glucose tolerance appears to be impaired, and the effect is different, depending on whether the youngster had passed its intrauterine life in a mildly or in a severely diabetic mother. When the maternal hyperglycemia was mild and resulted in fetal hyperinsulinemia, the induced increase in amino acid turnover was maintained in adulthood, and the β-cell response to glucose stimulation was deficient, while the insulin receptor system appeared to be unaffected[71-73]. When the maternal hyperglycemia was severe and resulted in fetal hypoinsulinemia, the adult offspring not only displayed a deregulation of the stimulated insulin output, but also insulin resistance in the liver and the peripheral tissues[72,74]. When the mothers were malnourished during pregnancy, whether in a qualitative (protein deficiency) or a quantitative (50% restriction) way, glucose tolerance was also impaired in the offspring[75,76].

Pregnancy causes a considerable stress on the glucose and insulin metabolism of the mother and implies important adaptations of the endocrine pancreas at the structural and functional level. The mass of islet tissue doubles and the activity of the β-cells is enhanced[77]. Normal pregnancy is associated with hyperinsulinemia and insulin resistance. When these youngsters of diabetic or malnourished mothers, with impaired glucose tolerance, become pregnant, they develop gestational diabetes[71,78,79]. This implies that their fetuses also will develop in an abnormal intrauterine milieu and have to adapt to it. Indeed, they display the typical features of fetuses from mildly diabetic mothers, and when they become adult they develop impaired glucose tolerance and gestational diabetes[71,78]. A diabetogenic tendency is thereby transmitted from one generation to another, without any genetic involvement, but as a result of the fact that the fetus developed in an abnormal intrauterine milieu.

In the human, a number of epidemiological studies also point to the importance of the intrauterine milieu for the development of the fetus. A higher incidence of non-insulin-dependent diabetes and of gestational diabetes is reported in children from diabetic mothers than from diabetic fathers[80], and a higher incidence of diabetes is present in the offspring from diabetic great-grandmothers via the maternal than via the paternal line[81]. Systematic treatment of diabetic mothers during pregnancy may result in a decreased incidence of diabetes in their children[82]. The most convincing data on the intrauterine transmission of the diabetogenic tendency in the human derive from the studies of Pettitt and co-workers on the Pima Indians, a population with a high incidence of diabetes[83]. Glucose tolerance is much more frequent in children from mothers who had diabetes during pregnancy than in children from mothers who developed diabetes only after that pregnancy. The difference is convincing: 33% vs. 1%[83]. Recent epidemiological studies, relating birth files from 50 years ago with the health condition of these people now, also demonstrate a significant relationship between body weight at birth, whether or not related to a known metabolic pathology of the mother, and the incidence of impaired glucose tolerance and diabetes in adulthood[84].

We can conclude that even a minor disturbance in maternal metabolism induces alterations in the fetal metabolism, with lasting consequences for the offspring, even over several generations. The effect is situated at the level of insulin secretion (number, sensitivity, synthesis and secretion of β-cells) and also at the level of the insulin receptor system (number and sensitivity of receptors and postreceptor mechanisms).

CONCLUSION

At the beginning of the century a large number of diabetic women died before the age of reproduction or were too unwell to ovulate. When pregnancy occurred, maternal morbidity and mortality were high and only a few children were born alive. The discovery of insulin was beneficial for the mother but perinatal survival was still rare. With improvements in diabetic care, perinatal mortality improved but remained very high. Clinical and fundamental research showed that, for the treatment of the fetus of a diabetic mother, normoglycemia is obligatory. To protect the fetus during conception, tight control is necessary before conception. This implies commitment from physician, obstetrician, neonatologist and non-medical personnel. The diabetic woman herself and her environment take the major responsibility for care and management.

The most important goals for the future are: the future reduction of congenital malformations, the early detection and prevention of pre-eclampsia, the prevention of diabetic complications during pregnancy and further investigation into the mechanisms of long-term effects.

References

1. Freinkel, N., Gable, S. G., Hadden, D. R. *et al.* (1985). Summary and recommendations of the second international workshop-conference on gestational diabetes mellitus. *Diabetes*, **34**, 123–6

2. Sepe, S. J., Connel, F. A., Geiss, L. S. and Teutsch, S. M. (1985). Gestational diabetes – incidence, maternal characteristics and perinatal outcome. *Diabetes*, **34**, 13–16

3. Gabbe, S. G. (1986). Gestational diabetes mellitus. *N. Engl. J. Med.*, **315**: 1025–6

4. Kühl, C., Hornnes, P. and Andersen, O. (1984). Aetiological factors in gestational diabetes. In Sutherland, H. W. and Stowers, K. M. (eds.) *Carbohydrate Metabolism in Pregnancy and the Newborn*, pp. 12–22. (Edinburgh: Churchill Livingstone)

5. Burt, R. L. and Davidson, L. W. F. (1974). Insulin half-life and utilization in normal pregnancy. *Obstet. Gynecol.*, **43**, 161–70

6. Bellmann, O. and Hartmann, E. (1975). Influence of pregnancy on the kinetics of insulin. *Am. J. Obstet. Gynecol.*, **122**, 829–33

7. Van Assche, F. A., Aerts, L. and De Prins, F. (1978). Morphological study of the endocrine pancreas in human pregnancy. *Br. J. Obstet. Gynaecol.*, **85**, 818–20

8. Cousins, L. (1987). Pregnancy complications among diabetic women. *Review* 1965–1985. *Obstet. Gynecol. Surv.*, **42**, 140–9

9. O'Sullivan, J. B. (1975). Long-term follow-up of gestational diabetics. In Camerini-Davalos, R. A. and Cole, H. S. (eds.) *Early Diabetes in Early Life*, pp. 503–10. (New York: Academic Press)

10. Stowers, J. M., Sutherland, H. W. and Kerridge, D. F. (1985). Long-range implications for the mother: the Aberdeen experience. *Diabetes*, **34**, 106–10

11. Grant, P. T., Oats, J. N. and Beischer, N. A. (1986). The long-term follow-up of women with gestational diabetes. *Aust. N.Z. J. Obstet. Gynaecol.*, **26**, 17–22

12. Mestman, J. H. (1988). Follow-up studies in women with gestational diabetes mellitus. The experience at Los Angeles County/University of Southern California Medical Center. In Weiss, P. A. M. and Coustan, D. R. (eds.) *Gestational Diabetes*, pp. 191–8. (New York: Springer-Verlag)

13. Oats, J. N., Beischer, N. A. and Grant, P. T. (1988). The emergence of diabetes and impaired glucose tolerance in women who had gestational diabetes. In Weiss, P. A. M. and Coustan, D. R. (eds.) *Gestational Diabetes*, pp. 199–207. (New York: Springer-Verlag)

14. Henry, O. A. and Beischer, N. A. (1991). Long-term implications of gestational diabetes for the mother. In Oats, J. N. (ed.) *Diabetes in Pregnancy*, pp. 461–83. (London: Baillière Tindall)

15. Jackson, W. P. U. and Woolf, N. (1958). Maternal prediabetes as a cause of the unexplained stillbirth. *Diabetes*, **7**, 446–8

16. Gabbe, S. G., Mestman, J. H., Freeman, R. K., Anderson, G. V. and Lowensohn, R. I. (1977). Management and the outcome of Class A diabetes mellitus. *Am. J. Obstet. Gynecol.*, **127**, 465–9

17. Merkatz, I. R., Duchon, M. A., Yamashita, T. S. and Houser, H. B. (1980). A pilot community based screening program for gestational diabetes. *Diabetes Care*, **3**, 453–7

18. Pettitt, D. J., Knowler, W. C., Baird, H. R. and Benett, P. H. (1980). Gestational diabetes: infant and maternal complications of pregnancy in relation to third-trimester glucose tolerance in Pima Indians. *Diabetes Care*, **3**, 458–64

19. Acker, D. B., Sachs, B. P. and Friedmann, E. A. (1985). Risk factor for shoulder dystocia. *Obstet. Gynecol.*, **66**, 762–68

20. Spellacy, W. N., Miller, S., Winegar, A. and Peterson, P. Q. (1985). Macrosomia – maternal characteristics and infant complications. *Obstet. Gynecol.*, **66**, 158–61

21. Martin, A. O., Simpson, J. L., Ober, C. and Freinkel, N. (1985). Frequency of diabetes mellitus in mothers of probands with gestational diabetes: possible maternal influence on the predisposition to gestational diabetes. *Am. J. Obstet. Gynecol.*, **151**, 471–5

22. Cousan, D. R. (1991). Screening and diagnosis of gestational diabetes. In Oats, J. N. (ed.) *Diabetes in Pregnancy*, pp. 293–313. (London: Baillière Tindall)

23. Hadden, D. R. (1985). Geographic, ethnic, and racial variations in the incidence of gestational diabetes. *Diabetes*, **34**, 21–3

24. Landon, M. B., Cembrowski, G. S. and Gabbe, S. G. (1986). Capillary blood glucose screening for gestational diabetes: a preliminary investigation. *Am. J. Obstet. Gynecol.*, **155**, 717–21

25. Weiner, C. P., Faustich, M. W., Burns, J., Fraser, M., Whitaker, L. and Klugman, M. (1987). Diagnosis of gestational diabetes by capillary blood samples and a portable reflectance meter. Derivation of threshold values and prospective validation. *Am. J. Obstet. Gynecol.*, **156**, 1085–9

26. Landon, M. B., Gabbe, S. G. and Sachs, L. (1990). Management of diabetes mellitus and pregnancy: a survey of obstetricians and maternal-fetal specialists. *Obstet. Gynecol.*, **75**, 635–40

27. Cefalu, W. T., Prather, K. L., Chester, D. L., Wheeler, C. J., Biswas, M. and Pernoll, M. L. (1990). Total serum glycosylated proteins in detection and monitoring of gestational diabetes. *Diabetes Care*, **13**, 872–5

28. O'Sullivan, J. B. and Mahan, C. M. (1964). Criteria for the oral glucose tolerance test in pregnancy. *Diabetes*, **13**, 278–85

29. Carpenter, M. W. and Coustan, D. R. (1982). Criteria for screening tests for gestational diabetes. *Am. J. Obstet. Gynecol.*, **144**, 768–73

30. Lind, T. and Philips, P. R. (1989). A prospective multicentre study to determine the influence of pregnancy upon the 75-g oral glucose tolerance test (OGTT). In Sutherland, H. W., Stowers, J. M. and Pearson, D. W. M. (eds.) *Carbohydrate Metabolism in Pregnancy and the Newborn IV*, pp. 209–26. (New York: Springer)

31. McCance, D. R. (1996). Classification and diagnosis of diabetes in pregnancy. In Dornhorst, A. and Hadden, D. R. (eds.) *Diabetes and Pregnancy: An International Approach to Diagnosis and Management*, pp. 23–42. (New York: John Wiley and Sons)

32. Kitzmiller, J. L., Gavin, L. A. and Gunderson, E. (1991). Preconception counseling: rationale for evaluation and management of diabetes prior to pregnancy. In Lee, R. V., Barron, W. M., Cotton, D. V. and Coustan, D. R. (eds.) *Current Obstetric Medicine*, pp. 1–16. (St Louis: Mosby Year Book)

33. Gabbe, S. G. (1977). Congenital malformations in infants of diabetic mothers. *Obstet. Gynecol. Surv.*, **32**, 125–32

34. Pedersen, J. (1977). *The Pregnant Diabetic and Her Newborn*, 2nd edn. (Baltimore: Williams & Wilkins)

35. Cousins, L. (1983). Congenital anomalies among infants of diabetic mothers: etiology, prevention, diagnosis. *Am. J. Obstet. Gynecol.*, **41**, 333–8

36. Lowy, C., Beard, R. W. and Goldschmidt, J. (1986). Congenital malformations in babies of diabetic mothers. *Diabetic Med.*, **3**, 458–62

37. Reece, E. A. and Hobbins, J. C. (1986). Diabetic embryopathy: pathogenesis, prenatal diagnosis and prevention. *Obstet. Gynecol. Surv.*, **41**, 325–35

38. Mills, J. L., Knopp, R. H., Simpson, J. L. *et al.* (1988). Lack of relation of increased malformation rates in infants of diabetic mothers to glycemic control during organogenesis. *N. Engl. J. Med.*, **318**, 671–6

39. Kucera, J. (1971). Rate and type of congenital anomalies among offspring of diabetic women. *J. Reprod. Med.*, **7**, 73

40. Freinkel, N., Cockroft, D. L., Lewis, N. J. *et al.* (1986). Fuel-mediated teratogenesis during early organogenesis: the effects of increased concentrations of glucose, ketones, or somatomedin inhibitor during rat embryo culture. *Am. J. Clin. Nutr.*, **44**, 896–995

41. Hanson, U., Persson, B. and Thunell, S. (1990). Relationship between haemoglobin A_{1c} in early Type 1 (insulin dependent) diabetic pregnancy and the occurrence of spontaneous abortion and fetal malformation in Sweden. *Diabetologia*, **33**, 100–4

42. Rashbass, P. and Ellington, S. K. L. (1988). Development of rat embryos cultured in serum prepared from rats with streptozotocin-induced diabetes. *Teratology*, **37**, 51–61

43. Eriksson, R. S. M., Thunberg, L. and Eriksson, U. J. (1989). Effects of interrupted insulin treatment on fetal outcome of pregnant diabetic rats. *Diabetes*, **38**, 764–72

44. Fuhrmann, K., Reiher, H., Semmler, K. *et al.*, (1983). Prevention of congenital malformations in infants of insulin-dependent diabetic mothers. *Diabetes Care*, **6**, 219–23

45. Damm, P. and Mølsted-Pedersen, L. (1989). Significant decrease in congenital malformations in newborn infants of an unselected population of diabetic women. *Am. J. Obstet. Gynecol.*, **161**, 1163–7

46. Goldman, J. A., Dickerd, D., Feldberg, D. *et al.* (1986). Pregnancy outcome in patients with insulin-dependent diabetes mellitus with preconceptual diabetic control: a comparative study. *Am. J. Obstet. Gynecol.*, **155**, 193–7

47. Steel, J. M., Johnstone, F. D., Hepburn, D. A. *et al.* (1990). Can prepregnancy care of diabetic women reduce the risk of abnormal babies? *Br. Med. J.*, **301**, 1070–4

48. Kitzmille, R. J. L., Gavin, L. A., Gin, G. D. *et al.* (1991). Pre-conception management of diabetes continued through early pregnancy prevents the excess of major congenital anomalies

in infants of diabetic mothers. *J. Am. Med. Assoc.*, **265**, 731–6

49. Miodovnik, M., Mimouni, F., Dignan, P. S. *et al.* (1988). Major malformations in infants of IDDM women: vasculopathy and early first-trimester poor glycemic control. *Diabetes Care*, **11**, 713–18

50. Pampfer, S., De Hertogh, R., Vanderheyden, I. *et al.* (1990). Decreased inner cell mass proportion in blastocysts from diabetic rats. *Diabetes*, **39**, 471–6

51. Steel, J. M. (1996). Pre-pregnancy care. In Dornhorst, A. and Hadden, D. R. (eds.) *Diabetes and Pregnancy: An International Approach to Diagnosis and Management*, pp. 101–19. (New York: John Wiley and Sons)

52. Hadden, D. R. (1991). Medical management of diabetes in pregnancy. In Oats, J. N. (ed.) *Diabetes in Pregnancy*, pp. 369–94. (London: Baillière Tindall)

53. Gabbe, S. G. (1985). Diabetes mellitus in pregnancy – how to manage. *Am. J. Obstet. Gynecol.*, **153**, 824

54. Weiss, P. A. M., Hofmann, H., Winter, R., Pürstner, P. and Lichtenegger, W. (1985). Amniotic fluid glucose values in normal and abnormal pregnancies. *Obstet. Gynecol.*, **65**, 333–9

55. Langer, O. (1991). Prevention of macrosomia. In Oats, J. N. (ed.) *Diabetes in Pregnancy*, pp. 333–47. (London: Baillière Tindall)

56. Aerts, L. and Van Assche, F. A. (1992). Islet transplantation in diabetic pregnant rats normalizes glucose homeostasis in their offspring. *J. Dev. Physiol.*, **17**, 283–7

57. Landon, M. B. and Gabbe, S. G. (1990). Antepartum fetal surveillance and delivery timing in diabetic pregnancies. *Clin. Diabetes*, **8**, 34–46

58. Pedersen, J. F. and Mølsted-Pedersen, L. (1979). Early growth retardation in diabetic pregnancy. *Br. Med. J.*, **I**, 18–19

59. Landon, M. B., Mintz, M. C. and Gabbe, S. G. (1989). Sonographic evaluation of fetal abdominal growth: predictor of the large-for-gestational-age infant in pregnancies complicated by diabetes mellitus. *Am. J. Obstet. Gynecol.*, **160**, 115–21

60. Coustan, D. R. (1988). Delivery timing mode and management. In Reece, E. A. and Coustan, D. R. (eds.) *Diabetes Mellitus in Pregnancy: Principles and Practices*, pp. 525–33. (New York: Churchill Livingstone)

61. Campbell, S. and Thomas, A. (1977). Ultrasound measurement of the fetal head to abdomen circumference ratio in the assessment of growth retardation. *Br. J. Obstet. Gynaecol.*, **84**, 165–74

62. Garner, P. R., D'Alton, M. E., Dudley, D. K., Huard, P. and Hardie, M. (1990). Preeclampsia in diabetic pregnancies. *Am. J. Obstet. Gynecol.*, **163**, 505–8

63. Van Assche, F. A., Spitz, B., Hanssen, M. *et al.* (1992). Increased thromboxane formation in diabetic pregnancy as a possible contributor to preeclampsia. *Am. J. Obstet. Gynecol.*, **168**, 84–7

64. Kitzmiller, J. L., Gavin, L. A., Gin, G. D. *et al.* (1988). Managing diabetes and pregnancy. *Curr. Probl. Obstet. Gynecol. Fertil.*, **11**, 107–66

65. Barss, V. A. (1989). Obstetrical complications. In Hare, J. W. (ed.) *Diabetes Complicating Pregnancy*, pp. 125–34. (New York: Alan R. Liss)

66. Diamond, M. P., Salyer, S. L., Vaughn, W. K., Cotton, R. and Boehm, F. H. (1987). Reassessment of White's classification and Pedersen's prognostically bad signs of diabetic pregnancies in insulin-dependent diabetic pregnancies. *Am. J. Obstet. Gynecol.*, **156**, 599–604

67. Coustan, D., Berkowitz, R. and Hobbins, J. (1980). Tight metabolic control of overt diabetes in pregnancy. *Am. J. Med.*, **68**, 845–52

68. Maresh, M. and Beard, R. W. (1989). Screening and management of gestational diabetes mellitus. In Sutherland, H. W., Stowers, J. M. and Pearson, D. W. M. (eds.) *Carbohydrate Metabolism in Pregnancy and the Newborn IV*, pp. 201–8. (London: Springer-Verlag)

69. Oats, J. N. (1991). Obstetrical management of patients with diabetes in pregnancy. In Oats, J. N. (ed.) *Diabetes in Pregnancy*. pp. 395–411. (London: Baillière Tindall)

70. Aerts, L. and Van Assche, F. A. (1981). Endocrine pancreas in the offspring of rats with experimentally induced diabetes. *J. Endocrinol.*, **88**, 81–8

71. Ktorza, A., Gauguier, D., Bihoreau, M. T. *et al.* (1990). Adult offspring from mildly hyperglycemic rats show impairment of glucose regulation and insulin secretion which is transmissible to the next generation. In Shafrir, E. (ed.) *Frontiers of Diabetes Research. Lessons from Animal Diabetes III*. pp. 555–60. (London: Smith-Gordon)

72. Aerts, L., Sodoyez-Goffaux, F., Sodoyez, J. C. *et al.* (1988). The diabetic intrauterine milieu has a long-lasting effect on insulin secretion by β-cells and on insulin uptake by target tissues. *Am. J. Obstet. Gynecol.*, **5**, 1287–92

73. Susa, J. B., Boylan, J. M., Seghal, P. and Schwartz, R. (1992). Persistence of impaired insulin secretion in infant rhesus markers that had been hyperinsulinemic *in utero*. *J. Clin. Endocrinol. Metab.*, **75**, 265–9

74. Holemans, K., Aerts, L. and Van Assche, F. A. (1991). Evidence for an insulin resistance in the

adult offspring of pregnant steptozotocin-diabetic rats. *Diabetologia*, **34**, 81–5

75. Dahri, S., Snoeck, A., Reusens-Billen, B. *et al.* (1991). Islet function in offspring of mothers on low-protein diet during gestation. *Diabetes*, **40**, 115–20

76. Holemans, K., Verhaeghe, J., Dequeker, J. and Van Assche, F. A. (1995). Insulin sensitivity in adult female rats subjected to malnutrition during perinatal period. *J. Soc. Gynecol. Invest.*, **3**, 71–7

77. Van Assche, F. A. and Aerts, L. (1975). Morphologic and ultrastructural modifications in the endocrine pancreas of pregnant rats. In Davlos, C. (ed.) *Early Diabetes in Early Life*, pp. 333–41. (New York: Academic Press)

78. Aerts, L., Holemans, K. and Van Assche, F. A. (1990). Maternal diabetes during pregnancy: consequences for the offspring. *Diabetes Metab. Rev.*, **6**, 147–67

79. Holemans, K., Van Bree, R., Verhaeghe, J. *et al.* (1993). *In vivo* glucose utilization by individual tissues in virgin and pregnant offspring of severely diabetic rats. *Diabetes*, **42**, 530–6

80. Martin, A. O., Simpson, J. L., Ober, C. and Freinkel, N. (1985). Frequency of diabetes mellitus in probands with gestational diabetes: possible maternal influence on the predisposition to diabetes. *Am. J. Obstet. Gynecol.*, **151**, 471–3

81. Dörner, G., Plagemann, A. and Reinagel, H. (1987). Familial diabetes aggregation in type 2 diabetics: gestational diabetes as apparent risk factor for increased diabetes susceptibility in the offspring. *Exp. Clin. Endocrinol.*, **89**, 84–90

82. Dörner, G., Steindel, E., Thoelke, H. and Sehliak, V. (1984). Evidence for decreasing prevalence of diabetes mellitus in childhood apparently produced by prevention of hyperinsulinism in the foetus and newborn. *Exp. Clin. Endocrinol.*, **84**, 134–42

83. Pettit, D. J., Aleck, K. A., Baird, H. R. *et al.* (1988). Congenital susceptibility to NIDMM. Role of intrauterine environment. *Diabetes*, **37**, 622–8

84. Phipps, K., Barker, D. J. P., Hales, C. N. *et al.* (1993). Fetal growth and impaired glucose tolerance in men and women. *Diabetologia*, **36**, 225–8

Venous thrombosis in pregnancy   21

I. A. Greer

INTRODUCTION

Pulmonary thromboembolism (PTE) remains a major cause of maternal death, and was the leading cause with 35 deaths in the most recent Report on Confidential Enquiries into Maternal Death in the United Kingdom[1]. This represents a substantial fall from the 1950s. The major component of this fall in incidence has been a reduction in deaths from PTE following vaginal delivery. Over this same period, there has been little change in the incidence of deaths occurring in the antenatal/intrapartum period and only a modest fall in deaths following Cesarean section, although it should be noted that the incidence of Cesarean section has increased substantially over this same period. Substandard care has been demonstrated to occur in many of these deaths, in particular, symptoms and signs suggestive of PTE or deep venous thrombosis (DVT) are ignored; clearly evident clinical risk factors for thromboembolism are ignored; and there is often inadequate diagnosis by way of objective assessment. Clearly there is a need for increased awareness of the condition and its risk factors in those caring for women in pregnancy.

PULMONARY THROMBOEMBOLISM AND DEEP VENOUS THROMBOSIS

Pulmonary thromboembolism invariably arises from DVT. In pregnancy DVT has features which differ significantly from that occurring in a non-pregnant individual. First, it should be noted that only 25–50% of patients with clinical signs suggestive of a DVT have such a diagnosis on objective investigation, thus emphasizing the need for accurate diagnosis. When symptoms do occur, they are most commonly leg swelling and pain. In heavily pregnant women such symptoms can be commonplace and it is important to remain vigilant to the possibility of underlying DVT in women at risk. In pregnancy, it is very common for the DVT to be left-sided, with left-sided DVT occurring in around 85% of cases in pregnancy compared to 55% in the non-pregnant. Furthermore, these thromboses when they do occur, tend to be iliofemoral rather than popliteofemoral with 72% being iliofemoral in pregnancy compared to around 9% in the non-pregnant. This is important because DVTs which are most likely to predispose to PTE are proximal, often in the iliofemoral region, suggesting that DVT in pregnancy may place the patient at higher risk of PTE than in the non-pregnant situation. A further associated feature seen in pregnant individuals with DVT is lower abdominal pain. This can cause some degree of diagnostic confusion but should not disuade the clinician from considering a diagnosis of DVT. Such abdominal pain may be due to thrombosis of the ovarian venous plexus or diversion of blood through the collateral circulation in the region of the ovary.

Deep venous thrombosis is not hazardous simply because of the risk of PTE alone. The diagnosis of DVT will place the patient at risk of further DVT with around 25% of women having a further deep venous thrombosis over a median follow-up period of 10 years. There is also a high frequency of venous insufficiency even after treated DVT. Around two-thirds of women will suffer from deep venous insufficiency. This is significantly greater than that which occurs following DVT in the non-pregnant patient. Around 80% of women will have long-term symptoms ranging from leg swelling to varicose veins and venous ulcerations[2].

The incidence of non-fatal venous thrombosis in pregnancy has been hard to gauge in the past due to screening difficulties, as techniques such as radioactive iodine-labelled fibrinogen and X-ray venography are not suitable for use in pregnancy. However, using non-invasive techniques and surveys of medical records, the incidence of DVT during pregnancy appears to be around or below 1/1000 maternities with a substantial increase in risk should the woman be aged over 35 years[3]. The risk is also substantially increased by operative delivery and emergency Cesarean section carries the highest level of risk, particularly in women over the age of 35[3].

The pathophysiology of venous thrombosis in pregnancy is similar to that in the non-pregnant situation and Virchow's triad is equally true for both situations. This triad of factors, proposed by Virchow in the late 19th century, of hypercoagulability, venous stasis and vascular endothelial damage still holds true today. Pregnancy is associated with increased coagulability combined with suppression of fibrinolysis in preparation for the hemostatic challenge of delivery[4]. There is significant change in the venous system with substantial reduction in venous flow which can be seen from the early part of the second trimester reaching a nadir at term, and taking several weeks to return to non-pregnant levels of venous flow[5,6]. Furthermore, differences can be seen in venous diameter between the left and the right with greater venous dilatation on the left postpartum, in keeping with the higher incidence of left-sided DVT. Vascular damage to pelvic veins can occur as the fetal head passes through the pelvis or in the course of operative vaginal or abdominal delivery.

RISK FACTORS FOR THROMBOEMBOLIC DISEASE

Risk factors can be identified for thromboembolic disease in pregnancy, the majority of which are clearly evident clinically. These are: increasing age, particularly age over 35 years; high parity; obesity; pre-existing pre-eclampsia; a past history of thrombosis, or underlying congenital or acquired thrombophilia; prolonged labor; dehydration; and operative delivery. These risk factors should be well known and have been documented on many occasions in the Confidential Enquiries into Maternal Deaths. However, in a recent survey of consultant obstetricians in the United Kingdom, Greer and de Swiet[7] found that only 15% of consultant obstetricians felt that age over 35 years was a risk factor of DVT and only 7% felt that emergency Cesarean section was a risk factor. Clearly there was an increased need for greater awareness of this condition and for institution of prophylaxis, and this has been met by the recent Royal College of Obstetricians and Gynaecologists' Guidelines on Thromboprophylaxis[8].

SCREENING FOR THROMBOPHILIA

It is becoming increasingly evident that women with a past history of DVT or with a current DVT should be screened for underlying thrombophilia. It is important to take a family and past medical history and to screen for the major congenital thrombophilias, i.e. antithrombin III, protein-C and protein-S deficiencies and activated protein-S resistance or factor V Leiden. Screening for acquired thrombophilia in the form of lupus anticoagulant and anticardiolipin antibody syndrome should also be performed. While antithrombin III deficiency, protein-C and protein-S deficiency are relatively uncommon, it is becoming increasingly apparent that activated protein-C resistance or factor V Leiden is a very common congenital defect in women with thromboembolic complications. This defect has only recently been described and it is due to inherited resistance to activated protein C. Protein C in its active form inhibits coagulation by proteolytic cleavage of activated factor V and activated factor VIII. This congenital resistance to activated protein C is due to a defect in the structure of factor V reflecting a single missense mutation in the gene at the factor V cleavage site where activated protein C would act. This leads to normal factor V coagulant activity but resistance to activated protein C (so-called factor V Leiden). Thus, there is a resultant hypercoagulable state. The background prevalence of factor V Leiden in the population is around 4% in Western Europe and activated protein-C resistance has been found in 21–50% of patients with previously unexplained thromboses, in contrast to a 5% incidence of other thrombophilias in patients with such a history, emphasizing the importance of this defect. In pregnancy, one study has shown that 59% of women with a DVT or PTE in pregnancy are resistant to activated protein C and of these 70% had thrombotic problems antenatally[9]. Thus, it is clear that it is important to screen for these congenital thrombophilias. Expert management in conjunction with a hematologist is required for such patients who will have particular needs for thromboprophylaxis during pregnancy and the puerperium.

THROMBOPROPHYLAXIS

Pregnancy and postpartum

Antenatal thromboprophylaxis will be required in many patients with thrombophilia and will usually be employed in patients with recurrent thrombotic events. Where a patient has had a past history of one thrombotic event either within or outwith pregnancy, there is some controversy over the management of such patients. Clearly these women should be screened for underlying thrombophilia which may influence management. However, in the absence of additional risk factors other than the previous event, there are two schools of thought – one which would withhold long-term antenatal therapy with low-dose heparin, and the other which would employ low-dose or low-molecular weight heparin therapy on a prophylactic basis through the antenatal period dating from around the mid-part of pregnancy or 6 weeks or so prior to the time of a thrombotic event in a previous pregnancy. When it comes to the postpartum situation there is unanimity of agreement that all patients should receive thromboprophylaxis for a minimum period of 6 weeks. This controversy in antenatal management for patients with a single episode of DVT emanates from the problems of long-term use of heparin and warfarin. Warfarin is a known teratogen and can cause the problem of warfarin embryopathy if the fetus is exposed between 6 and 9 weeks' gestation. The incidence of this condition may be around 4%. It takes the form of chondrodysplasia punctata which consists of nasal and midface hypoplasia, frontal bossing, short stature and stippled chondral calcification. This problem is potentially preventable with heparin substitution[10]. The problems with warfarin, however, are not simply related to warfarin embryopathy. In late pregnancy, close to labor, abruption and intracerebral bleeding in the fetus can occur. In the mid-part of pregnancy, owing to the immaturity of the fetal liver, therapeutic doses of warfarin in the mother will result in over-anticoagulation in the fetus as warfarin readily crosses the placenta. This may provoke spontaneous intracerebral hemorrhage. Thus, it would appear that heparin may be a better choice of antithrombotic therapy in pregnancy. Heparin does not cross the placenta or the breast; however, it too is associated with problems. These include heparin-induced osteoporosis, heparin-induced thrombocytopenia and allergic reactions. Heparin-induced osteoporosis has been shown to occur with long-term use of unfractionated heparin, and over 30% of women on prolonged heparin therapy will lose ≥ 10% of their bone mass with around 2% having symptomatic vertebral fractures[11]. Recently, low-molecular weight heparins have been introduced which may require only once daily administration and be associated with less hemorrhagic risk and possibly better antithrombotic effect than conventional unfractionated heparin. These agents may have a reduced risk of osteoporosis and undoubtedly do have a reduced risk of heparin-induced thrombocytopenia[12]. Heparin-induced thrombocytopenia is due to heparin-dependent IgG antibodies. It tends to occur more than 5 days after the initiation of therapy, provoking a paradoxically severe thrombotic event due to antibody-induced platelet activation. Platelet counts should be monitored regularly in patients on long-term heparin therapy in pregnancy. Heparin allergy can cause significant skin irritation but may be overcome by switching between types of heparin, although cross-reactivity commonly occurs. Therefore, it can be seen that neither heparin nor warfarin are ideal for use in the pregnant situation, but for the antenatal period heparin and possibly low-molecular weight heparins represent the best option. As neither warfarin nor heparin cross the breast in any significant amount, both are safe to use postpartum. An alternative antithrombotic agent for use around the time of delivery is dextran. While this offers effective thromboprophylaxis, there is a risk of anaphylactic and anaphylactoid reactions occurring. Recently anaphylactoid reactions have been documented at Cesarean section and these have been associated with uterine hypertonus, profound fetal distress, perinatal death and severe neurological damage. Thus, dextran should be avoided, or if it is to be used, delayed until after the fetus has been delivered. As there are now many alternatives, there is little place for the use of dextran in modern obstetric practice. Thromboembolic deterrent stockings may also be of value in preventing antenatal and postpartum DVT. Although their mechanism of action is unclear[13], they undoubtedly do influence the disease process and can be used either alone or in combination with other agents, such as low-dose or low-molecular weight heparin for high-risk patients.

Cesarean section

A particular situation where thromboprophylaxis should be involved is following Cesarean section. Patients should undergo a risk assessment[8]. Low-risk patients are those having an uncomplicated elective Cesarean section; moderate-risk patients are those with features such as an emergency Cesarean section in labor or other risk factors discussed above; and those at high risk will be women with multiple risk factors or major risk problems such as Cesarean hysterectomy, thrombophilia or paraplegia. Low-risk patients require no specific thromboprophylaxis. Moderate-risk patients should usually be treated with subcutaneous low-dose unfractionated or low-molecular weight heparins or mechanical methods such as thromboembolic deterrent stockings if heparin is contraindicated. For high-risk patients subcutaneous unfractionated heparin or low-molecular weight heparin combined with thromboembolic deterrent stockings should be used. A minimum duration of therapy should be 5 days but longer if the patient is at continued risk[8].

CONCLUSIONS

In conclusion, pregnancy and the puerperium require special considerations regarding the management of thromboembolism for both the mother and the fetus. In particular, it is important for the clinician to remain vigilant to the possibility of thrombosis in order to guide prompt objective diagnosis and appropriate management. There is also a need to consider the presence of risk factors for thrombosis and provide adequate thromboprophylaxis. Hopefully with such measures, the morbidity and mortality from venous thromboembolic disease in pregnancy can be reduced.

References

1. Department of Health, Welsh Office, Scottish Office Home and Health Department, Department of Health and Social Services Northern Ireland (1996). *Report on Confidential Enquiries into Maternal Deaths in the United Kingdom 1991–1993.* (London: HMSO)
2. Bergqvist, D., Bergqvist, A., Lindhagen, A. and Matzsch, T. (1992). Long term outcome of

patients with venous thromboembolism during pregnancy. In Greer, I. A., Turpie, A. G. G. and Forbes, C. D. (eds.) *Haemostasis and Thrombosis in Obstetrics and Gynaecology*, pp. 349–60. (London: Chapman and Hall)

3. Macklon, N. S. and Greer, I. A. (1996). Thromboembolism in obstetrics and gynaecology; the Scottish experience. *Scot. Med. J.*, **1**, 83–6

4. Forbes, C. D. and Greer, I. A. (1992). Physiology of haemostasis and the effect of pregnancy. In Greer, I. A., Turpie, A. G. G. and Forbes, C. D. (eds.) *Haemostasis and Thrombosis in Obstetrics and Gynaecology*, pp. 1–26. (London: Chapman and Hall)

5. Macklon, N. S., Greer, I. A. and Bowman, A. W. (1997). An ultrasound study of gestational and postural changes in the deep venous system of the leg in pregnancy. *Br. J. Obstet. Gynaecol.*, in press

6. Macklon, N. S. and Greer, I. A. (1997). An ultrasound study of the proximal deep veins in the puerperium. *Br. J. Obstet. Gynaecol.*, in press

7. Greer, I. A. and de Swiet, M. (1993). Thrombosis prophylaxis in obstetrics and gynaecology. *Br. J. Obstet. Gynaecol.*, **100**, 37–40

8. Royal College of Obstetricians and Gynaecologists Working Party on Prophylaxis Against Thromboembolism in Gynaecology and Obstetrics (Shaw, R. W., Bonnar, J., Greer, I. A., Harper, M. A. and Kakkar, V. V.) (1995). *Report of the RCOG Working Party on Prophylaxis Against Thromboembolism in Gynaecology and Obstetrics.* (London: RCOG)

9. Hellgren, M., Svensson, P. G. and Dahlback, B. (1995). Resistance to activated protein C as a basis for venous thromboembolism associated with pregnancy and oral contraceptives. *Am. J. Obstet. Gynecol.*, **173**, 210–13

10. Ginsberg, J. S. (1992). Fetal abnormalities and anticoagulants. In Greer, I. A., Turpie, A. G. G. and Forbes, C. D. (eds.) *Haemostasis and Thrombosis in Obstetrics and Gynaecology*, pp. 361–70. (London: Chapman and Hall)

11. Dahlman, T. C. (1993). Osteoporotic fractures and the recurrence of thromboembolism in pregnancy in the puerperium in 184 women undergoing thromboprophylaxis with heparin. *Am. J. Obstet. Gynecol.*, **168**, 1265–70

12. Nelson-Piercy, C. (1997). Hazards of heparin; bleeding, allergy, heparin induced thrombocytopaenia, osteoporosis. In Greer, I. A. (ed.) *Baillière's Clinical Obstetrics and Gynaecology, Venous Thromboembolism in Obstetrics and Gynaecology.* (London: Baillière, Tindall), in press

13. Macklon, N. S. and Greer, I. A. (1995). Compression stockings and posture: a comparative study of their effects on the proximal deep veins of the legs at rest. *Br. J. Radiol.*, **68**, 515–18

Epilepsy, anticonvulsants and pregnancy

22

E. Guthrie and M. J. Brodie

INTRODUCTION

Women with idiopathic or cryptogenic epilepsy, irrespective of seizure type, age at onset, or family history of epilepsy, are only about one-third as likely to become pregnant as their unaffected siblings[1]. Those who do face conflict. They have to choose to continue medication in a society where popular opinion indiscriminately supports the axiom that all drugs should be avoided during pregnancy. This dilemma is not helped by the fact that animal and human research has shown that all established antiepileptic drugs (AEDs) are potential teratogens[2]. We do not yet know enough about the newer AEDs to be wholly reassured regarding their lack of teratogenic potential.

EFFECTS OF PREGNANCY ON EPILEPSY

Changes in seizure frequency can occur during pregnancy, but cannot be predicted for an individual woman. Good or poor control in one pregnancy does not guarantee a similar pattern in a subsequent one. About one-third of women have more and one-third less frequent seizures. The remaining third experience no change in control. Alterations in seizure frequency do not always correlate with changes in AED levels[3]. Seizures during labor occur in 1–2% of epileptic women[4]. Status epilepticus is uncommon, affecting less than 1% of pregnancies in women with epilepsy[5].

Changes in seizure frequency have been ascribed to a variety of factors. Increased volume of distribution, decreased protein binding and accelerated hepatic metabolism and more efficient renal excretion of drugs can lead to a progressive fall in the circulating concentrations of some AEDs as pregnancy advances[6]. Total drug levels are commonly measured, but unbound (free) levels may also fall, although by not as much. Women may cut back on their medication as a protective behavior towards the baby[7]. Increased tiredness or sleep deprivation, together with hormonal changes in pregnancy, can be provocative factors.

The fetus appears to be relatively resistant to the deleterious effects of tonic–clonic seizures[8]. There are, however, a few anecdotal cases of fetal death after single seizures. Slowing of heart rate during generalized tonic–clonic but not partial seizures has been reported. First trimester seizures have been associated with an increased risk of fetal malformation[9]. High seizure frequency in the mother during pregnancy has also been suggested to have a modest impact on the child's developmental outcome[10].

EFFECTS OF EPILEPSY ON THE PREGNANCY

Pregnancy in women with epilepsy is considered to be at high risk, although the rates of published complications are conflicting[11]. Methods of delivery have been reviewed recently by Hiilesma[12], who found that induction rates were four times higher and Cesarean delivery was at least twice as common as in non-epileptic women. He questioned the need for this increased level of intervention.

TERATOGENESIS

This is the most emotive issue that complicates the pregnancies of women with epilepsy. In the general population the overall rate of malformation is between 2 and 3%. The incidence in children born to mothers with epilepsy is about 6%. The risk of abnormality increases with the number of drugs taken: 3% with one drug, 5% with two, 10% with three, and over 20% with four[13]. Dravet and co-workers[14] reported a 16% rate of abnormality with polytherapy and 6% in babies exposed to AED monotherapy. Although there are no specific teratogenic effects[15], abnormalities can be grouped as minor or major. The position of the newer drugs (vigabatrin, lamotrogine, gabapentin and topiramate) is uncertain[16].

Minor anomalies

These include digital and craniofacial anomalies and have been reported with all established AEDs[17]. Reported incidence rates vary between 5% and 45% of exposed infants[4]. Methods of ascertainment are suspect as in some studies the doctors examining the babies were not blinded. In a prospective study of 121 children of mothers with epilepsy and 105 controls examined in a blinded fashion at age 5½ years for 80 minor physical anomalies, including nine typical features previously reported characteristic of fetal hydantoin syndrome, only hypertelorism and digital hypoplasia were associated with phenytoin exposure[18]. A significant excess of minor anomalies considered characteristic of hydantoin syndrome was observed in the children of mothers with epilepsy and in the mothers themselves, compared with the controls, indicating a genetic link to epilepsy, rather than a consequence of AED ingestion[18]. Minor anomalies (hypertelorism, distal digital hypoplasia) harmonize or disappear during childhood[15], as does early postnatal growth retardation[19].

Major abnormalities

Published studies report major anomalies occurring with *all* established AEDs, including phenobarbitone, primidone, phenytoin, sodium valproate and carbamazepine[20]. The incidence of facial clefts and heart disease has been estimated at 18 per 1000 live births compared with 2 and 5 per 1000, respectively, for the rest of the population[6]. Lindhout and Omtzigt[21] have divided the established AEDs into two groups:

(1) Phenobarbitone, phenytoin and primidone were linked to congenital heart defects, cleft lip and palate, dysmorphic syndromes and, less often, skeletal anomalies and closure defects of the neural tube; and

(2) Carbamazepine and sodium valproate were associated particularly with a higher incidence of neural tube defects, specifically spina bifida aperta.

These syndromes were reported more commonly during a period when polytherapy with phenobarbitone, phenytoin or primidone was much more common than is currently the case. Changes in prescribing pattern as well as different study design may explain in part the inconsistencies in reporting over the years.

ESTABLISHED ANTIEPILEPTIC DRUGS

Barbiturates

An increased incidence of cleft palate and cardiac malformations has been reported with phenobarbitone and primidone, particularly when they are used in combination with phenytoin[5]. Phenobarbitone has been associated with a 0.3–0.4% risk of spina bifida aperta[21].

Phenytoin

The fetal hydantoin syndrome, consisting usually of minor craniofacial and digital anomalies, was first reported in 1973[22]. It occurs in around 10% of exposed fetuses[23]. Facial clefts, congenital heart disease and microcephaly are less common. Fetal susceptibility may correlate with the level of the microsomal detoxifying enzyme, epoxide hydrolase. A 0.3–0.4% risk of spina bifida aperta has also been observed[21].

Sodium valproate

Neural tube defects are estimated to occur in 1–2% of pregnancies at risk[24]. Other recorded abnormalities include hypospadias, craniofacial defects and skeletal anomalies[25].

Carbamazepine

There is an increased incidence of neural tube defects amounting to 0.5–1% in the babies of carbamazepine-treated women[26,27]. Other possible abnormalities include craniofacial defects, fingernail hypoplasia, and developmental delay, although the evidence for these is largely anecdotal[26].

Benzodiazepines

There appears to be an increased risk of growth retardation, dysmorphic features and neurological dysfunction, although the evidence in support of this is weak[5].

Ethosuximide

As this drug is seldom used in adults, little is known about its teratogenic potential.

NEWER ANTIEPILEPTIC DRUGS

These drugs have been introduced worldwide over the last 7 years. By the next millenium, we can expect to see the addition of further new agents[28].

Vigabatrin

Given in high doses to rabbits, vigabatrin has been shown to induce cleft palate in their offspring. The safety of vigabatrin in pregnancy and lactation in humans has not been established[29]. Prior to the end of June 1996, information was available on 77 pregnancies worldwide in women receiving vigabatrin in addition to other AEDs (data on file, Marion Merrell Dow). Defects noted after pregnancies in which mothers have taken vigabatrin included one baby with hypospadias, one with dysmorphic features and another with a diaphragmatic hernia[21].

Lamotrogine

This drug has not shown any evidence of teratogenesis in animal studies. Information to the end of September 1996 on 81 pregnancies is available, again using the drug as additional therapy (data on file, GlaxoWellcome).

Gabapentin

This drug has not been shown to be teratogenic in animal studies. Prior to the end of June 1996, outcome data were available for ten pregnancies in which gabapentin was used as an additional AED (data on file, Parke Davis).

Oxcarbazepine

High doses of this drug have been associated with malformations in rodents, but no strong evidence exists for teratogenicity in man. Oxcarbazepine use has been recorded in 29 documented pregnancies to the end of September 1996 (data on file, Ciba).

Topiramate

Topiramate has been found to be teratogenic in mice, rats and rabbits[16]. Information about ten pregnancies is currently available to the end of June 1996 (data on file, Janssen-Cilag).

Use in pregnancy for any of these drugs is not recommended in the Data Sheets. However, some women who have found them beneficial in controlling seizures have chosen to continue treatment during pregnancy. The established drugs are all known to be teratogens; perhaps this next generation of AEDs may offer a safer option for the pregnant woman with epilepsy and her baby. We need to collect data as quickly and as efficiently as possible.

FACTORS IMPLICATED IN TERATOGENESIS

Is the critical issue the AEDs taken by the pregnant woman or the genes which caused the mother's epilepsy[30]? To study the multifactorial etiology of congenital defects requires consideration of many factors, including family history, maternal age, concomitant disease, other drugs, diet, smoking, change in partner, environmental pollution, etc.[31]. Untreated women with epilepsy show a small increase above the general population of abnormalities such as cleft palate and spina bifida[4]. A well designed, prospective, non-intervention study of 225 singleton pregnancies found a correlation between the prevalence of abnormal pregnancy outcome and duration of epilepsy and AED treatment[32]. Nakane and his colleagues[13] concluded that for most birth anomalies or malformations the most likely etiological factor was antiepileptic medication. First trimester seizures have also been associated with an increased risk of malformation: 12.3% against 4% for babies exposed to maternal seizure at other times[9].

Evidence for a relationship between total daily dosage of sodium valproate and risk of spina bifida comes from work in rodents and a single clinical study[33,34]. The tentative conclusion is that there is a correlation between higher doses of valproate and its teratogenic effect. Whether it is total daily dose or peak concentration that is the major influence is unclear. However, this has led to the recommendation that valproate should be given at least three times daily and in the lowest possible dose[21]. It must be remembered, however, that dose is only a relative risk factor. Normal infants have been born to women who have received valproate in amounts exceeding 2400 mg per day, while spina bifida has occurred when the maternal dose was only 600 mg per day[9].

Birth defects in neonates exposed to AEDs tend to cluster in the same family. Individual genetic susceptibility to a teratogen is supported by twin studies[9]. Pharmacogenetic differences among offspring of different mothers, as well as among offspring of the same mothers, are probably involved[21]. Genetic predisposing factors for neural tube disorders may operate independently of the maternal epileptic genotype[9].

MANAGEMENT OF EPILEPSY IN PREGNANCY

This should start well *before conception*. If a woman with epilepsy has been seizure-free for more than 2 years and there is no evidence of an underlying anatomical lesion, she could be offered withdrawal of treatment. This also depends on the epilepsy syndrome. Patients with juvenile myoclonic epilepsy, for instance, often relapse[17]. If treatment is considered necessary:

(1) Review the regimen, aiming for monotherapy (if possible).

(2) Treat with the lowest effective dose.

(3) Split the dose into two or more increments or use a sustained-release formulation.

(4) Discuss the risks with the patient and her partner.

(5) Ensure that potential mothers appreciate that when pregnancy is confirmed, the time for teratogenesis is over and so the best way to protect the baby is to ensure optimal seizure control by good compliance with medication.

(6) Discuss available antenatal screening.

(7) Prescribe preconceptual folic acid and continue until at least 13 weeks gestation. Current recommendations are 5 mg of folic acid per day for women who have had a previous pregnancy complicated by a neural tube defect and 0.4 mg daily for all other women[35]. It seems appropriate to recommend the higher dose for all women with epilepsy[17]. Nevertheless, epidemiological studies offer no proof that folic acid deficiency is by itself the sole mechanism of AED-induced teratogenesis, nor that high dose folic acid is protective in this patient population[21].

(8) Discuss the chance of the baby developing epilepsy. Children born to mothers (but not fathers) with epilepsy have a three-fold increased risk of later seizures[36].

During pregnancy, women with epilepsy should be seen regularly by their general practitioner, obstetrician, and epileptologist. It is important that all professionals should communicate effectively with the patient and with each other. At these reviews checks should be made of seizure frequency and changes in drug dosage. The decision to act on falling drug levels must include awareness of the clinical situation. If a seizure-free patient with a driving licence has shown a large drop in phenytoin level, it might be in her best interests to increase the dose by a 25 mg increment. If the AED dose was increased during pregnancy, this may need to be reduced postnatally to prevent toxicity[6]. Serum AED levels will have stabilized by 8–10 weeks after delivery.

PROBLEMS WITH THE BABY

All established AEDs cross the placenta, and so can theoretically cause central nervous depression in the neonate. In practice, this is the most likely with phenobarbitone, primidone and the benzodiazepines[5]. A mild abstinence syndrome can occur in babies exposed to primidone or phenobarbitone, who may present with vomiting and suckling difficulties. Symptoms also include overactivity, restlessness, insomnia, hyperreflexia, and diarrhea. These can take a month or two to resolve.

A bleeding tendency can develop in the first few days of life in babies whose mothers take enzyme-inducing AEDs (carbamazepine, phenytoin, phenobarbitone, or primidone) as levels of vitamin K-dependent clotting factors are reduced[37]. Vitamin K should be given intramuscularly immediately after delivery to these babies. Recent studies have refuted concerns about its safety[38,39]. This evidence should put an end to all fears and doubts. This is important as newborn infants have been recommended previously to receive vitamin K orally[40], which will protect them from early but not late hemorrhagic disease[37,41].

Any malformation or retardation that occurs after prenatal AED exposure must be examined by pediatric, dysmorphologic, and clinical genetic analyses to exclude other causes. This will help determine the risk of recurrence[21]. Losche and colleagues[10] found that children with prenatal exposure to AED polytherapy had significantly lower scores than controls for a large number of psychological tests. In addition to polytherapy, there were even stronger effects of socioeconomic status. Among epilepsy variables, only the mother's seizure frequency during pregnancy had a modest impact on the child's development. Prospective studies have shown that any growth difference between AED exposed and control children is small and usually disappears at follow-up examinations by the age of 5.5 years[2].

BREAST FEEDING

All drugs are excreted in breast milk, but in lower concentrations than in maternal plasma[42]. The vast majority of infants will receive a subtherapeutic dose. In addition, all babies will have been exposed to similar AED concentrations *in utero* to those in the mother's plasma. As a general rule, therefore, breast feeding should be encouraged for all the usual reasons. However, mothers receiving AEDs tend to choose formula feeding. Even when they do breast feed, its duration is shorter than in non-epileptic women[43]. As yet there is no published information about excretion of gabapentin, lamotrogine, topiramate or vigabatrin into breast milk. However, women taking these drugs should not be debarred from breast feeding.

CONCLUSIONS

Women with epilepsy have a greater than 90% chance of a normal pregnancy and a healthy baby. In the future their care may be improved by:

(1) Balancing better the risks of medication and seizure control;

(2) Individualizing the management program;

(3) Employing less interventional methods of delivery; and

(4) Collecting high quality prospective data about new antiepileptic drugs.

References

1. Schupf, N. and Ottman, R. (1994). Likelihood of pregnancy in individuals with idiopathic/cryptogenic epilepsy: social and biologic influences. *Epilepsia*, **35**, 750–6
2. Yerby, M. S. (1993). Epilepsy and pregnancy, new issues for an old disorder. *Neurol. Clin.*, **11**, 777–86
3. Lander, C. M. and Eadie, M. J. (1991). Plasma antiepileptic drug concentrations during pregnancy. *Epilepsia*, **32**, 257–66
4. Crawford, P. (1993). Epilepsy and pregnancy. *Seizure*, **2**, 87–90
5. Brodie, M. J. (1989). Epilepsy, anticonvulsants and pregnancy. *Prescribers J.*, **29**, 251–7
6. Brodie, M. J. (1990). Management of epilepsy during pregnancy and lactation. *Lancet*, **336**, 426–7
7. Schmidt, D., Canger, R., Avanzini, G., Battino, D. and Cusi, C. (1983). Change of seizure frequency in pregnant epileptic women. *J. Neurol. Neurosurg. Psychiatr.*, **46**, 751–5
8. Hiilesma, V. K., Bardy, A. and Teramo, K. (1985). Obstetric outcome in women with epilespsy. *Am. J. Obstet. Gynecol.*, **152**, 499–504
9. Lindhout, D., Meinardi, H., Meijer, J. W. A. and Nau, H. (1992). Antiepileptic drugs and teratogenesis in two consecutive cohorts: changes in prescription policy paralleled by changes in pattern of malformations. *Neurology*, **42**, 94–110
10. Losche, G., Steinhausen, H. C., Koch, S. and Helge, H. (1994). The psychological development of children of epileptic parents. II. The differential impact of intrauterine exposure to anticonvulsant drugs and further influential factors. *Acta Paediatr.*, **83**, 961–6
11. Yerby, M. S. (1996). Contraception, pregnancy and lactation in women with epilepsy. In Brodie, M. J. and Treiman, D. M. (eds.) *Modern Management of Epilepsy, Baillière's Clinical Neurology*, pp. 887–908. (London: Baillière Tindall)
12. Hiilesma, V. K. (1992). Pregnancy and birth in women with epilepsy. *Neurology*, **42**, 8–11
13. Nakane, Y., Okuma, T., Takahashi, R., Sato, Y., Wada, T., Sato, T., Fukushima, Y., Kumashiro, H., Ono, T., Takahashi, T., Adki, Y., Kazamat-suri, H., Inami, M., Komai, S., Seino, M., Miyakoshi, M., Tanimura, T., Hazami, H., Kawahara, R., Otsuki, S., Hosokawa, K., Inanaga, K., Nakazawa, Y. and Yamamoto, K. (1980). Multi-institutional study on the teratogenicity and fetal toxicity of antiepileptic drugs: a report of a collaborative study group in Japan. *Epilepsia*, **21**, 663–80
14. Dravet, C., Julian, C., Legras, C., Magaudda, A., Guerrini, R., Genton, P., Soulayrol, S., Giraud, N., Mesdjian, E., Trentin, G., Roger, J. and Ayme, S. (1992). Epilepsy, antiepileptic drugs, and malformations in children of women with epilepsy: a French prospective cohort study. *Neurology*, **42**, 75–82
15. Janz, D. (1994). Are antiepileptic drugs harmful when taken during pregnancy? *J. Perinat. Med.*, **22**, 367–77
16. Dichter, M. A. and Brodie, M. J. (1996). New antiepileptic drugs. *N. Engl. J. Med.*, **334**, 1503–90
17. Brodie, M. J. and Dichter, M. A. (1996). Antiepileptic drugs. *N. Engl. J. Med.*, **334**, 168–75
18. Gaily, E., Granstrom, M. L., Hiilesma, V. and Bardy, A. (1988). Minor anomalies in offspring of epileptic mothers. *J. Pediatr.*, **112**, 520–9
19. Gaily, E. and Granstrom, M. J. (1989). A transient retardation of early postnatal growth in drug-exposed children of epileptic mothers. *Epilepsy Res.*, **4**, 147–55
20. Delgado-Escueta, A. V. and Janz, D. (1992). Consensus guidelines: preconception counselling, management, and care of the pregnant woman with epilepsy. *Neurology*, **42**, 149–60
21. Lindhout, D. and Omtzigt, J. (1994). Teratogenic effects of antiepileptic drugs: implications for the management of epilepsy in women of childbearing age. *Epilepsia*, **35**, 19–28
22. Loughnan, P. M., Gold, H. and Vance, J. C. (1973). Phenytoin teratogenicity in man. *Lancet*, **1**, 70–2
23. Buehler, B. A., Rao, V. and Finnell, R. H. (1994). Biochemical and molecular teratology of fetal hydantoin syndrome. *Neurol. Clin.*, **12**, 741–8
24. Editorial (1988). Valproate, spina bifida, and birth defect registries. *Lancet*, **ii**, 1404–5

25. Koch, S., Losche, G., Jager-Roman, E., Jacob, S., Rating, D., Deichl, A. and Helge, H. (1992). Major and minor birth malformations and antiepileptic drugs. *Neurology*, **42**, 83–8

26. Jones, K. J., Lacro, R. V., Johnson, K. A. and Adams, J. (1989). Patterns of malformations in children of women treated with carbamazepine during pregnancy. *N. Engl. J. Med.*, **320**, 1661–6

27. Rosa, F. W. (1991). Spina bifida in infants of women treated with carbamazepine during pregnancy. *N. Engl. J. Med.*, **324**, 674–7

28. Brodie, M. J. (1996). Antiepileptic drugs, clinical trials and the marketplace. *Lancet*, **347**, 777–9

29. Srinivasan, J. and Richens, A. (1994). A risk-benefit assessment of vigabatrin in the treatment of neurological disorders. *Drug Saf.*, **10**, 395–405

30. Homes, L. B., Harvey, E. A., Brown, K. S., Hayes, A. M. and Khoshbin, S. (1994). Anticonvulsant teratogenesis: 1. A study design for newborn infants. *Teratology*, **49**, 202–7

31. Milunsky, A. (1996). Congenital defects, folic acid and homoebox genes. *Lancet*, **348**, 419–20

32. Steegers-Theunissen, R. P. M., Reiner, W. O., Borm, G. F., Thomas, C. M. G., Merkus, H. M. W. M., Op de Coul, D. A. W., De Jong, P. A., van Geijn, H. P., Wouters, M. and Eskes, T. K. A. B. (1994). Factors influencing the risk of abnormal pregnancy outcome in epileptic women: a multi-centre prospective study. *Epilepsy Res.*, **18**, 261–9

33. Nau, H. (1985). Teratogenic valproic acid concentrations: infusion by implanted minipumps vs conventional injection regimen in the mouse. *Toxicol. Appl. Pharmacol.*, **80**, 243–50

34. Omtzigt, J. G. C., Los, F. J., Grobbee, D. E., Pijpers, L., Jahoda, M. G. J., Brandenburg, H., Stewart, P. A., Gaillard, H. L. J., Sachs, E. S., Wladimiroff, J. W. and Lindhout, D. (1992). The risk of spina bifida after first-trimester exposure to valproate in a prenatal cohort. *Neurology*, **42**, 119–25

35. Department of Health (1992). *Folic Acid and the Prevention of Neural Tube Defects*, Report from an Expert Advisory Group. (Heywood, United Kingdom: Department of Health Publications Unit)

36. Annegers, J. F., Hauser, W. A., Elveback, L. R., Anderson, V. E. and Kurland, L. T. (1978). Congenital malformations and seizure disorders in the offspring of parents with epilepsy. *Int. J. Epidemiol.*, **7**, 241–7

37. Zipursky, A. (1996). Vitamin K at birth. *Br. Med. J.*, **313**, 179–80

38. Von Kries, R., Gobel, U., Hachmeister, A., Kaletsch, U. and Michaelis, J. (1996). Vitamin K and childhood cancer: a population based case-control study in Lower Saxony, Germany. *Br. Med. J.*, **313**, 199–230

39. Ansell, P., Bull, D. and Roman, E. (1996). Childhood leukaemia and intramuscular vitamin K: findings from a case-control study. *Br. Med. J.*, **313**, 204–5

40. Croucher, C. and Azzopardi, D. (1994). Compliance with recommendations for giving vitamin K to newborn infants, *Br. Med. J.*, **308**, 894–5

41. Von Kries, R. and Hanawa, Y. (1993). Neonatal vitamin K prophylaxis. Report of scientific and standardization subcommittee on perinatal haemostasis. *Thromb. Haemost.*, **69**, 293–5

42. Nau, H., Kuhnz, W., Egger, H. -J., Rating, D. and Helge, H. (1982). Anticonvulsants during pregnancy and lactation: transplacental, maternal and neonatal pharmacokinetics. *Clin. Pharmacokinet.*, **7**, 508–43

43. Ito, S., Moretti, M., Liau, M. and Koren, G. (1995). Initiation and duration of breast-feeding in women receiving antiepileptics. *Am. J. Obstet. Gynecol.*, **172**, 881–6

Renal disease in pregnancy

23

J. M. Davison and J. E. C. Milne

INRODUCTION

This chapter reviews management, obstetric course and long-term prognosis in women with a variety of renal problems, focusing on the most recent literature to highlight some of the current controversies.

RENAL CHANGES IN NORMAL PREGNANCY

The kidneys enlarge because both vascular volume and interstitial space increase, and there is a 70% overall rise in renal volume by the third trimester[1]. Marked dilatation of the calyces, renal pelves and ureters occurs, and is evident in 90% of women by the third trimester, especially on the right side.

Glomerular filtration rate (GFR) and renal flow increase by 50–70% above pregnancy values. Glomerular filtration rate, as measured by 24-h creatinine clearance, increases immediately in early pregnancy, and serum levels of creatinine and urea decrease. Therefore, values for creatinine of 75 μmol/l (0.85 mg/dl) and for urea of 4.5 mmol/l (27 mg/dl), which are acceptable in non-pregnant women, would be suspect in pregnancy. Caution is, however, necessary when assessing renal function on the basis of serial serum creatinine levels alone (especially in the presence of renal disease), because even when up to 50% of renal function has been lost, the serum creatinine level can still be less than 130 mmol/l (145 mg/dl).

CHRONIC RENAL DISEASE PATIENTS

Fertility and the ability to sustain an uncomplicated pregnancy generally relate to the degree of functional impairment and the presence or absence of hypertension rather than to the renal lesion. Women can be arbitrarily considered in three categories[1,2]:

(1) Those with preserved or only mildly impaired renal function (serum creatinine ≤ 125 μmol/l or ≤ 1.4 mg/dl) and no hypertension;

(2) Those with moderate renal insufficiency (serum creatinine 125–250 μmol/l or 1.5–3 mg/dl (some use 221 μmol/l or 2.5 mg/dl as the upper limit)); and

(3) Those with severe renal insufficiency (serum creatinine ≥ 250 μmol/l or 2.5 mg/dl), usually with hypertension.

Women in the first category usually have successful obstetric outcomes and pregnancy does not appear to affect adversely the underlying disease; perinatal mortality in this group is now less than 3% and irreversible renal function loss in the mother is negligible[3–5]. This generalization, however, may not hold true for certain kidney diseases: for instance, patients with scleroderma and periarteritis nodosa, disorders often associated with hypertension, do poorly, and pregnancy in such women is best discouraged[3]. Women with lupus nephritis do not do as well as patients with primary glomerulopathies, especially if the disease has flared within 6 months of conception. Although there is still some controversy about whether or not pregnancy adversely affects the natural history of immunoglobulin A (IgA) nephritis, focal glomerular sclerosis, membranoproliferative nephritis and reflex nephropathy, the current view is that there is little supporting evidence for an ill-effect.

In general, across the three categories described, the message is that the worse the renal dysfunction, with or without hypertension, the worse the outcomes[3,6] (Table 1).

A 1996 analysis[6] of 67 women/82 pregnancies with moderate and severe disease from tertiary centers is important. Whilst maternal complications occurred in 70% and pregnancy related renal function loss in almost 50% (of whom 10% progressed rapidly to end-stage failure), the infant survival rate was over 90%, presumably reflecting the specialist obstetric and neonatal care in those centers.

Renal function

If, at any stage of pregnancy, renal function deteriorates significantly, then reversible causes, such as urinary infection, subtle dehydration and/or electrolyte imbalance (occasionally precipitated by inadvertent diuretic therapy) should be sought. Near term, as in normal pregnancy, a decrease in function of 15–20%, which affects serum creatinine minimally, is permissible[1]. Failure to detect a reversible cause of a significant decrement is a reason to deliver. When proteinuria occurs and persists, but blood pressure is normal and renal function preserved, pregnancy can be allowed to continue[3].

Blood pressure

During pregnancy, most of the specific risks of hypertension appear to be related to superimposed pre-eclampsia[7]. The true incidence of superimposed pre-eclampsia in women with pre-existing renal disease is difficult to establish because diagnosis cannot be made with certainty on clinical grounds alone; hypertension and proteinuria may be manifestations of the underlying renal disease. Treatment of mild hypertension (diastolic blood pressure below 95 mmHg in the second trimester or less than 100 mmHg in the third) is not necessary during normal pregnancy[8], but many would treat women with underlying renal disease more aggressively, believing that this preserves kidney function[9].

Fetal well-being and timing of delivery

Serial fetal surveillance is essential since renal disease can be associated with intrauterine growth retardation and, when complications do arise, the judicious moment for intervention must be judged in relation to fetal status (the same also applies to dialysis and transplant patients). Current technology should minimize the incidence of intrauterine fetal death as well as neonatal morbidity and mortality. Preterm delivery may be needed if there is evidence of impending intrauterine fetal death, if renal function deteriorates substantially, or if uncontrollable hypertension or eclampsia supervenes.

DIALYSIS PATIENTS

Despite reduced libido and relative infertility, women on hemodialysis and peritoneal dialysis can conceive and must therefore use contraception if they wish to avoid pregnancy[10]. Although conception is not common (an incidence of 1

Table 1 Severity of renal disease and prospects for pregnancy. Estimates are based on 2310 women/3425 pregnancies (1973–1995) and do not include collagen diseases. Numbers in parentheses refer to prospects when complication(s) develop before 28 weeks gestation (reference 1 and Davison, J. M. and Baylis, C., unpublished data)

Prospects	Renal disease category		
	Mild	Moderate	Severe
Pregnancy complications (%)	26	47	86
Successful obstetric outcome (%)	96 (85)	90 (59)	25 (71)
Long-term sequelae (%)	< 3 (9)	25 (71)	53 (92)

153

in 200 patients has been quoted), its true frequency is unknown because most pregnancies in dialyzed patients probably end in early spontaneous abortion and there is a high therapeutic abortion rate in this group. Pregnancy is 2–3 times less common in peritoneal dialysis patients than in hemodialysis patients[11].

Some women do achieve delivery of a viable infant and indeed some authorities think of childbearing as a goal of rehabilitation rather than a disconcerting accident[8]. Others, however, do not advise attempts at pregnancy or its continuation if present when the woman has severe renal insufficiency. These women are prone to volume overload, severe exacerbations of their hypertension and/or superimposed pre-eclampsia as well as polyhydramnios. They also have high fetal wastage at all stages in pregnancy. Even when therapeutic terminations are excluded, the live birth outcome at very best is 40–50%[1].

Women frequently present for care in advanced pregnancy because pregnancy was not suspected. Irregular menstruation is common in dialysis patients and missed periods are usually ignored. Urine pregnancy tests are unreliable (even if there is any urine available). Ultrasound is needed to confirm and to date the pregnancy.

It could be argued that if dialysis is used in pregnancy, then peritoneal dialysis is the method of choice because theoretically it should maintain a more stable environment for the fetus in terms of fluid and electrolyte homeostasis and cardiovascular stability[12]. Whatever the route, the dialysis strategy involves a 50% increase in hours and frequency and several aims[13,14]:

(1) Maintain serum urea < 20 mmol/l (120 mg/dl); some would argue < 15 mmol/l (90 mg/dl), as intrauterine death is more likely if levels are much in excess of 20 mmol/l. Success has occasionally been achieved despite levels of 25 mmol/l (150 mg/dl) for many weeks.

(2) Avoid hypotension during dialysis, which could be damaging to the fetus. In late

pregnancy the uterus and the supine posture may aggravate this by decreasing venous return.

(3) Ensure strict control of blood pressure.

(4) Avoid rapid fluctuations in intravascular volume, by limiting interdialysis weight gain to about 1 kg until late pregnancy.

(5) Scrutinize carefully for preterm labor, as dialysis and uterine contractions are associated.

(6) Watch calcium levels closely to avoid hypercalcemia.

Dialysis patients are usually anemic, which is invariably aggravated further in pregnancy. Blood transfusion may be needed, especially before delivery. Caution is necessary because transfusion may exacerbate hypertension and impair the ability to control circulatory overload, even with extra dialysis. Treatment of anemia with low dose synthetic erythropoietin (rHuEpo) has been used in pregnancy without ill-effect[15] and, indeed, requirements may double or triple.

KIDNEY TRANSPLANT PATIENTS

After transplantation, women's renal, endocrine and sexual functions return rapidly. About one in 50 women of child-bearing age with a functioning transplant becomes pregnant. Of the conceptions, 35% do not go beyond the first trimester because of spontaneous or therapeutic abortion. However, over 90% of pregnancies that do continue past early pregnancy end successfully[16] (Table 2).

A woman should be counselled from the time the various treatments for renal failure and the potential for optimal rehabilitation are discussed. Couples who want a child should be encouraged to discuss all the implications, including the harsh realities of maternal survival prospects[17,18]. In most, a wait of 18 months to 2 years post-transplant is advised. By then, the patient will have recovered from the surgery, graft function will have stabilized and immuno-

Table 2 Renal transplant patients and prospects for pregnancy. Estimates based on 3690 women in 4680 pregnancies which attained at least 28 weeks gestation (1961–1996). Figures in parentheses refer to implications when complication(s) developed prior to 28 weeks gestation (Davison, J. M. and Baylis, C., unpublished data)

Problems in pregnancy	Successful obstetric outcome	Problems in long-term
49%	94% (70%)	12% (25%)

suppression will be at maintenance levels. Also, if function is well maintained at 2 years, there is a high probability of allograft survival at 5 years. A suitable set of guidelines is given here, but the criteria are only relative:

(1) Good general health for about 2 years post-transplant;

(2) Stature compatible with good obstetric outcome;

(3) No or minimal proteinuria;

(4) No hypertension;

(5) No evidence of graft rejection;

(6) No pelvicalcyeal distension on a recent intravenous urography and/or ultrasound;

(7) Stable renal function with serum creatinine of 180 μmol/l (2 mg/dl) or less (preferably less than 125 μmol/l (1.4 mg/dl)); and

(8) Drug therapy reduced to maintenance levels: prednisone 15 mg/day or less and azathioprine 2 mg/kg body weight/day or less. Safe doses of cyclosporin-A have not yet been established because of limited clinical experience, but nowadays 5 mg/kg body weight/day or less has been advised. More information will be needed with the advent of the new oral cyclosporin preparation, Neoral[TM] (Sandoz), which has better bio-

availability and more stable pharmacokinetics[19].

The recent literature endorses key facts[1,20–24]. In most women, renal function is augmented during pregnancy, but permanent impairment occurs in 15% of pregnancies. In some there may be transient deterioration in late pregnancy (with or without proteinuria). Despite an overall complication rate of 46%, the chances of success exceed 90% (Table 2). If complications (usually hypertension, renal deterioration and/or rejection) occur before 28 weeks, then successful obstetric outcome is reduced by 20%. There is a 30% chance of developing hypertension, pre-eclampsia or both. Preterm delivery occurs in 46–60% and intrauterine growth retardation in at least 20–40% of pregnancies. Despite its pelvic location, the transplanted kidney rarely produces dystocia and is not injured during vaginal delivery. Cesarean section should be reserved for obstetric reasons only.

Neonatal complications include respiratory distress syndrome, leucopenia, thrombocytopenia, adrenocortical insufficiency and infection. More information is needed about the intrauterine effects and neonatal aftermath of immunosuppression which, at maintenance levels, is apparently harmless.

On balance, the latest data available indicate that pregnancy does not compromise long-term renal prognosis[25–27]. There is also good evidence that repeated pregnancies do not adversely affect graft function and/or fetal development, provided renal function is well preserved prior to pregnancy[24]. Also in the long-term, these patients, like all others on immunosuppression, have a malignancy rate many times greater than normal and the genital tract is no exception[18,28]. The only viable means of studying all types of outcome with post-transplant pregnancies will involve the establishment of a United Kingdom National Registry[29].

References

1. Bayliss, C. and Davison, J. M. (1997). The urinary system. In Broughton Pipkin, P. and Chamberlain, G. V. P. (eds.) *Clinical Physiology in Obstetrics.* (London: Blackwell Publications), in press

2. Jungers, P., Houillier, P., Forget, D., Labrunie, M., Skkiri, H., Giatras, I. and Discamps-Latscha, B. (1995). Influence of pregnancy on the course of primary chronic glomerulonephritis. *Lancet,* **346**, 1–22

3. Lindheimer, M. D. and Katz, A. I. (1994). Gestation in women with kidney disease: prognosis and management. *Bailliere's Clin. Obstet. Gynaecol.,* **8**, 387–404

4. Abe, S. (1996). Pregnancy in glomerulonephritic patients with decreased renal function. *Hypertens. Pregn.* **15**, 305–12

5. Holley, J. L., Bernardini, J., Quadri, K. H. M., Greenberg, A. and Laifer, S. A. (1996). Pregnancy outcomes in a prospective matched control study of pregnancy and renal disease. *Clin. Nephrol.,* **45**, 77–82

6. Jones, D. C. and Hayslett, J. P. (1996). Outcome of pregnancy in women with moderate or severe renal insufficiency. *N. Engl. J. Med.,* **335**, 226–32

7. Lindheimer, M. D. (1996). Pre-eclampsia-eclampsia 1996 preventable? Have the disputes on its treatment been resolved? *Curr. Opin. Nephrol. Hypertens.,* **5**, 452–8

8. Sibai, B. M. (1996). Treatment of hypertension in pregnant women. *N. Engl. J. Med.,* **335**, 257–64

9. Bakris, G. L. (1996). Is the level of arterial pressure reduction important for preservation of renal function. *Nephrol. Dial. Transplant.,* **11**, 2383–97

10. Hou, S. H. (1994). Pregnancy in women on haemodialysis and peritoneal dialysis. *Bailliere's Clin. Obstet. Gynaecol.,* **8**, 481–500

11. Hou, S. H. (1996). Pregnancy in women treated with peritoneal dialysis: viewpoint. *Peritoneal Dial. Int.,* **16**, 442–3

12. Redrow, M., Chereum, L., Elliott, J., Managlet, J., Mishler, R. E., Bennett, W. M., Lutz, M., Sigala, J., Byrnes, J., Philippe, M., Hou, S., Schon, D. (1988). Dialysis in the management of pregnant patients with renal insufficiency. *Medicine,* **67**, 199–208

13. Souqiyyeh, M. Z., Huraib, S. O., Saleh, A. G. M. and Aswad, S. (1992). Pregnancy in chronic hemodialysis patients in the Kingdom of Saudi Arabia. *Am. J. Kidney Dis.,* **19**, 235–8

14. Amoah, E. and Aras, H. (1991). Pregnancy in a hemodialysis patient with no residual renal function. *Am. J. Kidney Dis.,* **17**, 585–7

15. McGregor, E., Stewart, G., Junor, B. J. R. and Rodger, R. S. C. (1991). Successful use of recombinant human erythropoietin in pregnancy. *Nephrol. Dial. Transplant.,* **6**, 292–3

16. Davison, J. M. (1994). Pregnancy in renal allograft recipients: problems, prognosis and practicalities. *Bailliere's Clin. Obstet. Gynaecol.,* **8**, 501–25

17. Davison, J. M. (1995). Towards longterm graft survival in renal transplantation: pregnancy. *Nephrol. Dial. Transplant.,* **10** (Suppl. 1), 85–9

18. London, N., Farmery, S. M., Will, E. J., Davison, A. M. and Lodge, J. P. A. (1995). Risk of neoplasia in renal transplant patients. *Lancet,* **346**, 403–6

19. Holt, D. W., Mueller, E. A., Kovarik, J. M., Vanbree, J. B. and Kutz, K. (1994). The pharmacokinetics of Sandimuun Neoral: a new oral formulation of cyclosporine. *Transplant Proc.,* **26**, 2935–9

20. Ahlswede, K. M., Armenti, V. T. and Morkritz, M. J. (1992). Premature births in female transplant recipients: degree and effect of immunosuppressive regimen. *Surg. Forum,* **443**, 524–5

21. Armenti, V. T., Stefanosky, E. V., Cater, J. R., McGory, C. H., Radomski, J. S. and Moritz, M. J. (1995). Pregnancy in transplant recipients. *J. Transpl. Coord.,* **5**, 130–6

22. Armenti, V. T., Ahlswede, B. A., Moritz, M. J. and Jarrell, B. E. (1993). National Transplantation Registry: analysis of pregnancy outcomes of female kidney recipients with relation to time interval from transplantation to conception. *Transplant Proc.,* **25**, 1036–7

23. Gaughan, W. J., Moritz, M. J., Radomski, J. S., Burke, J. F. and Armenti, V. T. (1996). National Transplantation Pregnancy Registry – Report on outcomes in cyclosporine-treated female recipients with an interval from transplant to pregnancy of greater than 5 years. *Am. J. Kidney Dis.,* **28**, 266–9

24. Ehrich, J. H. H., Loirat, C., Davison, J. M., Rizzoni, G., Wittkop, B., Selwood, N. H. and Mallick, N. P. (1996). Repeated successful pregnancies after kidney transplantation in 102 women. *Nephrol. Dial. Transplant.,* **11**, 1314–22

25. Salmela, K. T., Kyllonen, L. E. J., Holmberg, C. and Granhagen-Riska, C. (1993). Impaired renal function after pregnancy in renal transplant recipients. *Transplantation,* **56**, 1372–5

26. First, M. R., Combs, C. A., Weiskittel, P. and Miodovinik, M. (1995). Lack of effect of pregnancy on renal allograft survival or function. *Transplantation*, **59**, 472–7

27. Sturgiss, S. N. and Davison, J. M. (1995). Effect of pregnancy on long-term function of renal allografts. *Am. J. Kidney Dis.*, **26**, 54–6

28. Opelz, G. (1996). Are post-transplant lymphomas inevitable? *Nephrol. Dial. Transplant.*, **11**, 1952–5

29. Davison, J. M. and Redman, C. W. G. (1997). Pregnancy post-transplant: the establishment of a UK Registry. *Br. J. Obstet. Gynaecol*, in press

Postnatal screening for inherited metabolic disorders

24

A. Green

INTRODUCTION

Neonatal screening for phenylketonuria (PKU) and congenital hypothyroidism (CHT) is an established service in most developed countries. Most programs use capillary blood collected as dried blood within the first week of life. Although it is possible to screen for many other inherited metabolic disorders (IMD) using this same specimen, there has not been widespread or uniform introduction of additional testing. The range of disorders which can be screened are listed in Table 1. Many European countries and states of the United States screen for galactosemia, homocystinuria, maple syrup urine disease and biotinidase deficiency. In contrast in the UK, only screening for PKU and CHT are provided universally with coverage for other disorders being patchy.

Table 1 Disorders which can be detected by existing neonatal screening programs

Phenylketonuria
Congenital hypothyroidism
Cystic fibrosis
Galactosemia
Maple syrup urine disease
Homocystinuria
Tyrosinemia
Congenital adrenal hyperplasia
Biotinidase deficiency
Muscular dystrophy
Hyperlipidemia
Sickle cell disease (β thalassemia)
Glucose-6-phosphate dehydrogenase deficiency

SCREENING CRITERIA

The decision to introduce programs for particular disorders has largely been influenced by the extent to which the screening criteria published in 1968 by Wilson and Jungner[1] are satisfied.

The availability of suitable (i.e. robust, capable of automation for large specimen numbers and realistic cost) screening technology and treatment which has a demonstrable effect on morbidity/mortality are of particular significance in assessing the case for screening for each particular disorder.

SCREENING TECHNOLOGIES

To date, screening technologies have largely been based on microbiological, chromatographic or chemical techniques. In particular, development of immunoassays with radioisotopic, enzymatic or fluorescence end-points has contributed to the development of new programs. Some commercially available systems have the potential to perform more than one assay simultaneously in a single dried blood spot.

Molecular biology

More recently, molecular biology-based methods have become applicable to dried blood spots[2–4] and have opened up enormous possibilities. For most disorders, however, it is likely that primary DNA screening will be limited due to the relatively high cost of this technology, and the time consuming nature of the techniques which do not lend themselves readily to large scale automation. Only for those disorders where there is a single mutation responsible for the majority of cases is it feasible to use DNA testing (e.g. G895 for medium-chain acyl-CoA dehydrogenase deficiency) as the primary screen. As a secondary tier, then DNA testing is useful (e.g. cystic fibrosis) and this approach is likely to be extended in a limited way for other disorders. An issue arising from disease screening by DNA analysis is how to deal with the consequence of diagnosing carriers of the disease, i.e. the need for genetic counselling and family testing.

Tandem mass spectrometry

The major technological advance which is likely to influence neonatal screening in the near future is tandem mass spectrometry (MS-MS). This allows the analysis of complex mixtures and a significant advance has been its application to biological fluids for the diagnosis of IMD. Use of this technique for quantitation of amino acids and acyl carnitines in small volume dried blood spots was first described in 1991[5]. More recently, the ability to use this technique for the specific diagnosis of certain amino acid and organic acid disorders has been described by the same group[6–8].

Tandem mass spectrometry has the capability for automation and use for large scale screening. The analytes are ionized by a soft ionization technique which minimizes fragmentation. The molecular ions are selected in the first mass spectrometer quadrupole and undergo collision induced fragmentation in a second mass spectrometer. Selection of appropriate scanning functions enables daughter ions of a specific molecular ion to be detected and quantified.

Tandem mass spectrometry is highly specific even in complex biological mixtures, and, by computer control, multiple analyses of several chemical classes (e.g. amino acids, acyl carnitines) in the same specimen can be achieved in less than 2 min per specimen. Accurate methods have been developed by Chace and Millington[6–8] in Pennsylvania, USA, and newborn screening tandem mass spectrometry has been introduced and is used in a limited setting in the USA. Disorders capable of being detected by MS-MS are listed in Table 2.

Table 2 Diagnosis of inherited metabolic disorders using tandem mass spectrometry for newborn screening

Chemical class	Diseases capable of detection
Amino acid	phenylketonuria maple syrup urine disease argininosuccinic aciduria tyrosinemia type 1 homocystinuria ornithine carbamoyltransferase deficiency and other urea cycle defects (by secondary increase in glutamine and alanine) citrullinemia hyperornithinemias
Acylcarnitine	propionic acidemia methylmalonic acidemias isovaleric acidemia glutaric acidemia type 1 glutaric acidemia type 2 3-hydroxy-3-methylglutaryl-CoA lyase deficiency 3-methylcrotonyl-CoA carboxylase deficiency branched-chain ketothiolase deficiency medium-chain acyl-CoA dehydrogenase deficiency 3-hydroxy long-chain acyl-CoA dehydrogenase deficiency carnitine palmitoyltransferase type 2 deficiency

Additional applications for the future include the possibility of diagnosis of disorders presenting as liver dysfunction in the neonate (e.g. biliary atresia) by analysis of bile acid conjugates/conjugated bilirubin.

TREATMENT FOR METABOLIC DISORDERS

The treatment approaches for metabolic disorders have developed considerably over recent years. In particular, transplantations (liver/bone marrow) are now significant options for certain disorders[9]. Implantation of fetal cells *in utero* and gene therapy are exciting possibilities for the future.

The prospects for treating IMD are enormous and to optimize the potential for such treatments early diagnosis will be important. The case for early diagnosis means that newborn screening will become even more important.

The impact of new screening technologies and new treatment modalities are illustrated by reference to two disorders – medium-chain acyl-CoA dehydrogenase (MCAD) deficiency and tyrosinemia type 1.

Medium-chain acyl-CoA dehydrogenase deficiency

Medium-chain acyl-CoA dehydrogenase (MCAD) is a key enzyme in the energy-producing pathway for the oxidation of fatty acids[10]. Deficiency results in blockage of fatty acid oxidation with resultant hypoglycemia. The disorder usually manifests in infancy following a prolonged fast or increased energy demands due to infection/stress/excessive exercise. Some babies show signs shortly after birth[11]. At its mildest the disease may be a self-limited hypoglycemia episode from which there is full recovery. More usually there are severe abnormalities, often suggestive of Reye's syndrome. In some, death occurs suddenly and unexpectedly.

The treatment of MCAD deficiency is directed towards preventing fasting and providing frequent feeds in time of stress. No special diet is needed. The outlook appears to be good.

Possible screening methods have been developed based on both metabolites analysis and specific mutation analysis[4,12,13]. Recently tandem mass spectrometry for acyl carnitines has been established in the USA[14].

Medium-chain acyl-CoA dehydrogenase deficiency fulfills all the main criteria for a screening program. The main concern is that a proportion of individuals with MCAD deficiency will never experience any ill-effects and there is no way of predicting which individuals these will be. If neonatal screening is introduced, all medium-chain acyl-CoA dehydrogenase deficient babies detected must therefore be treated as being at risk. The treatment is not difficult but the need to carefully monitor intercurrent illnesses for the first few years of life is bound to provoke anxiety for the family. It may be that some of these individuals would otherwise have been well throughout life and gone undetected.

Whole population neonatal screening for medium-chain acyl-CoA dehydrogenase deficiency is at present performed only as part of a supplementary program in Pittsburgh, USA. Pilot studies of tandem mass spectrometry screening, which include medium-chain acyl-CoA dehydrogenase deficiency, have recently started in centers in the UK.

Tyrosinemia type 1

Tyrosinemia type 1 (Tyr 1) is due to deficiency of fumarylacetoacetase (FA) and results in accumulation of characteristic metabolites, particularly succinyl acetone[15]. Patients with Tyr 1 may present with acute liver failure in infancy or with a more chronic disease resulting in hepatocellular carcinoma. For many years a diet low in tyrosine (and phenylalanine) has been the only form of treatment[16]. Such treatment may be life-saving in the acute form of the disease and may 'hold' the disorder for several years. Dietary restriction does not, however, prevent progressive liver damage and development of hepatoma.

Recently, liver transplantation before malignancy develops has proved to be successful[17,18]. Approximately 70 cases have been transplanted with overall success rates of 70–100% from different centers.

NTBC (2- (2-nitro-4-trifluoromethyl benzoyl)-1,3,cyclohexadione

This is a relatively new drug which inhibits 4-hydroxyphenylpyruvate dioxygenase, thereby preventing the formation of the toxic intermediary metabolites which accumulate in Tyr 1. Oral administration of NTBC has proven beneficial clinical effects in this condition[19]. It is now being used to treat approximately 120 patients worldwide. It is not yet known whether NTBC will prevent rather than simply delay the onset of malignancy and whether there are any long term side-effects of the drug itself.

This drug may prove to be the optimal treatment for tyrosinemia, in which case commencement of treatment immediately after birth may be important to totally prevent liver disease. If transplantation becomes the preferred option, then short term (e.g. for 3–6 months) treatment with NTBC may still be important, i.e. until liver transplantation is feasible. Whichever option is chosen, early diagnosis, i.e. via neonatal screening, is likely to be important to enable early treatment and thereby prevent development of significant liver and renal disease.

DISCUSSION

There is no doubt that advances in both technology and treatment are placing new pressures on the case for neonatal screening for several IMDs, with a challenge to the conventional criteria.

This potential for expansion of newborn screening programs is not without its problems and raises many issues.

Which disorders should be screened for?

Disorders can now be screened for which, as yet, have variable outcome (e.g. methylmalonic acidemia) and treatment remains unproven. The early diagnosis of such disorders can lead to genetic counselling and prenatal diagnosis options for subsequent pregnancies and family counselling which might otherwise not have been possible. Early diagnosis can reduce hospitalization and parental anxiety arising from the search for a diagnosis. Is there a case for screening for such disorders?

Information for parents

How much detail about each individual disorder should be provided? The screening principle that the test must be acceptable to the population assumes that there is informed choice. If screening is extended to say 10–20 different disorders which have different treatment potential, management regimens and outcomes, how realistic is it for parents to make *informed* consent to screening for all these different disorders? The sensitivity of the screening program will differ for each disorder. Some cases of particular disorders will be missed by screening and in such situations it is important that parents appreciate the fallibility of such programs.

Specimen collection

The optimal age for screening will not be the same for all disorders; for some, the earlier the better, whereas for others, sensitivity and specificity are optimized by testing later, e.g. 6–10 days. Age at screening will be a compromise for some disorders, resulting in a percentage of cases being missed by the screening process.

Laboratory organization

Provision of new services, i.e. MS-MS, will need to be considered in the context of economies of provision (i.e. centralization to maximize cost effectiveness vs. the advantages of local arrangements). Whatever, it will be important to link screening with diagnosis as a 'seamless' service.

The development of new technology will require careful introduction with protocols for follow-up and quality assurance.

Clinical services

Detection of a whole range of metabolic disorders will impact on the need for clinical services. This will include physician, clinical biochemist and dietetic services. There may be an increased workload overall if cases are detected which would otherwise have been missed. However, for the majority, the cases will simply be detected earlier and a few years after introduction of screening, the service, i.e. diagnosis, start of treatment, will simply have been moved forward from the age of clinical presentation to the first week of life, i.e. diagnosis following screening.

Funding

The funding of such services will require careful consideration by purchasers of healthcare. The costs of the additional screening and the costs and benefits of earlier treatment have to be considered in the context of costs and outcome of late diagnoses.

ACKNOWLEDGEMENTS

I am grateful to Mrs Narinder Virdi for help with the references and to Mrs Sheila Preston for preparation of this manuscript.

References

1. Wilson, J. M. G. and Jungner, G. (1968). *Principles and Practice of Screening and Disease*, pp. 26–39. (Geneva: World Health Organisation),
2. McCabe, E. R. (1994). DNA techniques for screening of inborn errors of metabolism. *Eur. J. Pediatr.*, **153** (7, Suppl. 1), S84–5
3. Seltzer, W. K., Accurso, F., Fall, M. Z., Van Riper, A. J., Descartes, M., Huang, Y. and McCabe, E. R. B. (1991). Screening for cystic fibrosis: feasibility of molecular genetic analysis of dried blood specimens. *Biochem. Med. Metab. Biol.*, **46**, 105–9
4. Seddon, H. R., Gray, G., Pollitt, R. J., Iitiä, A. and Green, A. (1997). Population screening for the common G985 mutation causing medium-chain acyl-CoA dehydrogenase deficiency using europium-labelled oligonucleotides and the DELFIA system. *Clin. Chem.*, in press
5. Millington, D. S., Kodo, N., Terada, N., Roe, D. and Chace, D. H. (1991). The analysis of diagnostic markers of genetic disorders in human blood and urine using tandem mass spectrometry. *Int. J. Mass Spectrom. Ion Process.*, **111**, 211–28
6. Chace, D. H., Millington, D. S., Terada, N., Kahler, S. G., Roe, C. R. and Hofman, L. F. (1993). Rapid diagnosis of phenylketonuria by quantitative analysis for phenylalanine and tyrosine in neonatal blood spots by tandem mass spectrometry. *Clin. Chem.*, **39** (1), 66–71
7. Chace, D. H., Hillman, S. L., Millington, D. S., Kahler, S. G., Roe, C. R. and Naylor, E. W. (1995). Rapid diagnosis of maple syrup urine disease in blood spots from newborns by tandem mass spectrometry. *Clin. Chem.*, **41**, 62–8
8. Chace, D. H., Hillman, S. L., Millington, D. S., Kahler, S. G., Adam, B. W. and Levy, H. L. (1996). Rapid diagnosis of homocystinuria and other hypermethioninemias from newborns' blood spots by tandem mass spectrometry. *Clin. Chem.*, **42**, 349–55
9. Mowat, A. P. (1992). Orthoptic liver transplantation in liver-based metabolic disorders. *Eur. J. Pediatr.*, **151** (Suppl.1), S32–8
10. Roe, C. R. and Coates, P. M. (1995). Mitochondrial fatty acid oxidation disorders. In Scriver, C. R., Beaudet, A. L., Sly, W. S. and Valle, D. (eds.) *The Metabolic and Molecular Bases of Inherited Disease*, 7th edn., pp. 1501–33. (New York: McGraw-Hill)
11. Wilcken, B., Carpentier, K. H. and Hammond, J. (1993). Neonatal symptoms in medium chain acyl coenzyme A dehydrogenase deficiency. *Arch. Dis. Child.*, **69**, 292–4
12. Tuchman, M., McCann, M. T., Johnson, P. E. and Lemieux, B. (1991). Screening newborns for multiple organic acidurias in dried filter paper urine samples: method development. *Pediatr. Res.*, **30** (4), 315–21
13. Bennett, M. J., Regni, M. C., Ostfeld, R. J., Santer, R. and Schmidt-Sommerfeld, E. (1994).

Population screening for medium chain acyl-CoA dehydrogenase deficiency: analysis of medium chain fatty acids and acylglycines in blood spots. *Ann. Clin. Biochem.*, **31**, 72–7

14. Chace, D. H. and Millington, D. S. (1994). Neonatal screening for inborn errors of metabolism by automated dynamic liquid secondary ion tandem mass spectrometry. In Farriaux, J.-P. and Dhondt, J.-L. (eds.) *New Horizons in Neonatal Screening*, pp. 373–6. (Amsterdam: Elsevier Science)

15. Lindblad, B., Lindstedt, S. and Steen, G. (1977). On the enzymic defects in hereditary tyrosinaemia. *Proc. Natl. Acad. Sci. USA*, **74**, 4641–5

16. Michaels, K., Matalon, R. and Wong, P. W. K. (1978). Importance of methionine restriction.

Dietary treatment of tyrosinaemia type 1. *J. Am. Diet. Assoc.*, **73**, 508

17. Paradis, K., Weber, A., Seidman, E. G., Larochelle, J., Garel, L., Lenaerts, C. and Roy, C. C. (1990). Liver transplantation for hereditary tyrosinaemia: the Quebec experience. *Am. J. Hum. Genet.*, **47**, 338–42

18. Wijburg, F. A., Reitsma, W. C. C., Sloof, M. J. H., Van Spronsen, F. J., Koetse, H. A., Reijngoud, D. J., Smit, G. P. A., Berger, R. and Bijleveld, C. M. A. (1995). Liver transplantation in tyrosinaemia type 1: the Groningen experience. *J. Inher. Metab. Dis.*, **18**, 115–18

19. Holme, E., Lindstedt, S. and Lock, E. A. (1995). Treatment of tyrosinaemia type 1 with an enzyme inhibitor (NTBC). *Int. Pediatr.*, **10**(1), 41–3

Pre- and postnatal diagnosis and management of lysosomal disorders

25

W. Endres

Lysosomes are membrane-bound organelles of the cytoplasm. Their main task is the digestion of macromolecules. Most of the lysosomal disorders are due to inherited enzymopenias of the intermediary metabolism within these organelles. In contrast, there are also lysosomal diseases such as cystinosis and the sialic acid storage disorders which are characterized by an impaired transport of acids across the lysosomal membrane.

The purpose of this paper is to give an overview of the diagnostic possibilities of these rather rare diseases *in utero* as well as in early infancy (Table 1), to mention therapeutical attempts (Tables 1 and 2), and to give an idea about their frequency (Table 3). However, it will not be possible to present the enormous clinical variability and biochemical details of these abnormalities[1].

Clinical signs in patients suffering from lysosomal disorders are not pathognomonic, although some features such as progressive neurological and mental deterioration, skeletal deformities, coarse facies and hepatosplenomegaly are found relatively often.

It has to be emphasized that only in a few cases will it be possible to recognize a lysosomal disorder clinically at birth. In most cases an early diagnosis based on clinical signs is most difficult since these signs are non-specific or appear in later childhood. Moreover, in none of these diseases has a routine newborn screening test been established, although some pilot screening studies for certain disorders and their respective carriers have been performed, e.g. for hexosaminidase A deficiency (Tay-Sachs disease)[2]. Most of these diseases must be detected by suspicion and following selective screening.

The mode of inheritance in all these diseases is autosomal recessive, except in mucopolysaccharidosis type II (Hunter disease)[3] and Fabry disease[4] where it is X-linked recessive.

In some disorders it would be advantageous to know the correct diagnosis in early infancy since symptomatic (e.g. cystinosis[5]) or specific therapies (e.g. Gaucher disease[6] and some mucopolysaccharidoses[3]) could be tried and have in part been proved to be effective (Table 2).

In general, the success of treatment in patients suffering from lysosomal disorders appears to be rather limited. Nevertheless, with respect to genetic counselling, the early diagnosis of the index case in a family is desirable before further children are born. If there is an index case in a family the situation is quite different in that for most lysosomal diseases a prenatal diagnosis is possible. There are only a few lysosomal disorders for which prenatal diagnosis (Table 1) is not possible, e.g. in carbohydrate-deficient glycoprotein syndrome[7], or can be carried out only under certain conditions, e.g. in Niemann-Pick disease type C[8], or has not yet been performed but should be possible, e.g. in α-*N*-acetylgalactosaminidase deficiency (Schindler disease)[9].

Most of the lysosomal disorders are very rare (Table 3). However, in distinct ethnic groups certain diseases appear with a higher frequency. For example, in the French province of Brittany the incidence of cystinosis[5] is 1 in 26 000, whereas elsewhere it is less than 1 in 100 000. The incidence of mucopolysaccharidosis type II (Hunter disease)[3] in Israel is 1 in 36 000 and in the Netherlands 1 in 24 000 compared to incidences of around 1 in 100 000 in other countries, and compared to the occurrence of 1 in

Table 1 Diagnosis and therapy in lysosomal diseases

Disease	Prenatal diagnosis	Postnatal diagnosis	Therapy
Lysosomal membrane transport disorders			
Cystinosis	+	+	cysteamine, renal transplantation
Sialic acid storage disorders			
Infantile free sialic acid storage disease	+	+	—
Salla disease	+	+	—
Lysosomal storage disorders			
Glycogenosis type II	+	+	(BMT?) [10,11]
Mucopolysaccharidoses	+	+	BMT
Mucolipidoses II and III	+	+	—
Glycoprotein degradation disorders			
Fucosidosis	+	+	—
α-Mannosidosis	+	+	—
β-Mannosidosis	+	+	—
Aspartylglycosaminuria	+	+	—
Sialidosis	+	+	—
Carbohydrate-deficient glycoprotein syndrome	−	+	—
Wolman disease and cholesteryl ester storage disease	+	+	diet, HMG-CoA reductase inhibitors, liver transplantation
Farber lipogranulomatosis	+	+	corticosteroids, BMT
Niemann-Pick disease types A and B	+	+	BMT
Niemann-Pick disease type C	(+)*	+	cholesterol-lowering drugs
Krabbe disease	+	+	—
Metachromatic leukodystrophy	+	+	eventually BMT
Multiple sulfatase deficiency	+	+	—
Gaucher disease	+	+	alglucerase, ev. splenectomy, BMT
Fabry disease	+	+	analgesia, renal transplantation
G_{M2} gangliosidoses	+	+	(BMT ?)
β-Galactosidase deficiency			
G_{M1} gangliosidosis	+	+	trihexyphenidyl
Morquio B disease	+	+	—
Galactosialidosis	+	+	—
α-*N*-acetylgalactosaminidase deficiency	(+)**	+	—

+, available; −, not available; BMT, bone marrow transplantation; *, restricted to families in which the index case has very low esterification levels; **, should be possible but not yet performed

Table 2 Lysosomal diseases with more or less promising therapies

Disease	Therapy
Cystinosis	symptomatically (Fanconi syndrome), cysteamine, renal transplantation, eventually thyroxine, insulin, pancreatic enzymes, testosterone
Gaucher disease	alglucerase (Ceredase®), partial splenectomy, joint replacement, BMT
Mucopolysaccharidoses	BMT (types I, II, III, IV, VI), (ER and GT in animal models with types I, II, VII)

BMT, bone marrow transplantation; ER, enzyme replacement; GT, gene transfer

Table 3   Incidence of lysosomal diseases[1]

Disease	Incidence (per number of inhabitants or live births, or number of cases known)
Lysosomal membrane transport disorders	
Cystinosis	1 in 100 000–326 440
Sialic acid storage diseases	113 cases from 76 families
Lysosomal storage disorders	
Glycogenosis type II	1 in 50 000–100 000
Mucopolysaccharidoses	1 in 32 300–38 500
Mucolipidoses	a few cases
Glycoprotein degradation disorders	at least 438 cases
Acid lipase deficiencies	at least 90 cases
Farber lipogranulomatosis	43 cases
Niemann-Pick disease types A and B	1 in 40 000–80 000 Ashkenazi Jews
Niemann-Pick disease type C	1 in 40 000–80 000
Krabbe disease	1 in 50 000–200 000
Metachromatic leuko-dystrophy	1 in 40 000–130 000
Multiple sulfatase deficiency	at least 50 cases
Gaucher disease	1 in 10 000
Fabry disease	1 in 40 000
G_{M2} gangliosidoses	1 in 360 000
β-Galactosidase deficiency	
$\quad G_{M1}$ gangliosidosis	some dozen cases
$\quad$Morquio B disease	15 cases from 9 families
Galactosialidosis	65 cases from 53 families
α-*N*-acetylgalactosaminidase deficiency	3 cases from 2 families

30 000 to 1 in 40 000 of all mucopolysaccharidoses together. If we calculate the overall incidence of lysosomal disorders from the respective incidences, excluding those data which reflect just 'number of cases known' (Table 3), we obtain a figure of 1 in 3500–4800, i.e. we have to expect one infant suffering from a lysosomal disorder among about 4000 newborns. This means that even in larger obstetrical units less than one case can be expected per year.

In summary, a routine newborn screening for these diseases is not available. An early diagnosis on a clinical basis is most difficult. Clinical symptoms of many of these diseases are severely progressive. Effective therapies are restricted to a rather modest number of diseases. For almost all abnormalities, prenatal diagnosis is possible.

References

1. Scriver, C. R., Beaudet, A. L., Sly, W. S. and Valle, D. (eds.) (1995). *The Metabolic and Molecular Bases of Inherited Disease*, 7th edn. (New York: McGraw-Hill Inc.)
2. Gravel, R. A., Clarke, J. T. R., Kaback, M. M., Mahuran, D., Sandhoff, K. and Suzuki, K. (1995). The G_{M2} gangliosidoses. In Scriver, C. R., Beaudet, A. L., Sly, W. S. and Valle, D. (eds.) *The Metabolic and Molecular Bases of In-herited Disease*, 7th edn., pp. 3763–97. (New York: McGraw-Hill Inc.)
3. Neufeld, E. F. and Muenzer, J. (1995). The mucopolysaccharidoses. In Scriver, C. R., Beaudet, A. L., Sly, W. S. and Valle, D. (eds.) *The Metabolic and Molecular Bases of Inherited Disease*, 7th edn., pp. 2465–94. (New York: McGraw-Hill Inc.)
4. Desnick, R. J., Ioannou, Y. A. and Eng, C. M. (1995). Alpha-galactosidase A deficiency: Fabry

disease. In Scriver, C. R., Beaudet, A. L., Sly, W. S. and Valle, D. (eds.) *The Metabolic and Molecular Bases of Inherited Disease,* 7th edn., pp. 2741–84. (New York: McGraw-Hill Inc.)

5. Gahl, W. A., Schneider, J. A. and Aula, P. P. (1995). Lysosomal transport disorders: cystinosis and sialic acid storage disorders. In Scriver, C. R., Beaudet, A. L., Sly, W. S. and Valle, D. (eds.) *The Metabolic and Molecular Bases of Inherited Disease,* 7th edn., pp. 3763–97. (New York: McGraw-Hill Inc.)

6. Beutler, E. and Grabowski, G. A. (1995). Gaucher disease. In Scriver, C. R., Beaudet, A. L., Sly, W. S. and Valle, D. (eds.) *The Metabolic and Molecular Bases of Inherited Disease,* 7th edn., pp. 2641–70. (New York: McGraw-Hill Inc.)

7. Thomas, G. H. and Beaudet, A. L. (1995). Disorders of glycoprotein degradation and structure: alpha-mannosidosis, beta-mannosidosis, fucosidosis, sialidosis, aspartylglucosaminuria, and carbohydrate-deficient glycoprotein syndrome. In Scriver, C. R., Beaudet, A. L., Sly, W. S. and Valle, D. (eds.) *The Metabolic and Molecular Bases of Inherited Disease,* 7th edn., pp. 2529–61. (New York: McGraw-Hill Inc.)

8. Pentchev, P. G., Vanier, M. T., Suzuki, K. and Patterson, M. C. (1995). Niemann-Pick disease type C: a cellular cholesterol lipidosis. In Scriver, C. R., Beaudet, A. L., Sly, W. S. and Valle, D. (eds.) *The Metabolic and Molecular Bases of Inherited Disease,* 7th edn., pp. 2625–39 (New York: McGraw-Hill Inc.)

9. Desnick, R. J. and Wang, A. M. (1995). Alpha-*N*-acetylgalactosaminidase deficiency: Schindler disease. In Scriver, C. R., Beaudet, A. L., Sly, W. S. and Valle, D. (eds.) *The Metabolic and Molecular Bases of Inherited Disease,* 7th edn., pp. 2509–28 (New York: McGraw-Hill Inc.)

10. Watson, J. G., Gardner-Medwin, D., Goldfinch, M. E. and Pearson, A. D. J. (1986). Bone marrow transplantation for glycogen storage disease type II (Pompé's disease). *N. Engl. J. Med.,* **314**, 385

11. Hirschhorn, R. (1995). Glycogen storage disease type II: acid alpha-glucosidase (acid maltase) deficiency. In Scriver, C. R., Beaudet, A. L., Sly, W. S. and Valle, D. (eds.) *The Metabolic and Molecular Bases of Inherited Disease,* 7th edn., pp. 2443–64. (New York: McGraw-Hill Inc.)

The neonatal diagnosis and management of inherited metabolic disease

26

J. E. Wraith

INTRODUCTION

Inherited metabolic disease (IMD) is an important cause of neonatal morbidity and mortality, but it is a diagnosis often regarded as a last resort in the sick neonate. Failure to make a diagnosis and start appropriate therapy may lead to severe brain damage or death in the affected patient. In addition the genetic risk to the family is not identified and further affected infants may be born until the cause of the problem is finally identified.

Individual disorders are rare and experience is important if diagnosis and treatment are to proceed smoothly. Expert laboratory services are essential and should be available to all regions. In addition results need interpretation by clinicians specialising in IMD, and prompt clinical consultation is urged to ensure that the diagnosed infant receives the best care. A policy of very aggressive investigation and management is advocated. Some clinicians are uncomfortable with this approach and are concerned about the risk of keeping alive a grossly handicapped infant. In my experience this is very rarely a problem. After a short period of very aggressive treatment one can generally judge the prognosis accurately. If the prospect of return to normal cerebral function is poor, one can be very conservative during a subsequent episode of acute deterioration. The episodic nature of most IMD ensures that treatment can be reassessed at frequent intervals. There will always be a risk of producing survivors with mild to moderate cerebral damage, but this is true of all acute neonatal illnesses, especially those affecting the central nervous system, e.g. neonatal meningitis or symptomatic hypoglycemia.

The detailed management of individual IMD is beyond the scope of this review and only general principles will be discussed. Those who wish further information about individual disorders are directed to the excellent textbook edited by Scriver and colleagues[1].

THE PRESENTATION OF IMD IN THE NEONATAL PERIOD

In the newborn period IMD can come to notice in a number of ways:

(1) As a result of newborn screening, e.g. phenylketonuria. This will not be considered further in this review.

(2) As an acute, severe non-specific illness often associated with acidosis and encephalopathy. These disorders will form the bulk of this review.

(3) With dysmorphic features or multiple congenital anomalies.

CLUES TO THE DIAGNOSIS OF AN IMD

The most important aspect of diagnosis is for the neonatologist to have a high index of suspicion of the possibility of an IMD in a seriously ill neonate. A number of clues can be obtained from the history, examination and simple bedside tests. The assessment begins with a careful scrutiny of the antenatal notes.

The following questions must always be considered.

(1) Is there a history of previous neonatal death or stillbirth?

(2) Are the parents related?

(3) Was there a period of normality after birth?

(4) Has there been a change of feed since birth?

(5) Is there any evidence of infection?

(6) Has the baby been subjected to a fast or a surgical procedure?

(7) Did the baby improve when milk feeds were discontinued?

(8) Was there a relapse on restarting feeds?

With one or two important exceptions (e.g. ornithine transcarbamylase (OTC) deficiency), inheritance is autosomal recessive and a family history of previous neonatal death or parental consanguinity can be important clues. In OTC deficiency there may be a history of male deaths on the maternal side of the family.

Most affected infants are born normally at term, have a normal birth-weight and usually remain well for the first few days of life. This intrauterine protection is due to several mechanisms including the natural fetal anabolic state, the hemodialysis provided by the placenta and the fact that the fetus is not in contact with dietary protein. Following birth there is a period of intense catabolism as well as the onset of protein-containing feeds and together these unmask the metabolic lesion in affected infants. For some disorders primarily affecting the central nervous system, placental protection does not occur, and these disorders, e.g. non-ketotic hyperglycinemia or primary disorders of pyruvate metabolism, will produce symptoms and signs *in utero*, e.g. structural brain malformations or intrauterine seizures as well as severe intrauterine growth retardation.

CLINICAL FEATURES OF IMD PRESENTING ACUTELY IN THE NEONATAL PERIOD

In general the clinical signs and symptoms are non-specific and it is rare to be able to make an exact diagnosis on clinical examination. Rarely the typical odor of maple syrup urine disease, isovaleric acidemia or glutaric aciduria may be noted and infants with classical galactosemia may have cataracts, but with other disorders one is usually faced with a neurologically abnormal infant who rapidly becomes comatose and in whom one is faced with increasing biochemical disturbance.

METABOLIC INVESTIGATIONS IN THE SICK NEONATE

It is urged that the metabolic investigations proceed rapidly in parallel with other tests aimed at detecting infection and other common causes of acute neonatal illness. Simple bedside tests may help. The finding of a very heavy ketonuria in the newborn period is unusual and should be followed by urgent urinary organic acid analysis. The calculation of the plasma anion gap $(Na^+ + K^+) - (Cl^- + HCO_3^-)$, normal 12–16 mmol/l) can be helpful. In those infants in whom it is raised, and especially in those with values > 25 mmol/l a specific organic acid disorder is very likely.

The sample requirements for specific metabolic tests will vary between laboratories. Depending on the clinical presentation investigations as summarized in Tables 1 and 2 are indicated. Before sending samples for detailed metabolic investigations the infant's clinical condition should be discussed with the

Table 1 First-line metabolic investigations in the sick neonate

Full blood count
Urea and electrolytes
Liver function tests
Blood gas
Urine reducing substances
Urine ketones

Table 2 Second line metabolic investigations in the sick neonate

Unexplained encephalopathy or neurological
deterioration
Urine amino acids
Urine organic acids
Plasma amino acids
Blood ammonia
Blood and cerebrospinal fluid (CSF) lactate
Plasma carnitine

Metabolic acidosis
Urine amino acids
Urine organic acids
Plasma amino acids
Blood lactate
Plasma carnitine

Persistent hypoglycemia
Urine amino acids
Urine organic acids
Plasma amino acids
Plasma insulin, C-peptide, cortisol
DNA analysis for medium-chain acyl-CoA dehydro-
genase deficiency (MCAD)
Beutler test (for galactosemia)
Plasma carnitine
If all normal think of possibility of glycogen
storage disease

Liver disease
Urine amino acids
Urine organic acids
Plasma amino acids
Blood lactate
Beutler test
Urine organic acids for succinyl acetone
(tyrosinemia type I)

metabolic consultant. The laboratory should always be telephoned in advance to indicate the urgency of the samples and appropriate rapid transport to the laboratory should be arranged.

MANAGEMENT AT FIRST PRESENTATION WHILST AWAITING RESULTS

The severity of symptoms dictates the aggressiveness of management. For infants with severe symptoms active treatment will be required, and the patient should be transferred to the specialist metabolic unit for management. The principles of management can be summarized as follows:

(1) Supportive care;

(2) Reducing load on affected pathways;

(3) Removal of toxic metabolites;

(4) Stimulation of residual enzyme activity.

Neonatal intensive care will be required, and arterial and central venous lines should be inserted. Respiratory support with early ventilation is advocated with close attention being paid to temperature control, hydration, circulatory support and blood glucose levels. Cerebral edema is often present and should be treated with mannitol. Significant metabolic acidosis (pH < 7.15) should be treated with intravenous (IV) sodium bicarbonate (0.5–2 mmol/h), but careful monitoring of plasma Na^+ will be necessary to avoid hypernatremia.

To reduce the load on affected pathways all exogenous protein should be discontinued. To try to reverse catabolism, insulin (0.05 (U/kg)/h) should be given with dextrose (5–10 (mg/kg)/min) aiming to keep the blood glucose between 7 and 10 mmol/l.

To remove toxic metabolites it is important to try to maintain an adequate urine output although this is often very difficult in the sick neonate. Dialysis (either continuous venovenous hemofiltration or peritoneal dialysis) should be started early especially in those infants with resistant acidosis or significant hyperammonemia (> 400 µmol/l) not responding to IV sodium benzoate (250 mg/kg bolus followed by 250–500 (mg/kg)/day infusion). Intravenous carnitine 100 (mg/kg)/day should be given in either three divided dosages or as a continuous infusion.

Some metabolic disorders respond to vitamin therapy, e.g. vitamin B_{12}-responsive methylmalonic acidemia. In a metabolic crisis, however, the blind use of multi-vitamin cocktails is unlikely to be successful. It is better to wait for the result of the metabolic screening tests and use the specific vitamin once a diagnosis has been established.

MANAGEMENT WHEN DEATH SEEMS INEVITABLE OR THE INFANT DIES DESPITE TREATMENT

Aggressive treatment is still indicated even if no diagnosis is established as some defects will be transient, e.g. transient hyperammonemia of prematurity. If death is inevitable, it is important to obtain as much information about the child as possible. Plasma, urine and/or cerebrospinal fluid (CSF) should be collected and frozen prior to death and a sample of blood should be obtained for DNA extraction. Autopsy is essential, and thought should be given to which tissues should be collected for biochemical studies. If the infant is dysmorphic, photographs should be taken and a skeletal survey performed.

LONG-TERM MANAGEMENT

The detailed management of individual disorders is beyond the scope of this review. In most disorders of intermediary metabolism, management will involve specialist medical, dietary and biochemical services and will consist of:

(1) A dietary regimen tailored to the particular condition;

(2) Continuation of drugs, e.g. sodium benzoate in urea cycle defects as well as vitamins in vitamin responsive disorders;

(3) Carnitine in disorders known to be associated with secondary carnitine deficiency, e.g. organic acidemias;

(4) The provision of a clearly worded emergency regimen giving the parents clear instructions on how to deal with intercurrent infections in an attempt to prevent metabolic decompensation;

(5) Open access to the metabolic ward and advice from the specialist dietician and metabolic consultant.

IMD AS A CAUSE OF DYSMORPHIC FEATURES OR MULTIPLE CONGENITAL ANOMALIES

Many metabolic disorders are associated with dysmorphic manifestations and a metabolic work up should be considered in any undiagnosed infant with multiple congenital anomalies or dysmorphic appearance.

In glutaric aciduria type II, congenital anomalies include a 'Potter-like' facial appearance, abnormal kidneys and genitalia, and anterior abdominal wall defects.

Inherited disorders of peroxisomal biogenesis such as Zellweger's syndrome and rhizomelic chondrodysplasia punctata produce a characteristic syndromic appearance that can be confirmed biochemically.

Deficiency of 3-hydroxyisobutyryl-CoA deacylase and 3-hydroxyisobutyric aciduria are associated with brain dysgenesis due to migrational defects as well as other congenital anomalies. In both of these disorders of valine metabolism a build up of a teratogenic intermediary compound may be responsible for the defects. In other disorders a deficiency of an essential end-product may cause the anomalies. This is seen most dramatically in disorders of central energy metabolism, e.g. primary disorders of pyruvate metabolism, where cystic malformation and structural cerebral defects are common. In the Smith–Lemli–Opitz syndrome, a block in the synthetic pathway of endogenous cholesterol metabolism leads to a disorder characterized by a distinctive facial appearance, cleft palate, hypospadias, polydactyly and often multiple internal malformations. It is likely that many other similar disorders will be shown to have an underlying biochemical basis.

Reference

1. Scriver, C. R., Beaudet, A. L., Sly, W. S. and Valle, D. (eds.) (1995). *The Metabolic and Molecular Bases of Inherited Disease,* 7th edn. (New York: McGraw-Hill)

The pathology of brain damage 27

R. N. Laurini

INTRODUCTION

The aim of this paper is to discuss the morphological findings in the fetal brain that can be of use in helping to decide different forms of clinical management aimed at protecting the perinatal brain. In this context it is important to bear in mind that a growing body of evidence suggests that a significant number of neurohandicaps may be the consequence of prenatal brain damage[1]. Therefore when discussing perinatal brain damage we must remember that the period between conception and 1 year of postnatal life represents a biological continuum. In effect, pathological events occurring early in pregnancy can both influence and/or express themselves in the perinatal as well as the postnatal period.

The main forms of perinatal brain pathology are represented by two major groups of lesions; hemorrhagic and non-hemorrhagic pathology. Moreover, these two major forms of brain damage are frequently combined. The hemorrhagic lesions are commonly represented by subarachnoid hemorrhage (SAH), germinal matrix hemorrhage (GMH), intraventricular hemorrhage (IVH) and other hemorrhagic lesions such as periventricular venous pathology. The non-hemorrhagic pathology consists chiefly of periventricular leukomalacia (PVL) and gray matter necrosis. Notwithstanding, the development of all these lesions will be influenced by the fetal condition at the time of the insult[2] (Table 1). In effect the prognostic significance of any form of brain damage will depend on whether it depicts a truly acute lesion (*de novo*) or whether the damage develops in an already compromised fetal condition (e.g. intrauterine growth retardation, IUGR). Consequently, a neuropathological examination of perinatal brains must try to define the brain condition before any major lesion occurs; that is to say, whether there are any tissue markers present that indicate a possible ancient damage occurring in early pregnancy, or the result of a sustained fetal distress or secondary to a subacute fetal distress that took place shortly before the development of a major form of brain damage[2]. Such an evaluation plays a major role when trying to time brain damage. Indeed, the subject of antenatal as opposed to perinatal origin for postnatal neurohandicap remains controversial. Experience with diagnostic routine suggests that events occurring during the last intrauterine week before birth have a major influence on the perinatal condition. In this context, the morphological findings in the placenta and brain can help time these pathological events. Pathology of the fetoplacental circulation can demonstrate the existence of changes secondary to acute, subacute or chronic fetal distress. Lesions of the uteroplacental circulation usually represent tissue markers of prolonged placental ischemia. A correlation between these placental morphological findings with those of the brain, as well as clinical data (ultrasound, magnetic resonance imaging, Doppler and cardiotocography), will allow for a better timing of the events, in particular of the brain damage.

In addition, it is as important to clearly define the lesions that are associated with major forms of brain damage[2]. In effect, these associate lesions can play a major role in defining the prognosis of the case in terms of an eventual postnatal neurohandicap (Figure 1). Hence when assessing perinatal brain pathology, one must take into consideration the main pathology of the fetus or the newborn and its correlation with the pathology of the placenta and of the brain in the same case. Table 1 shows a series of 28 preterm cases where the common forms of neonatal main pathology were seen in association with two main groups of placental pathology (ischemia and chorioamnionitis) as well as acute, subacute and chronic brain pathology. The large total number of observed brain lesions clearly illustrates that different forms of pathology can be present in the same case. Only this type of correlation allows for a complete assessment of the individual case. Furthermore, it illustrates once again the importance of chorioamnionitis in terms of prematurity and related perinatal brain damage.

A detailed morphological examination of the perinatal brain by a specialized pathologist confirms that major forms of brain pathology, such as GMH and PVL frequently occur in combination with other significant forms of brain damage, such as periventricular venous lesions, pathological gliosis and even abnormal corticacation[2]. A recent review of 30 perinatal brains showed, in total, the presence of 16 GMH/IVH, 11 periventricular venous lesions, four PVL, 13 pathological gliosis and four abnormal cortication.

Furthermore, there is much to gain from a routine correlation between the morphological patterns seen with sonography and those encountered at postmortem. In the hands of specialized professionals, there is a good correlation between ultrasound and morphological findings with regard to hemorrhagic lesions such as GMH, IVH and parenchymal hemorrhage. The correlation can be less evident for

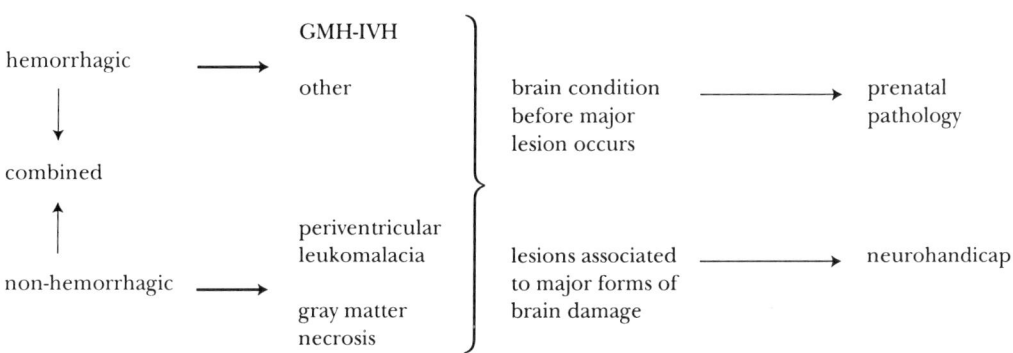

GMH, germinal matrix hemorrhage; IVH, intraventricular hemorrhage

Figure 1   Perinatal brain pathology (from reference 2)

Table 1   Morphological findings in 28 preterm infants (six pairs of twins). Number in parentheses refer to total number of observed lesions

Main pathology	Placenta (n = 20)	Brain (n = 28)
Hyaline membrane disease	ischemia (6)	acute (23) (hemorrhages)
Bronchopulmonary dysplasia		
Pulmonary hemorrhage	chorioamnionitis (12)	
Acute interstitial pulmonary emphysema		subacute/chronic (12)
Lung hypoplasia	normal (2)	(periventricular leukomalacia 3)
Lung immaturity		(gliosis 9)
Necrotizing enterocolitis		
Others		

Table 2 Main types of brain hemorrhages

Falx/tentorium
Meningeal congestion
Subdural hemorrhage
Subarachnoid hemorrhage
Subpial hemorrhage
Germinal matrix hemorrhage
Intraventricular hemorrhage
Choroid plexus hemorrhage
Periventricular venous congestion
Periventricular venous infarction
Hemorrhagic periventricular leukomalacia
Cerebellar hemorrhage

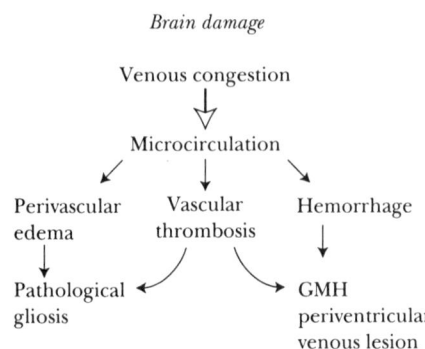

Figure 2 Effects of venous congestion on the microcirculation. GMH, germinal matrix hemorrhage

certain hemorrhagic lesions such as isolated germinal matrix hemorrhage, isolated or peripherally situated parenchymal hemorrhage and choroid plexus hemorrhage. Nevertheless, there is a poor correlation when dealing with microscopic areas of PVL and pathological gliosis.

Although the major forms of hemorrhagic lesions are well known, it is still important to make allusion to the number of different forms of hemorrhagic lesions that can be observed, in addition to germinal matrix and intraventricular hemorrhage (Table 2). In this context, I would like to underline the importance of the frequent finding of periventricular venous lesions in the form of periventricular radial venous congestion (PVVC), periventricular radial venous hemorrhage (PVVH) and periventricular venous infarction (PVVI). Little attention is usually paid to the existence of these periventricular venous lesions that can occur as isolated lesions or, frequently, accompany other major forms of brain pathology such as GMH and IVH. Moreover, foci of periventricular radial venous congestion can represent the morphological equivalent of the transient periventricular echodensities seen on ultrasound. Nowadays there is sufficient evidence to confirm a relationship between periventricular venous lesions and different forms of neurohandicap[3]. As a matter of fact, even transient periventricular echodensities can have clinical significance

in terms of neurohandicap, as recently shown by Levene and colleagues[4].

Much has been published on the pathogenesis of brain damage following a reduction in cerebral perfusion. However, there is also a need to define the way venous congestion, a common event in asphyxia, can influence the development of different forms of brain damage. Figure 2 illustrates the way venous congestion affects the microcirculation, giving rise to hemorrhagic lesions, vascular thrombosis and perivascular edema. The development of perivascular edema represents an important complication because it helps to destroy the blood/brain barrier, giving rise to focal perivascular white matter destruction. The author has previously postulated that this lesion plays a major role in the development of pathological gliosis[1]. Moreover, experimental work also shows that the destruction of the brain/blood barrier gives rise to pathological gliosis[5,6].

Pathological gliosis represents an important form of hypoxic-ischemic brain damage. It is characterized by the presence of reactive astrocytes which are hypertrophic glial cells with thick fibrillary processes and an increased expression of glial-fibrillary-acidic protein (GFAP). The main sites of pathological gliosis in the perinatal brain are: subpial, centrum semiovale, basal ganglia, germinal matrix, granular ependymitis and cerebellum.

The importance of pathological gliosis rests on the fact that it replaces myelination gliosis and therefore gives rise to migration defects and delayed myelinization. Essentially, radial glia transform into pathological glia, affecting their capacity to direct neuronal migration and this reduces the number of glial cells available for myelination.

In the context of pathological gliosis, it is important to bear in mind that there can be a transient form as well as a permanent form. In effect, if pathological gliosis develops without structural damage, it can represent a transitory phenomenon[5]. On the other hand, if there is structural brain damage, gliosis can persist in the form of a glial scar.

Pathological gliosis, PVL and granular ependymitis are important tissue markers of hypoxic–ischemic events in the fetal, perinatal and postnatal brain. Their presence is a sign that one or several episodes of fetal distress were serious enough to cause brain damage. Although a number of brain lesions can be timed within a given range[2], one must be aware that pathological gliosis can be difficult to time, mainly because it is not necessarily associated with a chronic condition. It can also develop after an episode of asphyxia and/or hypoperfusion severe enough to give rise to brain damage[1]. This concept is of cardinal importance in view of the frequent and undiscriminating use of the terms 'acute', 'subacute' and 'chronic'. A hemorrhage is not always purely an acute phenomenon (e.g. hemorrhagic PVL) and gliosis is not a chronic lesion by definition (e.g. pathological gliosis 3 days after an episode of fetal asphyxia).

Periventricular leukomalacia represents a necrosis of the white matter with a hypoxic–ischemic character and is preferentially localized to the border zones of the main arterial territories, in the boundary between ventriculofugal and ventriculopetal cerebral arteries. When hemorrhage develops in an area of PVL, it is diffuse and not distinctly perivascular. In this context, it is of clinical importance to distinguish between periventricular venous infarction and hemorrhagic PVL. In effect, periventricular venous infarction is characterized by the absence of underlying ischemic lesions and the presence of perivascular hemorrhage with white matter damage limited to the surrounding cerebral tissue, and absence of diffuse pathological gliosis as seen surrounding areas of PVL.

Recent work has demonstrated that infected amniotic fluid syndrome, with chorioamnionitis as its morphological expression, is frequently associated with prematurity and its complications[7]. This association is further shown in Table 1, confirming the significant incidence of chorioamnionitis in perinatal pathology. In addition, Leviton[8] has recently proposed a correlation between infected amniotic fluid syndrome (chorioamnionitis) and the development of PVL. In effect, a fetomaternal infection can be associated with an increase in prostaglandins as well as tumor necrosis factor, both of which can play a major role in the development of hemorrhagic and non-hemorrhagic brain damage. In my view, the frequent association between chorioamnionitis and fetal brain hemorrhage results from the biochemical cascade, including prostaglandins, released by the inflammatory process. The hemorrhagic brain damage present in these fetuses is identical with that observed after the use of prostaglandins for termination of pregnancy[1].

A recent review of 55 brain hemorrhages, in the period between 23 weeks gestation and term, showed a significant relationship with chorioamnionitis and/or positive microbiology. Table 3 summarizes these findings. Moreover, if

Table 3 Review of 55 brain hemorrhages, from 23 weeks gestation to term, and their relationship with chorioamnionitis and/or positive microbiology

	With chorioamnionitis	With positive microbiology	Without chorioamnionitis or positive microbiology
All hemorrhages	26	17	12
Major forms	21	10	12

Table 4 Relationship between non-hemorrhagic brain damage and chorioamnionitis or only positive microbiology

	With chorioamnionitis	*Only positive microbiology*	*Without chorioamnionitis or positive microbiology*	*Total*
Pathological gliosis	4	4	1	9
Periventricular leukomalacia	—	1	1	2

Table 5 Relationship between non-hemorrhagic brain damage and abruptio placentae

	*With abruptio placentae** ($n = 19$)	*Without abruptio placentae* ($n = 30$)
Pathological gliosis	2 (10.5%)	7 (23.3%)
Periventricular leukomalacia	1 (5.3%)	1 (3.3%)

*14/19 cases showed a chorioamnionitis or a positive microbiology

we considered only the major forms (SAH, GMH, IVH, PVVI and hemorrhagic PVL) of brain hemorrhages, we observed that this significant relationship between brain hemorrhage and chorioamnionitis–positive microbiology was still present.

Furthermore, a detailed study of these 55 perinatal brains by means of GFAP staining has shown that pathological gliosis is significantly associated with the presence of chorioamnionitis and positive microbiology (Table 4). Interestingly enough, this group of perinatal cases included 20 abruptio placentae, 14 of which were associated with chorioamnionitis–positive microbiology. Nevertheless, we were not able to confirm recent results[9] that placental abruption is a significant antenatal risk factor for the development of PVL and extensive periventricular hemorrhage (Table 5). Notwithstanding, one must bear in mind that abruptio placentae can be the result of an acute process (e.g. an infection) or a terminal complication of a chronic process (e.g. decidual vasculopathy)[10].

The former can be too acute for brain damage to develop, while the latter is at a higher risk for the development of brain lesions.

Finally, I would like to comment on the concept of the brain-sparing effect as representing a protective mechanism against brain damage during asphyxia. In the view of this author, the mere existence of such a redistribution already indicates the presence of a pathological condition.

Although it is agreed that this mechanism can reduce the deleterious effect of hypoxia, it is no guarantee that it will prevent tissue damage. Recent work[11] suggests that morphological markers of brain damage can develop despite the existence of a brain-sparing effect. Birth asphyxia may therefore be better defined if end-organ damage is added to the other parameters such as Apgar score and pH. In effect, the presence of an organ lesion and dysfunction is what permits confirmation of the pathological character of the condition.

References

1. Laurini, R. N. (1994). Fetal brain pathology. In Kurjak, A. and Chervenak, F. A. (eds.) *The Fetus as a Patient*, pp. 89–106. (New York and London: The Parthenon Publishing Group)

2. Laurini, R. N. (1993). The perinatal postmortem. In Spencer, J. A. D. and Ward, R. H. T. (eds.) *Intrapartum Fetal Surveillance*, pp. 199–212. (London: RCOG Press)

3. Volpe, J. J. (1989). Intraventricular hemorrhage and brain injury in the premature infant. *Clin. Perinatol.*, **16**(2), 361–86

4. Levene, M., Dowling, S., Graham, M., Fogelman, K., Galton, M. and Philips, M. (1992). Impaired motor function (clumsiness) in 5 year old children: correlation with neonatal ultrasound scans. *Arch. Dis. Child.*, **67**, 687–90

5. Goodlett, C. R., Leo, T. J., O'Callaghan, P. O., Mahoney, J. C. and West, J. R. (1993). Transient cortical astrogliosis induced by alcohol exposure during neonatal brain growth spurts in rats. *Dev. Brain Res.*, **72**, 85–97

6. Norton, W. T., Aquino, D. A., Hozumi, I., Chiu, F.-C. and Brosnan, C. F. (1992). Quantitative aspects of reactive gliosis: a review. *Neurochem. Res.*, **17**, 877–85

7. Romero, R., Sirtori, M., Oyarzun, E., Avila, C., Mazor, M., Callahan, R., Sabo, V., Athanassiadis, A. P. and Hobbins, J. C. (1989). Infection and labor. V. Prevalence, microbiology, and clinical significance of intraamniotic infection in women with preterm labor and intact membranes. *Am. J. Obstet. Gynecol.*, **161**, 817–24

8. Leviton, A. (1993). Preterm birth and cerebral palsy: is tumor necrosis factor the missing link? *Dev. Med. Child Neurol.*, **35**, 549–58

9. Gibbs, J. M. and Weindling, A. M. (1994). Neonatal intracranial lesions following placental abruption. *Eur. J. Ped.*, **153**, 195–7

10. Laurini, R. N. (1996). Abruptio placentae: from early pregnancy to term. In Chervenak, F. A. and Kurjak, A. (eds.) *Current Perspectives on the Fetus as a Patient*, pp. 433–44. (New York and London: The Parthenon Publishing Group)

11. Akalin-Sel, T., Bewleys, S., van Geijn, H. P., Laurini, R. N. and Nicolaides, K. H. (1993). The significance of MCA Doppler assessment in preterminal decompensation of the severely growth retarded fetus. Presented at the *2nd World Congress of Perinatal Medicine*, September, Rome

Protection of the fetal/infant brain: free radicals and antioxidants

28

O. D. Saugstad

INTRODUCTION

Birth asphyxia still represents a major cause of brain impairment. Globally more than 3% of live births (approximately 4 million) suffer moderate to severe birth asphyxia annually. Of these, approximately one million will die and another million develop sequelae such as mental retardation, cerebral palsy, epilepsia and learning disabilities[1]. A number of mechanisms may injure the perinatal brain and in recent years there has been an increasing interest in the role of free radicals and antioxidants.

Oxygen free radicals can be generated by a number of sources during, for instance, metabolism of hypoxanthine, catecholamines and arachidonic acid, and they can be produced by activated phagocytes, and in mitochondriae during reduction of oxygen to water in the respiratory chain[2].

Free radicals have a number of characteristics and a few of them are listed in Table 1. Many free radicals have a half-life of only a fraction of a second. They are highly reactive and may initiate chain reactions, so although each free radical is short lived their effects might well last over a longer period of time. They injure cellular membranes by lipid peroxidation and are also capable of oxidizing proteins. They can injure DNA and there are also accumulating data demonstrating a role in apoptosis or programmed cell death.

FREE RADICALS AND APOPTOSIS/ PROGRAMMED CELL DEATH

It has been shown that both the presence of oxygen radicals and depletion of antioxidants can initiate programmed cell death (PCD), which also can be inhibited by antioxidants. It seems that free radicals play a role in the activation phase of PCD where both oxygen radical dependent and independent pathways have been described. Of interest is the fact that B cell lymphoma leukemia-2 (Bcl-2), a major inhibitor of PCD, is also a powerful antioxidant. The execution phase of PCD seems to be independent of free radicals (for review see reference 3). This new knowledge concerning a possible relationship between free radicals and PCD could explain why apoptosis seems to occur in brains exposed to hypoxia–reoxygenation.

ROLE OF HYPOXANTHINE– XANTHINE OXIDASE

The hypoxanthine–xanthine oxidase system, together with activated phagocytes, have been especially highlighted in the discussion of hypoxia–reoxygenation injury. It has been known for more than 20 years that hypoxanthine accumulates in hypoxia[4] and also in the brain[5]. Xanthine oxidase is, however, not present in the brain in the human[6] (for review see

Table 1 Some characteristics of free radicals

Extremely short lived
Highly reactive
Initiate chain reactions
Injure cellular membranes
Inactivate enzymes
Degrade proteins
Injure DNA
Induce programmed cell death

reference 7). We have postulated that xanthine oxidase is released from the liver and intestine during hypoxia and shock[8,9] and several investigators have shown that this occurs[10–13]. In fact, quite recently, Supnet and colleagues[14] were able to demonstrate that xanthine oxidase is present in the blood of newborn infants. In infants with 'poor outcome', the xanthine oxidase activity, as well as the concentration of lipid peroxidation products, were significantly increased in infants with so-called poor outcome compared with normal controls at 4 h of age. These results only indicate that an interesting relationship between xanthine oxidase activity in blood, lipid peroxidation and outcome may exist.

Recently Feet and co-workers[15] could demonstrate by application of the microdialysis technique in newborn piglet brains that animals exposed to hypoxia and resuscitated with 100% oxygen had a slower normalization of brain hypoxanthine concentration than piglets resuscitated with room air. This might indicate an impairment of energy metabolism when 100% oxygen is used during resuscitation. A number of potentially harmful effects of 100% oxygen during resuscitation have been described both clinically and experimentally. Table 2 summarizes some of these[16].

DEFENSE AGAINST FREE RADICALS: ANTIOXIDANTS

A number of defense systems have been described. In the lung and kidney a maturation of antioxyenzymes such as superoxide dismutases, glutathione peroxidase and catalase seems to occur near term in animal fetuses[23,24].

Glutathione is a major intracellular antioxidant and is found in high concentrations (millimolar) in eukaryotic cells. Glutathione

Table 2 Some effects of using 100% oxygen during resuscitation (clinical and experimental data)

Reduced oxygen consumption[17,18]
Impaired intracellular energy production[15,19]
Reduced cerebral blood flow[20]
Reduced neurological survival[21,22]

is the substrate for glutathione peroxidase, which catalyzes oxidation of reduced to oxidized glutathione at the expense of hydrogen peroxide. Recently Vina and associates[25] found that the rate of glutathione synthesis from methionine is strongly reduced in preterm infants compared with term ones. In addition, Phylactos and colleagues[26] could demonstrate by using a sensitive technique that preterm infants with a gestational age of 29–34 weeks had only 50% of the activity of Cu/Zn superoxide dismutase in cord erythrocytes compared with term infants. These data therefore suggest that the intracellular defense against free radicals is also low in fetal life in the human infant. A preterm baby is therefore more vulnerable to attack from free radicals than a term baby. These recent data can therefore explain, at least partly, the high susceptibility of preterm infants to oxidative stress. Animal data from the brain, however, have not shown a developmental pattern such as that found in the lung. For instance, Mishra and Delivoria-Papadopoulos[27] could not find any change in brain superoxide dismutase activity in the fetal guinea pig.

FREE RADICALS AND NITRIC OXIDE DURING HYPOXIA AND REOXYGENATION

Quite recently Bågenholm and co-workers[28] showed that free radicals are produced in excess in the brain during ischemia–reperfusion. These investigators could detect a significant increase in the concentration of the stable free radical form of the trapping agent 2-ethyl-3 hydroxy-2, 4-trimethyloxazolidine (OXANOH) in the rat brain after reperfusion following 30 min of bilateral carotid ligation.

During hypoxia and reoxygenation, excitatory amino acids are released from the presynaptic neuronal membrane and calcium enters the neurons through glutamate activated channels. Calcium induces a number of enzymes in the neuron such as nitric oxide synthase. Thus the production of nitric oxide (NO) might increase. Nitric oxide reacts with superoxide

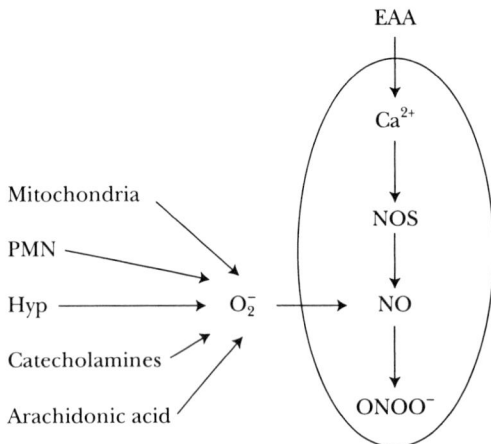

Figure 1 The superoxide radical O_2^- can be generated from a number of sources such as in mitochondrial respiration, activated polymorphonuclear leukocytes (PMN), oxidation of hypoxanthine (Hyp) and of catecholamines, and metabolism of arachidonic acid. In relation to hypoxia, excitatory amino acids (EAA) such as glutamate are released from the presynaptic membrane and activate glutamate receptors postsynaptically, resulting in an increased influx of calcium (Ca^{2+}), which induces a number of enzymes in the neuron, for instance nitric oxide synthase (NOS). The NO produced in this process may react with superoxide radicals and form peroxynitrite ($ONOO^-$) which is toxic in itself and also can decompose and form the toxic hydroxyl radical

radicals (Figure 1) and may generate the toxic peroxynitrite radical ($ONOO^-$)[29], which can decompose into the toxic hydroxyl radical. This can explain a close link between hypoxia and reoxygenation on the one hand, and the effect of excitatory amino acids on the neurons on the other hand. A close link between hypoxia/reoxygenation and neuronal cell injury can therefore now be established, at least theoretically. The clinical relevance of this is, however, not yet clarified.

CONSEQUENCES FOR BRAIN PROTECTION

This new knowledge has a number of possible therapeutic implications. We have shown that resuscitation can be carried out with room air just as efficiently as 100% oxygen both in experimental animal and human studies[30–33]. Perhaps the use of ambient air can reduce the production of free radicals in the reoxygenation period? Blockers of excitatory amino acids may be used in the future, as well as a number of antioxidants and free radical blockers. For instance, the xanthine oxidase blocker allopurinol also increases the adenosine level, which is brain protective; it might increase the adenine nucleotide pool in the brain, and it acts as an antioxidant *per se*.

CONCLUSION

Free radicals can be generated from a number of sources and they have numerous effects. In several organs in different species there seems to be an induction of antioxyenzymes at the end of fetal life. However, the situation in the brain is not very well characterized in this respect. Following asphyxia, excitatory amino acids activate, for instance, N-methyl-D-aspartate receptors so that calcium enters the neurons and an induction of enzymes such as nitric oxide synthase occurs with an increased production of nitric oxide. Oxygen radicals and nitric oxide can react and produce toxic metabolites such as peroxynitrite and the hydroxyl radical. A link between hypoxia/reoxygenation injury and neuronal damage caused by excitatory amino acids is therefore, at least theoretically, established. Knowledge of these mechanisms may produce a number of therapeutic consequences in the future.

References

1. World Health Organisation (1991). *Child Health and Development: Health of the Newborn.* (Geneva: World Health Organisation)
2. Saugstad, O. D. (1996). Mechanisms of tissue injury by oxygen radicals: implications for neonatal disease. *Acta Paediatr.*, **85**, 1–4
3. Jacobson, M. D. (1996). Reactive oxygen species and programmed cell death. *Trends Bioch. Sci.*, **243**, 83–6
4. Saugstad, O. D. (1975). Hypoxanthine as a measurement of hypoxia. *Pediatr. Res.*, **9**, 158–61
5. Saugstad, O. D. and Schrader, H. (1978). The determination of inosine and hypoxanthine in the rat brain during normothermic and hypothermic anoxia. *Acta Neurol. Scand.*, **57**, 281–8
6. Saksela, M. and Raivio, K. (1995). Expression of xanthine oxidase (XO) in relation to perinatal organ damage. *Pediatr. Res.*, **37**, 235 A
7. Saugstad, O. D. (1996). Role of xanthine oxidase and its inhibitor in hypoxia:reoxygenation injury. *Pediatrics*, **98**, 103–7
8. Saugstad, O. D. and Gluck, L. (1982). Plasma hypoxanthine levels in newborn infants: a specific indicator of hypoxia. *J. Perinat. Med.*, **10**, 266–72
9. Saugstad, O. D. (1985). Oxygen radicals and pulmonary damage. *Pediatr. Pulmonol.*, **1**, 167–75
10. Grum, C. M., Ragsdale, R. A., Ketai, L. H. and Simon, R. H. (1987). Plasma xanthine oxidase in patients with adult respiratory distress syndrome. *J. Crit. Care*, **2**, 22–6
11. Yokoyma, Y., Beckman, J. S., Beckman, T. K., Wheat, T. K., Cash, T. G., Freeman, B. A. and Parks, D. A. (1990). Circulating xanthine oxidase: potential mediators of ischemic injury. *Am. J. Physiol.*, **258**, G564–70
12. Friedl, H. P., Smith, D. J., Till, G. O., Thompson, P. D., Louise, D. S. and Ward, P. A. (1990). Ischemia-reperfusion in humans. Appearance of xanthine oxidase activity. *Am. J. Pathol.*, **136**, 491–5
13. Rootwelt, T., Almaas, R., Øyasaeter, S., Moen, A. and Saugstad, O. D. (1995). Release of xanthine oxidase to the systemic circulation during resuscitation from severe hypoxemia in newborn pigs. *Acta Paediatr.*, **85**, 507–11
14. Supnet, M. C., David-Cu, R. and Walther, F. J. (1994). Plasma xanthine oxidase and lipid hydroperoxide levels in preterm infants. *Pediatr. Res.*, **36**, 283–7
15. Feet, B. A., Xiang-Quing, Y., Øyasæter, S., Rootwelt, T. and Saugstad, O. D. (1996). Effects of hypoxia and resuscitation with 21% and 100% O_2 in newborn piglets: extracellular hypoxanthine (Hx) in brain cortex and femoral muscle. *Pediatr. Res.*, **39**, 208A
16. Saugstad, O. D. (1996). Resuscitation of newborn infants: do we need new guidelines? *Prenat. Neonat. Med.*, **1**, 26–8
17. Lodato, R. F. (1989). Decreased O_2 consumption and cardiac output during normobaric hyperoxia in conscious dogs. *J. Appl. Physiol.*, **67**, 1551–9
18. Reinhart, K., Bloos, F., Konig, F., Bredle, D. and Hannemann, L. (1991). Reversible decrease of oxygen consumption by hyperoxia. *Chest*, **99**, 690–4
19. Goplerud, J. M., Kim, S. and Delivoria-Papadopoulos, M. (1995). The effect of postasphyxial reoxygenation with 21% vs. 100% oxygen on Na^+, K^+-ATPase activity in striatum of newborn piglets. *Brain Res.*, **696**, 161–4
20. Lundstrøm, K., Pryds, O. and Greisen, G. (1995). Oxygen at birth and prolonged cerebral vasoconstriction in preterm infants. *Arch. Dis. Child.*, **73**, F81–6
21. Mickel, H. S., Vaishnav, Y. N., Kempski, O., Von Lubitz, D., Weiss, J. F. and Feuerstein, G. (1987). Breathing 100% oxygen after global brain ischemia in Mongolian gerbils results in increased lipid peroxidation and increased mortality. *Stroke*, **18**, 426–30
22. Zwemer, C. F., Whitesall, S. E. and D'Alecy, L. G. (1994). Cardiopulmonary-cerebral resuscitation with 100% oxygen exacerbates neurological dysfunction following nine minutes of normothermic cardiac arrest in dogs. *Resuscitation*, **27**, 159–70
23. Frank, L. and Groseclose, E. E. (1984). Preparation for birth into an O_2-rich environment: the antioxidant enzymes in the developing rabbit. *Pediatr. Res.*, **18**, 240–4
24. Hayashibe, H., Asayama, K., Dobashi, K. and Kato, K. (1990). Prenatal development of antioxidant enzymes in the developing rabbit lung. *Pediatr. Res.*, **27**, 472–5
25. Vina, J., Vento, M., Garcia-Sala, F., Puertes, I. R., Gasco, E., Sastre, J., Asensi, M. and Pallardo, F. V. (1995). L-cysteine and glutathione metabolism are impaired in premature infants due to cystathionase deficiency. *Am. J. Clin. Nutr.*, **61**, 1067–9
26. Phylactos, A. C., Leaf, A. A., Costeloe, K. and Crawford, M. A. (1995). Erythrocyte cupric/zinc superoxide dismutase exhibits reduced activity

in preterm and low birthweight infants at birth. *Acta Paediatr.*, **84**, 1421–5

27. Mishra, O. P. and Delivoria-Papadopoulos, M. (1988). Anti-oxidant enzymes in fetal guinea pig brain during development and the effect of maternal hypoxia. *Brain Res.*, **470**, 173–9

28. Bågenholm, R., Nilsson, U. A., Goteborg, C. W. and Kjellmer, I. (1996). Free radicals are formed in the brain of the fetal sheep during reperfusion after cerebral ischemia. In Bågenholm, R. (ed.) Hypoxic ischemic brain damage in the immature animal. PhD Thesis, Goteborg University

29. Beckman, J. S. (1991). The double-edged role of nitric oxide in brain function and superoxide-mediated injury. *J. Dev. Physiol.*, **15**, 53–9

30. Poulsen, J. P., Øyasæter, S. and Saugstad, O. D. (1993). Hypoxanthine, xanthine and uric acid in newborn pigs during hypoxemia followed by resuscitation with room air or 100% oxygen. *Crit. Care Med.*, **21**, 1058–65

31. Rootwelt, T., Løberg, E. M., Moen, A., Øyasæter, S. and Saugstad, O. D. (1992). Hypoxemia and reoxygenation with 21% or 100% oxygen in newborn pigs: changes in blood pressure, base deficit, and hypoxanthine and brain morphology, *Pediatr. Res.*, **32**, 107–13

32. Rootwelt, T., Odden, J.-P., Hall, C., Ganes, T. and Saugstad, O. D. (1993). Cerebral blood flow and evoked potentials during reoxygenation with 21% or 100% O_2 in newborn pigs. *J. Appl. Physiol.*, **75**, 2054–60

33. Ramji, S., Ahuja, S., Thirupuram, S., Rootwelt, T., Rooth, G. and Saugstad, O. D. (1993). Resuscitation of asphyxic newborn infants with room air or 100% oxygen. *Pediatr. Res.*, **34**, 809–12

Non-invasive investigation of cerebral oxygenation

29

J. S. Wyatt

INTRODUCTION

Despite improvements in perinatal care, hypoxic–ischemic injury to the brain remains an important cause of death and permanent neurodevelopmenal impairment in both term and preterm infants. Near infrared spectroscopy (NIRS) has the potential to provide non-invasive assessment of cerebral oxygenation and perfusion in the sick infant undergoing intensive care and in the fetus during labor. The aim of this article is to review recent findings from the clinical application of NIRS and to assess the likely implications of future technical developments in this rapidly changing area.

PRINCIPLES OF NIRS

The relative transparency of biological tissue to light in the near infrared part of the spectrum (700–1000 nm) enables photons to be detected following passage through tissue at distances of up to 8 cm. As the light passes through the head it is attenuated due to a combination of absorption and scattering. The only near infrared absorbers (chromophores) which are present in variable concentrations are oxy- and deoxyhemoglobin, and the oxidized form of the copper A moiety of cytochrome oxidase, the terminal member of the mitochondrial respiratory chain (see Figure 1).

During continuous transillumination of the brain, any changes in attenuation must be due to changes in the concentration of one or more of the chromophores, provided that the distance travelled by the photons (the optical pathlength) is constant. By obtaining attenuation data at several different wavelengths, it is possible to convert attenuation changes into concentration changes, provided that the optical pathlength is known[1].

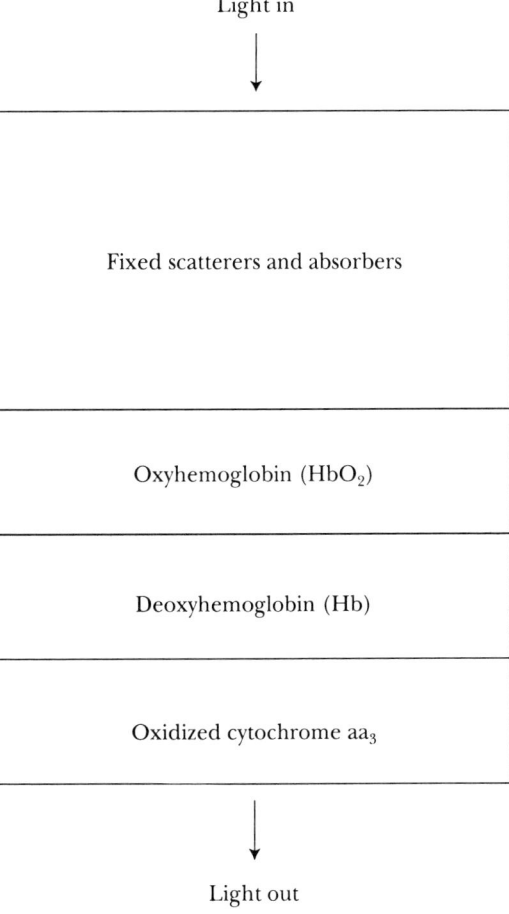

Figure 1 Schematic diagram of scatterers and absorbers within brain tissue

Until recently it was not possible to measure the optical pathlength directly at the bedside. Quantitative NIRS therefore depended on the use of a calibration constant (called the differential pathlength factor) obtained from previous 'time of flight' measurements in postmortem infants[2,3]. An estimate of optical pathlength is obtained by multiplying the distance between the transmitting and receiving optical fibers by this constant.

NIRS STUDIES IN NEWBORN INFANTS

Using this approach, a number of groups have obtained quantitative measurements from the brain in newborn infants undergoing intensive care[4-7]. Techniques have been developed for the measurement of a number of important hemodynamic variables including global cerebral blood flow (CBF), cerebral blood volume (CBV), its response to changing arterial carbon dioxide tension and mixed cerebral venous saturation[8-12].

Measurements of CBF in very preterm infants undergoing intensive care have been shown a remarkably wide range of values, from 5 to 30 ml $100g^{-1}$ min^{-1}. This degree of biological variability is consistent with data obtained using the intravenous ^{133}Xe technique[13]. In one recent study, no relationship between CBF and mean arterial blood pressure was found, suggesting that autoregulation of cerebral perfusion remained intact at arterial blood pressures between 24 and 30 mmHg[14]. Although it remains likely that there is a critical lower limit of CBF required to maintain cellular integrity, in follow-up studies no clear relationship between CBF measurements and long-term neurodevelopmental outcome has as yet been demonstrated. In one recent study, however, infants who went on to develop major periventricular hemorrhage had lower CBF on the first day of life compared with controls[15]. Appropriately grown very preterm infants demonstrated a consistent rise in CBF over the first 3 days of life, probably representing a normal adaptive response of the cerebral circulation to delivery[16]. By contrast,

there was no evidence of a similar consistent pattern in a group of infants with objective evidence of intrauterine growth failure. Some of these growth retarded infants had an elevated CBF on the first day of life, possibly indicating cerebral vasodilatation secondary to prolonged intrauterine hypoxia[16].

Although NIRS has obvious potential as a research tool for investigating cerebral hemodynamics, concerns remain about errors in the estimation of optical pathlength and the possibility that pathlength changes during NIRS measurements may lead to significant inaccuracies[17,18]. New techniques capable of measuring optical pathlength continuously will be required to address these issues (see below).

NIRS STUDIES IN THE FETUS

A number of preliminary studies have demonstrated the feasibility of obtaining quantitative information about cerebral oxygenation in human fetuses undergoing labor[19,20]. Using a specially designed flexible probe which may be inserted through the dilated cervix following rupture of the amniotic membranes, continuous measurements of oxy- and deoxyhemoglobin may be obtained throughout labor. The probe is maintained in position on the fetal scalp by suction.

Large changes in cerebral hemoglobin concentration are observed during uterine contractions, due to the effect of the mechanical forces of labor on the fetal cranium[19]. Mean cerebral saturation ($SmcO_2$) may be estimated from the ratio of oxy- and deoxyhemoglobin in the blood entering and leaving the field of illumination. In a study of 31 infants undergoing uncomplicated labor, $SmcO_2$ measured within 30 min of delivery had a wide range of 22–73%[21]. However, a close correlation with umbilical cord acid–base measurements at delivery was observed (see Figure 2). These preliminary observations suggest that measurement of $SmcO_2$ during labor may be of value for intrapartum fetal surveillance, provided that the reliability of these observations is validated in large scale clinical trials.

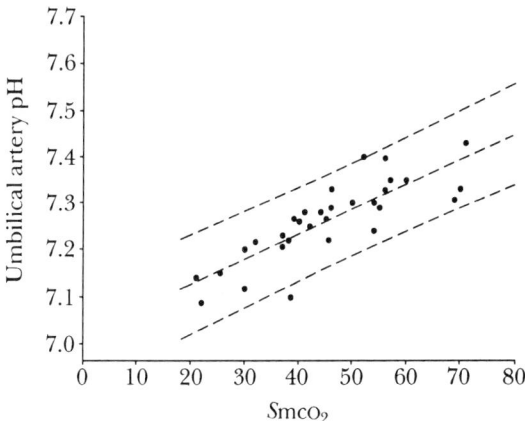

Figure 2 Correlation between fetal mean cerebral saturation ($SmcO_2$) measured within 30 min of delivery and umbilical artery pH at birth. The regression line and 95% confidence intervals of the data points are shown (reprinted from reference 21)

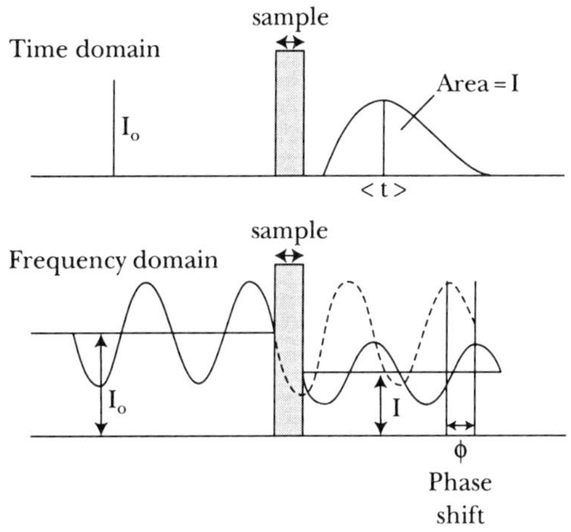

Figure 3 Principles underlying measurement of optical pathlength using time of flight method (upper panel) and phase shift method (lower panel)

RECENT TECHNICAL ADVANCES IN NIRS

Intensity modulated optical spectroscopy

Anxieties about the possibility that NIRS measurements during labor may be influenced by movement artefact have been expressed[22]. In order to investigate this issue we have employed new apparatus capable of continuous measurement of optical pathlength. This device, known as an intensity modulated optical spectrometer, uses very high frequency modulation of the incident light. By measuring the phase differences between the incident and transmitted light, as well as the amount of attenuation, it is possible to obtain simultaneous calculation of chromophore concentrations and optical pathlength[23] (see Figure 3). Preliminary observations in three fetuses have indicated that pathlength changes during uterine contractions are small (less than 5%) (unpublished observations). Although these results need to be verified in larger studies, they suggest that it is unlikely that major errors will result from movement of the optical probe or from pathlength changes during uterine contractions.

Wideband continuous wave spectroscopy

A white light source and a wideband spectrometer coupled to a sensitive light detector has recently been used for NIRS of the infant brain[24]. This technique has several advantages. First, because data are obtained simultaneously at more than 100 discrete wavelengths, curve fitting techniques can be used to improve the accuracy of chromophore measurements. This is particularly useful in determining changes in the redox state of cytochrome oxidase. Second, the optical pathlength can be measured continuously by second derivative spectroscopy using the absorption peak caused by tissue water. Third, by detecting the unique spectral features of the deoxyhemoglobin spectrum, it is possible to obtain absolute quantification of deoxyhemoglobin within the brain. Preliminary results in 19 newborn infants gave a mean differential pathlength factor of 3.91 ± 0.75 and a mean deoxyhemoglobin concentration of $14.6 \pm 4.0 \, \mu mol/l$[24].

By combining these measurements with the calculation of total hemoglobin concentration, the mean saturation of blood within the brain can be obtained, providing a useful and continuous index of the adequacy of cerebral oxygen delivery. Thus, this technique enables both cerebral oxygen saturation and blood volume to be measured continuously at the bedside, allowing the effects on the brain of clinical interventions such as changes in ventilator settings or inotrope infusions to be assessed in real time.

A similar technique has recently been applied to an experimental newborn animal model of delayed energy failure following transient hypoxia–ischemia[25]. Marked cerebral vasodilatation with a rise in mean cerebral saturation was seen during the development of delayed cerebral energy failure. A progressive decline in the redox state of cytochrome oxidase correlated very closely with simultaneous measurements of adenosine triphosphate concentrations obtained by phosphorus magnetic resonance spectroscopy. These data suggest that wideband NIRS may be capable of providing quantitative information on cerebral energetics as well as oxygenation.

NIRS imaging of the neonatal brain

Development of NIRS apparatus designed to obtain two-dimensional images of cerebral absorption and scattering is taking place very rapidly. Van Houten and co-workers[26] recently described the first use of an imaging spectrometer which was capable of providing a two-dimensional image of the neonatal brain, although the collection of a single image took several hours. Within the next few years it is likely that multichannel imaging spectrometers will become widely available, enabling detailed spatial information on cerebral oxygenation and perfusion to be obtained rapidly and conveniently at the bedside.

ACKNOWLEDGEMENTS

The author acknowledges the major contribution of colleagues in the Departments of Paediatrics, Medical Physics and Bioengineering, and Obstetrics and Gynaecology, University College London. This work is supported by the Medical Research Council, Wellcome Trust and Action Research.

References

1. Wray, S. C., Cope, M., Delpy, D. T., Wyatt, J. S. and Reynolds, E. O. R. (1988). Characterisation of the near infrared absorption spectra of cytochrome aa3 and haemoglobin for the non-invasive monitoring of cerebral oxygenation. *Biochem. Biophys. Acta*, **933**, 184–92
2. Delpy, D. T., Cope, M., van der Zee, P., Arridge, S. R., Wray, S. C. and Wyatt, J. S. (1988). Estimation of optical pathlength through tissue by direct time of flight measurement. *Phys. Med. Biol.*, **33**, 1433–42
3. Wyatt, J. S., Cope, M., Delpy, D. T., van der Zee, P., Arridge, S. R., Edwards, A D. and Reynolds, E. O. R. (1990). Measurement of optical pathlength for cerebral near infrared spectroscopy in newborn infants. *Dev. Neurosci.*, **12**, 140–4
4. Edwards, A. D., Wyatt, J. S., Richardson, C., Potter, A., Cope, M., Delpy, D. T. and Reynolds, E. O. R. (1991). Effects of indomethacin on cerebral haemodynamics in very preterm infants. *Lancet*, **335**, 1491–5
5. Pryds, O., Greisen, G., Skov, L. L. and Friis-Hansen, B. (1990). Carbon dioxide related changes in cerebral blood volume and cerebral blood flow in mechanically ventilated preterm neonates. Comparison of near infared spectrophotometry and 133 xenon clearance. *Pediatr. Res.*, **27**, 445–9
6. Livera, L.N., Spencer, S. A., Thorniley, M. S., Wickramsinghe, Y. A. B. D. and Rolfe, P. (1991). The effects of hypoxaemia and bradycardia on neonatal cerebral haemodynamics. *Arch. Dis. Child.*, **66**, 376–80
7. Bucher, H. U., Edwards, A. D., Lipp, A. E. and Duc, G. (1993). Comparison between near infrared spectroscopy and xenon clearance for estimation of cerebral blood flow in critically ill preterm infants. *Pediatr. Res.*, **33**, 56–60

8. Edwards, A. D., Wyatt, J. S., Richardson, C., Delpy, D. T., Cope, M. and Reynolds, E. O. R. (1988). Cotside measurement of cerebral blood flow in ill newborn infants by near infared spectroscopy. *Lancet*, **2**, 770–1

9. Wyatt, J. S., Cope, M., Delpy, D. T., Richrdson, C., Edwards, A. D., Wray, S. C. and Reynolds, E. O. R. (1990). Quantitation of cerebral blood volume in newborn infants by near infrared spectroscopy. *J. Appl. Physiol.*, **68**, 1086–91

10. Wyatt, J. S., Edwards, A. D., Cope, M., Delpy, D. T., McCormick, D. C., Potter, A. and Reynolds, E. O. R. (1991). Response of cerebral blood volume to changes in arterial carbon dioxide tension in preterm and term infants. *Pediatr. Res.*, **29**, 553–7

11. Skov, L., Pryds, O., Greisen, G. and Lou, H. (1993). Estimation of cerebral venous saturation in newborn infants by near infrared spectroscopy. *Pediatr. Res.*, **33**, 52–5

12. Yoxall, C. W., Weindling, A. M., Dawani, N. H. and Peart, I. (1995). Measurement of cerebral venous oxyhaemoglobin saturation in children by near infared spectroscopy and partial jugular venous occlusion. *Pediatr. Res.*, **38**, 319–23

13. Skov, L., Pryds, O. and Greisen, G. (1991). Estimating cerebral blood flow in newborn infants: comparison of near infared spectroscopy and ^{133}Xe clearance. *Pediatr. Res.*, **30**, 570–3

14. Tyszczuk, L., Meek, J. H. and Wyatt, J. S. (1995). Cerebral blood flow measured by near infrared spectroscopy in hypotensive preterm infants (abstract). *Proceedings Neonatal Society*, London June

15. Meek, J. H., Tyszczuk, L. and Wyatt, J. S. (1996). Low cerebral blood flow is a risk factor for severe intraventricular haemorrhage (abstract). *Pediatr. Res.*, **40**, 542A

16. Meek, J. H., Elwell, C. E., Reynolds, E. O. R. and Wyatt, J. S. (1995). Effect of intrauterine growth retardation on postnatal cerebral haemodynamics (abstract). *Pediatr. Res.*, **38**, 443A

17. Brun, N. C. and Greisen, G. (1994). Cerebrovascular responses to carbon dioxide as detected by near infrared spectrophotometry: comparison of three different measures. *Pediatr. Res.*, **36**, 20–4

18. Skov, L. and Greisen, G. (1994). Apparent cerebral cytochrome aa3 reduction during cardiopulmonary bypass in hypoxaemic children with cogenital heart disease. A critical analysis of *in vivo* near infrared spectrophotometric data. *Physiol. Meas.*, **15**, 447–57

19. Peebles, D. M., Edwards, A. D., Wyatt, J. S., Bishop, A. P., Cope, M., Delpy, D. T. and Reynolds, E. O. R. (1992). Changes in human fetal cerebral hemoglobin concentration and oxygenation during labour measured by near-infrared spectroscopy. *Am. J. Obstet. Gynecol.*, **166**, 1369–73

20. Faris, F., Doyle, M., Wickramsinghe, Y. A. B. D, Houston, R., Rolfe, P. and O'Brien, S. (1994). A noninvasive optical technique for intrapartum fetal monitoring: preliminary clinical studies. *Med. Eng. Phys.*, **16**, 287–91

21. Aldrich, C J., D'Antona, D., Wyatt, J. S., Spencer, J. A. D., Peebles, D. M. and Reynolds, E. O. R. (1994). Fetal cerebral oxygenation measured by near infrared spectroscopy shortly before birth and acid-base status at birth. *Obstet. Gynecol.*, **84**, 861–6

22. Hamilton, R. J., O'Brien, P. M. S., Wickramsinghe, Y. A. B. D. and Rolfe, P. (1995). Intrapartum fetal cerebral near infrared spectroscopy: apparent change in oxygenation demonstrated in a non-viable fetus. *Br. J. Obstet. Gynaecol.*, **102**, 1004–7

23. Duncan, A., Whitlock, T. L., Cope, M. and Delpy, D. T. (1993). A multiwavelength, wideband, intensity modulated optical spectrometer for near infrared spectroscopy and imaging. *Proc. Soc. Photo-optical Instrument. Eng.*, **1888**, 248–57

24. Cooper, C. E., Elwell, C. E., Meek, J. H., Matcher, S. J., Wyatt, J. S., Cope, M. and Delpy, D. T. (1996). The noninvasive measurement of absolute cerebral deoxyhemoglobin concentration and mean optical pathlength in the neonatal brain by second derivative infrared spectroscopy. *Pediatr. Res.*, **39**, 32–8

25. Springett, R., Tyszczuk, L., Penrice, J., Amess, P., Cooper, C., Delpy, D. T. and Wyatt, J. S. (1996). Cytochrome oxidase redox state correlates with the severity of delayed cerebral energy failure following transient hypoxia-ischemia in the newborn piglet (abstract). *Pediatr. Res.*, **40**, 553A

26. van Houten, J. P., Benaron, D. A., Spilman, S. and Stevenson, D. K. (1996). Imaging brain injury using time- resolved near infrared light scanning. *Pediatr. Res.*, **39**, 470–6

Blood–brain barrier in the neonatal period

30

P. Temesvári

Perinatal brain damage occurs frequently in cardiovascularly compromised, distressed and infected newborn infants. Both circulatory and metabolic changes seriously affect the brain microvasculature, the blood–brain barrier playing a fundamental role in the pathogenesis of secondary edema and bleeding. Blood–brain barrier permeability changes during neonatal diseases lead to marked alterations in the extracellular fluid space of the brain, resulting in an abnormal perineuronal milieu and neuronal cell death. Still, many questions remained to be experimentally tested. Because there is a distinct paucity of *in vivo* observations on the effects of cardiorespiratory collapse and bacterial components on the blood–brain barrier in the newborn period, we followed the permeability changes of cerebral microvessels intravitally during the early phases of experimentally induced pneumothorax and of meningeal bacterial infection in piglets and 14-day-old rats. 'Open cranial window' technique was used to visualize the piglets' pial-arachnoidal microvessels by fluorescein dyes of different molecular weight. These microvessels correspond in many respects (permeability and vasoreactivity) to the intraparenchymal ones, and recent evidence indicates that the microvasculature of piglets' brains is an excellent model for examining microvascular changes during the newborn period. Moreover, pneumothorax and bacterial meningitis remain the commonest clinical complications of neonatal distress, leading to death even in spite of the most modern therapeutic interventions. Different mediators taking part in brain edema formation were also experimentally tested.

RESULTS OBTAINED IN PIGLETS WITH EXPERIMENTALLY INDUCED PNEUMOTHORAX

Pial-arachnoidal microvessels (diameters 30–210 μm) were intravitally studied by fluorescent microscopy and compared to the hypoxanthine (HX) level of cisternal cerebrospinal fluid (CSF) in the course of pneumothorax, using low (sodium-fluorescein, molecular weight 376) and large molecular weight (fluorescein-labelled dextran, molecular weight 40 000) fluorescent tracer molecules at different stages of the clinical conditions: basal (B; physiological laboratory values); critical (C; severe acidosis, bradycardia, arterial hypotension and hypoxemia); and recovery (R; mild metabolic acidosis, tachycardia, arterial hypotension)[1–3]. At stage B neither low nor large molecular weight tracers penetrated the blood–brain barrier. The low molecular weight tracer passed the blood–brain barrier as a spotty leakage at stage C and diffuse fluorescein penetration was seen at stage R. Large molecular weight tracer escaped from the brain microvasculature only at stage R. The HX content in the CSF was significantly elevated at stage C. At stage R, it proved to be lower than at stage C, but still remained elevated.

RESULTS OBTAINED IN PIGLETS AND RATS WITH EXPERIMENTAL MENINGEAL BACTERIAL INFECTIONS

Piglets

Escherichia coli lipopolysaccharide given intracisternally

Newborn piglets were given 20 or 200 ng endotoxin into the cisterna cerebellomedullaris[4].

188

Spotty sodium fluorescein extravasations occurred in both groups after the endotoxin injections (time elapsed: 20 ng, 70.5 min; 200 ng, 55.2 min, mean values). A dose-dependent increase in sodium fluorescein uptake was also found by fluorescence spectrophotometry in different brain regions. Endotoxin-treated piglets had developed pleiocytosis, whereas there was no change in the white blood cell (WBC) count of peripheral blood samples. Sixty minutes after the intracisternal injection, endotoxin content measured by *Limulus* amebocyte lysate assay was mildly elevated in the CSF in both animal groups.

Elastase (EC 3.4.21.37) given intracisternally

The porcine enzyme elastase (dose 1.0 μg) resulted in spotty sodium fluorescein extravasation in pial venules in all treated animals 78 min (mean value) after the challenge. The concentration of elastase-α1-proteinase inhibitor complex increased significantly in CSF samples 4 h after the injection, while it did not change in sera. Pleiocytosis and leukocytosis were also observed[5].

14-day-old rats

Cerebrospinal fluid was obtained from the cisterna cerebellomedullaris and 200 ng/kg body weight of *Escherichia coli* endotoxin was given intracisternally. Four hours later cisternal CSF was sampled and WBC and protein concentration were determined. Vasopressin levels in plasma and CSF (measured by radioimmunoassay), plasma and urine osmolality were also measured. Expression of the vasopressin messenger RNA (mRNA) in the nucleus supraopticus (NSO) and paraventricularis (NPV) was investigated on brain cryostat sections by *in situ* hybridization analyses. A highly significant pleiocytosis and elevation of CSF protein concentration developed 4 h after the challenge. Significantly increased vasopressin mRNA levels were observed in the NSO. There were no significant differences in vasopressin mRNA levels in the NPV, and in the vasopressin and osmolality values measured in CSF, plasma and urine[6].

CONCLUSION

Our animal models detailed above seem to be useful for studying further the disturbed transport processes across the blood–brain barrier in the neonatal period of life.

References

1. Temesvári, P., Ábrahám, Cs., Joó, F., Kovács, J., Baranyi, Zs. and Rácz, K. (1990). Disturbed brain purine metabolism results in a gross opening of the blood–brain barrier in newborn piglets following experimental pneumothorax. *Neurosci. Lett.*, **113**, 163–8
2. Temesvári, P., Ábrahám, Cs. and Kovács, J. (1995). Tension pneumothorax in newborn piglets. *Crit. Care Med.*, **23**, 1446–8
3. Temesvári, P., Joó, F., Kovács, J. and Ábrahám, Cs. (1995). Ischemia-reperfusion-induced alternations of blood–brain barrier transport in newborn pigs. *Am. J. Physiol. (Heart Circ. Physiol.)*, **269**, H750–1
4. Temesvári, P., Ábrahám, Cs., Speer, C. P., Kovács, J. and Megyeri, P. (1993). *Escherichia coli* O111 B4 lipopolysaccharide given intracisternally induces blood–brain barrier opening during experimental neonatal meningitis in piglets. *Pediatr. Res.*, **34**, 182–6
5. Temesvári, P., Ábrahám, Cs., Gellén, J. Jr, Speer, C. P., Kovács, J. and Megyeri, P. (1995). Elastase given intracisternally opens blood–brain barrier in newborn piglets. *Biol. Neonate*, **67**, 59–63
6. Temesvári, P., Szöke, L., Boros, A., Ábrahám, Cs., Vecsernyés, M., Laczi, F., Pintér, S. and Gulya, K. (1996). Bacterial meningitis results in enhanced vasopressin gene expression in the supraoptic but not in the paraventricular nucleus in 14-day-old rats. *Pediatr. Res.*, **39**, 381A

N-methyl-D-aspartate receptor-related mechanisms in hypoxic-ischemic brain damage in the immature

31

E. Gilland and H. Hagberg

NMDA RECEPTOR-RELATED MECHANISMS IN HYPOXIA-ISCHEMIA

During the last 10 years, evidence has accumulated supporting claims that glutamate receptor-related mechanisms in general, and the N-methyl-D-aspartate (NMDA) receptor in particular, contribute to the process of continuing brain damage in the reperfusion phase after an hypoxic-ischemic insult in the immature brain. The NMDA receptor has a high permeability to calcium ions (Ca^{2+}) and a complex pharmacology, i.e. it requires binding of agonists to both its glycine and glutamate sites concomitant with cellular depolarization to become fully activated[1].

The NMDA receptor is important during development of the central nervous system (CNS). During ontogeny there are windows of vulnerability when the brain is especially prone to neural damage[2]. Receptors for NMDA are expressed in higher densities in the immature rat and human brain than in the adult. In the immature brain, the NMDA receptor is more easily excited, is less dependent on membrane depolarization for its activation and is considerably more susceptible to injections of excitotoxins than the adult brain[2,3].

Treatment with the non-competitive NMDA receptor antagonist dizocilpine maleate (MK-801) before[4–6] or after[7–9] the hypoxic-ischemic insult provides neuroprotection in immature rats, beagle puppies and fetal sheep, but one study with pre-ischemic administration in newborn pigs did not show a reduction of pathological score[10].

HARMFUL EFFECTS OF NMDA RECEPTOR ANTAGONISTS

In adult rodents, NMDA receptor antagonists cause increased glucose utilization, neural vacuolization and neural necrosis in certain areas of the limbic system[11,12]. Even though NMDA receptor antagonists do not have these side-effects in immature rats[13,14], and the non-competitive NMDA receptor antagonists magnesium sulfate and dextrometorphan have been given to infants[14,15], there are fears of deleterious neurodevelopmental effects of prolonged or repetitive administration of NMDA receptor antagonists[15]. Irrespective of these uncertainties concerning the clinical use of NMDA receptor blockers, the NMDA receptor plays a crucial role in the neurochemical cascade leading to perinatal brain injury. Therefore, in the search for new strategies of neuroprotection, it is important to consider and understand the mechanisms of NMDA receptor toxicity during and after hypoxia-ischemia.

NMDA RECEPTOR ACTIVATION DURING HYPOXIA-ISCHEMIA

During hypoxia-ischemia there are increases in the extracellular concentrations of excitatory amino acids among which glutamate predominates[16–19]. The magnitude of increase of excitatory amino acids is less pronounced during the insult in the immature than in the adult brain[16–21]. Treatment before but not after hypoxia-ischemia with the voltage-gated sodium channel blockers/glutamate release inhibitors phenytoin or BW1003C87 reduces subsequent brain damage[22,23]. Pretreatment with NMDA receptor antagonists affords a nearly complete protection from hypoxic-ischemic damage[7,24] while post-treatment attenuates cerebral infarction somewhat less (by 70%)[7,8,25]. These data indicate the existence of an intra-ischemic component of NMDA receptor toxicity. However, the absolute levels of extracellular amino acids during hypoxia-ischemia, although difficult to calculate, are much lower than what is required to cause acute toxicity in cortical cultures or slices[26–28]. There is no evidence that excitatory amino acids evoke ionic shifts during hypoxia-ischemia in the immature brain. On the contrary, the extracellular changes of excitatory amino acids follow a different time course as compared to extracellular Ca^{2+}, and administration of NMDA receptor antagonists does not affect the transmembrane movement of Ca^{2+} [19,29,30]. In addition, the acute biochemical changes in energy metabolites, reduction in glucose, adenosine triphosphate (ATP) and phosphocreatine (PCr), and increase in lactate, measured by magnetic resonance spectroscopy during hypoxia-ischemia, differ considerably from what is found after injection of glutamate analogs into the brain[31]. This information suggests that intra-ischemic events are different from a pure hyperstimulation of the NMDA receptors with subsequent Na^+ and/or Ca^{2+} overload of the cells.

NMDA RECEPTOR ACTIVATION DURING THE REPERFUSION PHASE

In the clinical situation of cerebral hypoxia-ischemia secondary to birth asphyxia, treatment after the insult is more likely to occur than treatment before the insult. Antagonizing NMDA receptors after hypoxia-ischemia affords a marked neuroprotection in animal models[7,8,25], and in the immature rat the extracellular levels of excitatory amino acids in the reperfusion phase, but not during hypoxia-ischemia, correlate with histological damage[32]. Clearly,

the NMDA receptor-dependent mechanisms in the reperfusion phase are important for the development of brain damage.

In adult focal ischemia, the protective action of NMDA receptor antagonists has been attributed to a reduction of peri-infarct depolarizations, or spreading depressions. Such ionic shifts may threaten tissue viability due to inability to respond with an increased blood flow in the region surrounding the infarct[33–35]. There are, however, several factors that differ between adult focal ischemia and the Rice-Vannucci model of hypoxia-ischemia in the immature rat. First, there is a near complete reperfusion in the immature rat up to 24 h after hypoxia-ischemia[36,37] (as is found in children after severe asphyxia), which would allow neurons to respond to the increased metabolic demands of spreading depressions. Second, spreading depressions are not easily elicitable in the immature rat[38], nor have we seen any temporary increases in intracellular Ca^{2+} regionally on the cortical surface as measured with Rhod-2 fluorescence after hypoxia-ischemia (Puka-Sundvall, Takita, Miyakawa and Hagberg, preliminary data). Moreover, energy utilization, measured by the changes in energy metabolites after decapitation, is not increased but rather tends to be decreased after hypoxia-ischemia[39]. This contradicts the idea of *increased* excitatory activity in the reperfusion phase.

However, burst-suppression patterns on electroencephalogram (EEG) have been recorded after hypoxia-ischemia in the immature rat[40] and suppression of postischemic epileptiform activity with MK-801 improves neural outcome in fetal sheep[9]. Slightly elevated or normal levels of excitatory amino acids during reperfusion[32] may be associated with a substantial influx of extracellular Ca^{2+} due to changes in the function of NMDA receptors[41–45]. In fact, in the immature rat model of hypoxia-ischemia there exist areas with markedly increased glucose utilization, as measured by the 2-deoxyglucose method, surrounding infarcted and hypometabolizing tissue in the first hours after hypoxia-ischemia (Figure 1)[36].

MITOCHONDRIAL DYSFUNCTION DURING RECIRCULATION

In the cerebral cortex of the immature rat, the early recovery period after hypoxia-ischemia is characterized by an incomplete restitution of ATP and PCr, a persistent increase in lactate levels, decreased nicotinamide adenine dinucleotide (NAD+)/NADH ratio, normal to increased glucose utilization and decreased energy utilization[36,39,46,47], despite normal cerebral blood flow[36,37]. These findings have been

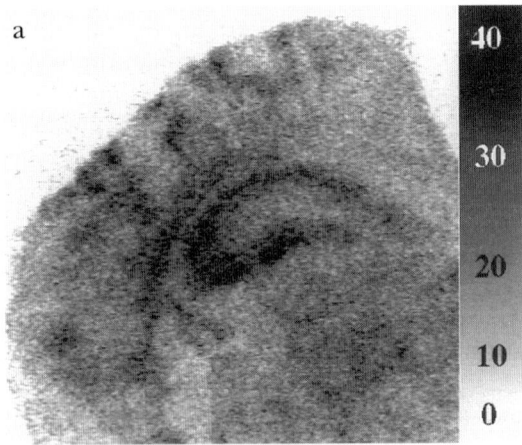

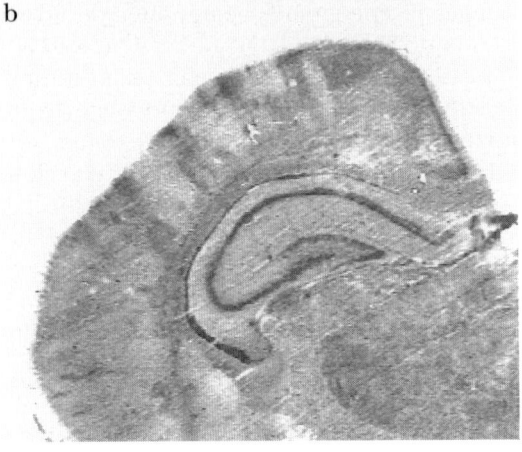

Figure 1 Regionally increased glucose utilization after hypoxia-ischemia. (a) 2-[^{14}C]deoxyglucose autoradiogram from the brain of a 7-day-old rat 5 h after hypoxia-ischemia. Glucose use is calibrated in μmol 100 g^{-1} min^{-1}. (b) Hematoxylin-eosin staining of the same section. Areas with increased glucose use, which appear histologically intact, surround hypometabolic areas that appear to be infarcted

interpreted as signs of impaired mitochondrial metabolism. In fact, a reduction in the activity of cytochrome aa₃ (cytochrome c oxidase), the final component of the electron transport chain, is found early after hypoxia-ischemia in the immature rat[48]. In newborn lambs there is a reduction in ADP-dependent mitochondrial activity after asphyxia[49], and in fetal sheep a progressive fall in oxidized cytochrome aa₃ occurs after transient cerebral ischemia[50]. These data match clinical data from infants with hypoxic ischemic encephalopathy. The discovery of brain regions with enhanced 18-fluoro-deoxyglucose uptake on positron emission tomography scans, i.e. increased glucose use, is associated with brain damage[51]. In addition, accumulation of brain lactate[52] or secondary fall of the phosphocreatine/orthophosphate (PCr/Pi) quotient[53], both analyzed with magnetic resonance spectroscopy, predicts an unfavorable outcome.

In adult models of global ischemia, the earliest perturbations separating tissue destined for infarction from tissue destined to recover is decreased activity of the pyruvate dehydrogenase complex and of pyruvate supported mitochondrial respiration[54]. Similarly, in adult focal ischemia with reperfusion, a secondary deterioration of the bioenergetic state is caused by mitochondrial injury[55]. The cause of this mitochondrial injury is unknown. Mitochondriae sequester intracellular Ca^{2+} during early recirculation, but this also takes place in undamaged areas[54]. In focal ischemia, the neuronal damage is ameliorated by treatment with N-tert-butyl-α-phenylnitrone (PBN), a free radical spin trap[56], which implicates oxidative damage.

ENERGY IMPAIRMENTS AND NMDA RECEPTOR TOXICITY

There is now evidence supporting the hypothesis that an impairment of energy metabolism may underlie delayed excitotoxic cell death[57–59]. In a situation with decreased high-energy phosphate stores and deteriorating membrane potential, the voltage-sensitive Mg^{2+} block of NMDA receptors is relieved, allowing the receptors to be persistently activated by endogenous concentrations of glutamate. Subtoxic amounts of the succinate dehydrogenase inhibitor malonate, combined with subtoxic amounts of either glutamate or NMDA, caused the formation of large lesions in rat striatum, which was blocked by administration of MK-801[60]. In the immature rat, 'penumbral' areas, i.e. areas surrounding infarcted tissue, that appear to be histologically intact and show increased glucose use despite normal cerebral blood flow (Figure 1), probably reflect tissue with impaired mitochondrial metabolism. This is further supported by a positive correlation between lactate levels and rate of glucose utilization[36]. The size of areas with increased glucose utilization is reduced (by 66%) by treatment with a neuroprotective dose of MK-801 given after hypoxia-ischemia[36]. The exact mechanisms involved are unknown but there are several possibilities.

First, the reduction in the hyper-glucose utilizing areas might be due to the possibility that NMDA receptor antagonists reduce the energy requirements of the cells through reduction of the influx of Na^+ and Ca^{2+}. More than half of the energy used by neurons is for maintenance of ionic gradients over the cell membrane[61]. In cells with impaired energy production, this might allow the cell to stabilize its internal environment and survive. In fact, recently we found that MK-801 reduced the energy utilization in the parietal cortex after hypoxia-ischemia by 40%, as determined by changes in energy metabolites after decapitation (Gilland and Hagberg, unpublished data).

Second, stimulation of NMDA receptors might cause mitochondrial damage through elevation of intracellular Ca^{2+}, release of nitric oxide (NO·) and production of free radicals[54,62] (Figure 2). NMDA receptor stimulation induces nitric oxide synthesis[63] and the specific neural nitric oxide synthase inhibitor, 7-nitroindazole, protects against excitotoxic striatal damage induced by either injections of NMDA or the metabolic inhibitors malonate or 3-nitropropionic acid[64]. Nitric oxide can react with

the superoxide radical to produce peroxynitrite, a freely diffusible substance which can oxidize sulfhydryl groups or form the highly reactive hydroxyl radical (·OH)[65]. Treatment of striatal excitotoxic lesions with 7-nitroindazole attenuate increases of hydroxyl radical and peroxynitrite formation[64]. Stimulation of the NMDA receptor can also induce free radical production in other ways, e.g. through activation of phospholipase A_2 (for review see Coyle and colleagues[66]), and treatment with either of the free radical scavengers S-PBN or PBN attenuates excitotoxic striatal damage induced by either injections of NMDA or the metabolic inhibitors 1-methyl-4-phenylpyridinium (MPP^+), malonate or 3-acetylpyridine[67].

Hypothetically, there is a vicious circle involving mitochondrial damage, making the cell more susceptible to excitotoxicity, which in turn further impairs the mitochondrial function through increases in intracellular Ca^{2+}, NO· formation and free radical production (Figure 2). In fetal sheep, extracellular citrulline, a marker of NO· formation, increases several hours after an ischemic insult, followed by rises in the excitotoxic index (extracellular excitatory amino acids) and epileptic seizures[68].

There is also a possibility that NMDA receptor antagonists might be protective at a very late time point. After adult ischemia, hypothermia in combination with MK-801 administered 3, 5 and 7 days after the insult resulted in permanent neuroprotection[69] which was not the case with hypothermia alone. This might be mediated by inflammatory cells, which appear in the neonatal brain after hypoxia-ischemia[70] and have been shown to produce molecules which stimulate glutamate receptors[71]. Moreover, glutamate receptor antagonists have been able to block the toxicity of tumor necrosis factor-α (TNF-α)[72,73], and TNF-α potentiates glutamate neurotoxicity, an effect which can be blocked by MK-801[74].

THERAPEUTIC IMPLICATIONS

It is possible to overcome/bypass the blocks in the mitochondrial respiration. Administration

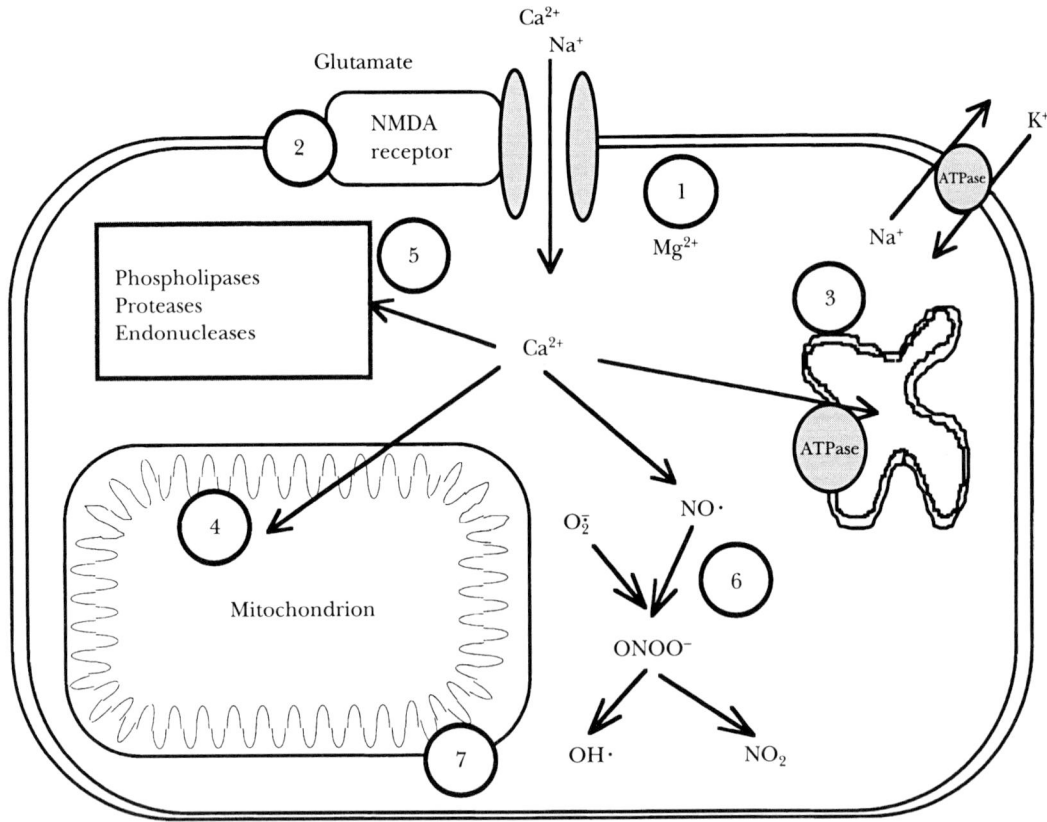

Figure 2 Injury mechanisms related to the *N*-methyl-D-aspartate (NMDA) receptor during reperfusion after hypoxia-ischemia. (1) Depolarization relieves the Mg^{2+} block of the NMDA receptor and (2) changes of the receptor characteristics are associated with an increased influx of Ca^{2+} and Na^+. (3) Due to impaired energy metabolism, Na^+ and Ca^{2+} cannot be extruded from the cell or recaptured into the endoplasmatic reticulum. (4) The mitochondria will accumulate Ca^{2+} instead of producing ATP. The increased intramitochondrial Ca^{2+} content leads to further impairment of mitochondrial function. (5) Ca^{2+} activates phospholipases, proteases and endonucleases which cause breakdown of the cellular membranes, cytoskeleton and DNA. As a consequence, there will be an increased release of oxygen free radicals. (6) Nitric oxide (NO) and superoxide (O_2^-) will form peroxynitrite ($ONOO^-$) which may increase the production of hydroxyl ($OH\cdot$) radicals. (7) Peroxynitrite and hydroxyl radicals attack the sulfhydryl groups of important metabolic enzymes and activate lipid peroxidation with impairment of mitochondrial membranes

of 1,3-butanediol, a substance which increases circulating ketone bodies, 24 h after ischemia in adult rats ameliorates neural damage[75]. Immature rats that have increased levels of ketone bodies after fasting, have reduced brain damage after hypoxia-ischemia compared to non-fasted controls[76] and glucose supplementation immediately after hypoxia-ischemia reduces brain damage in immature rats[77].

Non-specific inhibitors of nitric oxide synthase appear to ameliorate brain damage when administered before but not after the hypoxic-ischemic insult in the immature rat[78,79]. There is evidence that specific inhibition of neural nitric oxide synthase in adult ischemia models affords neuroprotection[80,81], and inhibition of inducible, calcium-independent, nitric oxide synthase, believed to be expressed in cells of the inflammatory system, reduces brain damage when administered even 24 h after ischemia in adult rats[82]. Neither of these specific drugs has been studied in immature models of cerebral hypoxia-ischemia.

Oxygen free radicals have been extensively studied in immature animal models of asphyxia and are reviewed elsewhere[83-85]. The xanthine oxidase inhibitors, allopurinol and oxypurinol[86,87], the iron chelator deferoxamine[88] and the lipid peroxidation inhibitor tirilazad[89], all reduce brain damage when administered after hypoxia-ischemia in the immature rat, but it is unclear whether these drugs exert their effect only in the vascular compartment, since none of them penetrates the blood–brain barrier very efficiently, and they might primarily affect inflammatory reactions at the endothelium and endothelial and microvascular patency. Possibly more lipophilic substances, like PBN, are needed to interfere with the mitochondrial-excitotoxic mechanisms outlined above.

CONCLUSION

The neurodeleterious mechanisms related to the NMDA receptor in the reperfusion phase after hypoxia-ischemia in immature animals are complex, possibly involving a combination of epileptical activity, altered NMDA receptor properties, mitochondrial dysfunction, nitric oxide production, free radical formation and inflammatory reactions.

ACKNOWLEDGEMENTS

This work was supported by the Swedish Medical Research Council (grant no. 9455), the 1987 Foundation for Stroke Research, the Sven Jerring Foundation, the Åke Wiberg Foundation, the Åhlén Foundation, the Magnus Bergwall Foundation, the Frimurare Barnhus Foundation, the Göteborg Medical Society, the First-of-May Flower Annual Campaign, the Linnéa och Josef Carlsson Foundation, the Swedish Society for Medical Research and the Medical Faculty of Göteborg, University of Göteborg.

References

1. Wong, E. H. F. and Kemp, J. A. (1991). Sites for antagonism on the N-methyl-D-aspartate receptor channel complex. *Annu. Rev. Pharmacol. Toxicol.*, **31**, 401–25

2. Johnston, M. V. (1995). Neurotransmitters and vulnerability of the developing brain. *Brain Dev.*, **17**, 301–6

3. McDonald, J. W. and Johnston, M. V. (1990). Physiological and pathophysiological roles of excitatory amino acids during central nervous system development. *Brain. Res. Rev.*, **15**, 41–70

4. Ford, L. M., Sanberg, P. R., Norman, A. B. and Fogelson, M. H. (1989). MK-801 prevents hippocampal neurodegeneration in neonatal hypoxic-ischemic rats. *Arch. Neurol.*, **46**, 1090–6

5. McDonald, J. W., Silverstein, F. S. and Johnston, M. V. (1987). MK-801 protects the neonatal brain from hypoxic-ischemic damage. *Eur. J. Pharmacol.*, **140**, 359–61

6. Ment, L. R., Stewart, W. B., Petroff, O. A. C., Duncan, C. C. and Montoya, D. (1989). Beagle puppy model of perinatal asphyxia: blockade of excitatory neurotransmitters. *Pediatr. Neurol.*, **5**, 281–6

7. Hattori, H., Morin, A. M., Schwartz, P. H., Fujikawa, D. G. and Wasterlain, C. G. (1989). Posthypoxic treatment with MK801 reduces hypoxic-ischemic damage in the neonatal rat. *Neurology*, **39**, 713–18

8. Hagberg, H., Gilland, E., Diemer, N. H. and Andiné, P. (1994). Hypoxia-ischemia in the neonatal rat brain: histopathology after posttreatment with NMDA and non-NMDA receptor antagonists. *Biol. Neonate*, **66**, 206–13

9. Tan, W. K. M., Williams, C. E., Gunn, A. H., Mallard, C. E. and Gluckman, P. D. (1992). Suppression of postischemic epileptiform activity with MK-801 improves neural outcome in fetal sheep. *Ann. Neurol.*, **32**, 677–82

10. LeBlanc, M. H., Vig, V., Smith, B., Parker, C. C., Evans, O. B. and Smith, E. E. (1991). MK-801 does not protect against hypoxic-ischemic brain injury in piglets. *Stroke*, **22**, 1270–5

11. Olney, J. W. (1994). Neurotoxicity of NMDA receptor antagonists: an overview. *Psychopharmacol. Bull.*, **30**, 533–40

12. Edvinsson, L., MacKenzie, E. T. and McCulloch, J. (1993). *Cerebral Blood Flow and Metabolism*, pp. 487–91, (New York: Raven Press)

13. Farber, N. B., Wozniak, D. F., Price, M. T., Labruyere, J., Huss, J., St. Peter, H. and Olney, J. W. (1995). Age-specific neurotoxicity in the rat associated with NMDA receptor blockage: potential relevance to schizophrenia? *Biol. Psych.*, **38**, 788–96

14. Gilland, E., Bona, E., Levene, M. and Hagberg, H. (1996). The NMDA receptor antagonists dizocilpine and magnesium do not increase glucose utilization, nor induce heat shock protein 72 expression in the limbic system of the immature rat. *Prenat. Neonat. Med.*, 1 (Suppl. 1), 49 (abstract)

15. Constantine-Paton, M. (1994). Effects of NMDA receptor antagonists on the developing brain. *Psychopharmacol. Bull.*, **30**, 561–5

16. Hagberg, H., Andersson, P., Kjellmer, I., Thiringer, K. and Thordstein, M. (1987). Extracellular overflow of glutamate, aspartate, GABA and taurine in the cortex and basal ganglia of fetal lambs during hypoxia-ischemia. *Neurosci. Lett.*, **78**, 311–17

17. Gordon, K. E., Simpson, J., Statman, D. and Silverstein, F. S. (1991). Effects of perinatal stroke on striatal amino acid efflux in rats studied with *in vivo* microdialysis. *Stroke*, **22**, 928–32

18. Silverstein, F. S., Naik, B. and Simpson, H. (1991). Hypoxia-ischemia stimulates hippocampal glutamate efflux in perinatal rat brain: an *in vivo* microdialysis study. *Pediatr. Res.*, **30**, 587–90

19. Andiné, P., Sandberg, M., Bågenholm, R., Lehmann, A. and Hagberg, H. (1991). Intra- and extracellular changes of amino acids in the cerebral cortex of the neonatal rat during hypoxia-ischemia. *Dev. Brain Res.*, **64**, 115–20

20. Benveniste, H., Drejer, J., Schousboe, A. and Diemer, N. H. (1984). Elevation of extracellular concentrations of glutamate and aspartate in rat hippocampus during transient cerebral ischemia monitored by intracerebral microdialysis. *J. Neurochem.*, **43**, 1469–74

21. Globus, M. Y.-T., Busto, R., Dietrich, W. D., Martinez, E., Valdes, I. and Ginsberg, M. D. (1988). Effect of ischemia on the *in vivo* release of striatal dopamine, glutamate, and gamma-aminobutyric acid studied by intracerebral microdialysis. *J. Neurochem.*, **51**, 1455–64

22. Gilland, E., Puka-Sundvall, M., Andiné, P., Bona, E. and Hagberg, H. (1994). Hypoxic-ischemic injury in the neonatal rat brain: effects of pre- and post-treatment with the glutamate release inhibitor BW1003C87. *Dev. Brain Res.*, **83**, 79–84

23. Hayakawa, T., Hamada, Y., Maihara, T., Hattori, H. and Mikawa, H. (1994). Phenytoin reduces neonatal hypoxic-ischemic brain damage in rats. *Life Sci.*, **54**, 387–92

24. Nozaki, K. and Flint Beal, M. (1992). Neuroprotective effects of L-kynurenine on hypoxia-ischemia and NMDA lesions in neonatal rats. *J. Cereb. Blood Flow Metab.*, **12**, 400–7

25. Andiné, P., Lehmann, A., Ellrén, K., Wennberg, E., Kjellmer, I., Nielsen, T. and Hagberg, H. (1988). The excitatory amino acid antagonist kynurenic acid administered after hypoxic-ischemia in neonatal rats offers neuroprotection. *Neurosci. Lett.*, **90**, 208–12

26. Lehmann, A. and Jacobson, I. (1991). Ion dependence and receptor mediation of glutamate toxicity in the immature rat hippocampal slice. *Eur. J. Neurosci.*, **2**, 620–8

27. Choi, D. W. (1985). Glutamate toxicity in cortical cell culture is calcium dependent. *Neurosci. Lett.*, **58**, 293–7

28. Garthwaite, G., Williams, G. D. and Garthwaite, J. (1992). Glutamate toxicity: an experimental and theoretical analysis. *Eur. J. Neurosci.*, **4**, 353–60

29. Stein, D. T. and Vanucci, R. C. (1988). Calcium accumulation during the evolution of hypoxic-ischemic brain damage in the immature rat. *J. Cereb. Blood Flow Metab.*, **8**, 834–42

30. Puka-Sundvall, M., Hagberg, H. and Andiné, P. (1994). Changes in extracellular calcium concentration in the immature rat cerebral cortex during anoxia is not influenced by MK-801. *Dev. Brain Res.*, **77**, 146–50

31. Young, R. S. K., Petroff, O. A. C., Aquila, W. J. and Yates, J. (1991). Effects of glutamate, quisqualate, and N-methyl-D-aspartate in neonatal brain. *Exp. Neurol.*, **111**, 362–8

32. Puka-Sundvall, M., Gilland, E., Bona, E., Lehmann, A., Sandberg, M. and Hagberg, H. (1996). Development of brain damage after neonatal hypoxia-ischemia: excitatory amino acids and cysteine. *Metab. Brain Dis.*, **11**, 109–23

33. Gill, R., Andiné, P., Hillered, L., Persson, L. and Hagberg, H. (1992). The effect of MK801 on cortical spreading depression in the penumbral zone following focal ischemia in the rat. *J. Cereb. Blood Flow Metab.*, **12**, 371–9

34. Mies, G., Kohno, K. and Hossman, K.-A. (1993). MK-801, a glutamate antagonist, lowers flow

threshold for inhibition of protein synthesis after middle cerebral artery occlusion of rat. *Neurosci. Lett.*, **155**, 65–8

35. Simon, R. P. and Shiraishi, K. (1990). *N*-methyl-D-aspartate antagonist reduces stroke size and regional glucose metabolism. *Ann. Neurol.*, **27**, 606–11

36. Gilland, E. and Hagberg, H. (1996). NMDA-receptor dependent increase of cerebral glucose utilization after hypoxia-ischemia in the neonatal rat. *J. Cereb. Blood Flow Metab.*, **16**, 1005–13

37. Mujsce, D. J., Christensen, M. A. and Vannucci, R. C. (1990). Cerebral blood flow and edema in perinatal hypoxic-ischemic brain damage. *Pediatr. Res.*, **27**, 450–3

38. Bures, J. (1957). The ontogenetic development of steady potential differences in the cerebral cortex in animals. *Electroenceph. Clin. Neurophysiol.*, **9**, 121–30

39. Vannucci, R. C., Yager, J. Y. and Vannucci, S. J. (1994). Cerebral glucose and energy utilization during the evolution of hypoxic-ischemic brain damage in the immature rat. *J. Cereb. Blood Flow Metab.*, **14**, 279–88

40. Chen, R., Silverstein, F. S., Aldrich, J. W. and Johnston, M. V. (1986). Evolution of acute cortical EEG changes in experimental perinatal hypoxic-ischemic encephalopathy. *Neurology*, **36** S86

41. Andiné, P., Jacobson, I. and Hagberg, H. (1988). Calcium uptake evoked by electrical stimulation is enhanced postischemically and precedes delayed neuronal death in CA1 of rat hippocampus: involvement of *N*-methyl-D-aspartate receptors. *J. Cereb. Blood Flow Metab.*, **8**, 799–807

42. Hammond, C., Crépel, V., Gozlan, H. and Ben-Ari, Y. (1994). Anoxic LTP sheds light on the multiple facets of NMDA receptors. *Trends Neurol. Sci.*, **17**, 497–503

43. Heurteaux, C., Lauritzen, I., Widmann, C. and Lazdunski, M. (1994). Glutamate induced overexpression of NMDA receptor messenger RNAs and protein triggered by activation of AMPA/kainate receptors in rat hippocampus following forebrain ischemia. *Brain Res.*, **659**, 67–74

44. Kohmura, E., Yamada, K., Hayakawa, T., Kinoshitsa, A., Matsumoto, K. and Mogami, H. (1990). Hippocampal neurons become more vulnerable to glutamate after subcritical hypoxia: an *in vitro* study. *J. Cereb. Blood Flow Metab.*, **10**, 877–84

45. Miyazaki, S., Katayama, Y., Furuichi, M., Kano, T., Yoshino, A. and Tsubokawa, T. (1994). *N*-methyl-D-aspartate receptor-mediated prolonged afterdischarges of CA1 pyramidal cells

46. Vannucci, R. C. (1990). Experimental biology of cerebral hypoxia-ischemia: relation to perinatal brain damage. *Pediatr. Res.*, **27**, 317–26

47. Yager, J. Y., Brucklacher, R. M. and Vannucci, R. C. (1991). Cerebral oxidative metabolism and redox state during hypoxia-ischemia and early recovery in immature rats. *Am. J. Physiol.*, **261**, H1102–8

48. Nelson, C. and Silverstein, F. S. (1994). Acute disruption of cytochrome oxidase activity in brain in a perinatal rat stroke model. *Pediatr. Res.*, **36**, 12–19

49. Rosenberg, A. A., Parks, J. K., Murdaugh, E. and Parker, W. D. (1989). Mitochondrial function after asphyxia in newborn lambs. *Stroke*, **20**, 674–9

50. Marks, K. A., Mallard, E. C., Roberts, I., Williams, C. E., Sirimanne, E. S., Johnston, B., Gluckman, P. D. and Edwards, A. D. (1996). Delayed vasodilation and altered oxygenation after cerebral ischemia in fetal sheep. *Pediatr. Res.*, **39**, 48–54

51. Blennow, M., Ingvar, M., Lagercrantz, H., Stone-Elander, S., Eriksson, L., Forsberg, H., Ericson, K. and Flodmark, O. (1995). Early [^{18}F]FDG positron emission tomography in infants with hypoxic-ischemic encephalopathy shows hypermetabolism during the post-asphyctic period. *Acta Paediatr.*, **84**, 1289–95

52. Groenendaal, F., Veenhoven, R. H. and Van der Grond, J. (1994). Cerebral lactate and *N*-acetyl-aspartate/choline ratios in asphyxiated full-term neonates demonstrated *in vivo* using proton magnetic resonance spectroscopy. *Pediatr. Res.*, **35**, 149–51

53. Roth, S. C., Edwards, A. D., Cady, E. B., Delpy, D. T., Wyatt, J. S., Azzopardi, D., Baudin, J., Townsend, J., Stewart, A. L. and Reynolds, E. O. R. (1992). Relation between cerebral oxidative metabolism following birth asphyxia and neurodevelopmental outcome and brain growth at one year. *Dev. Med. Child. Neurol.*, **34**, 285–95

54. Sims, N. R. and Zaidan, E. (1995). Biochemical changes associated with selective neuronal death following short-term cerebral ischaemia. *Int. J. Biochem. Cell Biol.*, **27**, 531–50

55. Kuroda, S., Katsura, K. -I., Tsuchidate, R. and Siesjö, B. K. (1996). Secondary bioenergetic failure after transient focal ischaemia is due to mitochondrial injury. *Acta Physiol. Scand.*, **156** 149–50

56. Zhao, Q., Pahlmark, K., Smith, M. -L. and Siesjö, B. K. (1994). Delayed treatment with the spin trap α-phenyl-*N*-tert-butyl-nitrone (PBN)

reduces infarct size following transient middle cerebral artery occlusion in rats. *Acta Physiol. Scand.*, **152**, 349–50

57. Beal, M. F., Hyman, B. T. and Koroshetz, W. (1993). Do defects in mitochondrial energy metabolism underlie the pathology of neuro-degenerative diseases? *Trends Neurol. Sci.*, **16**, 125–31

58. Novelli, A., Reilly, J. A., Lysko, P. G. and Henne-berry, R. C. (1988). Glutamate becomes neuro-toxic via the N-methyl-D-aspartate receptor when intracellular energy levels are reduced. *Brain Res.*, **451**, 205–12

59. Greene, J. G., Porter, R. H. P., Eller, R. V. and Greenamyre, J. T. (1993). Inhibition of succi-nate dehydrogenase by malonic acid produces an excitotoxic lesion in rat striatum. *J. Neuro-chem.*, **61**, 1151–4

60. Greene, J. G. and Greenamyre, J. T. (1995). Ex-acerbation of NMDA, AMPA, and L-glutamate excitotoxicity by the succinate dehydrogenase inhibitor malonate. *J. Neurochem.*, **64**, 2332–8

61. Hansen, A. J. (1985). Effect of anoxia on ion distribution in the brain. *Physiol. Rev.*, **65**, 101–47

62. Siesjö, B. K. (1992). Pathophysiology and treat-ment of focal cerebral ischemia. I: Pathophysi-ology. *J. Neurosurg.*, **77**, 169–84

63. Garthwaite, J., Garthwaite, G., Palmer, M. J. and Moncada, S. (1989). NMDA receptor activation induces nitric oxide synthesis from arginine in rat brain slices. *Eur. J. Pharmacol.*, **172**, 413–16

64. Schulz, J. B., Matthews, R. T., Jenkins, B. G., Fer-rante, R. J., Siwek, D., Henshaw, D. R., Cipolloni, P. B., Mecocci, P., Kowall, N. W., Rosen, B. R. *et al.* (1995). Blockade of neuronal nitric oxide synthase protects against excitotoxicity *in vivo*. *J. Neurosci.*, **15**, 8419–29

65. Beckman, J. (1991). The double-edged role of nitric oxide in brain function and superoxide-mediated injury. *J. Dev. Physiol.*, **15**, 53–9

66. Coyle, J. T. and Puttfarcken, P. (1993). Oxida-tive stress, glutamate, and neurodegenerative disorders. *Science*, **262**, 689–95

67. Schulz, J. B., Henshaw, D. R., Siwek, D., Jenkins, B. G., Ferrante, R. J., Cipolloni, P. B., Kowall, N. W., Rosen, B. R. and Beal, M. F. (1995). In-volvement of free radicals in excitotoxicity *in vivo*. *J. Neurochem.*, **64**, 2239–47

68. Tan, W. K. M., Williams, C. E., During, M. J., Mallard, C. E., Gunning, M. I., Gunn, A. J. and Gluckman, P. D. (1996). Accumulation of cyto-toxins during the development of seizures and edema after hypoxic-ischemic injury in late gestation fetal sheep. *Pediatr. Res.*, **39**, 791–7

69. Dietrich, W. D., Lin, B., Globus, M. Y. -T., Green, E. J., Ginsberg, M. D. and Busto, R. (1995). Ef-fect of delayed MK-801 (Dizocilpine) treatment with or without immediate postischemic hypo-thermia on chronic neuronal survival after global forebrain ischemia in rats. *J. Cereb. Blood Flow Metab.*, **15**, 960–8

70. McRae, A., Gilland, E., Bona, E. and Hagberg, H. (1995). Microglia activation after neonatal hypoxic-ischemia. *Dev. Brain. Res.*, **84**, 245–52

71. Giulian, D., Vaca, K. and Corpuz, M. (1993). Brain glia release factors with opposing actions upon neuronal survival. *J. Neurosci.*, **13**, 29–37

72. Gelbard, H. A., Dzenko, K. A., DiLoreto, D., del Cerro, C., del Cerro, M. and Epstein, L. G. (1993). Neurotoxic effects of tumor necrosis factor alpha in primary human neuronal cul-tures are mediated by activation of the glutamate AMPA receptor subtype: implications for AIDS neuropathogenesis. *Dev. Neurosci.*, **15**, 417–22

73. Talley, A. K., Dewhurst, S., Perry, S. W., Dollard, S. C., Gummuluru, S., Fine, S. M., New, D., Epstein, L. G., Gendelman, H. E. and Gelbard, H. A. (1995). Tumor necrosis factor alpha-induced apoptosis in human neuronal cells: protection by the antioxidant N-acetylcysteine and the genes bcl-2 and crmA. *Mol. Cell Biol.*, **15**, 2359–66

74. Chao, C. C. and Hu, S. (1994). Tumor necrosis factor-alpha potentiates glutamate neurotoxicity in human fetal brain cell cultures. *Dev. Neurosci.*, **16**, 172–9

75. Sims, N. R. and Heward, S. L. (1994). Delayed treatment with 1,3-butanediol reduces loss of CA 1 neurons in the hippocampus of rats follow-ing brief forebrain ischemia. *Brain Res.*, **662**, 216–22

76. Yager, J. Y., Heitjan, D. F., Towfighi, J. and Van-nucci, R. C. (1992). Effect of insulin-induced and fasting hypoglycemia on perinatal hypoxic-ischemic brain damage. *Pediatr. Res.*, **31**, 138–42

77. Hattori, H. and Wasteralin, C. G. (1990). Posthy-poxic glucose supplement reduces hypoxic-ischemic brain damage in the neonatal rat. *Ann. Neurol.*, **28**, 122–8

78. Hamada, Y., Hayakawa, T., Hattori, H. and Mikawa, H. (1994). Inhibitor of nitric oxide syn-thesis reduces hypoxic-ischemic brain damage in the neonatal rat. *Pediatr. Res.*, **35**, 10–14

79. Trifiletti, R. (1992). Neuroprotective effects of N-nitro-arginine in focal stroke in the 7-day old rat. *Eur. J. Pharmacol.*, **218**, 197–8

80. Huang, Z., Huang, P. L., Panahian, N., Dalkara, T., Fishman, M. C. and Moskowitz, M. A. (1994). Effects of cerebral ischemia in mice deficient in neuronal nitric oxide synthase. *Science*, **265**, 1883–5

81. Yoshida, T., Limmroth, V., Irikura, K. and Moskowitz, M. A. (1994). The NOS inhibitor, 7-nitroindazole, decreases focal infarct volume

but not the response to topical acetylcholine in pial vessels. *J. Cereb. Blood Flow Metab.*, **14**, 924–9

82. Iadecola, C., Zhang, F. and Xu, X. (1995). Inhibition of inducible nitric oxide synthase ameliorates cerebral ischemic damage. *Am. J. Physiol.*, **268**, R 286–92

83. Saugstad, O. D. (1996). Mechanisms of tissue injury by oxygen radicals: implications for neonatal disease. *Acta Pediatr.*, **85**, 1–4

84. Kjellmer, I. and Hagberg, H. (1994). Perinatal brain damage, excitatory amino acids and oxygen derived free radicals. In Van Geijn, H. P. and Copray, F. J. A. (eds.) *A Critical Appraisal of Fetal Surveillance*, pp. 604–14. (Amsterdam: Excerpta Medica)

85. Palmer, C. and Vannucci, R. (1993). Potential new therapies for perinatal cerebral hypoxia-ischemia. *Clin. Perinatol.*, **20**, 411–31

86. Palmer, C., Towfighi, J., Roberts, R. and Heitjan, D. F. (1993). Allopurinol administered after inducing hypoxia-ischemia reduces brain injury in 7-day-old rats. *Pediatr. Res.*, **33**, 405–11

87. Palmer, C. and Roberts, R. L. (1991). Reduction of perinatal brain damage with oxypurinol treatment after hypoxic-ischemic injury. *Neurology*, **29**, 362A

88. Palmer, C., Roberts, R. L. and Bero, C. (1994). Deferoxamine posttreatment reduces ischemic brain injury in neonatal rats. *Stroke*, **25**, 1039–45

89. Bågenholm, R., Andiné, P. and Hagberg, H. (1996). Effects of 21-aminosteroid tirilazad on brain damage and edema after perinatal hypoxia-ischemia in the rat. *Pediatr. Res.*, **40**, 404–9

Prediction, diagnosis and management of twin-to-twin transfusion syndrome

32

K. Nicolaides, N. Sebire and C. D'Ercole

INTRODUCTION

In monozygotic twin pregnancies, embryonic splitting within 3 days of fertilization occurs in about one-third of cases and results in two separate fetuses with independent placental circulations (monozygotic-dichorionic)[1,2]. Splitting after the 3rd day of fertilization is associated with vascular communications between the placentas; when cleavage is delayed beyond day 12, the fetuses are conjoint. In some monochorionic twin pregnancies, imbalance in the net flow of blood across the placental vascular communications from one fetus, the donor, to the other, the recipient, results in the clinical syndrome of twin-to-twin transfusion syndrome (TTS).

DETERMINATION OF CHORIONICITY

Prenatal determination of chorionicity by ultrasound, usually performed in the second and third trimesters, relies on assessment of fetal gender, number of placentas and characteristics of the dividing membrane[3-8]. Different-sex twins are always dizygotic and therefore dichorionic, but in about two-thirds of twin pregnancies the fetuses are of the same sex and these may be either monozygotic or dizygotic. Similarly, if there are two separate placentas the pregnancy is always dichorionic, but in the majority of cases the two placentas are adjacent to each other and there are often difficulties in distinguishing between dichorionic-fused and monochorionic placentas. Several studies have proposed that the inter-twin membrane is thicker and more echogenic in dichorionic than monochorionic pregnancies but this is a rather subjective criterion[3-6]. One study reported that dichorionicity is associated with an inter-twin septum thickness of 2 mm or more[7], but the reproducibility of this measurement is poor and is dependent on such technical aspects as the angle of insonation and gestational age[9].

Another feature of dichorionicity is the extension of placental tissue into the base of the inter-twin membrane, referred to as the twin peak sign or Λ sign[10,11]. In a study of 369 twin pregnancies prospectively evaluated at 10–14 weeks of gestation by transabdominal ultrasound, all monochorionic pregnancies resulted in same-sex twins and all different-sex twins were correctly classified as dichorionic[12]. Hence, chorionicity in twin pregnancies can be reliably determined by ultrasound at 10–14 weeks of gestation by looking for the presence or absence of extension in placental tissue into the base of the inter-twin membrane or the Λ-sign and T-sign, respectively (Figure 1).

FETAL LOSS ACCORDING TO CHORIONICITY

The risk of fetal or neonatal death in twin pregnancies is about five times greater than in singletons[13,14], and it is higher in identical than non-identical twins[15]. Postnatal, retrospective studies have reported that perinatal mortality is higher in like-sex than unlike-sex twins[16] and studies in which both zygosity and chorionicity were determined after birth reported that it is chorionicity

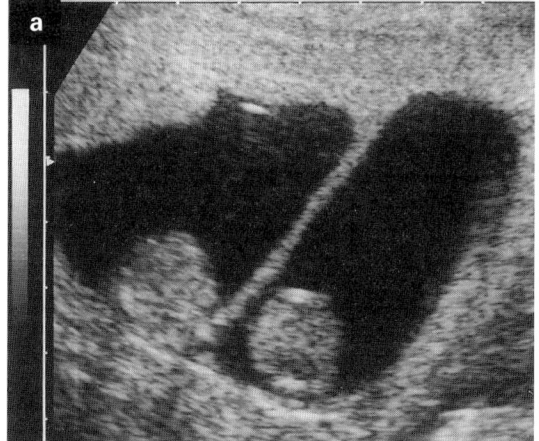

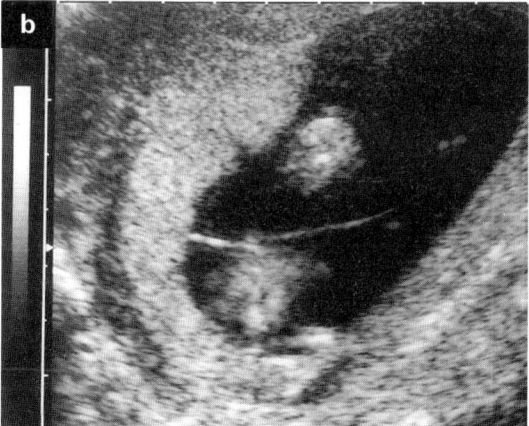

Figure 1 (a) Dichorionic twin pregnancy demonstrating extension of placental tissue into the base of the inter-twin membrane, or 'Λ sign', and (b) monochorionic twin pregnancy demonstrating the 'T-sign'

EARLY SONOGRAPHIC FEATURES OF TWIN-TO-TWIN TRANSFUSION SYNDROME

In singleton pregnancies at 10–14 weeks of gestation a sonographic sign that identifies fetuses at risk of chromosomal abnormalities, cardiac defects and a wide range of genetic syndromes is increased nuchal transluency thickness (Figure 2). In a continuing multicenter study involving more than 60 000 pregnancies, screening for trisomy 21 by a combination of maternal age and fetal nuchal translucency (NT) thickness identified 84% of affected pregnancies[19]. In fetuses from monochorionic twin pregnancies the prevalence of increased NT thickness is higher than in singletons and in dichorionic twins[20]. Increased NT thickness in one of the fetuses or increased inter-twin difference in NT in monochorionic pregnancies is an early ultrasonographic feature of the hemodynamic changes associated with TTS.

In our ongoing studies involving serial ultrasound scans in monochorionic twins it appears that the next manifestation of TTS is a substantial disparity in the amniotic fluid between the two sacs, manifested as a folding in the inter-twin membrane at 15–17 weeks of gestation (Figure 3). Such a fold is observed in about 25% of monochorionic twins and in about half of these cases there is progression to severe TTS with the

rather than zygosity that determines outcome[17,18]. In a continuing prospective ultrasound screening study at the Harris Birthright Research Centre for Fetal Medicine, all twin pregnancies scanned at 10–14 weeks are classified as dichorionic or monochorionic on the basis of the presence of the Λ-sign and T-sign, respectively. In more than 500 pregnancies the risk of miscarriage before 24 weeks of gestation and perinatal death after 24 weeks are about 12% and 3%, respectively, for monochorionic pregnancies and 2% and 2%, respectively, for dichorionic twins.

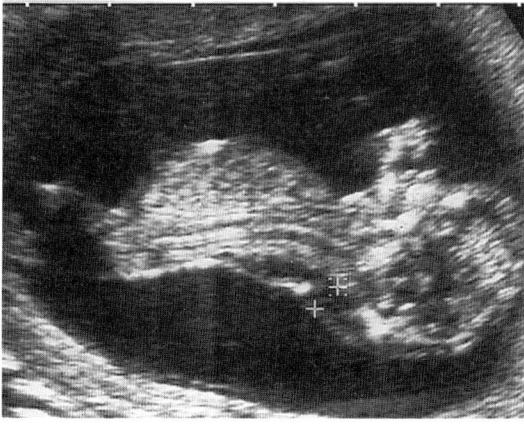

Figure 2 Sagittal view of a fetus at 12 weeks of gestation demonstrating increased fetal nuchal translucency thickness

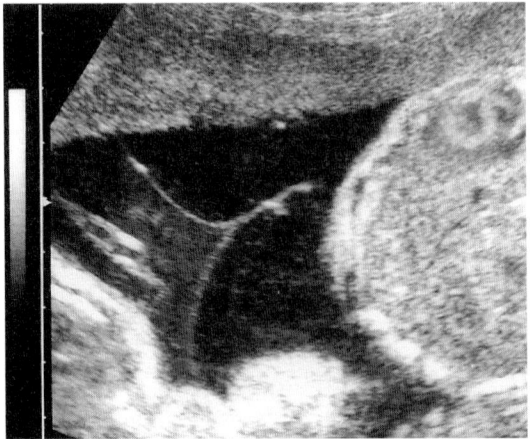

Figure 3 Folding of the inter-twin membrane at 15–17 weeks of gestation as an early manifestation of inter-twin disparity in amniotic fluid volume

amhydramnios/polyhydramnios sequence; in the other half of the cases there is a wide inter-twin disparity in amniotic fluid volume and fetal size but without the development of the anhydramnios/polyhydramnios sequence and the associated high risk of miscarriage and perinatal death. Similarly, the 75% of pregnancies without membrane folding at 15–17 weeks are not at increased risk for miscarriage or perinatal death.

CLINICAL FEATURES OF SEVERE TWIN-TO-TWIN TRANSFUSION SYNDROME

Traditionally, the diagnosis of TTS was made postnatally on the basis of an inter-twin disparity in birth weight of 20% or more[21,22]. These observations were made in live births and therefore the criteria may apply only to mild or moderate TTS since severe cases result in miscarriage or stillbirth.

Severe TTS presents with acute polyhydramnios during the second trimester of pregnancy. In such cases ultrasound examination demonstrates the anhydramnios/polyhydramnios sequence with or without large disparity in fetal size. The recipient fetus has a large bladder whereas the donor is anuric with a non-visible

bladder and is found 'stuck' and immobile at an edge of the placenta or the uterine wall where it is held fixed by the collapsed membranes. Additional sonographic findings may include the presence of a hypertrophic, dilated and dyskinetic heart in the recipient fetus. In the donor, the heart may be dilated and the bowel hyperechogenic; these fetuses are commonly seen in hypoxemic fetuses in pregnancies with severe uteroplacental insufficiency.

TREATMENT OPTIONS

In twin pregnancies with severe TTS the survival with expectant management is less than 10%[23]. Various therapies have been attempted to reduce this mortality, including indomethacin[24], surgical removal of one fetus[25], ultrasound-guided fetocide with intracardiac injection of potassium chloride[26–31], or insertion of thrombogenic coils[32], injection of thromboembolic material into the umbilical vein[33], or ultrasound-guided ligation of one umbilical cord[34]. However, with all such treatments, fetal survival remained at around only 25%.

Serial amniodrainage

An 18-gauge needle is introduced into the uterus under ultrasound guidance and the amniotic fluid is allowed to drain freely over a period of 40–120 min until there is subjective normalization of amniotic fluid volume on ultrasonographic examination. Improved survival of pregnancies presenting with acute polyhydramnios during the second trimester has been reported after treatment with serial amniocenteses and drainage of large volumes of amniotic fluid. This treatment presumably prevents the polyhydramnios-mediated risk of spontaneous abortion or very premature delivery[12,34–36]. In a study at the Harris Birthright Centre of 25 monozygotic twin pregnancies with acute polyhydramnios at less than 28 weeks of gestation, an average of three (range one to six) amniocenteses were performed and the total volume of amniotic fluid that was drained was 8410 ml (range 1000–20 500 ml)[35]. The total number of babies that survived was 16 of 50 (32%) and the number of pregnancies with at least one survivor was 11 of 25 (44%). Four (25%) of the survivors had cerebral palsy and brain scans demonstrated lesions compatible with intrauterine hypoxia/ischemia. Similarly, in studies published before 1991, amnio-drainage was associated with survival in 30–40% of the cases[35]. However, recent papers from three centers have reported survival of 72–83% of fetuses and the number of pregnancies with at least one survivor was 81–100%[36–40]. This apparent marked improvement in survival, compared to previous studies that used the same treatment protocols, could, at least in part, be the consequence of the inclusion of pregnancies with moderate TTS. Thus, the widespread use of routine ultrasound examination and the identification of monochorionic pregnancies with large inter-twin disparities in size and amniotic fluid volume could have stimulated physicians to undertake amniodrainage in pregnancies that may have resulted in live births even without such treatment.

Laser coagulation of the communicating placental vessels

An alternative method of treating severe TTS is endoscopic neodymium (Nd):YAG laser coagulation of the placental blood vessels that connect the circulations of the two fetuses. De Lia and colleagues[41] described a technique involving general or regional anesthesia in which the endoscope was introduced into the uterus after laparotomy, hysterotomy and the insertion of a purse-string suture to control bleeding and amniotic fluid leakage. This was attempted in 30 twin pregnancies and successful laser coagulation was achieved in 26; 18 of the pregnancies resulted in delivery of at least one live baby. However, despite the advantages of this approach, the technique has not gained widespread application, presumably because of its invasive nature.

Recently, Ville and co-workers[42,43] reported a sonoendoscopic technique performed under local anesthesia for successful separation of chorioangiopagus twins. Detailed ultrasound examination, including color flow mapping, is first performed to localize the placenta, the inter-twin amniotic membrane, the placental insertion of the umbilical cords and the communicating blood vessels on the chorionic plate[42]. The appropriate site of entry on the maternal abdomen is chosen to avoid injury to the placenta or fetuses and to allow access to the suspected area of vascular communications. Under continuous ultrasound visualization, a rigid 2-mm diameter fetoscope (field of vision 75°) housed in a 2.7-mm diameter cannula is introduced transabdominally into the amniotic cavity of the recipient twin. A 400-μm diameter Nd:YAG laser fiber is then passed down the side-arm of the cannula to 1 cm beyond the tip of the fetoscope. A combination of ultrasonographic and direct vision is used to examine systematically the chorionic plate along the whole length of the inter-twin membrane and identify the crossing vessels, which are coagulated by the administration of a total of 1000–4500 J delivered by 3-s shots using an output of 30–50 W at a distance of 1 cm[42]. Subsequently, amniotic fluid is drained through the fetoscope cannula over a period of 10–15 min to obtain subjective normalization of the amniotic fluid volume on ultrasonographic examination. The total procedure usually takes 30–45 min to complete. In 96 pregnancies at the Harris Birthright Centre, endoscopic laser coagulation was performed and there were 72% with at least one survivor and the total number of babies that survived was 52%.

The aim of systematic coagulation of all superficial placental vessels that cross or are adjacent to the inter-twin amniotic membrane is to interrupt the vascular communications between the circulations of the two fetuses. Arteriovenous anastomoses (which are thought to play the major role in the hemodynamic disturbance underlying feto–fetal transfusion) are found deep in common cotyledons but their afferent and efferent branches are superficial[1]. Although the inter-twin membrane does not necessarily overlie these common cotyledons[44], coagulation of all crossing vessels will inevitably include the afferent and efferent branches of these anastomoses.

Laser coagulation of communicating vessels potentially avoids many of the complications associated with severe TTS treated by other means. Cerebral palsy with preventricular leukomalacia is a well recognized complication of monochorionic twin pregnancies and is usually attributed to vascular accidents following the intrauterine death of one of the fetuses[45–47]. This complication is commonly seen in survivors after amniodrainage or other methods of treatment. Suggested mechanisms include a severe hypotensive episode due to hemorrhage from the survivor into the placenta of the dead fetus or disseminated intravascular coagulation after the release of thromboplastin from the dead twin. Laser coagulation of communicating vessels should potentially avoid these complications. However, brain damage observed in association with TTS does not occur only when one of the fetuses dies and in some cases it may be the consequence of intrauterine ischemic-hypoxic brain injury, in the donor fetus, hypoxia may be the consequence of hypovolemia and uteroplacental insufficiency, whereas in the recipient, hypoxia may be due to increased blood viscosity and hypervolemia-related congestive heart failure.

CONCLUSION

Twin pregnancies may be dichorionic (75%) or monochorionic (25%). The fetal loss rate in monochorionic pregnancies is much higher than in dichorionic twins, mainly due to twin-to-twin transfusion syndrome (TTS). The first manifestation of TTS is increased nuchal translucency thickness in one or both fetuses at 10–14 weeks of gestation. Subsequently, at 15–17 weeks, there is an inter-twin disparity in amniotic fluid manifested as folding of the inter-twin membrane. In about half of such cases with a membrane fold the large inter-twin disparities in amniotic fluid volume and fetal size persist throughout pregnancy but the outcome of such cases is usually good. In the other half, there is progression to severe TTS with the anhydramnios/polyhydramnios sequence and in these cases the survival with expectant management is less than 10%. Endoscopic laser ablation of the intercommunicating placental vessels is associated with survival of at least one of the babies in about 70% of pregnancies.

ACKNOWLEDGEMENT

Dr N. J. Sebire is supported by a grant from the Fetal Medicine Foundation (Charity No: 1037116).

References

1. Benirschke, K. and Kim, C. K. (1973). Multiple pregnancy. *N. Engl. J. Med.*, **228**, 1276–84
2. Hrubec, Z. and Robinette, D. (1984). The study if human twins in medical research. *N. Engl. J. Med.*, **310**, 435–41
3. Arts, N. F. T. and Lohman, A. H. M. (1971). The vascular anatomy of monochorionic diamniotic twin placentas and the trasnfusion syndrome. *Eur. J. Obstet. Gynecol.*, **3**, 85–93
4. Sekiya, S. and Hafez, E. S. E. (1977). Physiomorphology of twin transfusion syndrome. A study of 86 twin gestations. *Obstet. Gynecol.*, **50**, 288–92
5. Galea, P., Scott, J. M. and Goel, K. M. (1982). Feto-fetal transfusion syndrome. *Arch. Dis. Child.*, **57**, 781–94
6. Machin, G. A. and Still, K. (1995). The twin-twin transfusion syndrome: vascular anatomy of monochorionic placentas and their outcomes. In Keith, L. G., Papiernik, E., Keith, M. and Luke, B. (eds.) *Multiple Pregnancy*, pp. 367–93. (London: Parthenon Press)
7. Robertson, E. G. and Neer, K. J. (1983). Placental injection studies in twin gestation. *Am. J. Obstet. Gynecol.*, **147**, 170–4
8. Schatz, F. (1882). Eine besondere art von einseitiger polyhydramnie mit anderseitiger

oligohydramnie bei eineiigen zwillingen. *Arch. Gynakol.*, **19**, 329

9. Bajoria, R., Wigglesworth, J. and Fisk, N. M. (1995). Angioarchitecture of monochorionic placentas in relation to the twin-twin transfusion syndrome. *Am. J. Obstet. Gynecol*, **172**, 856–63

10. Finberg, H. J. (1992). The 'twin peak' sign: reliable evidence of dichorionic twinning. *J. Ultrasound Med.*, **11**, 571–7

11. Bessis, R. and Papiernik, E. (1981). Echographic imagery of amniotic membranes in twin pregnancies. In Gedda, L. and Parisi, P. (eds.) *Twin Research 3: Twin Biology and Multiple Pregnancy*, pp. 183–7. (New York: Alan R. Liss)

12. Sepulveda, W., Sebire, N. J., Hughes, K., Odibo, A. and Nicholaides, K. H. (1996). The lambda sign at 10–14 weeks of gestation as a predictor of chorionicity in twin pregnancies. *Ultrasound Obstet. Gynecol.*, **7**, 421–3

13. Botting, B. J., MacDonald Davis, I. and Macfarlane, A. J. (1987). Recent trends in the incidence of multiple births and associated mortality. *Arch. Dis. Child.*, **62**, 941–50

14. Gardner, M. O., Goldenberg, R. L., Cliver, S. P., Tucker, J. M., Nelson, K. G. and Copper, R. L. (1995). The origin and outcome of preterm twin pregnancies. *Obstet. Gynecol.*, **85**, 553–7

15. Chen, C. J., Wang, C. J., Yu, M. W. and Lee, T. K. (1992). Perinatal mortality and prevalence of major congenital malformations of twins in Taipei city. *Acta Genet. Med. Gemellol.*, **41**, 197–203

16. Rydhstrom, H. (1990). The effects of maternal age, parity and sex of the twins on twin perinatal mortality. A population based study. *Acta Genet. Med. Gemellol.*, **39**, 401–8

17. Machin, G., Bamforth, F., Innes, M. and Minichul, K. (1995). Some perinatal characteristics of monozygotic twins who are dichorionic. *Am. J. Med. Genet.*, **55**, 71–6

18. Dermon, R., Dermon, C. and Vlietinck, R. (1995). Placentation. In Keith, L. G., Papiernik, E., Keith, D. M. and Luke, B. (eds.) *Multiple Pregnancy*, pp. 113–28. (London: Parthenon Press)

19. Nicolaides, K. H., Sebire, N. J. and Snijders, R. J. M. (1997). Down's syndrome screening with nuchal transluency. *Lancet*, in press

20. Sebire, N. J., Snijders, R. J. M., Hughes, K., Sepulveda, W. and Nicolaides, K. H. (1996). Screening for trisomy 21 in twin pregnancies by maternal age and fetal nuchal translucency thickness at 10–14 weeks of gestation. *Br. J. Obstet. Gynaecol.*, **103**, 999–1003

21. Rausen, A. R., Seki, M. and Strauss, L. (1965). Twin transfusion syndrome. *J. Pediatr.*, **66**, 613–28

22. Tan, K. L., Tan, R., Tan, S. H. and Tan, A. M. (1979). The twin transfusion syndrome. Clinical observaions on 35 affected pairs. *Clin. Pediatr. Phila.*, **18**, 111–14

23. Saunders, N. J., Snijders, R. J. M. and Nicolaides, K. H. (1991). Twin-twin transfusion syndrome in the second trimester is associated with small inter-twin hemoglobin differences. *Fetal Diagn. Ther.*, **6**, 34–6

24. Jones, J. M., Sbarra, A. J., Dililklo, L., Cetrulo, C. L. and D'Altan, M. E. (1993). Indomethacin in severe twin to twin transfusion syndrome. *Am. J. Perinatol.*, **10**, 24–6

25. Urig, M. A., Simpson, G. F., Elliot, J. P. and Clewell, W. H. (1988). Twin twin transfusion syndrome: the surgical removal of one twin as a treatment option. *Fetal Ther.*, **3**, 185–8

26. Weiner, C. P. and Ludomirski, A. (1994). Diagnosis, pathophysiology, and treatment of chronic twin to twin transfusion syndrome. *Fetal Diagn. Ther.*, **9**, 283–90

27. Mahone, P. R., Sherer, D. M., Abramowicz, J. S. and Woods, J. T. (1993). Twin-twin tranfusion syndrome: rapid development of severe hydrops of the donor following selective feticide of the hydropic recipient. *Am. J. Obstet. Gynecol.*, **169**, 166–8

28. Wittmann, B. K., Farquharson, D. F., Thomas, W. D. S., Baldwin, V. J. and Wadsworth, L. D. (1986). The role of feticide in the management of severe twin transfusion syndrome. *Am. J. Obstet. Gynecol.*, **155**, 1023–6

29. Weiner, C. P. (1987). Diagnosis and treatment of twin to twin transfusion in the mid-second trimester of pregnancy. *Fetal Ther.*, **2**, 71–4

30. Chescheir, N. C. and Seeds, J. W. (1988). Polyhydramnios and oligohydramnios in twin gestations. *Obstet. Gynecol.*, **71**, 882–6

31. Donnenfield, A. E., Glazerman, L. R., Cutillo, D. M., Librizzi, R. J. and Weiner, S. (1989). Fetal exsanguination following intrauterine angiographic assessment and selective termination of a hydrocephalic, monozygotic co-twin. *Prenat. Diagn.*, **9**, 301–9

32. Bebbington, M. W., Wilson, R. D., Machan, L. and Wittmann, B. K. (1995). Selective fetocide in twin transfusion syndrome using ultrasound guided insertion of thrombogenic coils. *Fetal Diagn. Ther.*, **10**, 32–6

33. Dommergues, M., Mandelbrot, A. L. Delezoide, A. C. *et al.* (1995). Twin-to-twin transfusion syndrome: selective fetocide by embolisation of the hydropic fetus. *Fetal Diagn. Ther.*, **10**, 26–31

34. Lemery, D. J., Vanilieferinghen, P., Gasq, M., Finkeltin, F., Beaufrere, A. M. and Beytout, M. (1994). Fetal umbilical cord ligation under

ultrasound guidance. *Ultrasound Obstet. Gynecol.,* **4**, 399–401

35. Saunders, N. J., Snijders, R. J. M. and Nicolaides, K. H. (1992). Therapeutic amniocentesis in twin-twin transfusion syndrome appearing in the second trimester of pregnancy. *Am. J. Obstet. Gynecol.,* **166**, 820–4

36. Elliot, J. P., Urig, M. A. and Clewell, W. H. (1991). Aggressive therapeutic amniocentesis for treatment of twin-twin transfusion syndrome. *Obstet. Gynecol.,* **77**, 537–40

37. Reisner, D. P., Mahony, B. S., Petty, C N. *et al.* (1993). Stuck twin syndrome: outcome in thirty-seven consecutive cases. *Am. J. Obstet. Gynecol.,* **169**, 991–5

38. Pinette, M. G., Pan, Y., Pinette, S. G. and Stubblefield, P. G. (1993). Treatment of twin-twin transfusion syndrome. *Obstet. Gynecol.,* **82**, 841–6

39. Urig, M. A., Clewell, W. H. and Elliot, J. P. (1990). The twin transfusion syndrome. *Am. J. Obstet. Gynecol.,* **163**, 1522–6

40. Mahony, B. S., Petty, C. N., Nyberg, D. A., Luthy, D. A., Hickok, D. E. and Hirsch, J. H. (1990). The stuck twin phenomenon: ultrasonographic findings, pregnancy outcome and management with serial amniocentesis. *Am. J. Obstet, Gynecol.,* **163**, 1513–22

41. De Lia, J. E., Cruikshank, D. P. and Keye, W. R. (1990). Fetoscopic neodymium:YAG laser occlusion of placental vessels in severe twin-twin transfusion syndrome. *Obstet. Gynecol.,* **75**, 1046–53

42. Ville, Y., Hecher, K., Ogg, D., Warren, R. and Nicolaides, K. (1992). Successful outcome after Nd:YAG laser separation of chorioangiopagus-twins under sonoendoscopic control. *Ultrasound Obstet. Gynecol.,* **2**, 429–31

43. Ville, Y., Hyett, J., Hecher, K. and Nicolaides, K. Preliminary experience with endoscopic laser surgery for severe twin twin transfusion syndrome. *N. Engl. J. Med.,* **332**, 224–7

44. De Lia, J. E., Kuhlmaa, R. S., Cruikshank, D. P. and O'Bee, L. R. (1993). Placental surgery: a new frontier. *Placenta,* **14**, 477–85

45. Bejar, R., Vigliocco, G., Gramajo, H. *et al.* (1990). Antenatal origin of neurologic damage in newborn infants. II. Multiple gestations. *Am. J. Obstet. Gynecol.,* **162**, 1230–6

46. Bendon, R. W. and Siddiqi, T. (1989). Acute twin to twin *in utero* transfusion. *Pediatr. Pathol.,* **9**, 951–8

47. Fusi, L., MacOharland, P., Fisk, N., Nicolini, U. and Wigglesworth, J. (1991). Acute twin-twin transfusion: a possible mechanism for brain damaged survivors after intrauterine death of a monozygotic twin. *Obstet. Gynecol.,* **78**, 517–22

Abdominal wall defects: gastroschisis   33

P. A. M. Raine

INTRODUCTION

Abdominal wall defects fall into well recognised and defined groups of congenital anomalies[1,2]. However, their pathogenesis remains uncertain[3] and theories of common cause and development have been advanced. Nonetheless, following wide use and increasing sophistication of prenatal diagnosis, the importance of the differences between the lesions and their implications has become apparent.

Body stalk anomaly is rare and universally fatal. Gastroschisis and exomphalos (omphalocele) occur in intrauterine life with approximately equal frequency (1 : 4000)[4,5]. Exomphalos presents as failure of the fetal intestine to return to the abdominal cavity after the period of normal herniation into the yolk sac at about 10–12 weeks of fetal life: a membrane-covered umbilical herniation of varying amounts of viscera persists. Gastroschisis is a complete defect, almost always just to the right of a normal umbilical cord insertion, through which intestine extrudes into the amniotic fluid.

Chromosomal and other major congenital anomalies (cardiac, renal, limb) and syndromes (Beckwith-Wiedemann, pentalogy of Cantrell) are relatively common with exomphalos, whilst gastroschisis is almost always an isolated anomaly. The amount of extra-celomic intestine varies considerably in exomphalos and the presence or absence of liver in the hernia has a major bearing on the feasibility of surgical closure: the abdominal cavity is under-developed and has a relatively small capacity preventing primary surgical closure of major (liver extra-celomic) exomphalos. Minor exomphalos (defect less than 5 cm diameter) and hernia into the cord are at the other end of the spectrum. A large amount of intestine, though rarely the liver, is usually extra-abdominal in gastroschisis, and may be affected by ischemia, obstruction, stenosis or atresia, but primary surgical closure is often possible.

Prenatal diagnosis by anomaly ultrasound scan is indicated by a raised maternal serum α-fetoprotein level; by previous abnormality or by maternal or family history, and is now expected. Confusion of the ultrasonic appearance of the lesions is rare. Exclusion of chromosomal or other structural anomalies follows. Decisions regarding continuation of the pregnancy and the place, time and mode of delivery can be made in the early second trimester following detailed discussion between the involved professionals and the parents with their family and advisors.

Termination of pregnancy may be chosen for complicated and major exomphalos, for which survival of only 50% can be predicted. Uncomplicated minor exomphalos presents few difficulties or controversies in management and a very low risk of morbidity or mortality. Gastroschisis, on the other hand, presents a continuing challenge to make the most of the advantages of prenatal diagnosis and to reduce the residual morbidity due to poor early gut function, the need for prolonged parenteral nutrition, long hospital stay and the residual mortality of 10–15%. This paper concentrates on the current management and outcome of gastroschisis.

METHODS

Admissions of newborn babies with abdominal wall defects to the Neonatal Surgical Unit of the Royal Hospital for Sick Children in Glasgow between January 1983 and June 1996 were studied. Fetal deaths, stillbirths and early post-natal deaths prior to transfer were not included. Data was collected prospectively for all cases of gastroschisis.

The diagnosis of abdominal wall defects during this period was increasingly made pre-natally. Many pregnancies were referred to the regional Fetal Medicine Unit at the Queen Mother's Hospital in Glasgow for further man-agement. A raised maternal serum α-feto-protein level was usually the indicator for a detailed anomaly scan which revealed the de-fect. Differentiation between gastroschisis and exomphalos was almost always possible. Other anomalies (e.g. cardiac, renal and limb) were sought and chromosome analysis was per-formed, particularly for exomphalos. In the case of major exomphalos and exomphalos compli-cated by cardiac or chromosomal abnormality, the question of termination of pregnancy was discussed with parents.

Delivery at the Queen Mother's Hospital, ad-jacent to the Neonatal Surgical Unit, was advo-cated to facilitate speedy decisions and early surgery. Preterm delivery was necessary because of fetal distress in some cases and was thought desirable in others in which progressive bowel dilatation was noted. In the early part of the series some cases of gastroschisis underwent Cesarean section electively, but latterly it was reserved for fetal distress or maternal indica-tions. After birth the exposed bowel was pro-tected from cooling, drying, contamination and trauma by application of saline dressings or plas-tic membrane film, and the baby was assessed in detail. Surgery was performed as soon as possible.

Abdominal wall closure was achieved in a single stage (primary) whenever possible but, when the size of bowel relative to peritoneal cavity prevented this, either a membrane (dura mater or Vicryl collagen mesh) or a two-stage silastic 'silo' technique was used. Bowel atresia or stenosis was managed either by direct anasto-mosis or by enterostomy. Postoperatively a cen-tral venous catheter was inserted to allow parenteral nutrition. The baby remained para-lyzed with an endotracheal tube in place to permit intermittent positive pressure ventila-tion for a few days. When a 'silo' was used initially, skin closure was achieved at the second operation, usually within 8 days. Secondary surgery was also needed for closure of enteros-tomies. Enteral feeding was gradually intro-duced as intestinal function improved.

RESULTS

In the period January 1983 to June 1996, 72 neonates with gastroschisis were admitted. In the same period there were 35 cases of exom-phalos and hernia into the base of the umbilical cord. Of the 72 cases of gastroschisis, 40 were male and 32 female. A prenatal diagnosis was made in 58 (81%) cases. Ultrasound scans sug-gested bowel dilatation *in utero* in ten cases (14%).

Delivery was by the vaginal route in 36 (50%) cases and by Cesarean section in 36 (50%) cases of gastroschisis. Table 1 shows the indications for Cesarean section. The principal indication was fetal distress (at a mean gestation of 35.4 weeks) but maternal indications included pre-vious Cesarean section, breech presentation, failure to progress and ante-partum hemor-rhage. The mean gestation at birth for the whole group was 35.7 weeks and the mean birth weight was 2210 g; the babies were therefore in the 10th centile for weight.

Only four babies (6%) had an extra-intestinal anomaly (Table 2) and none had a chromo-somal abnormality. Associated gut abnormality occurred in 18 (25%) (Table 2).

The mean duration from birth to surgery was 3.3 h. Primary closure was performed in 47 (65%) and closure was achieved with use of a membrane in a further 12 (17%). Only 13

Table 1 Indications for Cesarean section (36 cases)

Indication	n
Emergency	24
maternal indications	3
fetal distress	21
Elective	12
maternal indications	2
fetal presence of gastroschisis	10

(18%) needed a two-stage 'silo' closure. Enterostomies were created in eight cases (seven with gut atresia and one with ischemia). Nine babies (12.5%) died; eight in the immediate postoperative period and one at 4 years due to microcephaly related to bowel ischemia following precipitate vaginal delivery at home. Details of these deaths are shown in Table 3. Ten other babies had complications as shown in Table 4, most of which were intestinal. Further surgery was needed in 19 cases, as also shown in Table 4. For the 63 (87.5%) survivors, the mean duration of parenteral nutrition was 30 days and the mean length of stay in hospital was 53 days.

To assess the significance of various factors, correlations were examined between the following pairs of factors.

(1) *Prenatal diagnosis and gestation/birth weight*
Babies with prenatal diagnosis were born at a mean gestation of 35.4 weeks compared with 36.8 weeks for those with no prenatal diagnosis.

Table 2 Anomalies occurring in the 72 babies with gastroschisis

Anomaly	n
Extra-intestinal anomalies	4
Severe intrauterine growth retardation	1
Partial amputation/syndactyly	1
Hydronephrosis	1
Amyoplasia of upper limbs	1
Associated gut abnormalities	18
Atresia (including multiple)	9
Stenosis	5
Obstruction (due to bands/adhesions)	3
Ischemia	1

Table 3 Details of neonatal and infant deaths (9 cases)

Birth weight (g)	Gestation (weeks)	Cause of death
1030	31	Persistent severe metabolic acidosis
1270	31	Volvulus/bowel ischemia
1400	31	Respiratory distress syndrome
2000	35	Bowel ischemia/adrenal hemorrhage
2020	38	Disseminated herpes simplex
2060	35	Bowel ischemia/necrosis
2200	36	Bowel ischemia
2340	35	Death at 4 years related to microcephaly
2980	40	Bowel ischemia/acute renal failure

Table 4 Complications following closure of gastroschisis, and indications for further abdominal surgery

	n
Complications following closure	10
Necrotizing enterocolitis	2
Malrotation obstruction	1
Bowel obstruction/fistula – hypothyroidism, cardiac anomaly	1
Duodenal obstruction	1
Obstruction related to adhesions to membrane	1
Adhesion obstruction – slow transit	1
Infected membrane – secondary ileal atresia	1
Anastomotic stricture	1
Hydrocephalus due to thrombosis	1
Indications for further abdominal surgery	19
Closure of enterostomies	7
Bowel obstruction	6
Exploration for volvulus/ischemia	3
Necrotizing enterocolitis	2
Malrotation	1

However, mean birth weight (2210 g) was the same for the two groups.

(2) *Prenatal diagnosis and survival* Survival following prenatal diagnosis was 51 of 58 (88%) compared with 12 of 14 (86%) without prenatal diagnosis.

(3) *Bowel dilatation in utero and gestation* The mean gestation at birth of the ten babies with bowel dilatation *in utero* was 34.5 weeks compared with 35.9 for the 62 without dilatation. Five of the ten with dilatation were delivered by elective Cesarean section on account of increasing dilatation.

(4) *Bowel dilatation in utero and gut atresia/stenosis* Of ten babies with bowel dilatation *in utero*, five (50%) had gut atresia stenosis; the other five had 'normal' bowel. Of the 62 babies with no dilatation *in utero*, nine (15%) had atresia/stenosis.

(5) *Bowel dilatation in utero and method of closure* Of the ten babies with bowel dilatation *in utero*, only one (10%) required two-stage 'silo' closure compared with 19% of the 62 babies with no dilatation.

(6) *Bowel dilatation in utero and survival* Of the ten babies with bowel dilatation *in utero*, nine (90%) survived compared with 87% survival for the 62 babies with no dilatation.

(7) *Method of delivery and survival* Of the 36 babies delivered by Cesarean section, four (11%) died compared with five (14%) of the 36 born by the vaginal route.

(8) *Gut atresia/stenosis and gestation/birth weight* The 14 babies with gut atresia/stenosis had a mean gestation of 35.4 weeks and a mean birth weight of 2340 g compared with 35.8 weeks and 2180 g, respectively, for the 58 without atresia/stenosis.

(9) *Gut atresia/stenosis and method of closure* The 14 babies with gut atresia/stenosis all underwent a primary (11) or membrane (three) closure, whereas 13 (22%) of the 58 without atresia/stenosis required a two-stage 'silo'.

(10) *Gut atresia/stenosis and survival* There were 11 (78%) survivors of the 14 babies with gut atresia/stenosis compared with 90% of the 58 without atresia/stenosis.

(11) *Method of closure and birth weight/gestation* For the 13 babies undergoing two-stage 'silo' closure, mean birth weight was 2168 g and mean gestation 36.1 weeks compared with 2217 g and 35.6 weeks, respectively, for the 59 undergoing primary and membrane closure.

(12) *Method of closure and duration of parenteral nutrition* The mean durations of parenteral nutrition for each group were: primary closure (47), 28 days; membrane closure (12), 34 days; and two-stage closure (13), 32 days.

(13) *Method of closure and length of hospital stay* The mean lengths of hospital stay for each group were: primary closure (47), 46 days; membrane closure (12), 70 days; and two-stage closure (13), 63 days.

(14) *Method of closure and survival* Survival following primary closure was 87%, following membrane closure was 92%, and following two-stage closure was 85%.

(15) *Survival and birth weight/gestation* The babies who died had a mean birth weight of 1920 g and a mean gestation of 34.6 weeks compared with 2250 g and 35.9 weeks, respectively, for survivors.

DISCUSSION

The prenatal diagnosis of gastroschisis is now standard when an anomaly scan follows a raised maternal α-fetoprotein level[5-7]. In the absence of this indicator (when the mother declines the test or books late), a routine scan may not pick up the anomaly. However, as anomaly scans become widely available in the early second trimester, prenatal diagnosis should approach 100%.

In this series the admission rate to a neonatal surgical unit for gastroschisis was twice that for exomphalos, despite the equal incidence

(1 : 4000) of the two lesions in the first trimester of pregnancy. This reflects the choice of termination for some cases of major exomphalos and exomphalos associated with other major anomaly or chromosomal abnormality for which expectation of uncomplicated survival is poor.

Prenatal diagnosis raises the possibility of elective Cesarean section but this has not been shown to improve either morbidity or mortality[8–12]. Nonetheless, readiness to perform emergency Cesarean section for fetal distress from about 35 weeks onwards is important in 30% of cases and serial biophysical assessment is necessary[13]. The prediction of those fetuses at potentially greater risk *in utero* has proved difficult; neither prenatal diagnosis itself nor bowel dilatation *in utero* was related to higher mortality although the latter was associated with shorter gestation at delivery. In addition, bowel dilatation *in utero* was not sensitive (36%) or specific (50%) for the presence of gut atresia/stenosis and did not relate to the method of closure and the need for a 'silo'. Ultrasonographic interpretation of bowel dilatation raises problems[14,15], and more detailed studies of gut wall thickness, in addition to dilatation, may be needed to improve prediction of gut abnormality.

Whilst it is likely that a longer interval between delivery and surgery has an adverse effect on abdominal wall closure in gastroschisis, this cannot be demonstrated in the present series which had a generally short interval. However, advantages for very early surgery have been noted[16] and further analysis of this factor is warranted. Surprisingly, babies with gut atresia/stenosis all had a primary or membrane closure; in part, this may reflect the desire by the surgeon to avoid a 'silo' in the presence of an enterostomy but also suggests that difficulty in primary closure is related more to thickening and matting of the exposed bowel than to dilatation of individual loops caused by obstruction.

The method of closure was not related to birth weight or gestation and survival was equally good for each method of closure. However, babies undergoing membrane closure had a longer duration of parenteral nutrition and a longer hospital stay than those having closure in two stages with a 'silo', and use of a membrane appeared to convey some disadvantage[9].

Survival for babies with gastroschisis was related to birth weight and gestation[17], and to a lesser degree to the presence of gut atresia/stenosis[17], but not to prenatal diagnosis[10], bowel dilatation *in utero*, or method of closure. The deaths could be grouped into those related principally to prematurity (respiratory distress syndrome and persistent metabolic acidosis), those unrelated to the gastroschisis defect (disseminated herpes simplex and microcephaly) and those related to bowel ischemia. The latter group are the most amenable to reduction through increased biophysical monitoring[13] and technical advances and the overall mortality from gastroschisis can be expected to drop progressively below 10%[18].

ACKNOWLEDGEMENTS

The author wishes to acknowledge the expertise, enthusiasm and skill of consultant colleagues and specialist nurses in both the Fetal Medicine Unit of the Queen Mother's Hospital and the Neonatal Surgical Unit of the Royal Hospital for Sick Children at Yorkhill, Glasgow.

References

1. Raine, P. A. M. (1991). Anterior abdominal wall defects. *Curr. Obstet. Gynaecol.*, **1**, 147–53
2. Langer, J. C. (1996). Gastroschisis and exomphalos. *Semin. Pediatr. Surg.*, **5**, 124–8
3. Kluth, D. and Lambrecht, W. (1996). The pathogenesis of omphalocele and gastroschisis – an unsolved problem. *Pediatr. Surg. Int.*, **11**, 62–6
4. MacKenzie, F., personal communication

5. Morrow, R. J., Whittle, M. J., McNay, M. R., Raine, P. A. M., Gibson, A. A. M. and Crossley, J. (1993). Prenatal diagnosis and management of anterior abdominal wall defects in the west of Scotland. *Prenat. Diagn.*, **13**, 111–13

6. Roberts, J. P. and Burge, D. M. (1990). Antenatal diagnosis of abdominal wall defects: a missed opportunity? *Arch. Dis. Child.*, **65**, 687–9

7. Dykes, E. H. (1996). Prenatal diagnosis and management of abdominal wall defects. *Semin. Pediatr. Surg.*, **5**, 90–4

8. Quirk, J. G., Fortney, J., Collins, H. B., West, J., Hassad, S. J. and Wagner, C. (1996). Outcomes of newborns with gastroschisis: the effects of mode of delivery, site of delivery, and interval from birth to surgery. *Am. J. Obstet. Gynecol.*, **174**, 1134–40

9. Novotny, D. A., Klein, R. L. and Boeckman, C. R. (1993). Gastroschisis: an 18-year review. *J. Pediatr. Surg.*, **28**, 650–2

10. Sipes, S. L., Weiner, C. P., Sipes, D. R., Grant, S. S. and Williamson, R. A. (1990). Gastroschisis and omphalocele: does either antenatal diagnosis or route of delivery make a difference in perinatal outcome? *Obstet. Gynecol.*, **76**, 195–9

11. Crabbe, D. C. G., Thomas, D. F. M., Beck, J. M. and Spicer, R. D. (1991). Prenatally diagnosed gastroschisis: a case for preterm delivery? *Pediatr. Surg. Int.*, **6**, 108–10

12. Moretti, M., Khoury, A., Rodriquez, J., Lobe, T., Shaver, D. and Sibai, B. (1990). The effect of mode of delivery on the perinatal outcome in fetuses with abdominal wall defects. *Am. J. Obstet. Gynecol.*, **163**, 833–8

13. Crawford, R. A. F., Ryan, G., Wright, V. M. and Rodeck, C. H. (1992). The importance of serial biophysical assessment of fetal wellbeing in gastroschisis. *Br. J. Obstet. Gynaecol.*, **99**, 899–902

14. Lenke, R. R., Persutte, W. R. and Nemes, J. (1990). Ultrasonographic assessment of intestinal damage in fetuses with gastroschisis: is it of clinical value? *Am. J. Obstet. Gynecol.*, **163**, 995–8

15. Babcock, C. J., Hedrick, M. H., Goldstein, R. B., Callen, P. W., Harrison, M. R., Adzick, N. S. and Filly, R. A. (1994). Gastroschisis: can ultrasonography of the fetal bowel accurately predict postnatal outcome? *J. Ultrasound Med.*, **13**, 701–6

16. Swift, R. I., Singh, M. P., Ziderman, D. A., Silverman, M., Elder, M. A. and Elder, M. G. (1992). A new regime in the management of gastroschisis. *J. Pediatr. Surg.*, **27**, 61–3

17. Luck, S. R., Sherman, J. O., Raffensperger, J. G. and Goldstein, I. R. (1985). Gastroschisis in 106 consecutive newborn infants. *Surgery*, **98**, 677–83

18. Eurenius, K. and Axelsson, O. (1994). Outcome for fetuses with abdominal wall defects detected by routine second trimester ultrasound. *Acta Obstet. Gynecol. Scand.*, **73**, 25–9

Investigation, treatment and outcome of fetal abnormalities: congenital heart disease

34

J. Le Bidois

Echocardiography of the fetus makes possible an accurate diagnosis of congenital heart disease, the most frequent of fetal malformations, with an incidence of 0.8% of live births. Ultrasonographic imaging of the fetal heart combines the use of M-mode, two-dimensional imaging and Doppler imaging, allowing a study of anatomy and physiology of the normal and the abnormal fetal heart. Detecting cardiac malformations in the fetus has major consequences. It allows optimal management during the perinatal period, particularly in the case of a newborn who needs an early infusion of prostaglandin E1 to maintain the patency of the ductus arteriosus. Detection of a cardiac malformation allows for the diagnosis of extracardiac malformations and chromosomal abnormalities which are often associated with cardiac malformations. It also offers the parents of the fetus as much information as possible concerning the treatment and outcome for the malformation so that they can take a decision whether to continue or terminate the pregnancy.

Indications for fetal echocardiography are many, but their relative yield is very variable. In 1993, Friedman and colleagues[1] reported that a family history of congenital heart disease, arrhythmias, maternal diabetes and teratogen exposure had a low yield (less than 3%) whereas extracardiac anomalies, aneuploidy and hydrops had a relative yield of 11–23%. Most importantly, a suspicious level 1 scan had the highest relative yield; 45% for the entire group of the study and 74% in 1992. This indicates clearly that every effort should be made to teach sonographers how to recognize the normal structures of the heart at the prenatal ultrasound screening at 18–24 weeks of gestation. That would allow for a better prenatal detection of congenital heart disease. In a multicenter study[2] the rate of antenatal diagnosis of congenital heart disease in patients referred for cardiac surgery within the first three months of life varied from 0% in England, Germany, The Netherlands and Israel to 15% in France. These rates are deceiving and should be improved. In France, a collaboration between pediatric cardiologists, sonographers and obstetricians has been implemented since the early 1980s[3]. Since then, pediatric cardiologists specially trained in fetal cardiology have taught a large proportion of sonographers to diagnose or at least suspect cardiac anomalies.

A level 1 scan, usually done around the 20th week of gestation, must include at least:

(1) A four-chamber view to confirm the presence of two atria, two ventricles, the presence of the intraventricular septum and of the ostium primum portion of the interatrial septum; and

(2) A view of the great vessels to rule out a transposition. This usually takes a very short time and allows the ruling out of the vast majority of severe cardiac malformation.

When this level 1 scan has shown an anomaly or has failed to show the aforementioned elements, an expert scan should be carried out by a specially trained sonographer, usually a pediatric cardiologist. This examination includes a precise description of the cardiac structures, the veins, the great arteries, the ductus arteriosus and the aortic arch. When a malformation is present, an assessment of the prognostic factors is made so that the parents can be informed as to whether the malformation is curable, amenable to palliative or curative surgery, or to interventional catheterization. They also need to be informed about whether there is a risk of fetal death, whether a specific perinatal management strategy needs to be planned, when surgery will be needed, and whether the child will be able to enjoy a normal life.

There are many classifications of cardiac malformations which are useful for the pediatric cardiologist or cardiac surgeon, but the only classification that is meaningful in the instance of prenatal diagnosis is a classification of curability. One usually considers curable a malformation with two normal-sized ventricles and two 'reasonably-sized' great arteries: this includes ventricular and atrial septal defects, tetralogy of Fallot, transposition of the great arteries, coarctation of the aorta, pulmonary valve stenosis and anomalous pulmonary venous drainage. At the other end of the spectrum are malformations with only one functional ventricle and/or with tiny pulmonary arteries, which at present are incurable. The main problems are those less clear-cut situations: for instance, where there is pulmonary atresia with an intact septum and a small right ventricle, there is no clear limit of ventricular size that tells you whether such a child will be cured or will live with a definitive palliation and a limited future. Similarly, it is often questioned whether a relatively small left ventricle at 20 weeks of gestation will become a hypoplastic left heart in the future, or a normal left ventricle after the repair of a coarctation of the aorta. In all these difficult cases, repeating the ultrasound examination after 3–4 weeks may allow a better assessment of the prognosis.

Good perinatal management is of the utmost importance in congenital heart diseases where survival depends on the patency of the ductus arteriosus, such as interruption of the aortic arch, or the foramen ovale, such as transposition of the great arteries. In these cases, delivery should occur in a multidisciplinary center with obstetrics, neonatal intensive care and pediatric cardiology. A fetal cardiac malformation is not by itself an indication for a Cesarean section. In ductal-dependent malformations, an infusion of prostaglandin E1 should be started promptly. In isolated transposition of the great arteries, an ultrasound examination should be carried out immediately after birth to assess the size of the foramen ovale and perform a Rashkind atrioseptostomy to enlarge it if necessary. A child with a transposition can die within its first hours if the foramen ovale is too small and does not allow satisfactory mixing of the oxygenated blood of the left heart and pulmonary artery and the hypoxemic blood of the right heart and aorta.

Neonatal surgery is needed in transposition of the great arteries, in total anomalous pulmonary venous drainage and often in coarctation of the aorta, as well as in malformations with deep cyanosis. Surgery is now replaced in some instances by interventional catheterization, particularly in cases of valvar stenoses, whether aortic or pulmonary. In other cases, surgery is usually delayed but there is a clear trend to early (first 6 months or 1 year) complete repair of cardiac malformations, except in complex cases where a preliminary palliative intervention may be necessary. Some cases are too complex to be amenable to conventional surgery so that the only possibility is a cardiac transplantation, which still carries the risk of numerous complications and early and late mortality.

In conclusion, it appears that a prerequisite for good antenatal diagnosis and management of congenital heart disease is the collaboration of obstetricians, sonographers, pediatric cardiologists, geneticists and neonatologists. Complete and sincere information should be given to the parents of an affected fetus when the diagnosis is made. When there is a doubt concerning the prognosis of a malformation, ultrasound examination should be repeated. Delivery and neonatal care should be prepared for in order to be ready to react promptly and efficiently to a potentially hazardous situation. Finally, emphasis should be made on the quality of the level 1 scanning without which there would be no prenatal cardiology.

References

1. Friedman, A. H., Copel, J. A. and Kleinman, C. S. (1993). Fetal echocardiography and fetal cardiology: indications, diagnosis and management. *Semin. Perinatal.*, **17**, 76–88

2. Lacour-Gayet, F., Brawn, W. J., Corno, A., Crupi, G., di Carlo, D., Ebels, T., Elliott, M., Horvath, P., Ilyin, V., Maruzewski, B., Rubay, R., Sairanen, H., Smolinsky, A., Stellin, G. and Ziemer, G. (European Congenital Surgeon Club) (1993). Multicenter European study on the influence of fetal diagnosis on neonatal cardiac surgery. *Cardiol. Young*, **3** (Suppl.), 62

3. Fermont, L., De Geeter, B., Aubry, M. C., Kachaner, J. and Sidi, D. (1986). A close collaboration between obstetricians and pediatric cardiologists allows antenatal detection of severe cardiac malformations by two-dimensional echocardiography. In Doyle, E. F., Engle, M. E. and Gersony, W. M. (eds.) *Pediatric Cardiology. Proceedings of the Second World Congress*, p.34. (New York: Springer-Verlag)

Nitric oxide in parturition

35

J. Norman

INTRODUCTION

Nitric oxide (NO) is a tiny molecule, whose biological importance was first outlined in 1987 when NO was identified as an endothelial-derived vasodilator[1]. Nitric oxide is derived from L-arginine by the action of nitric oxide synthase (NOS), which converts L-arginine to L-citrulline and NO. There are three main forms of NOS, encoded by three distinct genes (Table 1). Nitric oxide synthase-I and NOS-III are calcium dependent, and release small quantities of NO in response to stimuli such as acetylcholine, shear stress and endothelin. Nitric oxide synthase-II is independent of calcium and releases much larger quantities of NO when induced by stimuli such as lipopolysaccharide and γ-interferon. The production of NO by NOS can be competitively inhibited by analogs of L-arginine such as N^{ω}-nitro-L-arginine (L-NMMA) and N^{ω}-nitro-L-arginine methyl ester (L-NAME).

Over the last decade, it has become clear that NO is involved in a vast array of physiological and pathological processes throughout the body[2]. Nitric oxide is a smooth muscle relaxant in the vascular system, lungs and gastrointestinal tract, it is a neurotransmitter in the brain and in the peripheral nervous system and it is released from the immune system in large quantities as part of host defense. An increasing body of evidence indicates that NO may play a role in parturition. This paper will focus on two main areas; first, on a potential therapeutic role for NO donors in the treatment of preterm labor; and, second, on the putative role of endogenous NO synthesis in the control of the onset of parturition.

THERAPEUTIC ROLE FOR NO DONORS IN THE TREATMENT OF PRETERM LABOR

In vitro studies

The relaxant effect of NO on isolated myometrial strips was first demonstrated in rats[3]. Further studies have since shown that L-arginine (the precursor of NO synthesis), sodium nitroprusside (a NO donor), and cyclic guanosine monophosphate (cGMP; the second messenger through which NO exerts its actions) also inhibited contractility of rat myometrium[3–5]. The inhibitory effects of L-arginine were abolished by L-NAME and methylene blue, confirming that the observed effects were mediated specifically by NO acting via an increase in guanylate cyclase activity. Taken together, these data indicate that NO is a powerful inhibitor of rat myometrial contractility, and that this inhibition is effected predominantly by the production of cyclic GMP within the smooth muscle cells.

In vitro data on human myometrium are less extensive, and the effect of NO gas on myometrial contractility *in vitro* has not been investigated. Several studies have examined the effect of agents which release NO on contractility of isolated myometrial strips obtained from

Table 1 The three isoforms of nitric oxide synthase (NOS)

Name	Name	Location
NOS-I	bNOS	brain
		NANC neurons
NOS-II	iNOS	macrophages
		neutrophils
		vascular smooth muscle
NOS-III	eNOS	vascular endothelium

NANC; non-adrenergic, non-cholinergic

women undergoing Cesarean section[6–8]. Both the NO donors diethylamine/NO and streptozotocin, which releases NO in response to ultraviolet (UV) radiation, caused inhibition of spontaneous and oxytocin-induced activity when amplitude or force of contractions was measured. Studies with diethylamine/NO (concentrations up to 10^{-4} mol/l) showed that this drug achieved a maximum reduction in 'spontaneous' myometrial force to 20% of pretreatment values in myometrium removed prior to the onset of labor, and 40% of pretreatment values in myometrium removed from women in active labor. Streptozotocin, which releases NO in response to UV radiation, reduced the amplitude of contractions by 50% when applied in concentrations of 10^{-3} mol/l[8]. Initial contractile activity in this latter study was a mixture of 'spontaneous' and 'oxytocin- induced'. Both of these studies demonstrated that NO donors can reduce the amplitude and force of human myometrial contractions. Unfortunately, neither of the above agents is available in a form which could be administered *in vivo*. Our own group

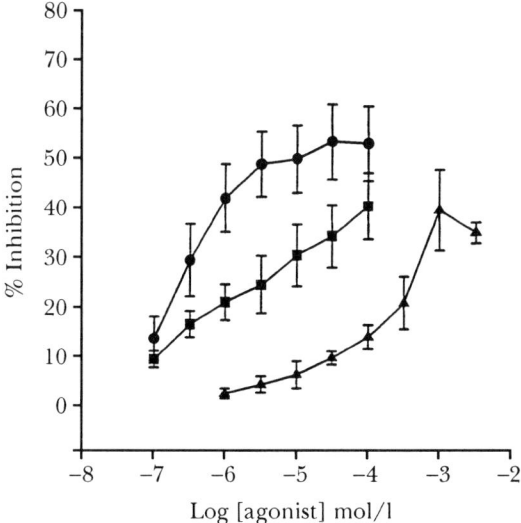

Figure 1 Effect of sodium nitroprusside (SNP, ●), glyceryl trinitrate (GTN, ■) and cyclic guanosine monophosphate (cGMP, ▲) *in vitro* on amplitude of contractions in myometrial strips obtained from women undergoing Cesearean section prior to the onset of labor

has studied the effect of two NO donors which are available for *in vivo* use, glyceryl trinitrate (GTN) and sodium nitroprusside (SNP)[7]. Glyceryl trinitrate reduced the amplitude of contractions by a maximum of 40% when applied in concentrations of 10^{-4} mol/l and SNP reduced contractions by 53% at 10^{-4} mol/l (Figure 1). Glyceryl trinitrate and SNP had differing effects on frequency: a 30% decrease in frequency was noted with 10^{-4} mol/l GTN whereas 10^{-4} mol/l SNP caused a 40% increase in frequency.

These studies indicate that NO donors may be useful clinically as tocolytic agents. However, large concentrations of NO are required to have a significant inhibitory effect on myometrial contractions, and the use of such agents may be limited by the profound hypotension these concentrations would induce *in vivo*. Controlled clinical studies are required to determine the efficacy of NO for the inhibition of preterm labor.

In vivo studies

A preliminary study on the effect of NO donors on myometrial contractility *in vivo* has recently been performed. Glyceryl trinitrate patches were administered to women with a diagnosis of preterm labor between 22 and 33 weeks' gestation[9]. Deponit 10 patches (which deliver a total of 10 mg GTN transdermally over 24 h) were applied to the abdomen to a maximum of two patches in the first hour, and then two patches at 24 h intervals thereafter. This regimen was followed for each of the 20 episodes of preterm labor in a total of 13 women. Only one of the women delivered prematurely, and in this case delivery was attributed to cervical incompetence. In the remaining women, pregnancy continued unaffected. Although the results of this study suggest that GTN may be effective in the treatment of preterm labor, the results of controlled studies should be awaited before widespread use.

We have recently studied the effect of NO donors on uterine contraction *in vivo* using a model of women undergoing therapeutic abortion in the second trimester[7]. The effect of

GTN on myometrial contractility was quantified objectively in these women. Each woman previously had been given mifepristone (200 mg) which stimulates myometrial contractions. Accurate measurements of uterine activity were made in these women using an intrauterine pressure catheter and calculated in Montevideo units. Compared with a placebo infusion of normal saline, a 15-min infusion of GTN at a dose of 20 µg/min had no significant effect on uterine contractions. The dose of GTN applied would be expected to generate plasma levels considerably in excess of those achieved by two patches, each releasing 10 mg GTN in 24 h.

Conclusion

Nitric oxide inhibits human myometrial contractility. *In vitro* studies indicate that NO donors may be useful in the treatment of preterm labor, and *in vivo* studies are in progress to determine their efficacy in clinical practice. If NO is found to be an effective tocolytic, it could have a major impact in the reduction of neonatal mortality and morbidity.

ROLE OF NITRIC OXIDE IN THE ONSET OF PARTURITION

Data from rat and rabbit studies indicate that NO may play a pivotal role in the onset of parturition. Nitric oxide is produced within the uterus during pregnancy, it acts as a myometrial relaxant, and the production of NO is attenuated at the time of the onset of labor (see reference 10 for review). Hence NO may promote myometrial quiescence during pregnancy, and a decline in NO synthesis may play a role in the control of the onset of paturition.

Since the etiology of parturition in the human is obscure, much interest has focused on whether NO may similarly control the onset of human labor. As shown above, NO clearly inhibits myometrial contractility. The production of NO itself from the pregnant human uterus has not been determined, partly due to the practical difficulties of measuring NO. However, a variety of studies have looked at other parts of the NO–cyclic GMP pathway. Pregnant human myometrium in culture generated nitrate/nitrite (the breakdown products of NO synthesis) and cyclic GMP (the second messenger through which NO exerts its actions[6]. Immunocytochemical techniques have identified NOS, the enzyme which generates NO, in both the syncytiotrophoblast and the vascular tissue of the placenta[11-15]. These studies all imply that NO is produced within the pregnant human uterus and may impact on myometrial function.

Since NO is produced within the pregnant human uterus, a change in this production may occur at the onset of parturition, and hence be responsible for the onset of labor. The most convincing evidence that a change in NO synthesis is responsible for the onset of labor comes from data showing that amniotic fluid nitrate concentrations were lower at the end of pregnancy (37–41 weeks) than in the second or first trimester[16]. None of these patients was in labor at the time of sampling. In addition, a lower myometrial content of cyclic GMP (the second messenger through which NO exerts its actions) was found in myometrium obtained from laboring compared with non-laboring women[6]. These results imply that NO production within the uterus gradually falls during the third trimester, and that a further fall occurs at the onset of labor, contributing to the mechanism of onset of human parturition.

Other groups have used different assays as an index of NO synthesis, and have failed to show a change in NO production at the time of labor. Several groups[17,18] have determined NO synthase activity in uterine tissues before and after the onset of labor by measuring the conversion of radiolabelled arginine to citrulline both in the presence and absence of calcium. Nitric oxide synthase activity (both calcium dependent and calcium independent) in placenta, myometrium, membranes and choriodecidua prior to the onset of labor is shown in Table 2. In contrast to animal data, *no* decrease in NOS activity was observed following the onset of labor. Indeed, a significant *increase* in NOS activity was observed in myometrium. Furthermore, in a study on myometrial generation of nitrate

Table 2 Nitric oxide synthase (NOS) activity as conversion of radiolabelled L-arginine to citrulline in tissues obtained from women prior to and following the onset of labor. Constructed from data in Di Iulio *et al.* 1996[17] and Ramsay *et al.* 1996[18]

Tissue	NOS activity before labor (nmol min^{-1} g^{-1})	NOS activity during labor (nmol min^{-1} g^{-1})
Myometrium[18]	0.02	1.39*
Placenta[18]	10	—
Placenta[17]	30.5	32
Amnion[17]	0.03	0.04
Chorio-decidua[17]	0.03	0.04

*$p = 0.048$

in culture, there was no difference in the ability of myometrium in the two groups to generate nitrate/nitrite[6]. Both these studies cast doubt on whether a fall in NO plays a major role in the onset of parturition, and further work is required to clarify this.

A decrease in sensitivity to the tocolytic effects of NO has been demonstrated following the onset of labor in humans. *In vitro* studies show that the median effective dose for inhibition of myometrial contractions is 15 times greater when tissue is removed from laboring patients, compared with the concentration required when tissue is removed prior to the onset of labor[6]. Even in the absence of a change in NO production, this decrease in sensitivity to the tocolytic effects of NO at the time of onset of labor will stimulate myometrial contractility. Hence, a reduction in myometrial sensitivity to NO may play a role in the control of the onset of parturition.

Conclusion

Changes in endogenous NO synthesis appear to play a role in the onset of labor in animals. Although NO is produced within the pregnant human uterus, evidence on whether NO pro-

duction changes at the time of the onset of labor is conflicting. However, a decrease in sensitivity to the tocolytic effect of NO may play a role in the initiation of paturition. Further work is required to determined the contribution of NO to the control of human parturition.

SUMMARY

Nitric oxide is a powerful myometrial relaxant and is produced within the human uterus during pregnancy. The role of nitric oxide in the treatment of preterm labor and in the control of the onset of labor at term remains to be established. If such roles are shown, nitric oxide will represent a powerful new agent for the reduction of preterm delivery and our understanding of the physiology of parturition will be significantly improved.

ACKNOWLEDGEMENTS

Grateful thanks are due to the following organizations who have funded this work: Well-being, The Medical Research Council (Grant no. G94 37277), Tenovus and the Yorkhill NHS Trust; and to Linda Ward for excellent technical help.

References

1. Palmer, R., Ferrige, A. and Moncada, S. (1987). Nitric oxide release accounts for the biological activity of endothelium-derived relaxing factor. *Nature (London)*, **327**, 524–6

2. Anggard, E. (1994). Nitric oxide: mediator, murderer, and medicine. *Lancet*, **343**, 1199–206

3. Yallampalli, C., Garfield, R. and Byam-Smith, M. (1993). Nitric oxide inhibits uterine contractility during pregnancy but not during delivery. *Endocrinology*, **133**, 1899–902

4. Yallampalli, C., Izumi, H., Byam-Smith, M. and Garfield, R. (1993). An L-arginine-nitric oxide-cyclic guanosine monophosphate system exists in the uterus and inhibits contractility during pregnancy. *Am. J. Obstet. Gynecol.*, **170**, 175–85

5. Izumi, H., Yallampalli, C. and Garfield, R. (1993). Gestational changes in L-arginine-induced relaxation of pregnant rat and human myometrial smooth muscle. *Am. J. Obstet. Gynecol.*, **169**, 1327–37

6. Buhimschi, I., Yallampalli, C., Dong, Y. -L. and Garfield, R. (1995). Involvement of a nitric-oxide guanosine monophosphate pathway in control of human uterine contractility during pregnancy. *Am. J. Obstet. Gynecol.*, **172**, 1577–84

7. Norman, J. E., Ward, L. M., Martin, W., Macklon, N. S., Cameron, A. D., MacLean, M. R., McGrath, J. C., Greer, I. A. and Cameron, I. T. (1997). Glyceryl trinitrate in the treatment of preterm labour – another placebo? In *The Biology of Nitric Oxide*, in press. (London: Portland Press)

8. Lee, J. and Chang, K. (1995). Different sensitivity to nitric oxide of human pregnant and nonpregnant myometrial contractility. *Pharm. Commun.*, **5**, 147–54

9. Lees, C., Campbell, S., Jauniaux, E., Brown, R., Ramsay, B., Gibb, D., Moncada, S. and Martin, J. F. (1994). Arrest of preterm labour and prolongation of gestation with glyceryl trinitrate, a nitric oxide donor. *Lancet*, **343**, 1325–6

10. Norman, J. (1996). Nitric oxide and the myometrium. *Pharm. Ther.*, **70**, 91–100

11. Eis, A., Brockman, D., Pollock, J. and Myatt, L. (1995). Immunohistochemical localisation of endothelial nitric oxide synthase in human villous and extravillous trophoblast populations and expression during syncytiotrophoblast formation *in vitro*. *Placenta*, **16**, 113–26

12. Buttery, L., McCarthy, A., Springall, D., Sullivan, M. H. F., Elder, M. G., Michel, T. and Polak, J. M. (1994). Endothelial nitric oxide synthase in the human placenta: regional distribution and proposed regulatory role at the feto-maternal interface. *Placenta*, **15**, 257–65

13. Conrad, K., Vill, M., McGuire, P., Dail, W. and Davis, A. (1993). Expression of nitric oxide synthase by syncytiotrophoblast in human placental villi. *FASEB J.*, **7**, 1268–76

14. Myatt, L., Brockman, D., Langdon, G. and Pollock, J. (1993). Constitutive calcium-dependent isoform of nitric oxide synthase in the human placenta. *Placenta*, **14**, 373–83

15. Myatt, L., Brockman, D., Eis, A. and Pollock, J. (1993). Immunohistochemical localization of nitric oxide synthase in the human placenta. *Placenta*, **14**, 487–95

16. Morris, N., Carroll, S., Nicolaides, K., Steer, P. and Warren, J. (1995). Exhaled nitric oxide concentration and amniotic fluid nitrite concentration during pregnancy. *Eur. J. Clin. Invest.*, **25**, 138–41

17. Di Iulio, J., Gude, N., King, R. and Brennecke, S. (1996). Human placental and fetal membrane nitric oxide synthase activity before, during and after labour and term. *Reprod. Fertil. Dev.*, **7**, 1505–8

18. Ramsay, B., Sooranna, S. and Johnson, M. (1996). Nitric oxide synthase activities in human myometrium and villous trophoblast throughout pregnancy. *Obstet. Gynecol.*, **87**, 249–53

Midwife-led care: an account of the implementation process at Southmead NHS Trust

36

R. J. Johnson

INTRODUCTION

English maternity services are subject to a new policy directive entitled *Changing Childbirth*[1] which challenges service providers to change radically many aspects of maternity care. The major thrust of the policy is that childbearing women should become the central focus of care and participate in decisions about their care. The main themes of policy are choice, continuity and control for women. The policy sets out clear objectives to guide the implementation process. Providers must meet national 'indicators of success' (Table 1) which form the basis of contracts with purchasers from 1995/96 and monitor implementation of the policy that should be completed by 1999.

The 'lead professional' is defined in *Changing Childbirth* as: 'The professional who will give a substantial part of the care personally, and who is responsible for ensuring that the woman has access to care from other professionals, as appropriate'. One of the main objectives is that by 1999: 'A woman with an uncomplicated pregnancy should, if she wishes, be able to book with a midwife as the lead professional for the entire episode of care including delivery in a general hospital'[1]. The 'indicators of success' relating to this objective are: 'At least 30% of women should have the midwife as the lead professional', and 'At least 30% of women delivered in a maternity unit should be admitted under the management of the midwife'.

This process involves a radical shift from the conventional medical model of care to 'midwife-led care'. The purpose of this paper is to discuss

Table 1 'Indicators of Success', as defined in *Changing Childbirth*, 1993[1]

All women should be entitled to carry their own notes

Every woman should know one midwife who ensures continuity of her midwifery care – the named midwife

At least 30% of women should have the midwife as the lead professional

Every woman should know the lead professional who has a key role in planning and provision of care

At least 75% of women should know the person who cares for them during their delivery

Midwives should have direct access to some beds in all maternity units

At least 30% of women delivered in a maternity unit should be admitted under the management of a midwife

The total number of antenatal visits for women with uncomplicated pregnancies should have been reviewed in the light of the available evidence and the Royal College of Obstetricians and Gynaecologists guidelines

All front line ambulances should have a paramedic able to support the midwife who needs to transfer a woman to hospital in an emergency

All women should have access to information about the services available in their locality

how Southmead Maternity Unit in Bristol has implemented this key objective of midwife-led care.

CONTEXT

A variety of models of midwife-led care have been described in the literature[2]. These include the Midwifery Development Unit in Glasgow[3], a separate midwifery unit at Ayrshire Central Hospital[4] that is adjacent to the consultant unit, a 'home from home scheme' within the Leicester Royal Infirmary[5] and a private midwifery unit in Southampton[6]. The location of planned midwife and general practitioner-led care has been controversial[7]. The Glasgow Midwifery Development Unit has undertaken an important randomized controlled trial of the effectiveness of midwife-led care that indicates, along with other similar studies[8], that midwife-led care is a safe option for women with low-risk pregnancies. Southmead Maternity Unit were spurred on to implement midwife-led care in accordance with *Changing Childbirth* to meet the policy directives and the contract specification of the local purchaser.

The environment of policy implementation is important[9] and some details about Southmead Maternity Unit are therefore included at this point. Southmead Maternity Unit provides care to approximately 5500 women a year and has a full range of obstetric care with on site access to neonatal intensive care, and anesthetic services. The service provides care to a mixed inner city, urban and rural population of all social classes. To improve service access for women within a wide geographical catchment area, all six consultant obstetricians continue to hold hospital and peripheral antenatal clinics. To meet the *Changing Childbirth* and other business targets the maternity services management board (a multidisciplinary group) prepared a 'Maternity Services Strategy' to guide it through the changes required over the next 5 years. Two community-based midwifery teams had already been implemented and a major part of the strategy is the implementation of more team midwifery. A number of models of team midwifery have been described[10]. The model at Southmead Maternity Unit[11] is a team of six to seven community-based midwives who hold a caseload of approximately 250 women a year, for whom they provide total care. Until 1995 women were either 'consultant booked' (96%), general practitioner booked (2%) or booked for a home birth (2%), with 'shared care' the

norm for the majority of women with uncomplicated pregnancies.

OBJECTIVES

The initial key objectives of implementing midwife-led care at Southmead Maternity Unit were:

(1) To meet the *Changing Childbirth* targets as required by the local health authority;

(2) To offer women greater choice of 'booking';

(3) To reduce the number of unnecessary consultant antenatal appointments for women;

(4) To reduce the number of women attending the consultant clinics;

(5) To allow more time for each consultation and reduce waiting time;

(6) To offer greater continuity of care to women; and

(7) To allow midwives to take professional responsibility for the entire pregnancy.

POLICY IMPLEMENTATION PROCESS

A meeting was held in the spring of 1995 between the author (maternity services manager and leader of this process) and all the consultants, to discuss implementing midwife-led care. Southmead Maternity Unit was actively developing several changes in the way the service was provided, i.e. additional community-based teams, a new midwifery hospital rotation, and a nationally funded 'Complicated Care Team' project, so an incremental approach to midwife-led care was agreed. The initial aim was to implement this new booking system in identified areas where continuity of carer had already been implemented and the midwife provided the majority of pregnancy care. The term 'midwife-led care' is politically sensitive. There was concern that the term might give women and general practitioners the impression that it excluded the involvement of the general practitioner and access to screening tests, neither of which was the intention. The term 'midwife booking' was adopted, which succinctly described the type of booking without implying any change to the woman/general practitioner relationship. It was planned that all midwives would potentially be involved with providing care to women who were midwife-booked, and no special ward or beds were allocated. Midwife-led care is part of the overall strategy to improve continuity of midwife care primarily by the implementation of community-based midwifery teams. The policy was ratified in September 1995. Although an incremental approach was planned, 22% of women (approximately 100 each month) are now initially a 'midwife booking', and approximately 150 women who were 'midwife bookings' have now delivered (July 1996).

Due to the potential number of midwives involved (approximately 175 midwives) very clear policy, guidelines and protocols were required to ensure safe practice. Midwifery has had an established model of professional supervision since 1902. The supervisors of midwives (who are also senior midwifery managers at Southmead Maternity Unit) agreed to take responsibility for compiling the first drafts of these documents for consultation. The debate amongst the five supervisors was at two levels. Firstly the theoretical principles of professional accountability and the appropriate extent of a midwife's role when she is practicing without medical supervision. Secondly the practical aspects of the systems that were required to ensure that care is appropriately provided. Midwives at Southmead Maternity Unit provide a range of 'medical interventions', e.g. cannulation and initiation of syntocinon within clear protocols. There was concern that the quality of the woman's care could be reduced rather than enhanced if midwives were no longer allowed to undertake these interventions without specific referral to a doctor. There were a number of similar instances that needed to be resolved, which is only possible within a well-functioning multidisciplinary team where there is mutual respect.

Ham and Hill[12] note that 'Conflicts cannot be resolved during the policy making stage', and 'little is known in advance about the actual impact of the new measures'. Within the context of implementing 'midwife bookings' it was important to *try* to foresee the impact of this development. Barrett and Fudge[13] have emphasized that: 'there is a need to consider implementation as a policy/action continuum in which an interactive and negotiative process is taking place over time between those seeking to put policy into effect and those upon whom action depends'. The 'bottom up' contribution of doctors, midwives and others working in each area with the manager was therefore perceived to be the key to successful implementation of the policy. Such radical policy development as midwives becoming the lead professional requires professional debate to define the midwife's role within the context of providing care in a large maternity unit. This debate included the aspects of care the midwife can provide on her own professional accountability, those tasks that require medically agreed protocols, and most importantly when care should be 'handed over' to a consultant team.

The other key to success is effective team working enabled by a culture of weekly multidisciplinary audit meetings to discuss the care provided to individual women. Doctors and midwives undertake case presentations of any women they care for (particularly if the case is unusual) and invite discussion about the care of the women. Examples of good, bad and questionable care, management or practice can be discussed rather than focusing on 'incidents'. This approach encourages open constructive criticism and a learning environment rather than negative covert criticism that can undermine effective team working.

The draft policy and guidelines were initially discussed and then further developed by the managers and staff who usually worked in each area. Their comments were invaluable in determining a workable system. Midwives generally wanted as little difference as possible in terms of policy between the 'midwife-booked' and 'consultant-booked' women, as they would be looking after both types of women. It was defining when medical advice should be sought that was considered important. Considering the experience of Chelsea and Westminster Hospital[14], it was envisaged that at least 30% of 'midwife-booked' women would transfer to consultant care during the pregnancy. Uncomplicated swift referral systems (midwife to consultant and referral back to the midwife) have been defined. The initial selection of women suitable for 'midwife booking' is undertaken by the community-based midwife. A 1-day 'time out' was held with these midwives to discuss with them and their manager the potential problems that they envisaged with the new system. Of critical importance were the selection criteria and the involvement, good working relationships and team work with general practitioners. Rather than using a 'risk' system, or defining women who are suitable for 'midwife booking', the criteria for women who must be referred to a consultant obstetrician (Table 2) were defined, adapted from those used by Chelsea and Westminster Hospitals[15]. All 'low-risk' women can continue to choose a 'consultant booking' if that is their preference. The criteria are not exhaustive as the midwife has to use her professional judgement about the appropriateness of not recommending a 'consultant booking'. If the midwife is uncertain she can discuss individual women with any member of the consultant team.

Following some debate, guidelines were produced for all stages of pregnancy. These allow midwives to provide care in 'normal pregnancy' as well as offering women a defined range of antenatal screening tests without referral to a consultant, e.g. ultrasound dating scans, fetal anomaly screening and scanning for presentation in late pregnancy. If abnormalities are found the woman is advised by the clinic staff to see the consultant and the midwife is informed. Referral to a consultant is required if women need antenatal admission. During intrapartum care, 'midwife-booked' women have access to epidural analgesia, and once delivered the baby is registered under the 'on call' consultant pediatrician and receives a full examination by a pediatrician before transfer home.

Table 2 Indications for medical consultation at booking

The woman's personal choice
Risk identified at booking
  Any complicating medical condition including
    Heart disease
    Hypertension
    Chest disease
    Renal disease
    Autoimmune disease
    Hepatitis B
    Human immunodeficiency virus
    Diabetes
    Epilepsy
    Deep vein thrombosis/embolism/blood disease
  Age under 16 years
  Relevant gynecological history including
    Infertility treatment this pregnancy
    Intrauterine contraceptive device *in situ*
    Known uterine anomaly
    Ovarian tumor
    Cervical disease
    Uterine scar/surgery
    Fibroids
  Family history
    Hereditary condition in family
  Psychiatric illness
  Relevant past obstetric history including
    Previous pregnancy loss after 14 weeks gestation
    Major postpartum hemorrhage
    Previous stillbirth or neonatal death
    Previous abnormal or handicapped baby
    Previous small baby (< 2.5 kg)
    Previous premature labor (< 35 weeks)
    Hypertensive disease of pregnancy
    Previous intrauterine growth retardation
    Multiple pregnancy
    Rhesus antibodies

All community-based midwives were provided with a personal copy of the policy and guidelines within a 'filo fax' that replaced their diary (copies are readily available in the hospital for all other midwives). Change rarely runs absolutely smoothly. In order to ensure safe practice, midwifery supervisors are currently notified of all 'midwife bookings' and are auditing the policy implementation. The existing perinatal audit mechanisms are monitoring the appropriateness of the guidelines and systems are available to update the guidelines if necessary and circulate them to all staff. A formal evaluation is planned to assess the satisfaction that women and professionals have with the system, as well as auditing clinical outcomes.

IMPLEMENTATION PROBLEMS

There were some problems encountered with implementing this system, but due to the approach of involving staff in the policy process these were fewer than expected. The majority were of a bureaucratic and organizational nature rather than related to clinical care. Some consultants were concerned that a disruption to the historical booking system combined with a number of women being referred to the consultant later in pregnancy would result in inequitable caseloads. Various systems were discussed to solve this potential problem. These included geographical boundaries, designated midwife and consultant links or a 'color code' on the notes to signify the consultant whom the woman should see if she required medical care. The system that was finally agreed was that the woman would be referred to consultants on a rotational basis unless the woman wanted to attend a local peripheral clinic. Women requiring intrapartum or postnatal consultant care are referred to the 'on call' consultant team. Other problems have related to the new systems required to ensure that test results and letters are forwarded to the midwife for action and filing in the patient records.

Southmead Maternity Unit uses the STORK maternity data system. This is a computer-based program with links to all departments, wards and community bases, and is used to record the initial booking history, the delivery and all in-patient care. The system of 'midwife booking' required new codes to be generated, to ensure audit and contract monitoring was possible. The information department were at first disbelieving that midwives could be responsible for in-patient care. A copy of *Changing Childbirth* and some negotiation was necessary to persuade the department that 'midwife bookings' were to be implemented. Once convinced, new 'codes' were allocated, and a process for recording the

type of booking and any change to the booking is available on the computer system and will facilitate accurate auditing.

IMPLEMENTATION SURPRISES

Concern was expressed by some general practitioners that they were being excluded from providing maternity care to their patients. If the community midwife or midwifery team was unable to answer their concerns, discussion meetings were arranged with the community midwifery manager to explain the philosophy of 'midwife bookings' and their relevance to *Changing Childbirth*. With increasing demands on the general practitioner's time, a diminishing number of general practitioners had been using the general practitioner booking system and these bookings accounted for only 2% of deliveries in 1994/95. Following the implementation of 'midwife bookings' the few general practitioners who undertook 'general practitioner bookings' decided to transfer all their patients to 'midwife bookings'. This enabled the general practitioner to be involved in antenatal care but freed from the commitment to be at the birth. The general practitioners were satisfied that they were welcome at the delivery if they were available and the woman particularly wanted them there but that the care could be adequately provided by midwives.

The change to 'midwife booking' is a major policy change. The experience so far is that midwives have welcomed the change because it more appropriately represents the way the service was already working and a major change in midwifery practice has not been required.

BENEFIT OF MIDWIFE-LED CARE

The process of data collection to evaluate this scheme is under way and preliminary results should be available in the spring of 1997. Anecdotal evidence would suggest that 'midwife bookings' may appropriately allow the consultant more time to manage the care of women with complicated pregnancy and more time for the training of junior medical staff. Midwives experience more satisfaction in providing continuity of care and in being responsible for the care of women with uncomplicated pregnancies. Women with uncomplicated pregnancies do not need to attend a consultant clinic. This reduces the number of professionals she meets in her pregnancy, potentially providing a more personalized service from known midwives and general practitioner. Should a complication develop at any time in the pregnancy, however, the woman has access to the full range of obstetric care.

CONCLUSIONS

The 'midwife booking' scheme has been smoothly and successfully introduced into a large maternity unit without extra expenditure or need for additional midwifery training. The policy implementation process was relatively uncomplicated due to the involvement of medical and midwifery staff at all stages of the policy formation. The implementation process is being continuously monitored by the midwifery supervisors and by regular review meetings between managers, midwives and doctors. The scheme has begun to make more time available for consultations with women who have complicated pregnancies. This model of midwife-led care has been introduced into a large maternity service without the need for additional midwifery staff, different accommodation or a 'separate' unit, and is a viable model for consideration when planning the implementation of midwife-led care.

References

1. Department of Health (1993). *Report of the Expert Advisory Group: Changing Childbirth*. (London: HMSO)
2. NHS Management Executive (1993). *A Study of Midwife- and GP-led Maternity Units*. (London: NHS Management Executive)
3. Turnball, D., Holmes, A., Shields, N. *et al.* (1996). Randomised, controlled trial of efficacy of midwife-managed care. *Lancet*, **348**, 213–18
4. The natural choice. Purpose-built midwifery unit opened at Ayrshire Central Hospital (Editorial). *Midwives*, **108**, 190
5. Morris-Thompson, P. (1993). A historical perspective on maternity services and the Leicester Royal Infirmary approach to the Winterton Report's recommendations. *J. Nurs. Management*, **1**, 31–7
6. Hobbs, L. (1994). Never say die – setting up a birth centre in Southampton. *MIDIRS Midwifery Digest*, **4**, 139–41
7. Campbell, R. and Macfarlane, A. (1994). *Where to be Born*. (Oxford: National Perinatal Epidemiology Unit)
8. Macvicar, J., Dobbie, G., Owen-Johnstone, L., Jagger, C., Hopkins, M. and Kennedy, J. (1993). Simulated home delivery in hospital: a randomised controlled trial. *Br. J. Obstet. Gynaecol.*, **100**, 316–23
9. Easton, D. (1965). *A Systems Analysis of Political Life*. (New York: Wiley)
10. Wraight, A., Ball, J., Seccombe, I. and Stock, I. (1993). *Mapping Team Midwifery*, Institute of Manpower Studies, Report Series 242. (Brighton: Institute of Manpower Studies)
11. Ward, P. and Frohlich, J. (1994). Team Midwifery in Bristol. *MIDIRS Midwifery Digest*, **14**, 149–51
12. Ham, C. and Hill, M. (1993). *The Policy Process in the Modern Capitalist State*, 2nd edn. (London: Harvester Wheatsheaf)
13. Barrett, S. and Fudge, C. (eds.) (1981). *Policy and Action* (London: Methuen)
14. Lewis, P. (1995). Developing a group practice approach to care. *MIDIRS Midwifery Digest*, **5**, 104–8
15. Lewis, P. (1995). Refining the model-group practice midwifery. *MIDIRS Midwifery Digest*, **5**, 219–23

The value of perinatal nursing in Europe

37

J. Robinson

INTRODUCTION

Evidence on the value of qualified nursing care to beneficial patient outcomes is slowly accumulating. The International Council of Nurses' publication *The Value of Nursing in a Changing World*[1] reviews the research on a global basis. Meeting the canons of hard science in the form of rigorously controlled trials of an intervention as diffuse as nursing care is notoriously difficult. Unsurprisingly, despite reporting some good studies in the United Kingdom and elsewhere, the largest number of controlled trials originate from North America where both financial resources and advanced skills in nursing research are in greater abundance than elsewhere.

Despite the impressive record of North American perinatal nurses in developing advanced practice, caution is needed in looking uncritically to the USA for our role models. The USA health system is the most expensive in the world[2] and, some might argue, excessively dependent on interventionist high technology. The ranking of the USA in international perinatal mortality fell progressively from third in the world in 1950 to 19th in 1990[3].

THE VALUE OF PERINATAL NURSING

A search of MEDLINE and CINAHL databases on perinatal nursing in Europe demonstrates a largely descriptive set of studies predominantly from Scandinavia and The Netherlands, with a number of case studies in England. We can learn from these providing that the caveats of caution over methods and wider generalization are observed. We carried out such a case study of neonatal services in Nottingham[4] and the following key findings will be used to explore issues concerning the value of perinatal nursing in Europe:

(1) Family care is central to perinatal nursing. Family care includes direct care, support and education, transitional care and bereavement care;

(2) Rigid job specification inhibits staff flexibility and limits opportunities for continuity of care; and

(3) Neonatal nurses are the 'glue' in the system, substituting for other workers as needed.

In the social sciences generalization is frequently achieved by the painstaking accumulation of evidence from small scale or non-statistical studies over time, with careful comparison of research objectives, methods and outcomes. In order to compare the findings of the Nottingham study with other contemporary studies, the content of the ten papers reported in the *Neonatal Nurses Yearbook* (1996) was reviewed. In summary, technical skill combined with family support, commitment and enthusiasm on the part of the neonatal nurse was apparent in six of the papers[5–10]; teamwork and/or extensive substitution for others was reported in four[6,8,10,11]; and the development of transitional care in one[8]. It would appear therefore that there is a high degree of correspondence between the findings of the Nottingham case study and those activities which are valued and expected of neonatal nursing by contemporary authors who

Table 1 Data on population, income and health expenditure in five European states in 1990

	Population (millions)	GNP ($ per capita)	Health expenditure 1990	
			% of GDP	$ per capita
Sweden	9	25 110	8.8	2343
Kazakhstan	17	2 470	2.6	54
Romania	23	1 390	3.9	63
United Kingdom	57	16 550	6.1	1039
Russia	148	3 220	3.0	157

are active in the field. Two further papers in the yearbook were indirectly concerned with perinatal nursing. The first described the need for parental support, counselling and education when parents' expectations of a perfect baby are not realized, and implied the crucial role of perinatal nursing in these activities[12]. The second, on the legal rights of infants and children[13], reminded readers of the United Nations Convention on Human Rights Article 24, which is as follows:

(1) Parties recognise the rights of the child to the highest attainable standards of health and to facilities for the treatment of illness and rehabilitation;

(2) Parties should strive to ensure that no child is deprived of his or her access to such health care service;

(3) Parties should pursue full implementation of this right and in particular it shall take appropriate measures to diminish infant and child mortality, ensure provision of medical assistance, combat disease and malnutrition, ensure proper prenatal and postnatal health care for mothers, ensure that all segments of society, in particular parents and children, are informed and have access to education, and develop preventative health care; and

(4) Parties should undertake, encourage, and promote international co-operation with a view to achieving progressively the full realization of the right recognised in the present article[13].

Table 2 Human resources for healthcare in five European states, 1988–92

	Doctors per 1000 population	Nurse to doctor ratio
Sweden	2.73	3.4
Kazakhstan	4.12	3.0
Romania	1.79	?
United Kingdom	1.40	2.0
Russia	4.69	?

FAMILY AND CHILD HEALTH, AND HEALTH SERVICES IN EUROPE

There is currently a fundamental question being asked as to how these human rights can be translated into action across Europe in order to deliver perinatal nursing care in the ways which are valued and which bring benefits to infants and their families. The World Health Organization (WHO) of Europe consists of fifty countries, including twenty-seven from the former Soviet Union. The countries vary widely in the size of their populations, level of economic development, and health status. Health inequities are increasing between western Europe and the countries of central and eastern Europe and the newly independent states. The rise of wars, poverty and violence has had a serious impact on the most vulnerable, frequently mothers and infants[14]. Sometimes the data for monitoring progress, or deterioration, of health issues in the Region is simply not available. Tables 1 and 2 show data on five of the most and least populous countries in the region: Sweden, Kazakhstan, Romania, the United

Table 3 Life expectancy, maternal and neonatal mortality in five European states in 1992

	Life expectancy at birth	Maternal mortality (per 100 000 births)	Neonatal mortality (per 1000 live births)
Sweden	78	0	3.14
Kazakhstan	69	56.85	?
Romania	70	60.29	9.32
United Kingdom	75	6.66	4.31
Russia	69	50.77	?

Kingdom and Russia. Table 1 shows data on their spending on health, and Table 2 gives their ratio of doctors per 1000 population and the ratio of nurses to doctors[2].

These data contain unexplained inequities. Kazakhstan and Russia appear to have an over-supply of doctors relative to the other three countries, and to their stage of economic development. The proportion of nurses to doctors in Romania and Russia is simply not available. The WHO recognizes a variety of factors which impede the delivery of nursing services in some countries in Europe. These include the virtual absence of nurses from policy-making and decision-making at all levels, shortages of well trained nurses, insufficient resources to support the work of nurses and midwives, and the undervaluation of nursing with its concomitant subordination to medicine. Yet, nursing is a part of the more general trend to increase the cost-effectiveness of health care delivery. As the evidence quoted above demonstrates, nursing has a valuable, and a valued contribution to make.

Tables 3 and 4 show data on available health indicators relative to the health of mothers and infants for the same five countries[2,15]. Life expectancy at birth in 1992 is indicative of the ageing population across the region, although the east-west differential is reported to be growing[14]. Reasons for concern over the health status of women and children in the newly independent states and central and eastern Europe may be deduced from the data on maternal and infant mortality in 1992 in Kazakhstan, Romania and Russia, and in the cases of diphtheria in 1994 in Russia and Kazakhstan[15]. Data for

Table 4 Infant mortality and diphtheria cases in five European states in 1992

	Infant mortality (per 1000 live births)	Diphtheria cases
Sweden	5.19	0
Kazakhstan	26.25	489
Romania	23.35	0
United Kingdom	6.58	4
Russia	18.40	39 703

neonatal mortality is incomplete, and for perinatal mortality not available.

CONCLUSION

It would appear from the evidence presented that the rights of the child to the highest attainable standards of health, with access to facilities for the treatment of illness and rehabilitation, are far from being realized in parts of Europe. Perinatal nurses, as members of health care teams, have demonstrated the value of their contribution to family care by providing direct and transitional care, support and education and bereavement care. Nurses from western Europe are trying in a number of ways to help their colleagues across Europe in the difficult times they face, and in the struggle to update their practice in order to reverse the adverse health circumstances which many families confront[16]. Nurses are trying also to meet the exhortation of the International Council of Nurses to demonstrate the value and cost-effectiveness of nursing to consumers, other providers and to policy makers at all levels[1]. It is now perhaps time for some governments, some politicians and some individuals to recognize that the perception of nursing as a low status occupation requiring minimal training, with the associated denial of the value of psycho-social elements of care, is a thing of the past and that nursing for the health of all children and their families is an activity to be celebrated and valued[14].

ACKNOWLEDGEMENTS

The author wishes to acknowledge with thanks the help received in preparing this paper from Sue Bradley, Wendy Stanton, Liz Potter and Dr David Wright.

References

1. International Council of Nurses (1996). *The Value of Nursing in a Changing World*. (Geneva: ICN)
2. The World Bank (1993). *World Development Report 1993 Investing in Health*. (New York: Oxford University Press)
3. US Department of Health and Human Services (1995). *Vital and Health Statistics Perinatal Mortality in the United States: 1985–91*. Series 20, publication no. (PHS) 95-1854. (Hyattsville, MD: DHSS)
4. James, N., Arthur, T. and Pittman, A. (1993). *Nursing Quality Counts: a case study of neonatal services 1990–1992*. Nursing Policy Studies 9. (Department of Nursing and Midwifery Studies, University of Nottingham)
5. Greenall, F. (1996). Synchronous ventilation in pre-term infants: the role of the nurse. In *Neonatal Nurses Yearbook* (Cambridge: CMA Medical Data)
6. Overington, S. (1996). The development of the neonatal nurse practitioner role in New Zealand. In *Neonatal Nurses Yearbook* (Cambridge: CMA Medical Data)
7. Byrne, B. and Hull, D. (1996). Is 100% breast milk possible in a neonatal environment? In *Neonatal Nurses Yearbook*. (Cambridge: CMA Medical Data)
8. Foden, P. (1996). Pre-term care in the community. In *Neonatal Nurses Yearbook*. (Cambridge: CMA Medical Data)
9. Padden, T. (1996). Development issues in neonatal nursing: utilising the Nidcap approach. In *Neonatal Nurses Yearbook*. (Cambridge: CMA Medical Data)
10. Redshaw, M. E. and Harris, A. (1996). What is the role of the advanced nurse practitioner in neonatal care? In *Neonatal Nurses Yearbook*. (Cambridge: CMA Medical Data)
11. Palframan, M. and Thorpe, H. (1996). The change to primary nursing in a two centre regional neo-natal service: is it worth it? In *Neonatal Nurses Yearbook*. (Cambridge: CMA Medical Data)
12. Brain, J. (1996). The importance of a perfect baby. In *Neonatal Nurses Yearbook*. (Cambridge: CMA Medical Data)
13. Urquhart, P. (1996). Legal rights of infants and children. In *Neonatal Nurses Yearbook*. (Cambridge: CMA Medical Data)
14. World Health Organization (1994). *Health in Europe*. WHO Regional Publications, European Series, no. 56. (Copenhagen: WHO Regional Office for Europe)
15. World Health Organization (1996). *WHO European Health for All Database*. World Wide Web
16. Jones, K. (1996). Child health in Moscow and changes in Russian nurse education. *Paediatr. Nursing*, **8(2)**, 10–12, and **8(3)**, 10–11

Practical neonatal transport

38

M. F. Whitfield

INTRODUCTION

This paper discusses practical issues in the provision of an integrated neonatal transport program within a regionalized neonatal perinatal health-care delivery system. It reflects experience with long-distance transports in all weathers using land vehicles and aircraft in Ontario and British Columbia.

INFRASTRUCTURE

The tertiary perinatal center functions as a resource to the smaller facilities it serves, with 24 h telephone access to experienced obstetric and neonatal specialists for telephone consultations from which decisions about transfers can be made and organized. The provision of facilities and trained personnel for maternal and neonatal transfer are the responsibility of the tertiary center. To support such a program, the necessary logistics of staffing, purchase and maintenance of patient transport equipment, access to appropriate vehicles/aircraft and consequent budgetary arrangements have to be worked out by the tertiary center with the appropriate health-care funding agencies. These arrangements have to be sufficiently detailed so that there are few circumstances that have not been foreseen (e.g. how much oxygen do the ambulances carry?, what electrical outlets are available on which aircraft at what voltage, and does the incubator adapter fit?).

Various combinations of personnel are used for neonatal transfer in different places. In general there need to be at least two staff for acute transfers, and more if there are twins or the patient is being transferred to an extracorporeal membrane oxygenation (ECMO) center. The skills required within each team must include a sophisticated ability to assess and care for sick neonatal patients, a high level of technical ability, an understanding of all functional aspects of the transport equipment and an ability to trouble-shoot in the event of failure. These skills may be provided by a combination of doctors, nurses, infant transport paramedics, or respiratory technologists.

DOES THE MOTHER/BABY REALLY NEED TO BE TRANSFERRED?

Transfer of mothers and babies from smaller centers to higher level perinatal facilities involves significant cost and dislocation to the family at a critical time in their lives. It may geographically separate the parents, or the parents from the baby and cause considerable social and economic disruption. Whether this disruption is justified depends on the likelihood and seriousness of the perinatal problem which may develop, and the capability of the facility close to where the parents live in coping with this. There is a risk factor involved in any patient transfer, both to the patients and the staff directly involved. Different hospitals are able to manage different levels of illness in mothers and babies. In order to use perinatal and neonatal beds optimally within a region there needs to be prior discussion and agreement about what sorts of cases should be cared for in which hospitals. Frequently, it is the availability of appropriately trained staff to provide sustained high level care which is the most important factor in the decision to transfer.

231

SHOULD THE BABY BE TRANSFERRED *IN UTERO?*

Neonatal transport is only one part of the complete package of regionalized perinatal/neonatal care. Wherever possible, babies and mothers requiring transfer to a larger center because of anticipated significant perinatal or neonatal problems should be transferred prior to delivery unless there are contraindications to maternal transfer. Principal contraindications to maternal transfer include advancing labor with threat of delivery in transit, severe pregnancy induced hypertension or active bleeding. There need to be established defined criteria for consultation regarding potential maternal transfer. Whether it is feasible to transfer prior to delivery requires careful assessment at the referring hospital and telephone discussion between the perinatal obstetrician in the tertiary perinatal center and the caregiver in the referring hospital. Sometimes the most appropriate solution is a combined maternal and neonatal transport team.

ARRANGEMENTS FOR TRANSPORT OF THE NEWBORN

The goals of neonatal transport are: transfer of the baby with as little physiological and emotional disturbance to baby and family as possible; maximum safety for both patients and staff; and cost effective use of resources.

Phase 1: preparation, assessment and initial stabilization

The first contact from the referring hospital alerts the perinatal center staff of the possible impending delivery of an infant likely to require a higher level of care than can be provided in the birth hospital. This initiates a discussion between the doctors at the referring hospital and obstetric and neonatology staff at the tertiary perinatal unit about mode of delivery, timing of delivery, antenatal steroids, anticipated problems, resuscitation and stabilization plans, equipment and staffing, etc. Not infre-

quently, deliveries which seem imminent to the staff in the referring hospital can be delayed with appropriate treatment and the baby transferred *in utero*. If the baby is to be delivered in the referring hospital, a plan for resuscitation and stabilization of the baby at delivery needs to be agreed upon beforehand.

The transport team is alerted that there may be a neonatal transport pending, arrangements are made to free up the appropriate staff, and equipment is checked. At the same time the ambulance provider needs to be warned that a potential neonatal transport is pending, so that appropriate arrangements can be made to provide a vehicle (helicopter, aircraft, etc.). When notified that the baby is born, a prompt response will be required. We do not usually send out our team until we have been notified that the baby is born and successfully resuscitated. This avoids unnecessary costs caused by transports which have to be aborted because the baby is either not viable, or is much larger and healthier than was expected and does not need to be moved. Moreover, it is not feasible or desirable for the transport team to serve as an infant resuscitation service for outlying hospitals. Adequate arrangements for infant resuscitation need to be made wherever babies are born.

Aircraft and helicopters are extremely expensive to use and are only justified where geography prevents anticipated arrival of the transport team at the referring hospital within 2 h from dispatch. Pressurized jet aircraft are far preferable to less sophisticated aircraft provided that safe landing facilities exist in reasonable proximity to the birth hospital. Pressurized aircraft are able to fly above the weather, well clear of the mountains, and provide the opportunity to adjust pressurization altitude to assist with oxygenation of a patient with lung problems (Table 1). It is difficult, but possible, to assess a patient in a jet during flight, and possible even to reintubate if necessary, but you cannot pull over to the side of the road to re-stabilize the baby as you can in an ambulance. In a helicopter, there is much vibration and noise making auscultation of the chest an almost fruitless exercise. It is therefore very difficult to

Table 1 Illustration of the effect of increasing altitude on the required fractional inspired oxygen concentration (FiO_2)

Required FiO_2 at sea level	Equivalent FiO_2 required by patient according to pressurization altitude (m)					
	600	1200	1800	2400	3000	3600
0.21	0.23	0.25	0.27	0.29	0.31	0.34
0.30	0.33	0.35	0.38	0.42	0.45	0.49
0.40	0.43	0.47	0.51	0.55	0.60	0.65
0.50	0.55	0.59	0.63	0.68	0.75	0.82
0.60	0.65	0.70	0.76	0.82	0.90	1.00
0.70	0.75	0.81	0.88	0.96	< 1.00	< 1.00
0.80	0.86	0.94	< 1.00	< 1.00	< 1.00	< 1.00
0.90	0.98	< 1.00	< 1.00	< 1.00	< 1.00	< 1.00

A pressurization altitude of 3600 m should be assumed on pressurized commercial jets unless the pilot states otherwise.
Data calculated from Liebman, J. *et al.* (1976). *Pediatrics*, **57**, 408–10

decide in flight if the baby has developed a pneumothorax since you started the return flight. You have to be completely dependent for your on-going assessment of the patient on monitor readings. Helicopters are more dangerous than fixed-wing aircraft. Helicopters are susceptible to changing weather and are particularly dangerous in the mountains. Helicopters are not pressurized. Most helicopters used for ambulance work these days have two engines and can stay airborne and land on one engine.

All personnel involved in transports using aircraft need to have been adequately trained in emergency procedures in the event of aircraft malfunction, and need to take adequate protective clothing, particularly in the winter. Sometimes the weather in the winter is such that it may not be possible to fly into a remote destination and the patient may have to be managed in the referring hospital for several days with telephone support from the tertiary neonatologist. Alternatively the transport team may get in through the weather to the patient, but be stuck there for several days caring for an acutely sick baby, unable to leave and rapidly becoming exhausted. It is important to remember that there have been accidents with loss of life of members of transport teams with or without the patient in helicopters, aircraft and ambulances. Careful thought needs to be given to safety issues before dispatching a transport team in bad weather to a remote destination for a baby of marginal viability.

Phase 2: dispatch of the transport team and telephone support for staff in the referring hospital

Once the tertiary neonatologist has been notified of the birth and status of the baby the transport team is dispatched promptly (within 20 min) with the best information about the baby's status. A continued dialog takes place between the neonatologist and the referring hospital to optimize stabilization of the baby. This may require telephone assistance of physicians unfamiliar with the use of neonatal equipment and the assessment of a small sick infant. There is an implicit progressive shift of responsibility for the patient as the tertiary center staff take on more of the treatment decision making. Updated information about the baby's condition is passed on to the transport team by radio so they will be prepared for the baby on arrival.

Phase 3: the transport team in the referring hospital

On arrival at the bedside the transport team assess the infant's condition, make the appropriate diagnoses and continue the process of stabilization. This will involve review of the baby's clinical condition, usually including a blood gas analysis if available, and an X-ray. Particular care needs to be taken over evaluation of ventilatory status, the possibility of apneic attacks during transport, and the adequate and accurate fixation of tubes. Blood pressure may need to be supported to improve perfusion. Consideration should be given to taking cultures and starting antibiotics if this has not been done already. Vascular access needs to be secured either as an intravenous infusion, or an arterial line or both, to maintain hydration and blood glucose and to provide a route for drugs if needed. The insertion of even an intravenous cannula is much easier in the controlled environment of the baby unit than in transit. Use of a portable pulse oximeter in addition to standard cardiorespiratory monitoring is a significant benefit. Ventilator settings should, if possible, provide some room for increase in mean airway pressure or inspired oxygen concentration to allow for potential deterioration in transit and the effects of decreased barometric pressure.

The presence or absence of a pneumothorax is particularly important, as reduction in barometric pressure will increase the volume of the pneumothorax and consequent intrathoracic pressure effects if it is not continuously adequately drained. A baby with an established pneumothorax will have to have the chest drain connected to a Heimlich chest drain valve and this will have to be aspirated regularly to ensure adequate drainage during transfer.

Babies with duct dependent cyanotic heart disease, diaphragmatic hernia, tracheo-esophageal fistula, gastroschisis/exomphalos, or persistent pulmonary hypertension of the newborn represent special situations requiring additional treatment methods beyond the scope of this paper.

The transport team must obtain a full perinatal history, documentation of progress of labor, condition at delivery, resuscitation details and subsequent management prior to arrival of the team. This is most quickly done by photocopying all of the baby's clinical charts, and obtaining permission to take the chest X-rays. A treatment consent form must be signed. A sample of maternal blood and the placenta should also be collected. Once the baby's situation has been adequately assessed, it is important that the transport team communicate with the neonatologist back at the tertiary unit about details of treatment, anticipated time of departure, and arrival at the tertiary unit.

When the baby is stabilized on the transport equipment and ready to go, it is very important that a visit is made to the parents if they are available, touching contact encouraged and the baby's condition discussed. The parents must have the telephone number of the unit where the baby is going for care. We usually take a Polaroid photograph of the baby to give to the parents before leaving.

Phase 4: transfer back to the tertiary unit

The focus of the trip back to the tertiary unit is stability, creating as little disturbance to the baby as possible, rather than getting there with all speed. The team monitor color, heart rate, respiratory rate, blood pressure, temperature, oximetry, gas and electrical supply and behavior of the ventilator. Up-adjustments may be required in inspired oxygen concentration. Alternatively lower altitude equivalent cabin pressurization may be requested, but this uses more fuel and is expensive.

Phase 5: arrival at the tertiary unit and hand-over

On arrival at the tertiary unit the patient is transferred to the in-house neonatal intensive care unit (NICU) equipment and details of the history and management and all documentation handed over to the staff who will be managing the baby. The transport team must telephone the parents in the referring hospital to confirm safe arrival of the baby and let them know who their contact person should be in the NICU. The neonatologist or social worker should also make arrangements for the parents to travel to be with their baby, and admission of the mother to the postnatal ward of the perinatal center. The transport equipment then needs to be cleaned and re-stocked as a matter of some urgency ready for the next transport.

STRESS AND RISK IN TRANSPORTATION OF HIGH-RISK INFANTS

Most individuals involved in intensive care activities enjoy the excitement of transport, but the process of transporting a sick baby, from the anticipation of going out on a transport to handing the baby over to the NICU staff involves considerable stress, which only becomes apparent when the pressure is off. Managing the same baby through the same procedures in the familiarity of the NICU setting is much easier because of the availability of help, advice and emotional support. There is an element of danger involved in picking up sick babies from remote locations or travelling at speed on overcrowded highways with the best interests of the baby uppermost in one's mind.

We lost a transport team in January 1995 on what seemed to be not an unusually hazardous, reasonably routine transport. Two pilots, one physician and two infant transport paramedics died. This event had serious ramifications for morale, and neonatal transports were covered by the two most senior neonatologists for 3 weeks until extensive team debriefings of all the people involved in any way had been worked through. Staff involved in neonatal transports need adequate 'down time' afterwards, of the type mandated for the pilots we fly with. Those of us who send others on neonatal transports need to be aware of the risks and not expect others to do what we would not be prepared to do ourselves in the prevailing conditions.

Further reading

1. Black, J. A. and Whitfield, M. F. (1991). *Neonatal Emergencies*, 2nd edn., pp. 64–70. (Oxford: Butterworth Heinemann Ltd.)
2. MacDonald, M. G. and Miller, M. K. (1989). *Emergency Transport of the Perinatal Patient*. (Boston: Little, Brown and Co.)
3. Day, S. E. and Chapman, R. A. (1992). Transport of critically ill patients in need of extracorporeal life support (Review). *Crit. Care Clin.*, **8**, 581–96
4. Kollee, L. A., Brand, R., Schreuder, A. M., Ens-Dokkum, M. H., Veen, S. and Verloove-Vanhorick, S. P. (1992). Five year outcome of preterm and very low birthweight infants: comparison between maternal and neonatal transport. *Obstet. Gynecol.*, **80**, 635–8
5. Shenai, J. P. (1993). Neonatal transport. Outreach education program. *Pediatr. Clin. N. Am.*, **40**, 275–85
6. Jain, L. and Vidyasagar, D. (1993). Cardiopulmonary resuscitation of newborns. Its application to transport medicine. *Pediatr. Clin. N. Am.*, **40**, 287–302

Neonatal transport

39

V. C. H. von Loewenich and K.-H. Vonderheit

INTRODUCTION

Perinatal centers are combinations of a maternity hospital with a children's hospital or, at least, with a service for sick newborn babies. The aim of this organization is to give uninterrupted care to sick newborn babies, for instance preterm infants, beginning immediately at birth. This idea is not as new as one might think. In Frankfurt am Main, during the middle of the last century, Doctor Theobald Christ joined a babies hospital to his maternity hospital. Unfortunately, this model had been given up in our century. The same occurred with the Kaiserin Auguste Victoria Haus in Berlin, where a maternity unit had been incorporated into a children's hospital. The separation of delivery hospitals and children's hospitals implicated the need for transport, guided by specialized nurses and doctors. Butterfield has given a very interesting historical overview of neonatal transport systems in the USA[1]. Lemburg at Dusseldorf in Germany, and Dangel at Zurich in Switzerland have been recognized as experts in neonatal transport in central Europe since the end of the 1960s. For obvious reasons there are no controlled studies to be found about the effectiveness of a medically guided transport, compared with an unguided transport. On the other hand there are many reports showing clearly that regionalization of high-risk deliveries into perinatal centers, i.e. with the prenatal transport of the infant *in utero*, is more effective in reducing the mortality and morbidity of high-risk infants than postnatal transport to a remote neonatal intensive care unit[2–16]. These reports are not at all new. There are only a few papers showing no differences in outcome between inborn and outborn infants[17].

The question remains open as to whether the reason for the worse outcome of transported infants is due to the transport itself or to the 'condition of being outborn', i.e. not being born in a perinatal centre. Boenisch and colleagues[13] showed that vertical accelerations in ambulances are potentially dangerous and that the infant's head may come into resonance (about 15 cps) with these accelerations. By analyzing data of the Hessische Perinatal Study we looked for differences between the results documented in perinatal centers (Perinatalzentrum) and in non-perinatal centers.

METHODS

We analyzed the data of all very-low-birth-weight infants, i.e. ≤ 1500 g birth weight, born in Hessen in 1994. Access to the data of the Hessische Perinatal and Neonatal Study is restricted due to the rather strict laws for data protection in Germany. Normally each participant gets the overall data for the state of Hessen together with the data from their own hospital. We asked for the cumulated data of nine perinatal centers, selected using personal knowledge of the author, and the cumulated data of all other maternity units, so anonymity was maintained. Statistical analysis was carried out using the χ^2 test, two-tailed.

RESULTS

Table 1 shows the results of the Hessische Perinatal Study in 1994, which show many significant differences between the perinatal centers and the non-perinatal centers. No differences

Table 1 Results of the 1994 Hessische Perinatal Study on very-low-birth-weight infants

	Perinatal centers	Non-perinatal centers	p
Total deliveries	440	197	
Liveborns	388	140	
Perinatal mortality	22%	43%	$< 10^{-6}$
Stillborn babies	12%	29%	$< 10^{-6}$
Pediatrician present during delivery			
all deliveries	78%	54%	$< 10^{-6}$
liveborns only	86%	73%	$< 10^{-4}$
Umbilical artery pH not measured	9%	31%	$< 10^{-6}$
Apgar score ≤ 4			
1 min	29%	42%	< 0.01
5 min	8%	18%	< 0.005
10 min	7%	16%	< 0.005
Mortality first week postnatally	12%	19%	<0.03

could be found between the two groups concerning the rate of infants born at less than 28 weeks of gestation, or with birth weights < 1000 g.

Ten years ago we analyzed our own data, comparing them with the remainder of all other very-low-birth-weight infants born in Hessen 1983–1985 ($n = 666$). The first-week mortality rate in our perinatal center was 14.6% (171 infants), compared with 30.9% (495 infants) in the remainder of the state ($p < 0.0001$). Saule and co-workers[14] published data from Bavaria in 1987; the first-week mortality rate in infants < 2000 g birth weight was 12% in perinatal centers, and 29% in other units ($p < 0.001$). Reiter[18] also analyzed the Hessische Perinatal Study from 1993 to 1995. He found in infants born at gestational ages of 29 to 31 weeks a perinatal mortality of 7% ($n = 683$) in perinatal centers compared with 20% ($n = 222$) in other units ($p < 10^{-6}$).

In 1981 we compared the incidence of intraventricular hemorrhage in very-low-birth-weight infants born in our institution (perinatal center) with those transported to our unit from outside; the incidences were 3% (1/33) and 50% (4/8), respectively. Although the numbers were very small, the difference was significant ($p = 0.04$; Fisher's exact test)[15]. We did not continue this study, because by means of these limited data we persuaded our obstetric colleagues to transfer high-risk pregnancies into our perinatal center. But cumulating these scarce data with those of two other comparable studies[16,19] ($n = 319$), the incidence rates (with 90% confidence limits) were as follows: perinatal centers, 18% ± 6%; non-perinatal centers, 50% ± 6%; $p < 10^{-6}$. This means that the incidence of intraventricular hemorrhage could be reduced by 1.8–4.7 times ($p = 0.025$) by avoiding birth outside a perinatal center[5]. In Saule's results from Bavaria, the rates were 14.6% and 40.4% ($p < 0.001$) for perinatal centers and other units, respectively, in babies with birth weights in the range 1000–1499 g (personal communication).

DISCUSSION

In our analysis of the results from 1994, the first surprise was the striking difference in the stillbirth rate between the two types of delivery unit. This can be explained only by differences in deciding who lives and who does not, and in different methods of treating the asphyxiated preterm infant. In this context it may be of interest that pediatricians were far less often present during the deliveries which took place in non-perinatal centers. The cause might be a different attitude towards the very immature infant. Absence of pediatricians possibly also means a different quality of primary care of the newborn. Presence of, and daily communication with, neonatologists on the other hand may modify the attitudes of obstetricians and midwives in perinatal centers towards these fragile infants. The lower interest in umbilical artery pH seen in non-perinatal centers seems also to reflect a different interest in the tiny baby. Finally, the very different evolution of the Apgar scores from 1 to 5 and 10 min shows rather clearly the different quality of primary care in the two types of unit. Whether this is due to different interests, attitudes or even skills, is not clear. One might speculate that in non-perinatal centers a very premature birth is a relatively rare event, so that routine care is inadequate. It is impressive that the rates of perinatal mortality and neonatal mortality, as well as the differences between the two types of unit, have remained nearly the same over more than a decade.

Obladen introduced a neonatal transport service in the Bochum region of Germany which would go to the referring maternity hospital and stabilize the infant before transporting him or her under conditions of more or less full intensive care. Indeed he lowered the neonatal mortality rate in all transported infants (preterm and term) from 9.8 to 3.5%, and the need for mechanical ventilation from 44 to 22%[20]. One possible side-effect of this success should not be overlooked: obstetricians may become reluctant to send high-risk mothers prenatally into perinatal centers, as has occurred in South Carolina[21]. However, the expenses for such a perfect service are a real burden: in Germany there is no reimbursement for this time-consuming activity, as it is declared as a pre-hospital treatment which is included in the hospital stay, in remarkable contrast to the rescue services for adults. The same applies in the USA[22]. We roughly calculated the time needed for the primary care of an inborn infant, compared with an outborn: about 1 h vs. 3 h, respectively, not forgetting the costs for the transport itself. If one

follows the concept of a resuscitation service, the time can easily be expanded up to 8 h, the neonatal team sitting at the bedside of the mother, waiting for the preterm delivery. Because hardly any neonatal intensive care units have extra personnel for this outside work, care of the patients in the units themselves will necessarily be diluted by the absence of experienced staff. Therefore in a time when financial resources are becoming smaller and smaller, it can no longer be justified to waste money and manpower by failing to send high-risk deliveries to perinatal centers in time. The strongest arguments, however, are the undoubtedly better results obtained in infants born and cared for in perinatal centers. There are good ethical and medical arguments, but also good economic reasons. It should no longer be accepted that worse medicine is done for more money, i.e. transporting the baby postnatally under mobile intensive care, instead of the mother prenatally in a simple ambulance, and with better results. It may be added that in the Rhein-Main region of Germany, regionalization of high-risk deliveries has been more or less the rule since 1981.

CONCLUSION

Better results are obtained in infants born in perinatal centers due to better primary care, immediately after delivery, as shown by the striking differences in perinatal mortality in infants born at 29–31 weeks gestational age[18]. The better results could also be due to greater interest of the attending personnel in small preterm infants, the availability of well-trained pediatricians, the low number of infants declared stillborn, and the nearly always measured umbilical artery pH in the perinatal centers. In comparison with these factors the transport process itself might possibly have a smaller impact on the outcome. The message has therefore to be that no very-low-birth-weight infant should be born outside a perinatal center.

References

1. Butterfield, L. J. (1993). Historical perspectives of neonatal transport. *Pediatr. Clin. N. Am.*, **40**, 221–39

2. Anderson, C., Aladjem, S., Ayuste, O., Caldwell, C. and Ismail, M. (1981). An analysis of maternal transport within a suburban metropolitan region. *Am. J. Obstet. Gynecol.*, **140**, 499–504

3. Boehm, F. H. and Haire, M. F. (1979). One-way maternal transport: an evolving concept. Inpatient services. *Am. J. Obstet. Gynecol.*, **134**, 484–9

4. Cordero, L., Backes, C. and Zuspan, F. (1982). Very low birthweight infant: I. influence of place of birth on survival. *Am. J. Obstet. Gynecol.*, **143**, 533–7

5. Harding, J. E. and Morton, S. M. (1993). Adverse effects of neonatal transport between level III centers. *J. Paediatr. Child Health*, **29**, 146–9

6. Harris, T. R., Isaman, J. and Giles, H. R. (1978). Improved neonatal survival through maternal transport. *Obstet. Gynecol.*, **52**, 294–300

7. von Loewenich, V., Bielicki, M., Halberstadt, E. and Grau, H. (1984). Wie weit ist die intraventrikulaere Blutung sehr unreifer Fruehgeborener vermeidbar? In Dudenhausen, J. W. and Saling, E. (eds.) *Perinatale Medizin X*, pp. 308–9. (Stuttgart and New York: G. Thieme Publ.)

8. McCormick, M. C., Shapiro, S. and Starfield, B.-H. (1985). The regionalization of perinatal services. Summary of evaluation of a national demonstration program. *J. Am. Med. Assoc.*, **253**, 799–804

9. Modanlou, H. D., Dorchester, W., Freeman, R. K. and Rommal, C. (1980). Perinatal transport to a regional perinatal center in a metropolitan area: maternal versus neonatal transport. *Am. J. Obstet. Gynecol.*, **138**, 1157–64

10. Riegel, K., Selbmann, H. K. and Oesterlund, K. (1985). *Perinatalrisiken und kindliche Mortalitaet und Morbiditaet. Arvo-Ylppoe-Studie. BPT-Bericht 5/85.* (Munich: Gesellschaft für Strahlen- und Umweltforschung)

11. Rosenblatt, R. A., Reinken, J. and Shoemack, P. (1985): Is obstetrics safe in small hospitals? Evidence from New Zealand's regionalized perinatal system. *Lancet*, **2**, 429–39

12. Usher, R. (1977). Changing mortality rates with perinatal intensive care and regionalization. *Semin. Perinatol.*, **1**, 309–19

13. Boenisch, H., Gaden, W., Mau, D., Gurbandt, U., Teuteberg, H. O., Braun, H. and Beermann, H. J. (1985). Mechanische Belastung Neugeborener bei Inkubatortransporten. *Mschr. Kinderheilk.*, **133**, 471–5

14. Saule, H., Riegel, K. and Beltinger, C. (1987): Effectiveness of neonatal transport systems. *J. Perinat. Med.*, **15**, 515–21

15. Bielicki, M., von Loewenich, V., Halberstadt, E. and Grau, H. (1984). Intraventrikulaere Blutungen bei sehr kleinen Fruehgeborenen. In S. Kowalewski (ed.) *Paediatrische Intensivmedizin VI*, pp. 150–2. (Stuttgart and New York: G. Thieme Publ.)

16. Clark, C. E., Clyman, R. I., Roth, R. S., Sniderman, S. H., Lande, B. and Ballard, R. A. (1981). Risk factor analysis of intraventricular hemorrhage in low birthweight infants. *J. Pediatr.*, **99**, 625–8

17. Kollee, L. A., Brand, R., Schreuder, A. M., Ens-Dokkum, M. H., Veen, S. and Verloove-van Horick, S. P. (1992). Five-year outcome of preterm and very low birth weight infants: a comparison between maternal and neonatal transport. *Obstet. Gynecol.*, **80**, 635–8

18. Reiter, H. L., Feldmann, R., Vonderheit, K.-H. and Rascher, W. (1996). Derzeitiger Stand der Regionalisierung von Risikogeburten – Daten der hessischen Perinatal- und Neonatalerhebung (HEPNE). *22 Sympos. Deutsch-Oesterreichischen Ges. Neonatologie Paediatr. Intensivmed.*, Dresden, Germany, September (Abstr.)

19. Garcia-Prats, J. A., Procianoy, R. S., Adams, J. M. and Rudolp, A. J. (1982). The hyaline membrane disease – intraventricular hemorrhage relationship in the very low birth weight infant. Perinatal aspects. *Acta Paediatr. Scand.*, **71**, 79–84

20. Obladen, M. (1985). Das Risiko, geboren zu werden. *Forum d. Kinderheilk.*, **1**, 17–22

21. Hulsey, T. C., Pittard, W. B. and Ebeling, M. (1991). Regionalized perinatal transport systems: association with changes in location of birth, neonatal transport, and survival of very low birth weight deliveries. *J. S. Carol. Med. Assoc.*, **87**, 581–4

22. Zwischenberger, J. B., Keeney, S., Raymond, G., Hanson, M. and Cox, C. S. (1992). Neonatal transport in Texas. *Tex. Med.*, **88**, 66–9

Advanced neonatal nurse practitioners: development of an educational program

40

E. Perks, S. Smith and M. Hall

INTRODUCTION

The purpose of this paper is to provide a brief historic perspective of the first nationally accredited course to educate advanced neonatal nurse practitioners in the United Kingdom, and to identify some of the issues arising from the development of the role.

BACKGROUND TO THE COURSE DEVELOPMENT

The ability to provide the optimal care and management of the sick newborn is dependent on the availability of personnel who have a specific education and training in neonatology. It was in the 1970s in the USA that experienced neonatal nurses were first offered the opportunity to undertake an educational course which enabled them to advance their role clinically, and assume a leading role in the care of the sick, newborn infant[1]. Interest in the concept of the advanced neonatal nurse practitioner (ANNP) in the United Kingdom developed in the former Wessex Region in the 1980s, when a working party comprising senior doctors and nurses was established with the primary aim of suggesting long term strategies for improving the standard and quality of neonatal care in the region. One of the recommendations of this group was that the role of the neonatal nurse could be developed and expanded. This suggestion was accepted and supported, and as a result a formal educational course was initiated which provided a firm educational base for role development and enhancement rather than simply 'extending the role'. A group of senior nurses and a neonatologist subsequently visited the USA in 1991, to evaluate both the educational courses for ANNPs, and their role in neonatal units. Following this visit a course management team consisting of pediatricians, senior nurses throughout the region, representatives of nursing and midwifery education, National Health Service management and the University of Southampton Science Faculty was established to plan a course of education and training for ANNPs in Wessex.

COURSE DETAILS

In 1991 the course was validated by the English National Board (ENB) and subsequently given the designation 'ENB A19'. The University of Southampton also accredited the course with 60 Credit and Accumulation Transfer (CAT) points at level 3 (degree level). Since the initiation of the course, continuous assessment and evaluations have been undertaken both by the course co-ordinators and students. This has led to further development of the academic content of the course, and redefinition of the learning outcomes. In November 1995 the length of the course was extended from 9 months to 12 months (52 weeks) following conjoint validation of the course by the University of Southampton and the ENB. This resulted in the award of a Bachelor of Science (Honours) degree in Neonatal Studies and the ENB A19 to successful students.

Experienced neonatal nurses who meet the stringent entry requirements, and are successful at interview are required to pass the entrance examination based on a bioscience learning package. The students normally have 10 weeks to undertake the self-directed learning package. In addition, tutorials are facilitated in Southampton prior to undertaking the examination. This package has proven to be an invaluable tool as it enables students to acquire an understanding of basic sciences, and in addition it ensures that they have attained a standard which prepares them to study at degree level.

The theoretical component of the course is undertaken at the University of Southampton, based in the School of Nursing and Midwifery. Students are also required to complete a period of clinical apprenticeship normally undertaken in their seconding unit. The first cohort of seven students in 1992 were from six units in the former Wessex Region. The following year's intake included a student from an adjacent region (Oxford), and subsequently students have been seconded from units throughout the United Kingdom. The course is in its fifth year and there are 46 qualified nurses who have undertaken the course in Southampton; it is anticipated that a further 18 will graduate later this year. Several other centres in England have now established Advanced Neonatal Nurse Practitioner courses.

The program continues to be designed specifically to meet the needs of suitably experienced and motivated neonatal nurses enabling them to develop and increase their theoretical and clinical expertize, in order to improve the standard and quality of neonatal care.

The general aims of the course are to develop advanced neonatal nurse practitioners capable of:

(1) Assuming a leading role in the immediate care and the subsequent management of the sick neonate and its family;

(2) Demonstrating problem-solving approaches to management of care by drawing upon an in-depth knowledge base;

(3) A greater responsibility for patient care initiating management; this will involve im-

mediate independent decision making involving clinical judgement, utilizing evidence-based research, and leadership skills; and

(4) Selecting and utilizing appropriate professional skills for the maximum benefit of the infant and its family.

The curriculum has been specifically designed to integrate biomedical sciences, behavioral sciences, and neonatal medicine with an advanced level of nursing expertize. The theoretical component of the course, comprising of 520 hours' teaching, is undertaken by lecturers from the University, consultant pediatricians, consultants from other specialties (for example genetics, pathology, radiology), senior nurses/midwives and qualified ANNPs. The course has five main modules: advanced neonatal nursing, applied neonatal nursing, applied neonatal care, behavioral sciences, biomedical sciences applied to the neonate, and principles of research in clinical practice. The modules are all inter-linked and integrated throughout the course and provide the opportunity to respond to educational, professional and practical initiatives, whilst further enhancing the academic and professional development of students. A variety of teaching methods are used during the course including lectures, seminars, workshops, practice-based clinical sessions and journal clubs. These sessions are all carefully planned and interwoven to ensure that wherever possible theoretical sessions are applied or linked with neonatal clinical practice and case management. There are a total of 16 study block weeks in Southampton, the remaining weeks being spent in the students' seconding base units. During the first 9 months it is anticipated that the students will spend the majority of time undertaking self-directed learning and consolidating their academic knowledge, undertaking practical skills, as well as beginning the process of role transition from senior neonatal nurse to ANNP. The final 3 months are defined as the clinical preceptorship and it is specifically during this period that the student is acquiring clinical skills and continuing to consolidate and integrate theory with practice.

Integration of theory and practice, and the acquisition of the clinical competencies requires a suitable learning environment. The teaching support system comes from medical and nurse mentors in the clinical area of the seconding unit. Students will undertake their clinical preceptorship normally in their own neonatal unit, under the clinical supervision of a neonatal consultant and ANNP. The clinical preceptorship is a key element of this course as the student has to achieve several clinical objectives, and demonstrate on completion of the course that they are able to function in the clinical area at the level required of an ANNP. It is therefore essential that the student receives a wide range of support, clinical teaching, supervision and assessment during this period. The range of clinical experience in the seconding unit is evaluated on application to undertake the course by completion of a unit profile. Prior to each student starting the course a mentorship visit by the course co-ordinators is undertaken to the seconding unit. The function of these informal visits is to disseminate information regarding the role and level of commitment of the medical and nurse mentors, and ensure consistency when using the assessment tools. These sessions also provide the opportunity for mentors to discuss potential problems or concerns not only in relation to assessment, but facilitating and supporting the student while they are undertaking role transition. These informal visits have also helped promote a consistent approach to student assessment.

There is a formative and summative component to the assessment of theory. Summative assessment determines the extent to which the student has achieved the outcomes of the course, and contributes to the final grade and classification of the degree. Progress on the course will depend upon successful completion of the continuous assessment of theoretical examinations and assignments, and the satisfactory completion of clinical assessments in accordance with the scheme of continuous assessment of practical competence.

PIONEERING THE NEW ROLE

This educational course has been developed in response to the challenging and ever-changing opportunities for neonatal nurses. Although the rationale for development of the role was, and continues to be, the improvement of the quality and standard of care, the introduction of changes to the staffing of neonatal units by junior doctors has implications for the provision of clinical services[2,3]. The motivation of nurses to accept new roles and responsibilities, and the continued support of consultants who acknowledge nurses as colleagues in an interdisciplinary team, are essential elements in the evolution of the role. The development of the course can be related to multiple factors, but the initial curriculum effectively expanded the knowledge base and level of clinical functioning of neonatal nurses. The ANNPs who are educated at the graduate level continue to retain a strong nursing identity, although it may be perceived by some professionals that the focus is on developing clinical skills. The interdependent collaboration needed in a neonatal unit requires preparation beyond that which focuses primarily on the acquisition of technical competence.

The inability of ANNPs to 'prescribe' continues to restrict their optimal functioning. Recent advice on prescribing from the Law Department of the Royal Pharmaceutical Society regarding the interpretation of the Medicine Act of 1968, states 'that the Society's view is that a protocol purporting to authorize the supply or administration of a prescription-only medicine in the absence of patient-specific written directions of a doctor or dentist does not comply with the Act'. The clinical implications of this advice in Southampton have resulted in ANNPs being unable to 'order' medications.

EVALUATION

The introduction of the ANNP requires collaboration between disciplines and it would be naive to believe that there would not be any resistance. Doctors may feel threatened by nurses who see themselves as 'equal partners' in care. Conversely nursing colleagues may feel threatened by the increased responsibility and accountability crucial to collaboration. The blurring of boundaries between medicine and nursing in the role of the ANNP has challenged ideas about who is ultimately accountable for the care of neonates. The General Medical Council's guidance to doctors[4] is that they can delegate medical care to nurses if they are sure that the nurse is competent to undertake the role, but overall responsibility for managing patient care remains with the doctor. ANNPs are subject to the United Kingdom Central Council's (UKCC) Guidance[5], and they are also accountable to their patients, employers and to the courts. In a recent article in the British Medical Journal, recommendations by Dowling and colleagues[6] summarized many issues surrounding accountability when nurses expanded their roles.

Many of these recommendations have implications for the development of the role of the ANNP. In the changing boundaries between professional groups, nurses must acknowledge their level of competence before accepting adjustments to their range of practice, and the regulating authorities for all professionals should work together to ensure that the guidance they give emphasizes partnership or teamwork rather than hierarchy. The complexity of neonatal care is such that no single profession can reasonably assume accountability or management responsibility for all care. Effective risk management strategies developed by provider units, based on guidance from statutory and government agencies, would enable employers to develop effective clinical guidelines

so that employees are able to exercise professional accountability.

Evaluation of the ANNP educational programme and the ANNP role has been undertaken by the ENB[7]. Many of the recommendations in their report have already been incorporated into the revised course, but the ENB also identified that many of the qualified practitioners do provide an advanced level of care. Evidence from Canada[8] indicates that the level of care provided is at least equivalent to that given by junior medical staff. A further evaluation study on the professional functioning of ANNPs, and their integration into neonatal units funded by the former Wessex Region, is expected to be published later this year.

SUMMARY

There are many elements that are essential if the role of the ANNP is to be successful. The introduction of the course has enabled experienced neonatal nurses to function at levels that incorporate both medical and nursing elements in their role. This has had an impact on both professions, and to establish collaborative practice continuous negotiation is necessary to define the responsibilities of all practitioners. This is an opportunity for experienced nurses to develop personally and professionally in the clinical environment, and have an influence on the standards and quality of neonatal care, not only by applying and integrating theoretical knowledge with nursing skills, but also by dissemination of this expertize to other members of the multiprofessional team.

References

1. Johnson, P., Jung, A. and Boros, S. (1979). Neonatal nurse practitioners: part 1 – a new expanded nursing role. *Perinatol. Neonatol.*, **3**, 34–6

2. Department of Health (1993). *Heads of Agreement: Ministerial Group on Junior Doctors' Hours.* (London: Department of Health)

3. Department of Health (1993). *Hospital Doctors: Training for the Future. The Calman Report of the Working Group on Specialist Medical Training.* (London: Department of Health)

4. General Medical Council (1995). *Duties of a Doctor: Guidance from the GMC.* (London: General Medical Council)

5. United Kingdom Central Council (1992). *Code of Professional Conduct for the Nurse, Midwife and Health Visitor*, 3rd edn. (London: United Kingdom Central Council)

6. Dowling, S., Martin, R., Skidmore, P., Doyal, L., Cameron, A. and Lloyd, S. (1996). Nurses taking on junior doctors' work: a confusion of accountability. *Br. Med. J.*, **312**, 1211–14

7. Redshaw, M. E. and Harris, A. (1995). *Breaking New Ground: an Exploratory Study of the Role of the Advanced Neonatal Nurse Practitioner and the Educational Programme of Preparation.* (London: ENB for Nursing Midwifery and Health Visiting)

8. Mitchell, A., Watts, J., Whyte, R., Blatz, S., Norman, G. R., Guyatt, G. H., Southwell, D., Hunsberger, M. and Paes, B. (1991). Evaluation of graduating neonatal nurse practitioners. *Pediatrics*, **88**, 789–94

Prenatal treatment of lung immaturity — 41

E. V. Cosmi, R. La Torre, J. Piazze, N. Lerro and L. Maranghi

INTRODUCTION

In spite of great advances in its prevention and treatment, i.e. antenatal glucocorticoids, postpartum surfactant replacement therapy and artificial ventilation, respiratory distress syndrome (IRDS) of the neonate remains a major cause of mortality and morbidity in preterm newborn infants. A retrospective analysis of the non-randomized use of corticosteroids from the database of the NIHCHD neonatal network has suggested that a treatment-to-treatment interval of < 24 h can decrease death and intraventricular hemorrhage (IVH) but not IRDS in steroid exposed preterm infants. There has been no prospective attempt to define the minimal interval from treatment to response in either animal models or clinically[1]. The results of the NIH Consensus Conference also state that maternal corticosteroid treatment should be considered unless preterm delivery is imminent[2]; in other words, maternal corticosteroid treatment should not be considered if preterm delivery is imminent. Although the impact of corticosteroids on neonatal mortality and on the reduction of IVH is unquestionable, they are not a panacea because about 10% of neonates exposed to them are still affected by IRDS[3].

The administration of supplementary surfactant to neonates affected by IRDS has become quite a common treatment for this condition, although repeated doses are often required because uniform distribution of the substance within the lung is seldom obtained. It seems therefore logical that the most rational approach would be the prevention rather than the treatment of IRDS and that the most natural way would be to instil supplementary surfactant into the fetal pulmonary liquid (FPL) compartment, i.e. at birth before the first breath or *in utero* by direct injection into amniotic fluid close to the fetal mouth and nostrils so that it will undergo uniform distribution within the FPL. The scientific basis for 'prophylactic' intra-amniotic fluid administration of surfactant spans three decades of research on the fluid dynamics and related biochemistry of the FPL and amniotic fluid compartments. Three lines of research have paved the way. First, Adams and co-workers[4,5] provided the first detailed and systematic studies of FPL. They defined the organic and inorganic composition, surface activity, fluid movement and comparison with other liquid compartments of the maternal–fetal complex. Second, Gluck and associates[6,7] presented meticulous studies of the chemical development of FPL and fetal pulmonary tissue. Then Scarpelli[8,9] proved the metabolic origin of FPL surfactant from pulmonary tissue and defined the lipid and protein gradients between FPL and amniotic fluid. From these data, he suggested that amniotic fluid phospholipids may be used to diagnose fetal lung maturity (FLM); Gluck and colleagues[10] later proved this concept to be correct. Collectively, these studies had established that FPL surfactants are the principal substrate for the formation of intra-alveolar bubbles at the onset of air-breathing at birth[11]. Surfactants form the ultrathin films of bubbles that carry air to the alveoli ('saccules') and establish normal gas exchange and alveolar stability. Even after successful therapeutic intratracheal instillation of surfactant to the postnatal infant – first reported in the pioneering study of Fujiwara and co-workers[12] – significant clinical intervention is required. Thus, the 'prophylactic' aspect of intra-amniotic fluid administration is to 'normalize' the transition to air-breathing at birth and thereby reduce or obviate the need for extended interventions (e.g. surfactant instillation, assisted/controlled ventilation) during the neonatal period.

Studies in baboons[13,14] have indicated that antenatal intra-amniotic instillation of surfactant may be as effective as post-delivery intratracheal administration for the prevention of IRDS. Petrikovsky and associates[15] have reported on the feasibility of intrauterine administration of surfactant by injection through a fiberoptic endoscope, which had been passed through the cervical canal during active preterm labor after spontaneous rupture of the membranes. The surfactant was injected into the mouth of the human fetus under direct vision through the endoscope. The authors found no fetal, maternal or neonatal complications in the three cases reported. However, queries remain about the efficacy of the procedure, e.g. regarding entry of the surfactant into the large pulmonary airways and regarding the role, if any, of fetal breathing movements (FBMs).

Intra-amniotic delivery of surfactant is subjected both to immediate dilution and fetal swallowing so that it may not enter the FPL compartment in sufficient concentrations. Our observation on fetal sheep that there is no net flux of FPL outwards or inwards through the trachea, particularly in the absence of FBMs[16,17],

and that aminophylline given to the mother induces and/or increases FBMs[18], has prompted us to combine antenatal administration of aminophylline with intra-amniotic fluid administration of natural supplementary surfactant with the hope that during FBMs it would reach the lower airways of the fetus. We have reasoned, therefore, that antenatal administration of aminophylline, when linked with specifically directed intra-amniotic fluid administration of natural surfactant[19–22], should result in the introduction of supplementary surfactant into the immature lung (i.e. FPL) of the fetus.

MATERIAL AND METHODS

Relevant characteristics of the six patients are outlined in Table 1. Fetal conditions were documented by cardiotocography and Doppler velocimetry. Three fetuses were affected by severe intrauterine growth retardation (IUGR). In two cases the conditions of the mother were rapidly deteriorating and in the sixth case tocolysis was suspended because of the intractable vaginal bleeding at 24 weeks gestation. The indication for Cesarean section in three cases was severe deterioration of the fetal condition, in two cases the mother was affected by HELLP (hemolysis, elevated liver enzymes, low platelets). The sixth case was affected by a severe vaginal bleeding of marked degree which

Table 1 Summary of cases treated with intra-amniotic supplementary natural surfactant prior to the administration of surfactant

Case	Gestation age (weeks)	Diagnosis	CTG	Doppler flow analysis[†]	Pre-surfactant injection		
					Shake test	L/S	PG
1	28	IUGR	n.r.	RED	neg.	1.8	absent
2	32	IUGR	r.	AED	neg.	2.0	absent
3	32	HELLP	r.	RI of uterine arteries	neg.	1.9	absent
4	28	IUGR	n.r.	RED	neg.	NA	NA
5	28	HELLP	r.	> PI umb.art.	neg.	2.0	absent
6	24	Preterm labor, uncontrollable vaginal bleeding	r.	Normal	neg.	1.0	absent

CTG = cardiotocography; [†] = umbilical artery; L/S = lecithin/sphyngomyelin; PG = phosphatidylglycerol; IUGR = intrauterine growth retardation; HELLP = hemolysis, elevated liver enzymes, low platelets; n.r. = non-reactive; r. = reactive; RED = reversed end-diastolic flow; AED = absent end-diastolic flow; RI = resistance index; PI = pulsatility index; neg. = negative; NA = not analyzed

contraindicated further tocolysis; because labor proceeded rapidly without signs of fetal distress and the presentation was cephalic, it was decided to deliver the fetus vaginally.

After obtaining informed consent, amniocentesis was performed under ultrasound guidance to collect amniotic fluid for testing FLM; the needle was directed near the fetal nostrils and mouth and was kept in place. Fetal lung maturity was assessed by a rapid test, the shake test, and later on by lecithin/sphyngomyelin (L/S) determination and phosphatidylglycerol measurement using the method of Gluck and colleagues[6,7]. If the shake test indicated FLM, a bolus of 240 mg of aminophylline was administered over 10 min to the mother followed by intravenous infusion at the rate of $0.02–0.1 \text{ mg kg}^{-1} \text{ min}^{-1}$. The fetus was continuously monitored by Doppler velocimetry; 5–15 min after the loading dose of aminophylline, FBMs appeared first as vortices through the fetal nostrils, then began at a rate of 10–12/min as documented both by chest wall movements and inspiratory and expiratory flows of amniotic fluid through the nostrils which were recorded continuously with color Doppler equipment. Natural surfactant (Curosurf, Chiesi Farmaceutici, Parma, Italy; 80 mg in 1 ml) was then instilled through the amniocentesis needle directed toward the fetal mouth and nostrils. Cesarean section was performed under epidural anesthesia 60–150 min after the administration of surfactant. Before the incision of amniotic membranes a sample of amniotic fluid was collected with a 10 ml syringe.

RESULTS

Table 2 shows relevant maternal, fetal and neonatal data of the six fetuses treated *in utero* with supplementary natural surfactant after maternal intravenous administration of aminophylline. Entry of the surfactant in the amniotic fluid compartment was seen by ultrasound as a sonolucent material that moved down the trachea and upper airways during FBMs, which had increased in depth and frequency during aminophylline infusion; some of supplementary surfactant was swallowed by the fetus. Following aminophylline infusion to the mother, fetal heart rate increased by 10–15 beats/min. Treatment with supplementary surfactant increased significantly the L/S, and the phosphatidylglycerol concentration in the amniotic fluid samples taken during the Cesarean section. Time to sustained respiration, Apgar score at 1 and 5 min, sex and weight are shown in Table 2.

The neonates were transferred to the neonatal ward; four of them (cases 1–4) followed an uneventful clinical course to the time of discharge from the hospital. Case No. 5 showed radiological signs of mild IRDS and 3 h

Table 2 Summary of cases treated with intra-amniotic supplementary natural surfactant after maternal intravenous administration of aminophylline. Post-surfactant tests were on amniotic fluid taken at Cesarean section

| Case | Mode of delivery | Post-surfactant | | | Weight (g) | Sex | T.S.R. (s) | Apgar at 1 and 5 min | Clinical outcome |
		Shake test	L/S	PG					
1	CS	pos.	5.0	present	1035	M	30	8/10	uneventful
2	CS	pos.	3.5	present	1650	M	25	8/9	uneventful
3	CS	pos.	2.5	present	1700	M	45	8/10	uneventful
4	CS	pos.	NA	NA	1095	M	30	7/10	uneventful
5	CS	pos.	2.4	present	970	M	20	5/8	mild IRDS*
6	VD	ND	ND	ND	630	F	35	6/8	IRDS†

L/S = lecithin/sphyngomyelin;   PG = phosphatidylglycerol;   T.S.R. = time to sustained respiration; CS = Cesarean section; VD = vaginal delivery; pos. = positive; NA = not analyzed; ND = not determined; IRDS = neonatal respiratory distress syndrome; *treated at birth with one dose of supplementary natural surfactant and extubated after 72 h; †the same as case 5, extubated after 13 days. Died at 35 days of life following a blood-borne cytomegalovirus infection

after birth received a dose of 120 mg of Curosurf. The infant was extubated 72 h later. Case No. 6 (birth weight = 630 g) was born at 24 weeks gestation in good condition and had administered (according to a protocol in use in the Neonatology Department for all babies weighing less than 900 g) a prophylactic dose of 120 mg of Curosurf. Artificial ventilation was required for 13 days before successful extubation. Unfortunately, at 35 days of life she died as the consequence of a disseminated cytomegalovirus infection acquired following blood transfusions for the treatment of anemia of prematurity.

DISCUSSION

The present study shows a successful outcome of prenatal administration of natural surfactant to the human fetus. We obviously were not able to demonstrate conclusively the distribution of surfactant into distal airways. However, several lines of evidence may suggest that effective intrapulmonary distribution of supplementary surfactant was achieved, including:

(1) The surfactant was injected at the mouth and nostrils level of the fetus and was seen to be distributed into the upper airways;

(2) Fetal breathing movements induced by intravenous administration of aminophylline to the mother were sustained and deep as documented by ultrasound and color Doppler, thus favoring entry into and distribution by diffusion throughout all potential airspaces, a process that is aided by the agitation produced by fetal breathing movements;

(3) It is also possible that smooth muscle relaxation induced by aminophylline may lower the resistance to the movement of supplementary surfactant through the airways;

(4) Some of the supplementary surfactant was seen to be swallowed by the fetus which was expected, particularly since gastric fluid at birth often reflects the surfactant content of the lung;

(5) Continued fetal breathing movements favor rapid dispersion and uniform distribution of the surfactant into the smallest airways and saccules, as suggested by our studies in the sheep fetus[16] and also by Adams and co-workers[4,5];

(6) Consequently, the previously surfactant-poor fetal pulmonary liquid (see first amniotic fluid L/S and phosphatidylglycerol analysis) had been enriched by the prophylactic surfactant at the sites required for successful adaptation to air-breathing at birth; and

(7) The uneventful clinical course of the newborn infants is consistent with the known role of fetal pulmonary liquid as the first substrate for normal surfactant function at birth[11].

Our results compel continued efforts for improving this method.

References

1. Wright, L. L., Verter, J., Younes, N., Stevenson, D., Fanaroff, A. A., Shankaran, S. *et al.* (1995). Antenatal corticosteroid administration and neonatal outcome in very low birth weight infants: the NICHD neonatal research network. *Am. J. Obstet. Gynecol.*, **173**, 269–74
2. NIH Consensus Development Conference (1995). Effects of corticosteroids for fetal maturation on perinatal outcomes, February 28–March 2, 1994. *Am. J. Obstet. Gynecol.*, **173**, 246–52
3. Crowley, P., Chalmers, I. and Keirse, M. J. N. (1990). The effects of corticosteroid administration before preterm delivery: an overview of the evidence from controlled trials. *Br. J. Obstet. Gynaecol.*, **97**, 11–25

4. Adams, F. H. and Fujiwara, T. (1963). Surfactant in the fetal lamb tracheal fluid. *J. Pediatr.*, **63**, 537–42

5. Adams, F. H., Fujiwara, T. and Rowshan, G. (1963). The nature and origin of the fluid in the fetal lamb lung. *J. Pediatr.*, **63**, 881–8

6. Gluck, L., Motoyama, E. K., Smits, H. L. and Kulovich, M. V. (1967). The biochemical development of surface activity in mammalian lung I. *Pediatr. Res.*, **1**, 237–46

7. Gluck, L., Scribney, M. and Kulovich, M. V. (1967). The biochemical development of surface activity in the mammalian lung II. *Pediatr. Res.*, **1**, 247–65

8. Scarpelli, E. M. (ed.) (1967). The lung tracheal fluid, and lipid metabolism of the fetus. *Pediatrics*, **40**, 951–61

9. Scarpelli, E. M. (1968). *The Surfactant System of the Lung.* (Philadelphia: Lea and Febiger)

10. Gluck, L., Kulovich, M. V., Borer, R. C. Jr, Brenner, P. H., Anderson, G. G. and Spellacy, W. N. (1971). Diagnosis of respiratory distress syndrome by amniocentesis. *Am. J. Obstet. Gynecol.*, **109**, 440–5

11. Scarpelli, E. M. (1978). Intrapulmonary foam at birth: an adaptional phenomenon. *Pediatr. Res.*, **12**, 1070–80

12. Fujiwara, T., Chida, S., Watabe, Y., Maeta, H., Morita, T. and Abe, T. (1980). Artificial surfactant therapy in hyaline membrane disease. *Lancet*, **1**, 155–9

13. Galan, H. L., Cipriani, C., Coulson, J. J., Bean, J. D., Collier, G. and Kuehl, T. J. (1993). Surfactant replacement therapy *in utero* for the prevention of hyaline membrane disease in the preterm baboon. *Am. J. Obstet. Gynecol.*, **169**, 817–24

14. Galan, H. L., Cipriani, C., Coalson, J. J., Bean-Lijewski, J. D., Collier, G. and Kuhel, T. J. (1996). Hyaline membrane disease surfactant prophylaxis in the preterm baboon: a comparison of postpartum versus *in utero* therapy. *Prenat. Neonat. Med.*, **1**, 122–30

15. Petrikovsky, B. M., Lysikiewicz, A., Markin, L. B. and Slomko, Z. (1995). *In utero* surfactant administration to preterm human fetuses by endoscopy. *Fetal Diagn. Ther.*, **10**, 127–30

16. Scarpelli, E. M., Condorelli, S. and Cosmi, E. V. (1975). Fetal pulmonary fluid I. Validation and significance of method for determination of volume and volume change. *Pediatr. Res.*, **9**, 190–5

17. Scarpelli, E. M., Condorelli, S. and Cosmi, E. V. (1975). Lamb fetal pulmonary fluid II. Fate of phosphatidylcholine. *Pediatr. Res.*, **9**, 195–201

18. Cosmi, E. V., Felli, F., Grossmann, G., Lachmann, B. and Robertson, B. (1979). Improved survival in the premature rabbit neonate following antenatal treatment with aminophylline. *IRCS Med. Sci.*, **7**, 115

19. Cosmi, E. V., La Torre, R., Di Iorio, R. and Anceschi, M. M. (1996). A novel treatment of fetal lung immaturity. Society for Perinatal Obstetricians, 16th Annual Meeting. *Am. J. Obstet. Gynecol.*, **174** (1(2)), 487 abstr. 653

20. Cosmi, E. V., La Torre, R., Di Iorio, R. and Anceschi, M. M. (1996). Surfactant administration to the human fetus *in utero*: a new approach to prevention of neonatal respiratory distress syndrome (IRDS). *J. Perinat. Med.*, **24**, 191–3

21. Cosmi, E. V., La Torre, R. and Di Iorio, R. (1996). Intraamniotic instillation of surfactant for prevention of neonatal respiratory distress syndrome (IRDS): a preliminary report. *Appl. Cardiopulm. Pathophysiol.*, **6**, 3–5

22. Cosmi, E. V. (1996). Prenatal administration of surfactant. *Prenat. Neonat. Med.*, **1**, 109–11

Perfluorocarbon liquid ventilation   42

A. Valls-i-Soler, M. A. Gómez, E. Gastiasoro and F. J. Alvarez

INTRODUCTION

In mammals, birth represents a transition from placental to pulmonary gas exchange. Then, atmospheric gas replaces the liquid present in the fetal lungs, and an air–liquid interface is established in the alveoli. If birth takes place at term, a successful transition does occur, because of the presence of a mature pulmonary surfactant system at the alveolar surface.

Pulmonary surfactant is a complex mixture of surface-active phospholipids (phosphatidyl-choline and -glycerol), proteins (surfactant-associated proteins, A, B, C and D), and neutral lipids. This surface-active material, by decreasing surface tension at the alveolar air–liquid interface, keeps the alveoli open and prevents their collapse during expiration. After birth, at end-expiration, a volume of gas remains in the lungs – the so-called functional residual capacity (FRC). This volume of gas is equal to the volume of pulmonary fluid present in the fetal lungs. The presence of the FRC facilitates the breathing cycle, by increasing lung compliance and decreasing work associated with breathing, thus facilitating extrauterine gas exchange.

In preterm deliveries, alveolar surfactant might be deficient, and an adequate FRC is therefore not established, leading to the development of respiratory distress syndrome (RDS). In spite of prevention of premature birth and the use of pharmacological induction of fetal lung maturity, some babies are born with immature lungs and develop a severe RDS.

If RDS is present, mechanical ventilation might be necessary, and the baby might go on to develop a form of chronic respiratory insufficiency, known as bronchopulmonary dysplasia (BPD). In this situation, prophylactic or rescue treatments with exogenous surfactant have been shown to be clinically effective. Short-term gas exchange is enhanced, complications such as air-leak are less frequent, and long-term outcome – survival without BPD – is improved.

In other neonatal respiratory diseases, like meconium aspiration syndrome, pneumonia, and congenital diaphragmatic hernia (CDH), surfactant dysfunction might contribute to the abnormal lung function found in these conditions. Furthermore, some newborn infants might develop an adult-type RDS, in which a surfactant dysfunction could also be present.

A different approach used to overcome the high alveolar surface tension found in these conditions, is to replace the alveolar air–liquid by a liquid–liquid interface, replacing nitrogen, the carrier gas, by a perfluorocarbon (PFC) liquid. The PFC is a family of synthetic compounds obtained by complete fluorination of hydrocarbons. The resulting C–F non-polar bonds make them extremely stable and non-reactive. They are immiscible with water, lipids or solvents, so do not affect the concentration or properties of endogenous alveolar surfactant[1]. Furthermore, some PFC liquids (Table 1) have a relatively low surface tension, high solubility for O_2 and CO_2, and a high vapor pressure range (31–230 mmHg at 25°C), that facilitate elimination by evaporation through the lungs. All these properties, and the lack of known toxicity, make them suitable for gas transport to the lungs.

EXPERIMENTAL LIQUID VENTILATION

In 1966, Clark and Gollan[2] showed that at atmospheric pressures, PFC could briefly support respiration in mammals; once removed from PFC, mice reassumed air-breathing and survived. Nevertheless, the high density and viscosity of PFC preclude its use in spontaneous respiration.

Later, several systems were designed to mechanically assist respiration[3,4], which were proven effective in supporting both oxygenation and CO_2 elimination. The idea, physiological application, and practice of total or tidal liquid ventilation (LV) was mainly pursued by Shaffer and co-workers, with more than a decade of experimental work[5–7].

Total LV has been extensively studied, and found to effectively enhance pulmonary gas exchange in immature[8,9] and adult[10,11] animals with normal or abnormal lungs. Nevertheless, questions about the clinical feasibility and implications, and the possible side-effects are still to be investigated. For all these reasons, total LV, a very promising technique, remains a research tool.

Recently, a simplified technique, called partial LV or PFC-associated gas exchange[12], has been developed. In partial LV, a volume of PFC,

equal to the estimated FRC, is introduced into the lungs, and then tidal volumes of gas from a conventional mechanical ventilator are delivered. This technique has been proven to be effective in several experimental models of respiratory failure in both immature and adult animals: meconium aspiration[13], CDH[14], gastric aspiration[15], surfactant deficiency induced by lung lavage[16,17], oleic acid injury[18], etc. The main differences between these two LV techniques are shown in Table 2.

The following briefly reviews our findings in experimental LV performed on very immature lambs at the Department of Physiology and Pediatrics, University of Temple, Philadelphia, USA, and performed on adult rats with acute respiratory failure (ARF) induced by repeated lung lavage, accomplished in our laboratory.

First, we studied the effects of rescue therapy with brief partial LV or tracheal instillation of modified porcine surfactant (Curosurf®) on lung mechanics, gas exchange and pulmonary structure in very immature lambs[8] (111 days). Results were compared with those obtained in lambs managed with gas and total LV. Gas

Table 1 Physical properties of air, water and some perfluorocarbon (PFC) liquids. FC-75 and FC-77 are industrial PFCs from 3M Corp., Rimar-101 from Miteni SPL and Liquivent from Alliance Pharmaceutical Corp.

	Air	Water	Rimar-101	FC-75	FC-77	Liquivent
Boiling point (°C)	—	100	101	102	97	143
Density (g/ml)*	0.0013	1.00	1.77	1.78	1.78	1.92
Dynamic viscosity (cP)*	0.02	0.67	0.89	0.80	0.80	NA
Vapor pressure (mmHg)†	—	47	64	63	85	11
Surface tension (dyn/cm)*	—	72	15	15	15	18
O_2 solubility (ml gas/100 ml liquid)*	20.95	3.0	52.0	52.0	50.0	53.0
CO_2 solubility (ml gas/100 ml liquid)†	0.03	57.0	160.0	160.0	198.0	210.0

*Data at 25°C; †data at 37°C; NA, data not available

Table 2 Differences and similarities between total and partial liquid ventilation (LV) and gas ventilation

	Gas ventilation	Total LV	Partial LV
Functional residual capacity	air	PFC	PFC
Tidal volume	air	PFC	air
Frequency (cycles per min)	unlimited	≤ 10	unlimited
Type of ventilator	conventional or HFV	experimental phase (special type)	conventional or HFV
Alveolar interface	air–liquid	liquid–liquid	liquid–liquid?

PFC, perfluorocarbon; HFV, high frequency ventilation

exchange and compliance improved in both rescued groups, but not reaching levels of total LV lambs (Figure 1). Lung histology showed uneven ventilation in all but the total LV group.

We have shown that total LV is an adequate technique to provide short term pulmonary gas exchange in adult rats with ARF, induced by lung lavage[10]. Rats with and without ARF had similar blood gases while on total LV, and a significantly higher PaO_2 and lower $PaCO_2$ than rats with ARF managed with conventional gas ventilation (Figure 2). Nevertheless, lavage rats needed a higher peak inspiratory pressure to achieve the same tidal volume than non-lavage rats (Figure 3). This finding supports the hypothesis that even in the absence of an air–liquid interface, high interfacial tension remains in the PFC–aqueous hypophase interface, in surfactant-deficient PFC-filled lungs.

Comparison of the effects of both LV methods[16], total and partial LV, in rats with ARF, showed gas exchange to be similarly improved over that found in rats with ARF managed with conventional gas ventilation (Figure 4).

The potential uses of PFC in respiratory therapy are not limited to partial or total liquid breathing, but include lung imaging and airway

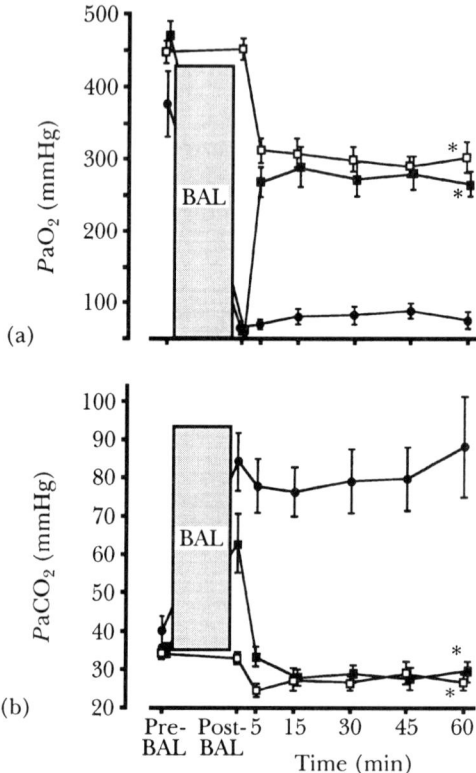

(a)

(b)

Figure 2 Pulmonary gas exchange in animals managed on gas ventilation and total liquid ventilation (LV). During LV, differences between groups managed with this technique were not observed (means ± SE). □, Normal animals managed on total LV; ■, rats with acute respiratory failure (ARF) managed on total LV; ●, rats with ARF managed on gas ventilation (*Anova, $p < 0.05$ vs. gas-ventilated animals). Vertical bar represents the bronchvoalveolar lavage process (BAL) in ARF groups only (■,●). After BAL, mean PaO_2 (a) showed a significant decrease in animals with ARF, but those managed on total LV demonstrated an increase in oxygenation, reaching similar values to normal animals on LV. An increase in mean $PaCO_2$ (b) was observed in ARF groups. Only after total LV started was a decrease of this parameter to baseline evident

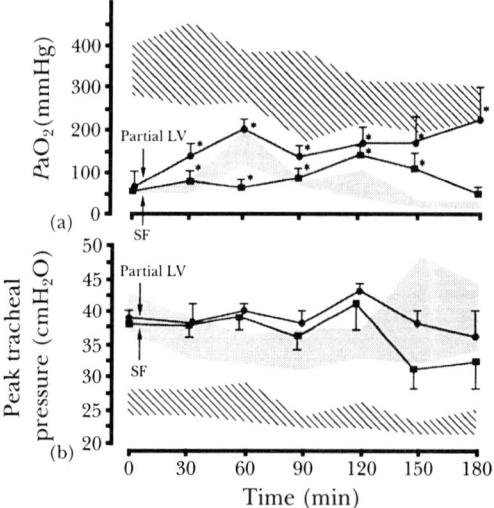

Figure 1 (a) Mean oxygen arterial pressure (PaO_2) and (b) peak tracheal pressures (PTP) before and for 180 min after surfactant (SF) and partial liquid ventilation (LV) rescue (means ± SE). Striped and grey areas represent means ± SE of lambs managed with total LV or gas ventilation from birth, respectively (*Student's t-test, $p < 0.05$ vs. baseline). Mean PaO_2 (a) improved after SF rescue and remained relatively constant until 150 min, to later decrease to the baseline. In partial LV lambs, there was an increase in PaO_2 and although values were higher than in SF lambs, differences were not statistically significant. PTP (b) was similar in both SF and partial LV lambs

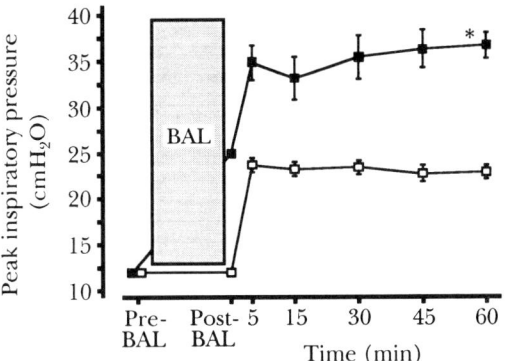

Figure 3 Mean peak inspiratory pressure (means ± SE). Both groups were managed on total liquid ventilation (LV), however, animals with acute respiratory failure (ARF) showed a significantly greater inspiratory pressure than normal rats. This finding supports the hypothesis that even in the absence of air–liquid interface, high interfacial tension remains in the surfactant (SF)-deficient perfluorocarbon (PFC)-filled lung. Perhaps exogenous SF administration, prior to LV, will produce better elastic pulmonary characteristics. □, Normal animals managed on total LV; ■, rats with ARF managed on LV (*Anova, $p < 0.05$ vs. normal LV group). Vertical bar represents the lavage process (BAL) in ARF group only

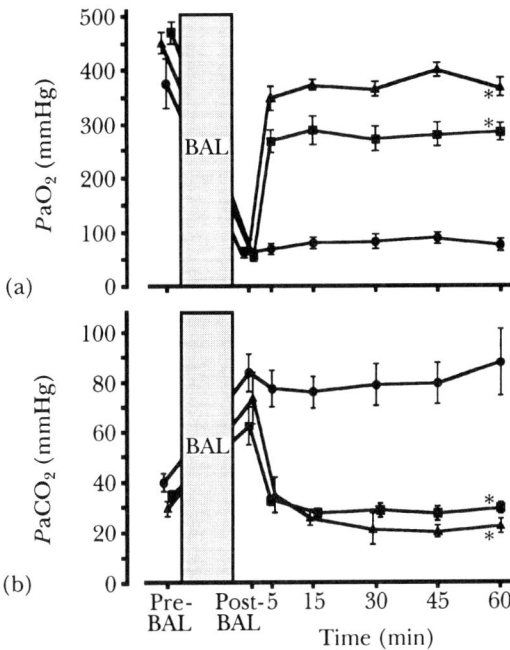

Figure 4 Pulmonary gas exchange in animals with acute respiratory failure (ARF) managed on gas ventilation, and total and partial liquid ventilation (LV). Differences between groups managed with any LV technique were not observed (means ± SE). ●, Gas-ventilated group; ■, total and ▲, partial LV groups (*Anova, $p < 0.05$ vs. gas-ventilated group). Vertical bar represents the lavage process (BAL) in all groups. After BAL, a sudden decrease of mean PaO_2 (a) was shown in all groups. However, those managed on total or partial LV demonstrated an increase in oxygenation. An increase in $PaCO_2$ (b) was observed in all groups. Only after total or partial LV started was a decrease of this parameter to baseline evident

lavage[19], pulmonary distribution of drugs[20], treatment of lung cancer, and its use as a surfactant-like substance[21,22].

INITIAL CLINICAL EXPERIENCES

In neonatal medicine, LV eventually might be proven to be clinically effective both in preterm infants with severe RDS failing surfactant therapy, and in full-term infants with severe pulmonary insufficiency caused by meconium aspiration, pulmonary hypertension or CDH.

Experience in patients with respiratory distress syndrome

In 1989, Greenspan and colleagues first reported the use of LV with a PFC in a human preterm infant[23]. Later, the same authors showed that LV was capable of briefly supporting gas exchange[24]. A short period of tidal LV with a PFC was used in three preterm infants with severe RDS, who failed conventional therapy. A brief period of 3–5 min of LV produced in all infants a marked increase in lung compliance, without deleterious effects on the cardiovascular system. All infants died, but oxygenation improved in two babies after the start of LV.

This original report, although anecdotal, clearly showed the feasibility, and the potential for clinical use of LV. It also greatly stimulated clinical research into the use of this therapeutic strategy in neonatal respiratory failure.

Later, the observational study[24] was expanded to include six critically ill preterm infants[25]. Those babies were included that were not candidates for other conventional therapies or where these had failed. All had unstable cardiovascular status, poor oxygenation and ventilation, and needed high ventilatory pressures. The PFC was given by a gravity-assisted technique. After 20–30 ml/kg of PFC were given, a few tidal volumes were also delivered before the infants were placed back in gas ventilation. All infants tolerated the procedures, experiencing a variable improvement of gas exchange, and a constant increase in lung compliance. Pressure–volume loops showed a decrease in peak tracheal pressure after PFC delivery. A transient improvement for up to 5 h was observed, and one infant survived. Chest X-ray showed a uniform lung distribution of the PFC, and presence of PFC in the pleura was not observed.

The uptake, distribution and elimination of PFC in infants have been studied[26]. Concentrations of PFC in blood, lung and other tissues, and expiratory gas samples showed that uptake and elimination are organ dependent. The PFC can cross the alveolar barrier in small quantities, be distributed in the body by the blood, and eliminated by evaporation through the lungs. The lungs had the highest mean concentration of PFC (9.33 ± 5.03 nl/g of tissue), but in the surviving infant, concentrations in the lung were greatly diminished[26].

The first pilot safety and efficacy study, performed in seven infants with severe RDS, also showed improvement in gas exchange[27]. The PFC used was perflubron (Liquivent®, Alliance Pharmaceutical Corp., San Diego, California), which has been approved by the US Food and Drug Administration (FDA) for clinical trials. The included babies (mean $\pm$ SD gestational age: 27.8 ± 1.3 weeks) had received two doses of exogenous surfactant at least, were less than 5 days of age, and thought to be at a high risk of dying. At enrollment, an FRC volume of PFC was given, and babies were placed back on mechanical ventilation with time-cycled pressure-limited machines. Two infants were managed with high frequency ventilation. Oxygenation index (45.1 ± 9.2 at baseline $vs.$ 11 ± 3.9 at 48 h), mean

airway pressure (16.4 ± 1.3 $vs.$ 12.4 ± 1 cmH$_2$0), $PaCO_2$ (71 ± 21 $vs.$ 46.8 ± 2.1 mmHg), and dynamic compliance (0.22 ± 0.05 $vs.$ 0.48 ± 0.19 ml/cmH$_2$0) all improved during partial LV[27]. Two patients survived (28.6%), and were in room air at 36 weeks' post-conceptional age. No adverse effects were seen.

The clinical and ventilatory course of a total of 13 cases similarly treated[27], were presented at the Society of Pediatric Research – American Pediatric Society (SPR-APS) meeting in San Diego last year (unpublished data). A 54% survival rate (7 of 13 babies) was reported.

A phase II, open label, FDA-approved clinical trial has started in several US units (J. Greenspan, principal investigator). A total of 50 infants with severe RDS will be included, and randomized to conventional management or partial LV, for a cumulative period of no more than 96 h. Primary assessment of clinical efficacy will be based on gas exchange and ventilatory data, and values for lung compliance.

Experience in term infant candidates for extracorporeal membrane oxygenation

The use of partial LV in conjunction with extracorporeal membrane oxygenation (ECMO) has also been reported[28,29]. Five term newborn infants, four children, and 10 adults were managed with partial LV to evaluate its effect on ECMO requirements. Four newborn babies had CDH, and one had pulmonary hypertension. Unfortunately, short-term effects (improvement of gas exchange), and complications (mucus plugs, and fluoro-thorax) for all patients occurred simultaneously. Of the 19 patients treated, 14 were weaned from ECMO, and 11 of these survived. An overall survival rate of 58% was reported. All survivors were said to be without evidence of pulmonary or systemic side-effects, 2–12 months after the therapy.

The chest X-ray appearance of an infant with CDH managed with partial LV, after 16 days on ECMO, has also been reported[30].

Another FDA-approved clinical trial (J. C. Jackson, principal investigator) is also recruiting term babies as candidates for ECMO. The primary outcome measures are need of ECMO, survival at discharge, and the incidence of BPD. A total of 72 infants are to be included in the trial who must meet the following entry criteria: gestational age ≥ 34 weeks; birth weight ≥ 2.0 kg; postnatal age < 30 days; failure of conventional ventilation ($FiO_2 \geq 0.8$, $f \geq 30$ breath/min, peak inspiratory and end-expiratory pressures of ≥ 30 and ≥ 4 cmH$_2$O, respectively); and an oxygenation index > 20.

CONCLUSIONS

In summary, partial LV with a PFC compound has already proceeded beyond the laboratory assessment period, and reached the status of an investigational clinical strategy in severe neonatal respiratory insufficiency. Early reports are encouraging, but it is hoped that there will be an intense and extended randomized evaluation, as for surfactant therapy, before the procedure is introduced in clinical practice. Its future role could be in the treatment of preterm infants with severe RDS unresponsive to other standard therapies, and in the treatment of term infants, who are possible candidates for ECMO.

ACKNOWLEDGEMENTS

The authors are grateful to Mr Ricardo Corres, laboratory technical assistant, for his technical assistance with the experimental procedures. These investigations were supported in part by grants 93/0151, 95/1332, and 95/1348 from the Fondo Investigaciones Sanitarias (FIS), Spanish Ministry of Health, and UPV 025.350-TA115/95 from the University of the Basque Country.

References

1. Modell, J. H., Gollan, F., Giammona, S. T. and Parker, D. (1970). Effect of fluorocarbon liquid on surface tension properties of pulmonary surfactant. *Chest*, **57**, 263–5
2. Clark, L. C. and Gollan F. (1966). Survival of mammals breathing organic liquids equilibrated with oxygen at atmospheric pressure. *Science*, **152**, 1755–6
3. Shaffer, T. H. and Moskowitz, G. D. (1974). Demand-controlled liquid ventilation of the lungs. *J. Appl. Physiol.*, **36**, 208–13
4. Matthews, W. H., Balzer, R. H., Shelburne, J. D., Pratt, P. C. and Kylstra, J. A. (1978). Steady-state gas exchange in normothermic, anesthetized, liquid-ventilated dogs. *Undersea Biomed. Res.*, **5**, 341–4
5. Shaffer, T. H., Rubenstein, D., Moskowitz, G. D. and Delivoria-Papadopoulos, M. (1976). Gaseous exchange and acid–base balance in premature lambs during liquid ventilation since birth. *Pediatr. Res.*, **10**, 227–31
6. Shaffer, T. H., Tran, N., Bhutani, B. K. and Sivieri, E. M. (1983). Cardiopulmonary function in very preterm lambs during liquid ventilation. *Pediatr. Res.*, **17**, 680–4
7. Wolfson, M. R., Greenspan, J. S., Deoras, K. S., Rubenstein, S. D. and Shaffer, T. H. (1992). Comparison of gas and liquid ventilation: clinical, physiological, and histological correlates. *J. Appl. Physiol.*, **72**, 1024–31
8. Valls-i-Soler, A., Wolfson, M. R., Kechner, N., Foust, R. and Shaffer, T. H. (1996). Comparison of natural surfactant and brief liquid ventilation rescue treatment in very immature lambs. Clinical and physiological correlates. *Biol. Neonate*, **69**, 275–83
9. Shaffer, T. H., Douglas, P. R., Lowe, C. A. and Bhutani, V. K. (1983). The effects of liquid ventilation on cardiopulmonary function in preterm lambs. *Pediatr. Res.*, **17**, 303–6
10. Valls-i-Soler, A., Alvarez, F. J., Gómez, M. A., López-Heredia, J., Gastiasoro, E., Arnaiz, A., Fernández, B. and Alfonso, L. F. (1995). Is surfactant (SF) needed in a perfluorocarbon filled lung? *Pediatr. Res.*, **37**, 354A
11. Koen, P. A., Wolfson, M. R. and Shaffer, T. H. (1988). Fluorocarbon ventilation: maximal expiratory flows and CO$_2$ elimination. *Pediatr. Res.*, **24**, 291–6
12. Fuhrman, B. P., Paczan, P. R. and DeFrancisis, M. (1991). Perfluorocarbon-associated gas exchange. *Crit. Care Med.*, **19**, 712–22
13. Foust, R., Tran, N., Greenspan, J. S., Miller, T., Cox, C., Wolfson, M. R. and Shaffer, T. H. (1995). Comparison of liquid assisted ventilation and exogenous surfactant therapy in the

management of acute meconium aspiration (MAS). *Pediatr. Res.*, **37**, 331A

14. Major, D., Cadenas, M., Cloutier, R., Fournier, L., Wolfson, M. R. and Shaffer, T. H. (1995). Combined gas ventilation and perfluorochemical tracheal instillation as an alternative treatment for lethal congenital diaphragmatic hernia in lambs. *J. Pediatr. Surg.*, **30**, 1178–82

15. Nesti, F. D., Fuhrman, B. P., Papo, M. C., Steinhorn, D. M., Hernan, L. J., Leach, C. L., Holm, B., Paczam, P. and Burak, B. (1993). Perfluorocarbon associated gas exchange (PAGE) in gastric aspiration. *Crit. Care Med.*, **21**, S157

16. Alvarez, F. J., Gómez, M. A., López-Heredia, J., Gastiasoro, E., Arnaiz, A., Alfonso, L. F. and Valls-i-Soler, A. (1995). Comparison of perfluorocarbon (PFC) tidal and partial liquid ventilation. *Pediatr. Res.*, **38**, 423

17. Tütüncü, A. S., Faithfull, N. S. and Lachmann, B. (1993). Comparison of ventilatory support with intratracheal perfluorocarbon administration and conventional mechanical ventilation in animals with acute respiratory failure. *Am. Rev. Respir. Dis.*, **148**, 785–92

18. Curtis, S. E., Peek, J. T. and Kelly, D. R. (1993). Partial liquid breathing with perflubron improves arterial oxygenation in acute canine lung injury. *J. Appl. Physiol.*, **75**, 2696–702

19. Calderwood, H. W., Modell, J. H., Ruiz, B. C., Brogden, J. E. and Hood, C. I. (1973). Pulmonary lavage with perfluorocarbon in a model of pulmonary edema. *Anesthesiology*, **38**, 141–4

20. Wolfson, M. R., Greenspan, J. S. and Shaffer, T. H. (1991). Pulmonary administration of vasoactive drugs (PAD) by perfluorocarbon liquid ventilation. *Pediatr. Res.*, **29**, 336A

21. Mercurio, M. R., Fiascone, J. M., Lima, D. M. and Jacobs, H. C. (1989). Surface tension and pulmonary compliance in premature rabbits. *J. Appl. Physiol.*, **66**, 2039–44

22. Gladstone, I. M., Ray, A. O., Salafia, A. M., Pérez-Fontán, J., Mercurio, M. R. and Jacobs, H. C. (1990). Effect of artificial surfactant on pulmonary function in preterm and full-term lambs. *J. Appl. Physiol.*, **69**, 465–72

23. Greenspan, J. S., Wolfson, M. R., Rubenstein, S. D. and Shaffer, T. H. (1989). Liquid ventilation of a preterm baby. *Lancet*, **1**, 1095

24. Greenspan, J. S., Wolfson, M. R., Rubenstein, S. D. and Shaffer, T. H. (1990). Liquid ventilation of human preterm neonates. *J. Pediatr.*, **117**, 106–11

25. Shaffer, T. H., Greenspan, J. S. and Wolfson, M. R. (1989). Liquid ventilation. In Boymton, B. R., Carlo, W. A. and Jobe, A. H. (eds.) *New Therapies for Neonatal Respiratory Failure. A Physiological Approach*, pp. 279–301 (Cambridge: Cambridge University Press)

26. Wolfson, M. R., Clark, L. C., Hoffman, R. E., Davies, S. L., Greenspan, J. S. and Shaffer, T. H. (1990). Liquid ventilation in neonates: uptake, distribution, and elimination of the liquid. *Pediatr. Res.*, **27**, 37A

27. Leach, C. L., Greenspan, J. S., Rubenstein, S. D., Shaffer, T. H., Wolfson, M. R., Jackson, J. C., deLemos, R. and Fuhrman, B. P. (1995). Partial liquid ventilation with Liquivent[®]: a pilot safety and efficacy study in premature newborns with severe respiratory distress syndrome (RDS). *Pediatr. Res.*, **37**, 220A

28. Hirschl, R. B., Pranikoff, T., Gauger, P., Schreiner, R. J., Dechert, R. and Bartlett, R. H. (1995). Liquid ventilation in adults, children, and full-tern neonates. *Lancet*, **346**, 1201–2

29. Hirschl, R. B., Parent, A., Tooley, R., McCracken, M., Johnston, K., Shaffer, T. H., Wolfson, M. R. and Bartlett, R. H. (1993). Liquid ventilation improves pulmonary function and gas exchange during extracorporeal life support. *FASEB J.*, **7**, A229

30. Gross, G. W., Greenspan, J. S., Fox, W. W., Rubenstein, S. D., Wolfson, M. R. and Shaffer, T. H. (1995). Use of liquid ventilation with perflubron during extracorporeal membrane oxygenation: chest radiographic appearance. *Radiology*, **194**, 717–20

The role of extracorporeal membrane oxygenation in the neonatal period

43

C. Davis

INTRODUCTION

Extracorporeal membrane oxygenation (ECMO) is a means of providing temporary life support for patients with potentially reversible respiratory or cardiac failure by the use of a modified cardiopulmonary bypass circuit. In the neonatal period, it is used for patients not responding to conventional treatment. Extracorporeal membrane oxygenation support facilitates healing and provides reliable oxygen delivery without some of the deleterious effects of conventional treatment.

The first neonate to be successfully supported by ECMO was in 1975[1]. Neonatal ECMO has been recognized as a standard treatment for mature infants in the United States since 1985. The Extracorporeal Life Support Organization (ELSO) maintains a worldwide Neonatal ECMO registry. All recognized ECMO centers in the UK are affiliated. Presently, almost 12 000 neonates are registered, with an overall survival of over 80% (Neonatal ECMO registry interim data January 1997). Most neonates supported by ECMO have underlying pulmonary hypertension from a variety of conditions (Table 1).

INDICATIONS FOR ECMO SUPPORT

Infants who receive ECMO support are those not responding to conventional management. The decision on when to introduce ECMO support is a difficult one as ECMO is an invasive technique and associated complications may cause severe consequences, especially hemorrhage. A number of criteria for instituting ECMO support have evolved (Table 2). The oxygenation index (OI) is the most widely used estimate of respiratory insufficiency. The formula is:

$$OI = \frac{P\text{aw} \times F\text{io}_2 \times 100}{P\text{ao}_2}$$

(*P*aw is mean airway pressure measured in cmH_2O; $P\text{ao}_2$ is postductal, measured in mmHg). In the early 1980s an OI > 40 for $\geq$ 3 h was associated with an 80% mortality[2].

Table 1 Extracorporeal Life Support Organization data on neonatal extracorporeal membrane oxygenation

Diagnosis	Patients (n)	Percentage of total	Survival (%)
MAS	4263	36	94
CDH	2451	20	59
Pneumonia/sepsis	1853	16	76
Primary pulmonary hypertension	1598	13	83
RDS	1166	10	82
Air leak syndrome	49	<< 1	69
Others	541	5	76

MAS, meconium aspiration syndrome; CDH, congenital diaphragmatic hernia; RDS = respiratory distress syndrome

Table 2 Neonatal extracorporeal membrane oxygenation (ECMO) selection criteria

Weight > 2000 g
34 weeks completed gestation
Not more than 10–14 days of high pressure ventilation
Unresponsive to maximal conventional management: OI > 40
No contraindication to ECMO support:
    evidence of congenital/acquired central nervous system abnormality
    irreversible cardiopulmonary disease
    period of asystole (outside postdelivery period)
No reason to question continuing conventional care:
    major congenital anomalies
    severe encephalopathy

PHYSIOLOGY OF EXTRACORPOREAL LIFE SUPPORT

Neonatal extracorporeal life support (ECLS) is achieved by gravity drainage of venous blood from the right atrium via a large cannula inserted through the internal jugular vein. The blood is pumped through the extracorporeal circuit with removal of carbon dioxide (CO_2) and addition of O_2 in the membrane lung, before returning the 'arterialized' blood via the carotid artery to the aortic arch (veno–arterial ECMO) or to the venous circulation (veno–venous ECMO). In veno–arterial ECMO the functions of both lungs and heart are partially or fully bypassed. Veno–venous ECMO returns the 'arterialized' blood to the right heart, allowing normal pulmonary blood flow, though a variable fraction of the returning extracorporeal blood will be 'recirculated' into the drainage cannula. Oxygen delivery is dependent on the extracorporeal flow rate and CO_2 clearance is dependent on the membrane lung capacity.

PATIENT MANAGEMENT ON ECMO

The infant is managed on an open bassinet. Cannulation is performed in the ECMO unit aided by high dose narcotics, muscle relaxation and local anesthetic infiltration. Because of anatomical considerations, the right side of the neck is the optimum site for cannulation in the neonate. A loading dose of heparin 50–100 U/kg is given. Large diameter catheters (8–14 F) are inserted into the vessels. Two separate cannulae are used in the case of veno–arterial ECMO, one via the internal jugular vein and one via the common carotid artery. A double-lumen cannula is inserted into the internal jugular vein for veno–venous ECMO with the 'arterial' return directed preferentially towards the tricuspid valve. The patient is connected to a preprimed extracorporeal circuit. Extracorporeal circulation is gradually increased to 100 ml kg^{-1} min^{-1} for veno–arterial ECMO and up to 120 ml kg^{-1} min^{-1} for veno–venous ECMO. Following institution of ECLS, the ventilator parameters are reduced to allow lung rest. There follows a variable period of time when the infant is dependent on ECMO because the native lungs lose gas exchange function. This is associated with a 'white-out' on chest radiograph. The reason for this is not fully understood but is associated with very low lung compliance[3].

Because of the extracorporeal element of blood flow, it is necessary to continue heparinization of the patient to prevent the blood clotting. Heparinization is carefully titrated to give an activated clotting time of 160–220 s depending on bleeding risk factors. Aprotinin, an antifibrinolytic agent, may be used in patients at high risk of bleeding.

As most infants are fluid overloaded at commencement of ECLS, fluid restriction with maximum calorie intake is the goal. Patients on ECLS support require less sodium and more potassium than normal. Because of ongoing platelet loss in the circuit, intermittent platelet transfusions are necessary to maintain a platelet count $\geq 100\,000 \times 10^{-9}$ l^{-1}.

Hemoglobin concentration is kept at 14–16 g dl^{-1} (hematocrit 40–50) to ensure adequate oxygen delivery to the tissues.

Cardiopulmonary support allows chest physiotherapy to be performed without the risk of patient hypoxia and cardiovascular destabilization that characterizes so many infants with pulmonary hypertension. This is an important aspect of management. As native lung function improves, lung compliance increases, gas exchange returns to normal and extracorporeal bypass can be gradually reduced. Once the lungs are shown to be capable of functioning without the need for extracorporeal life support, decannulation is undertaken. Most neonate patients are fit for extubation within 24 h of decannulation.

UK collaborative neonatal ECMO trial

Controversy surrounded the introduction of neonatal ECMO to the UK because of the view that there was less need for neonatal ECMO than in North America[4] and the lack of a formal prospective randomized trial[5,6]. A collaborative trial was undertaken to assess whether a policy of referral for ECMO had a beneficial effect on survival without severe disability when assessed at 1 year of age. During the period of the trial, those clinicians providing an ECMO service agreed to limit neonatal ECMO for eligible candidates to those entered in the trial. Candidates were eligible for trial entry when parameters of severity of lung disease (OI ≥ 40 or $PaCO_2$ ≥ 12 kPa) were met, providing there were no contraindications. The interim trial results have been published[7]. Data were analyzed on an intention to treat basis. Patients randomized to ECMO (84% actually received ECMO support) had an overall mortality of 32%. Those randomized to conventional care had an overall mortality of 59%. An OI ≥ 60 was associated with a worse prognosis in both treatment groups, though the rate was lower in the ECMO arm for both strata. The effects of an ECMO policy on known deaths is shown in Figure 1.

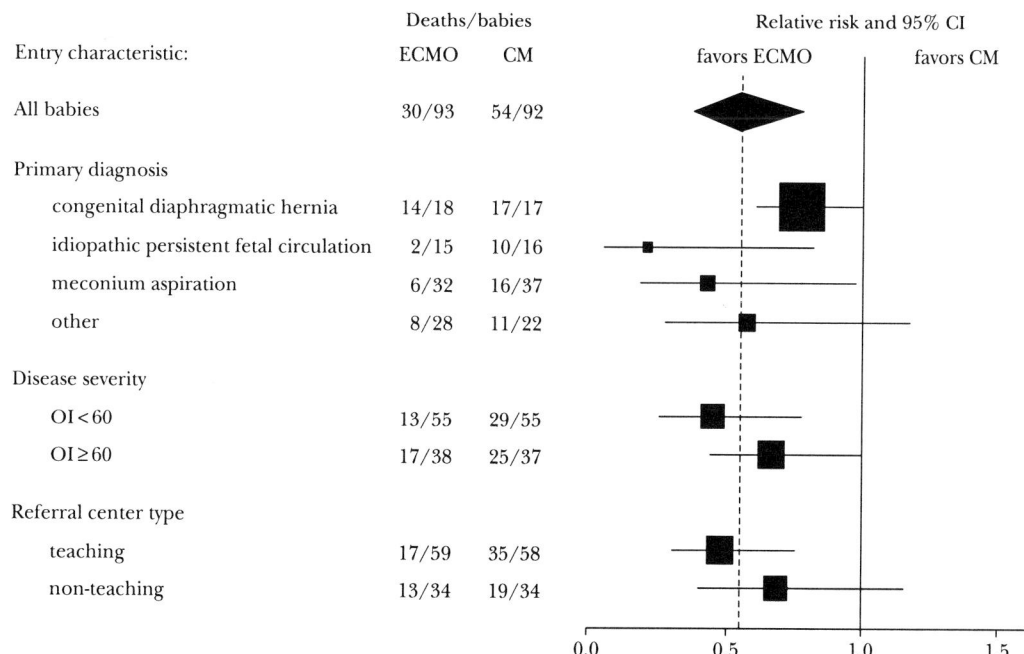

Entry characteristic:	Deaths/babies		Relative risk and 95% CI	
	ECMO	CM	favors ECMO	favors CM
All babies	30/93	54/92		
Primary diagnosis				
congenital diaphragmatic hernia	14/18	17/17		
idiopathic persistent fetal circulation	2/15	10/16		
meconium aspiration	6/32	16/37		
other	8/28	11/22		
Disease severity				
OI < 60	13/55	29/55		
OI ≥ 60	17/38	25/37		
Referral center type				
teaching	17/59	35/58		
non-teaching	13/34	19/34		

Figure 1 Effects of an extracorporeal membrane oxygenation (ECMO) policy on known deaths. CM, conventional management

Follow-up

Interim neurodevelopmental follow-up data form the UK collaborative neonatal ECMO trial comparing ECMO vs. conventional management, have shown no statistical difference in the incidence of severe impairment and disability (2% vs. 2%) or impairment not classed as severe (16% vs. 10%) in survivors at 1 year[7]. These ECMO data are comparable with other long-term studies[8]. The completed 1-year neurodevelopmental analysis is awaited. This will be the first formal comparison of conventional management and ECMO support. It is hoped to re-evaluate these cohorts during early school years for more subtle abnormalities, especially cognitive defects.

THE FUTURE

As veno–venous ECMO becomes more frequently utilized and as circuit anticoagulation problems are solved, it may be appropriate to consider ECMO in lower risk infants than at present. It may also be appropriate to consider infants weighing less than the present 2000 g limit[9].

The role of ECMO in an era of new treatment modalities, such as inhaled nitric oxide, high frequency ventilation and liquid ventilation, is an evolving one. The efficacy of neonatal ECMO has been verified and it may be useful as a safety net for the future randomized studies of these newer modalities.

One important concern associated with the widespread use of newer treatment modalities is the potential risk of delayed referral for ECMO and the associated increased morbidity and mortality attributable to transportation of these critically ill infants[10]. Criteria for early referral require definition in this changing scene.

References

1. Bartlett, R. H., Gazzaniga, A. B., Jefferies, M. R. et al. (1976). Extracorporeal membrane oxygenation cardiopulmonary support in infancy. Trans. Am. Soc. Artif. Intern. Organs, 22, 80–90
2. Beck, R., Anderson, K. D., Pearson, G. D. et al. (1986). Criteria for extracorporeal membrane oxygenation in a population of infants with persistent pulmonary hypertension of the newborn. J. Pediatr. Surg., 21, 297–302
3. Lotze, A., Short, B. L. and Taylor, G. A. (1987). Lung compliance as a measure of lung function in newborns with respiratory failure requiring extracorporeal membrane oxygenation. Crit. Care. Med., 15, 226–9
4. Editorial (1988). Persistent fetal circulation and extracorporeal membrane oxygenation. Lancet, ii, 1289–91
5. Bartlett, R. H., Roloff, D. W., Cornell, R. G. et al. (1985). Extracorporeal circulation in neonatal respiratory failure: a prospective randomized study. Pediatrics, 76, 479–87
6. O'Rourke, P. P., Crone, R. K., Vacanti, J. P. et al. (1989). Extracorporeal membrane oxygenation and conventional medical therapy in neonates with persistent pulmonary hypertension of the newborn: a prospective randomized study. Pediatrics, 84, 957–63
7. UK Collaborative ECMO Trial Group (1996). UK collaborative randomised trial of neonatal extracorporeal membrane oxygenation. Lancet, 348, 75–82
8. Glass, P., Miller, M. and Short, B. L. (1989). Morbidity in ECMO survivors: neurodevelopmental outcome at one year of age. Pediatrics, 83, 72–8
9. Hirschl, R. B., Schumacher, R. E., Snedecor, S. N. et al. (1993). The efficacy of extracorporeal life support in premature and low birth weight newborns. J. Pediatr. Surg., 28, 1336–41
10. Boedy, R. F., Howell, C. J., Kanto and W. P. Jr (1990). Hidden mortality associated with extracorporeal membrane oxygenation. J. Pediatr., 117, 462–4

Perinatal audit: report of the European Association of Perinatal Medicine Working Party, Florence, November 1993

44

P. M. Dunn

BACKGROUND

In 1990 the XII European Congress of Perinatal Medicine was held in Lyon. On that occasion the General Assembly drew attention to the lack of a standard approach across Europe in the way perinatal data were collected, analyzed and reported, and asked me if I would convene a Working Party to study the problem. As I had been involved in perinatal audit since the 1950s and had worked on this subject for both the World Health Organization (WHO) and the International Federation of Gynecology and Obstetrics (FIGO) for more than 20 years, I agreed to do so.

My first aim was to identify key workers in the field of perinatal audit from both obstetrics and pediatrics as well as epidemiology, statistics and public health from each European country. From this list I planned to select a representative and balanced Working Party that would meet and prepare a draft report. The next step would have been to have a European conference of all those interested to discuss this report, which after appropriate modification would then be published.

Although I made progress in identifying key potential collaborators in the field, the rest of my plan stalled due to lack of funding. In 1992 I reported the lack of progress to the General Assembly when it met in Amsterdam for the XIII Congress. I wanted to withdraw from the project, but Secretary/Treasurer Gian Carlo Di Renzo persuaded me to try again, and shortly afterwards he came up with the idea of hitching our proposed workshop to an International Conference on 'Improving the Standard of Perinatal Care' to be held in Florence in November, 1993. This Conference was organized by Professor Gian Paolo Donzelli of the Department of Pediatrics, University of Florence, with funding from an Italian company, Frater SpA, Pescara. We remain very grateful to Professor Donzelli for being such a splendid host to our Working Party which met for 4 days prior to the Conference.

EUROPEAN ASSOCIATION OF PERINATAL MEDICINE WORKING PARTY

The Working Party consisted of 14 people from nine countries, all distinguished for their interest in and contributions to perinatal audit. Obstetrics was represented by Gian Carlo Di Renzo (Italy), Bo Lindberg (Sweden), Michael Maresh (UK) and Zdenek Stembera (Czech Republic); pediatrics was represented by Lya den Ouden (The Netherlands), Umberto de Vonderweid and Gian Paolo Donzelli (Italy) and myself; epidemiology was represented by Leiv Bakketeig (Norway), Gerard Breart (France), Simone Buitendijk (The Netherlands) and both Ann Johnson and Alison Macfarlane from the National Perinatal Epidemiology Unit in Oxford (UK); public health was represented by Gillian McIlwaine (UK) and finally André

L'Hours represented the World Health Organization.

Prior to our meeting three working papers had been circulated: the first was on the perinatal audit of maternal, fetal and neonatal mortality by Gillian McIlwaine and myself, and then two papers on maternal and perinatal morbidity, respectively, by Ann Johnson and Michael Maresh. The Working Party rapidly agreed that our report should concentrate on trying to standardize the methodology of auditing perinatal outcome in terms of maternal, fetal and infant mortality and morbidity, and that whenever possible we should continue to use the nomenclature, definitions and classification already established by WHO[1,2] and FIGO[3]. We recognized, of course, that our efforts were only the beginning of a long journey towards achieving uniformity across Europe in all the many aspects of perinatal audit, and that our recommendations would undoubtedly be modified, extended and improved with the passage of time.

By the time we left Florence we had agreed a wide range of recommendations, but a great deal of work remained in order to weld them into a cohesive report. It was agreed that this should be undertaken by the UK members of the Working Party both for linguistic reasons and because they could continue to meet at small expense. At this point I want to express once more my gratitude to Gillian McIlwaine, Ann Johnson, Alison Macfarlane and Michael Maresh for taking on the daunting task of 'rapporteur'. In addition, André L'Hours was most helpful in checking the manuscript for errors, and in particular the coding.

Early in 1994 we received generous support from Milupa AG., Germany, to further the aims of the Working Party. We are immensely grateful to Professor Rudiger Ghraf and Dr Dagmar Lehwalder for this help which could not have come at a better time. The first draft of our report had been circulated to members of the Working Party and this funding enabled us to meet again, this time in Helsinki in June, 1994, during the XIV European Congress of Perinatal Medicine.

A second draft was completed, circulated internally and amended during the year that followed, and in 1995 the penultimate draft was sent to a number of distinguished clinicians throughout Europe with a request for their comments. They were: Simone Alexaniants of Armenia, Manuel Carrapato of Portugal, Forrester Cockburn of Scotland, Joachim Dudenhausen of Germany, Wolfgang Kunzel also of Germany and Karel Marsal of Sweden. The Working Party is most grateful to these referees for their comments.

Armed with our referees' warm approval and support we then sought publication. Without funding, this also presented a problem. It was eventually solved by the Editors of a new journal, *Prenatal and Neonatal Medicine*, Gian Carlo Di Renzo and Forrester Cockburn. They agreed to include it in the second issue[4] and circulate it to members of the European Association of Perinatal Medicine (EAPM). Our report has also been published as a separate booklet by Parthenon Publishing[5], and, thanks to funding by Milupa UK (Ms Niamh Rice, Scientific Division), we are able to distribute a limited number of copies throughout Europe.

Some time has been spent discussing why our report took 6 years to materialize. It may be that our experience will help others in the future. The key to achievement is undoubtedly having adequate initial funding, and we urge the EAPM to explore ways of making this possible.

To return to the report, our aim has not been to provide a comprehensive list of items to be audited, but rather to describe how perinatal audit might best be approached, while at the same time giving a few examples of how this might be done.

Professor Gerard Breart of INSERM will now take over the baton from me and will discuss what our Working Party tried to achieve. Few people could be better placed to do so. As a very distinguished epidemiologist he has been involved in the evaluation of perinatal care at the national, regional and institutional levels in France for very many years.

References

1. World Health Organization (1992, 1993). *International Statistical Classification of Diseases and Related Health Problems*, 10th revision, Vol. 1, Vol. 2. (Geneva: World Health Organization)
2. World Health Organization (1980). *International Classification of Impairments, Disabilities and Handicaps.* (Geneva: World Health Organization)
3. International Federation of Gynecology and Obstetrics (1982). *Report of the FIGO Committee on Perinatal Mortality and Morbidity on Monitoring and Reporting Perinatal Mortality and Morbidity.* (London: FIGO)
4. European Association of Perinatal Medicine (1996). Perinatal audit. Report of a Working Party, Florence, November 4–7th, 1993. *Prenat. Neonat. Med.*, **1**, 160–94
5. European Association of Perinatal Medicine (1996). *Perinatal Audit. Report of a Working Party, Florence, November 4–7th, 1993.* (Carnforth, UK: Parthenon Publishing)

Ethics and the neonatal nurse

45

H. E. McHaffie

INTRODUCTION

Over the past two decades the face of neonatology has changed almost out of recognition, but of course just improving our statistics on saving the lives of ever smaller, sicker babies is not the full story. What are we saving them for? What quality of life do they have thereafter? And what quality of life do their families have? Have we gone beyond what is compassionate? It is this ethical dilemma that I want to concentrate on in this paper.

A huge literature exists on the subject of non-treatment of infants. Much of it is anecdotal, or the wisdom of clinical experts, or based on large-scale questionnaire studies. We found there was a dearth of knowledge about what people intimately involved in these matters thought and how they practiced – not just the consultants, but all the other grades of doctors and neonatal nurses as well. So our study took a very different approach and this paper is based on data obtained from a 2-year enquiry completed recently[1]. Approximately 2 weeks were spent in each of six of the largest neonatal units (NICUs) throughout Scotland – four in University-based Hospitals and two in District General Hospitals. After a preliminary period building up trust and confidence, I carried out in-depth interviews with a stratified sample of doctors and nurses so that each grade was represented. As well as talking informally to many staff, I formally interviewed 57 doctors and 119 nurses.

Our sample consisted of 21 consultants, 23 registrars, 13 SHOs, six senior sisters/managers, 33 sisters and 80 staff midwives/nurses. We believe they are representative of staff working in NICUs in this country.

This paper concerns neonatal nurses and is therefore presenting only a small part of a much bigger study – just some of the preceptions of the neonatal nurses themselves. Inevitably this will result in an unbalanced picture and I want to emphasize that I am very much in sympathy with the consultants too. I was enormously impressed by their commitment and caring. However, I am using these findings of less than optimal practice in order to suggest ways to minimize unnecessary tension or conflict. The dilemmas for the neonatal nurse in the NICU are different from those facing the neonatologist.

BACKGROUND

Just to set a context, I want to make five general points.

Different categories of babies present dilemmas

Three main groups of infants present ethical dilemmas relating to withdrawal of treatment:

(1) The congenitally abnormal;

(2) The very premature;

(3) Those whose prognosis is poor but who are no longer dependent on medical intervention.

Some of the issues are common to all groups; some are peculiar to that situation.

However, it is important to note that when it comes to decision-making, staff perceive a difference between babies who are dying anyway and those who are not actually dying but their future looks bleak. In the second group, the decision about whether or not to treat hinges on quality of life. And when it comes to quality of life judgements, it is clear that individuals draw their lines at different points along the continuum from conditions which are incompatible with life (e.g. anencephaly or no intestine) to conditions where there is every prospect of a reasonably good quality of life (e.g. uncomplicated Down's syndrome). So the babies who might live but with major problems present more questions than those who will not live whatever we do for them.

Practice varies

Readiness to withdraw or withhold treatment varies considerably between units and between individuals. In general there is widespread agreement that withdrawing and withholding treatment in some circumstances is good medical practice.

Nevertheless, sometimes fear of repercussions compels people to pursue an aggressive course in an effort to minimize the risk of court action. Sometimes doctors are satisfied with nothing less than hard measurable data to show beyond doubt that treatment is medically futile. Then treatment may be withdrawn but by that time the baby is only hours from death anyway. The result of such compulsions is that overly burdensome treatment is sometimes inflicted on babies.

However, other clinicians operate quite differently. Where they feel the burdens far outweigh the benefits of treatment and there is no prospect of a reasonable quality of life, they are prepared to withdraw treatment much sooner. And there are those who are prepared to go further and take steps to hasten the death.

In between, all shades of opinion are represented.

Decision-making is complicated

I do not want to diminish the difficulty of making decisions about whether treatment is the best option for certain babies. We all recognize that the whole area is littered with uncertainties. Making prognoses for these neonates is an inexact science and babies have an uncom-

fortable knack of defying the very best predictions.

Opinions change over time and with experience

Seeing the outcome of what goes on in our NICUs can be sobering – babies we all thought were 'no-hopers' trotting off happily to normal school; babies who we persuaded the parents stood a good chance of intact survival, becoming a life-long dependent 'burden'.

One interesting finding to emerge from our study related to the influence of professional experience on staff's inclination to treat babies. We found that while doctors were fairly evenly divided, proportionately far more nurses became less keen to treat after working with babies in an NICU for a time (Figure 1).

Roles and responsibilities differ

The roles and responsibilities of the two disciplines are very different. Nurses are involved for long periods at the cotside and build up close relationships with the family. Doctors' involvement tends to be more spasmodic, and less intimate.

In general, doctors have more to lose when treatment fails or babies die. They generally

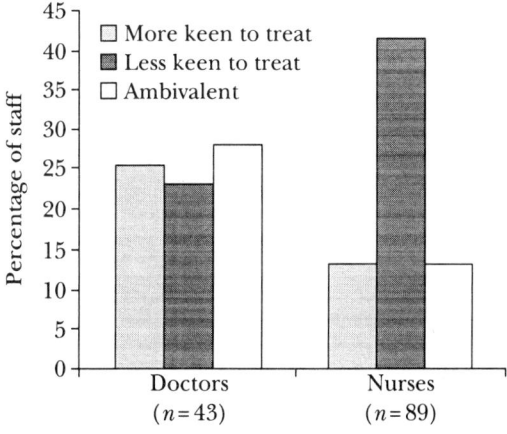

Figure 1 The effect of experience in a neonatal unit on inclination to treat

feels a strong compulsion to try to save lives, and find it hard to abandon efforts once they have started. Nurses, on the other hand, place greater emphasis on caring rather than curing. These tragic cases offer special opportunities for them to comfort and support families.

THE ISSUES

Regarding the neonatal nurses, there are five main issues which emerged from our enquiry.

Involvement in the discussion around withdrawal of treatment

In all except one of the study units, there were nurses who felt that nursing staff were insufficiently involved in the discussion and decision-making. They reported that some consultants made no effort at all to find out what they felt. Others went through the motions of asking but did not really listen to the answer – by the consultants' own admission as well as in the nurses' perceptions. Relatively few were seen to really take account of what the nurses caring for the baby thought was appropriate.

The nurses pointed out that if they are excluded, not only are they personally frustrated but the quality of their own care-giving suffers. It becomes difficult to reinforce and reinterpret medical messages, and difficult to tailor care sensitivity to parents' needs and wishes.

Consultants, however, are aware of the potential for conflict if more people are involved. Some told us about practical measures they adopted to avoid potential conflict, e.g. they made it known that such critical decisions were the responsibility of the consultant alone; or they limited other involvement to those colleagues whose opinions they knew and trusted. But nurses who were not so included resented this way of operating. Although they most definitely did not want the responsibility of the final decision, they felt that if they were trusted to care for the baby they should be involved in the discussion around his welfare. They believed that they had unique insights into the family dynamics and feelings, and could contribute a useful perspective.

There were other consultants, however, who made such decisions a matter entirely open to scrutiny and debate. They tended to work on the basis of achieving a consensus. The nurses mostly welcomed this approach although there were still misgivings reported about the relative weight of opinions offered. How much value *should* be attached to intuitive responses or to individual perceptions of parents' tolerances?

Implementation of the decision

Almost invariably it falls to the neonatal nurses to manage the case after a decision is made. But very few doctors appeared to recognize the dilemmas nurses face when they are dealing with someone else's decision.

The nurses in our study felt strongly that every effort should be made to ensure as good a dying as could be achieved. Indeed they went to great lengths to try to orchestrate things in tune with parental wishes. Sometimes they took on a deep personal commitment: staying on after their shift to cuddle a dying baby, or providing ongoing support for parents for a long time after the death.

However, their best endeavors can be thwarted by other people. Occasionally they feel the wrong decision has been made. More frequently they feel things are not timed appropriately. And very often they feel that communication has been less optimal and it falls to them to take on the remedial work.

In some units, the consultants do not agree amongst themselves and there are then real tensions for the team. It is very disturbing to be told in the morning that a baby is not for resuscitation if he collapses, and that same evening asked to escort the baby to a hospital miles away for 'experimental' surgery. How does the nurse explain that to the parents?

On top of all these team problems, there are some situations where the circumstances of the case pose particularly painful dilemmas. Take, for example, the severely birth-asphyxiated infant, so severely damaged that she does not have a sucking reflex. The practice in some units is to pass a nasogastric tube and wait for an infection or a sudden collapse to open a window of opportunity for non-treatment. Elsewhere the practice is to go through the motions of offering her a bottle. She does not suck but that is seen as concrete evidence that she lacks the wherewithal for basic survival. Either way the practical consequences are distressing for staff – especially the 'starving to death'. Nurses in our study became extremely upset remembering these cases even years after the event.

So even where they agree in principle that death is a preferable option for a given baby, the practical implications arising from the decision can cause real problems for the nurses who implement it. Ordering such a course of action is a very different matter from actually caring for

the infant while she dies slowly and miserably, but both carry a heavy burden. The law in this country precludes intervention actively to end her life, and medicine currently offers no acceptable alternative. So the decision is about choosing the least unacceptable option.

Timing of events

It is rare for nurses to disagree with the final decision to withdraw treatment; but the timing of events represents one of the single largest and most often cited problems for everyone as Figure 2 illustrates.

If the decision to withdraw is only ever made when a baby is inches from death, then staff are concerned about the protraction of suffering – for the baby and the parents. If the decision is

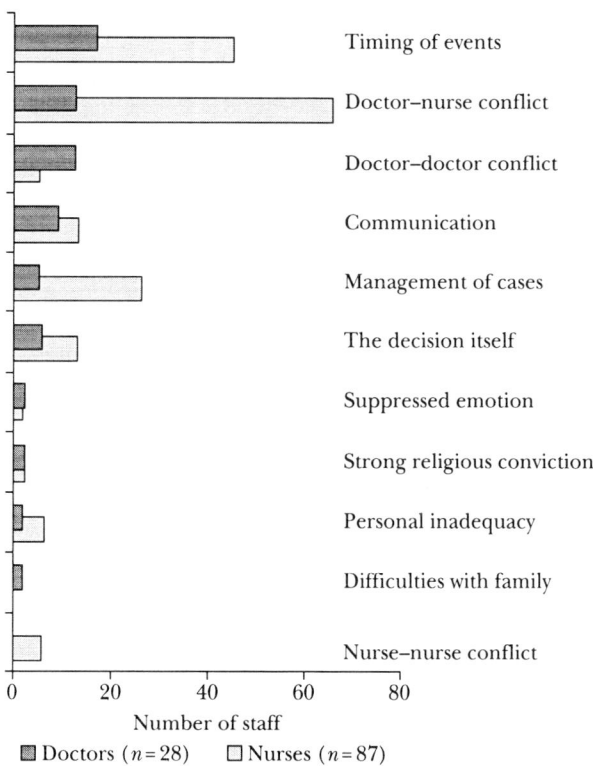

Figure 2 Sources of tension identified by doctors and nurses

267

made sooner, then concerns relate to the reasons for the withdrawal, the uncertainties of prognosis, and the means by which death is facilitated.

Overall nurses and junior doctors think consultants are too slow in deciding to stop treating. They get frustrated by procrastination and apparent indecisiveness. The consultants, on the other hand, think that nurses are too hasty and that they do not fully understand all the factors which have to be considered. It is interesting to find that each group thinks that they are in a strong position to know what best meets the parents' needs. But their perceptions of when parents are ready for this step differ greatly.

Communication

Communication is a thorny issue in so many areas of practice. When it comes to these delicate negotiations it becomes even more critically important.

With colleagues

As we have seen, nurses are sometimes left out of communications. But even where the practice is in principle to include them, they are sometimes left in the dark inadvertently. Doctors frequently discuss cases informally in the corridor, or over coffee. Someone suggests, 'Such-and-such might be worth a try', and the treatment changes direction again, but the message does not always filter down to the nurse actually caring for the baby. The change of plan appears to her to be a further example of medical inconsistency or indecision. In reality it might be a perfectly proper and wise delay but that is not how it is perceived by those at the sharp end.

Good communication within the team is essential if everyone is to work together and provide a consistent and clear picture for parents. Consultants may well hold different views about legal limits, or about where a life becomes intolerable, or when the administration of a large dose of opiates becomes euthanasia. But these differences should be settled away from the cotside, and other team members should not become pawns in battles of power. Communication with the junior doctors, the nurses and the parents needs to be careful and consistent. Where deviations from an agreed plan are necessary, knowing the reasons for the change can minimize misunderstanding and resentment, and improve overall care.

With parents

Nurses perceive medical communication with parents to be less than adequate. In all units they reported that they themselves repeatedly acted as interpreters in order to make information accessible to the parents, but few doctors acknowledged this problem.

Expert communicators do, however, exist and they are highly valued. Where the consultant informs the team wisely, shares his thinking with colleagues, but also listens attentively to their views and paces his communication sensitively, colleagues in their turn are more inclined to offer insights into family concerns and to share their personal reservations. The team then become mutually interactive and supportive. A more comprehensive picture of the family is built up and their needs can be met more effectively.

Documentation

Some doctors admitted they were lax about documentation. In addition, a small number said they were guarded in what they committed to paper. But whilst such a practice might protect the consultant, it could confuse the junior doctors and nurses. Other teams, however, operated in an open and comprehensive way, documenting discussions and decisions unambiguously. In these units staff believed such openness helped everyone to work harmoniously and with the minimum of tension.

THE WAY FORWARD?

These findings are only a small part of the whole picture we uncovered. But what can we conclude from them?

Team approach

If the best decision is to be made and the family managed in the most sensitive way possible there needs to be a team approach to both the decision-making and the management of the dying. To effect this both doctors and nurses should be actively involved in the discussions around these critical decisions. It requires mutual respect for each other's contribution if the complementary skills of each discipline are to be capitalized on. It also requires junior doctors and nurses to be more ready and able to justify their position and articulate their views clearly to others.

Sensitivity

Nurses accept that the consultant is the team leader. They do not envy him the task of deciding whether a baby lives or dies, but with the role of team leader, they believe, come special responsibilities:

(1) To be actively involved in the ongoing case;

(2) To communicate effectively with the staff and with the parents;

(3) To be consistent or to explain perceived inconsistencies;

(4) To listen sensitively to team members' beliefs and opinions;

(5) To pace events sensitively.

Insight and respect for others

It is not only the consultant who bears responsibility for good team effort. There is a need for each team member to gain insight into his or her own opinions, values and beliefs, to understand why he or she thinks and behaves in a certain way. Each individual must respect the views of colleagues and parents and treat those who hold opposing views with courtesy and kindness.

These are agonizing decisions and caring for the families is a stressful process. The doctors and nurses involved need support, not criticism, and these comments are offered in that spirit. We can and do all draw our lines at different places along the continuum from death to life but if we are to provide a consistent and harmonious service for families caught up in one of life's most profoundly sad experiences, we need to work together not in opposition, the skills of each discipline complementing those of the other.

ACKNOWLEDGEMENTS

We are greatly indebted to the doctors and nurses who contributed so generously to the reported study, sharing their pain and their doubts as well as their experiences. The research was funded by the Scottish Office Home and Health Department.

Reference

1. McHaffie, H. E. and Fowlie, P. W. (1996). *Life, death and decisions: Doctors and Nurses Reflect on Neonatal Practice*. (Hale: Hochland and Hochland)

Ethics and the perinatologist

46

J.-P. Relier

INTRODUCTION

Ethics in perinatology do not only concern questions treated by an ethical committee in life-threatening situations. Ethics include all the questions raised by one human being, the distressed fetus or neonate to another human being, the neonatologist, together with his team, so as to judge the optimal survival conditions for him/her and his/her surroundings, including parents, family and society. Actually, the main aspect which should be considered is the respect of this human being in its entire 'individuality', including different parts of its physical body (physical, mental and emotional) which have been barely fused during the fetal period and are at higher risk due to the fetal or perinatal distress. In this condition, the fundamental principle of ethics in perinatology is to do all that is possible to encourage the progress of this being, newly become a human being. The difficulty lies in the fact that each human being, even the fetus and newborn, has capacities and above all needs that are impossible to assess accurately and completely. Western civilization has tried to simplify the problem by making fetal and newborn individuals into complete citizens, with the rights and obligations of an often too narrow-minded, materialistic society, but a human being, even a fetus or newborn, is not just a citizen of a city, country or even the world. A human being is part of the evolution of the universe (or cosmos) and his particular life on earth is only a stage in this universal evolution. When one speaks of life starting at conception, one should think only of life of the physical body which progressively incorporates its soul or consciousness, at which time every capability will have been developed as regards his perception as well as his expression, resulting in the complete development of the brain and personality.

Recent important data in fetal behavior and fetal capabilities have demonstrated very well the very early onset of fetal perception and its importance in brain development, maturation and organization.

It is not the aim of this chapter to put forward philosophical views about human beings, but it should be accepted that the physical body, with its other psychological and mental capabilities, is the foundation of consciousness during this particular life. It should be accepted that after the death of this physical support, life does not end. Life is eternal, before conception and after death. Death is only one aspect of life, one step in this universal evolution.

According to this view, the distressed neonate can be considered as being at a cross-roads, since immediately after the almost complete fusion of the different parts of a being (physical, mental, emotional), any severe physical distress leads to a rapid separation of these parts, with the liberation of the consciousness. Dilemmas in perinatal care are situations in which what is best for this consciousness in its universal evolution will be discussed and not just what is best for this human being in this particular life. It is probable that the needs of this fetus or very tiny premature infant who has accepted to grow and live, are much more extensive than adults could imagine with their narrow-minded intelligence. It seems important to accept that every fetus, premature or newborn infant is an individual. Every human being in development has his/her specific heritage, memory and understanding that influence each step of this early development and for which we have the responsibility when, due to his/her illness, he or she comes into our care. This means that every fetus and newborn has a specific demand, depending on many items and circumstances, including family history, past events, evolution of pregnancy and sociocultural economic conditions, all events which cannot be judged and estimated by a theoretical ethical committee *complying with established rules.*

I have no time in this short chapter to consider in detail all the inconveniences of such a theoretical committee. The main criticism to this attitude, mainly in US committees, is that it considers the child as the parents' property.

Even the mother is not free to 'dispose' of her child as she wishes. The child ought to be considered as an individual with its own body and its own soul. As a result of its illness, the child is received into the care of a team of neonatal doctors, who have grater means of judgement, resulting from experience and access to persons who can be consulted for additional information.

Moreover, the perinatal team (medical and paramedical staff) is capable of assessing more accurately the progress of the illness because of continuous surveillance of the fetus or newborn and its parents through continual communication with them, and above all the personality of the child through a continued affective psycho-sensorial contact. It is therefore the perinatal care team that is best able to make the decisions that should be taken.

In ethical committees it is usual, at least in the USA, to obtain the consent of the parents either to continue or to discontinue resuscitation procedures. Such an approach seems to us to be completely inhuman. It is unthinkable that the parents can possibly take into account all the factors required by a decision to stop resuscitation, i.e. medical knowledge, the ability to reason without emotional stress and freedom of choice. In addition, it does not seem possible that the parents should have to bear for the rest of their lives the burden of having made the decision 'to kill their child'. Similarly, it is sometimes impossible to accept the request of parents to continue with resuscitative care when it is clear that the prognosis is hopeless.

This is the reason why it is much more important to approach these neonatal dilemmas in a climate of confidence and understanding rather than to try to deal with these ethical problems with the coldness and severity of an approach centered on constitutional and legal aspects.

The ideal situation would thus be to know exactly the elements of this specificity. Modern science, despite all its progress, does not permit this as yet. It is therefore necessary to limit ourselves to the means that we have available. Schematically two groups of factors are needed for the decision: the physical condition and that of the environment. If one considers all the factors which play a part in the decision-making process, one realizes that there cannot be a standardized decision made by an administrative ethical committee. Each fetus and each newborn should be the subject of a reflection, of a repeated and extensive discussion leading to a decision that is often initially partial, transitory, modifiable and modified. Three schematic types of situations of increasing difficulty will be considered.

SITUATIONS INVOLVING EASILY MADE DECISIONS

This is the case in irreversible cerebral damage in the neonate at term or above all in the premature infant with vital distress. It is not possible here to describe each of these conditions, which depends above all on the gestational age of the infant. It is sufficient just to remind ourselves that an experience of more than 30 years of neonatal intensive care, with long-term follow-up, has allowed us to assess as accurately as possible the seriousness of a given situation with the aid of the clinical, biological, electro-encephalographic and echographic data. When there is agreement between the different specialists, the unanimity of those in charge does not cause difficulties. It is occasionally necessary to wait for a confirmation diagnosis of one of the specialists. This decision is taken irrespective of the family environment given the irremediable seriousness of the case. The decision to interrupt resuscitation simply results in the sparing of a period of unnecessary suffering for a being that is in any case condemned.

SITUATIONS INVOLVING INTERMEDIATE DECISIONS

This applies to all cases of vital distress where cerebral function is not in jeopardy, i.e. all neonates with a normal brain following clinical, electroencephalographic and echographic investigation. In this group are neonates whose vital prognosis is threatened by irreversible organ damage, for example pulmonary (severe hypoplasia, total refractory hypoxia, fulminant subacute bronchopulmonary dysplasia) or gastrointestinal (severe enterocolitis with resection of the colon and ileum incompatible with enteral feeding).

For many years, cerebral integrity prevented all debate on cessation of resuscitation. At present, there is further discussion taking place. The decision is of course made taking into account all the medical facts but also, and above all, family factors: past history and family surroundings, all factors with a fundamental importance if a return home is hoped for, even after a long passage of time. It is evidently impossible to describe all these situations in detail. Each neonate is a new problem and referring to comparable situations in the past is only by way of example. We have never been able to deal with strictly identical cases.

SITUATIONS INVOLVING DIFFICULT DECISIONS

This is essentially the case with very premature babies and neonates of very low birth weight, with limits that increase over the years. Thus, in 1967, the date of the establishment of the center at Port-Royal, 78% of neonates weighing less than 1200 g died during their stay in the intensive care unit. Since 1984 more than 84% have survived. The problem at the present time concerns principally neonates weighing less than 1000 g. In 1986 a survey was carried out in six

centers in three European countries and one American state. Immediate survival varied from 40–70%, of which 10–40% was for neonates weighing less than 750 g. The results at 3–4 years of age varied from one center with absence of motor handicap and a mean IQ of 105 ± 15 without major sensory disturbance to another center with 50% of neurological sequelae, severe sensory disturbance and bronchopulmonary dysplasia requiring expensive care. The principle reason for these large differences was precisely the fact that resuscitative care could be stopped in situations beyond control, depending on the center. The team that reported the absence of major sequelae acknowledged that 80% of the deaths followed after discontinuation of intensive care decided on by a multidisciplinary team on clinical, ultrasonographic and electroencephalographic criteria. The other group that reported a 50% incidence of severe sequelae, was obliged 'by law' to continue to provide intensive care whatever the outcome.

Thus, this is a striking example of the difficulty of coming to a decision in different countries. Undoubtedly, the law is formally applied in all countries. However, the law requires that effective help be provided for any individual in danger. What then is effective help in respect of a newborn infant of 600 g whose outcome is hopeless, as judged by the experience of the neonatal care team, resulting either in rapid death or the occurrence of severe sequelae.

Again, it is only the team that can, by reason of its past experience, assess the prognosis based on the progress of the pregnancy, the hours following birth and the quality of the family environment. It is thus certainly the local team that should have the power to decide if intensive care be stopped.

OTHER SITUATIONS

It is also the local unit that should sometimes decide to refuse to care for a distressed very premature baby at 24–25 weeks gestational age that is at the limits of viability according to their own criteria of viability, which vary according to financial and material as well as human and affective factors.

Another important aspect which should be considered by the perinatologist is the attitude vis à vis some decisions in the matter of assisted reproduction. In some ways, one could compare the danger of maintaining at all costs the life of a newborn with profound and irreversible brain damage, with the desperate eagerness to create life as in some foolish indications for *in vitro* fertilization/intracytoplasmic spermatid injection or other reproductive technologies whatever the age of the woman or the socio-affective conditions of the parents.

When and how?

The last part of this chapter will discuss when and how action should be taken, when the decision is taken to interrupt pregnancy or intensive care.

The doctor and the team should thus leave their narrow intellectual bases of reference and try to assess the needs of this human being. Western man, faithful to his tradition of logic, knows at present that the consciousness of the neonate is not the same at 25–30 as at 36 weeks. It progresses as a function of its capabilities of perception, which is as much sensitive as sensorial and affective. However, more and more, influenced by oriental intuition, the pediatrician senses that it is the soul of this being in peril that has already decided all beforehand. Very often, as some psychologists are wont say, these neonates have not asked to live this time round, a life which appears to them much too difficult.

However, others would say that they know, these little beings, in being born at an exact moment, in this particular obstetrical and pediatric environment, that they offer themselves for a team decision which also has the means to help them to live, sometimes even under good conditions.

Thus, once again, it is for the local team to take its decision at the instant that seems most appropriate as much for the fetus/neonate, as for the parents and even for the team that should 'accompany' him in the most effective manner possible.

'How' then is the last worry. Here again, methods differ according to differences in perception. In fact, it is better to act as a being in full possession of all his capabilities of sensoriaffective perception so as to avoid the suffering and the anguish of this separation, even if the death of the physical body does not take place at the same level of consciousness for a premature baby of 25 or 30 weeks as for a newborn infant at term, a child or an adult.

CONCLUSION

This short contribution on the subject of ethics and perinatology cannot deal with all the problems of the fetus or neonate in life-threatening situations. The aim of these comments is to show how the intensive care team can approach this difficult problem, perhaps in an incomplete manner, but in any case in a much better way than a conventional ethical committee, which is often unable to assess adequately the immense dilemma of the sick fetus or newly born infant.

Prematurity: community-based prevention program

47

E. Saling, T. Al-Taie, A. Placht and W. Masur

INTRODUCTION

One of the most urgent tasks of modern obstetrics is to reduce the number of preterm deliveries, especially those with infants of less than 1500 g birth weight. These infants represent one of the largest groups of newborns demonstrating high mortality and morbidity rates. Neonatologists have achieved enormous success in keeping extremely premature infants alive, however, the number of children with long lasting or definite impairment is alarming. For instance Riegel and co-workers[1] in 1995 published a study in which they examined disabilities, structural impairments and functional impairments in children at 4 years of age who were admitted to a hospital in Southern Bavaria. These children had been born very prematurely and were compared to a representative sample of all children born in Southern Bavaria, including preterm and small for gestational age infants. Surprisingly, major impairments occurred 14 times more frequently; they were found in 31% in the very preterm group vs. 2.3% in the control group. The total frequency of any impairment amounted to 78% as opposed to 40% in the control group. The type of impairment varied but included impaired vision, defective hearing, epilepsy or motor deficits including cerebral palsy, and reductions of speech facilities, vocabulary and visual-motor integration.

In 1994, Hack and associates[2] conducted a follow-up study of school age children who had been born with very low birth weight (< 1500 g) or with extremely low birth weight (< 750 g). When compared to children who had been born at term, these children also demonstrate higher rates of impairment such as low intelligence, limited academic skills, poor visual motor function, poor gross motor function, poor adaptive functioning, behavioral problems, cerebral palsy, visual disability, hearing disability, subnormal weight, subnormal height and subnormal head size.

A number of factors are known to cause late spontaneous abortions and premature delivery. However, as far as effective preventive measures are concerned, we can limit ourselves to the knowledge that most of the avoidable causes are to be found among patients with ascending genital infections and that the correct diagnostic and therapeutic strategies are of decisive importance here. According to our initial results, when risk factors are detected early and suitable preventive measures are undertaken in good time, there is an excellent chance of preventing a high number of late abortions and very low birth weight newborns which has not been achievable in the past.

Concerning efforts to prevent prematurity, many publications and recommendations have been reviewed in the literature, such as that by Papiernik[3]. Most of them are based on the presumption that socioeconomic factors such as low social status, psychological stressors and physical stress are the main causes of premature birth. Some successes have been achieved with programs based on these aspects, particularly in model studies. However, the main obstacle preventing a consistent reduction in the number of very low birth weight infants on a broad scale concerns the amount of expense involved. Considerable organizational and personal expenses are necessary to realize such projects, and these resources are hardly available to such an extent in all countries. We began our activities to reduce the rate of premature births approximately 25 years ago[4,5]. However, our successes were only partially satisfactory, and 6 years ago we developed a new Prematurity Prevention Program which is based on the ascending infection origin[6]. Several reports on this program have been published already[7-10]. Its practical introduction into our clinical routine, and later into the clinical practice of colleagues in our area, has led to a considerable decrease in the number of very low birth weight infants. However, in spite of achieving a reduction rate of about 40% in our department and 50% in co-operation with practitioners, we had to admit that the practical employment of the program and the consequent application of preventive measures started at a relatively late stage of the whole prematurity pathogenetic process. Therefore, 3 years ago, we added another aspect to the program which employed the active co-operation of the pregnant patient herself. In this chapter, I will present to you the combination of both main parts of our program. This solution appears to be a quite different, relatively easy, more economic and more effective way to achieve considerable success in reducing the rate of very small and extremely small premature infants.

FIRST PART OF THE PREVENTION PROGRAM

Our general program relies on our knowledge that ascending infection is the main reason for very early prematurity. The decisive proof was that the most successful measure to prevent recurrent late abortions and early premature births was to perform in those patients an early total operative cervical occlusion, which leads to a total barrier in the lower genital tract. We introduced this operation in 1981[11] and noted that the success rate of achieving a surviving infant in such patients increased from less than 20% before, to about 80% after the operation[12]. This convincing experience, together with a retrospective evaluation in our department[7] and

similar results from placental pathology[13,14], confirmed that ascending infection is the most frequent cause of very early prematurity. The incidence of ascending infections as a cause of prematurity approaches 70% or even more[7]. Highly sophisticated biochemical and immunological studies later supported this hypothesis. One of the most often cited authors in this field is Roberto Romero and his co-workers[15].

Another interesting aspect is illustrated by our latest studies which have demonstrated concrete signs of impairment of the immune status, with respect to the cellular and humoral parameters of the immune system, in women with prematurity symptoms[18]. Sixty-five percent of them had stressful situations and we assume that ascending infections may be enhanced by such impairments. Furthermore, we concluded that those pregnant women living in a critical social status, and who therefore are more likely to have impaired immunity, can be helped earlier and more effectively through appropriate education and preventive medical measures started at a very early stage in the pregnancy. Our Prematurity Prevention Program offers more success in helping these patients than is possible through the complicated and necessarily expensive intensive care given by the social services.

In Table 1 are summarized our ideas about the stages of threatened prematurity, prophylactic and therapeutic measures depending on diagnostic findings and/or the presence of symptoms as well as chances of success and efficiency of countermeasures.

Stage 1 of endangerment is a potentially increased risk in cases with anamnestic load such as one or more prior late spontaneous abortions or very premature labor. The best prophylactic countermeasure is, as already mentioned, to perform an operative early total cervix occlusion at about 12 gestational weeks to create a barrier against the ascension of organisms.

The second early stage of increased risk is a disturbance of the vaginal milieu which can mostly be detected by simple pH measurement at the introitus. In such a case of so-called 'dysbiosis', a substitution with preparations of *Lactobacillus acidophilus* on its own is recommended.

Table 1 Stages of threatened prematurity, prophylactic and therapeutic measures, depending on diagnostic findings and/or the presence of symptoms as well as chances of success and efficiency of countermeasures

Stage of endangerment	Symptoms or findings	Prophylactic or therapeutic measures	Chances of success and efficiency of measures
1. Potentially increased risk	anamnestic risk average (1 miscarriage or 1 very small premature) high (≥ 2 miscarriages or very small prematures)	small early total cervix occlusion extensive early total cervix occlusion	best suitable stages with highest chances of success
2. Very early stage	disturbance of vaginal milieu without symptoms of ascension, but increased pH, 'dysbiosis' in native preparation no symptoms of prematurity	a substitution of *Lactobacillus acidophilus* should be the primary treatment here	
3. Early stage	still no symptoms of prematurity (a) Microscopically or culturally proven local vaginal infection, such as bacterial vaginosis (organisms such as anaerobes, *Candida*, *Trichomonas* and others); (b) Evidence of *Chlamydia* in the cervix and/or urethra; (c) Evidence of bacteria at lower egg-pole; (d) Significant bacteriuria;	local chemotherapy and/or antiseptic measures, local antibiotic therapy Systemic antibiotic therapy recommendation of rest, corroborant and relaxing measures among others for improving immunological conditions	still good chances of success after-treatment with *Lactobacillus* preparation in case pH increases
4. Late stage	with symptoms of prematurity (increased contractions (premature labor) and/or critical cervix state) (e) Microscopic or local infection proved by culture (vaginal and/or cervical or at lower egg-pole); (f) Symptoms of prematurity without microscopic or cultural proof of organisms, but positive CRP or positive fFN findings	calculated antibiotic therapy or specific antibiotic therapy	increasingly unsuccessful

CRP, C-reactive protein; fFN, fetal fibronectin

Both of these stages allow the best chances for success in the prevention of prematurity.

The third also relatively early stage of increased risk includes cases without symptoms of premature labor, but in which proven vaginal infection is present, such as bacterial vaginosis, *Chlamydia* infection of the cervical canal or urethra, infections of the lower egg-pole (which can be detected by our recently developed egg-pole lavage) or significant bacteriuria. In such cases, local chemotherapeutic, antiseptic measures, local antibiotic or systemic antibiotic therapy is recommended. The chances of success are still favorable. In both this and the next stage the patients concerned should be recommended rest, corroborant and physical as well as psychological relaxing measures to improve their immunological status.

The fourth and most progressed stage involves symptoms of prematurity such as apparent premature uterine contractions and/or critical findings of cervical change. Systemic antibiotic therapy is the method of choice, if organisms can be identified or laboratory parameters such as C-reactive protein (CRP) or fetal fibronectin (fFN) are positive.

In the last stage, the therapeutic measures are increasingly unsuccessful. In both of the last stages, an additional 'cure' with *Lactobacillus acidophilus* preparations is indicated because most of the therapeutic measures concerned disturb the biologically balanced vaginal milieu, which can be confirmed by increased vaginal pH values.

NEW COMMUNITY-BASED PART OF THE PREVENTION PROGRAM

After this introductory overview, we continue with the actual part of our prevention program, the, as we call it, 'prenatal care self-examination'. The main points are summarized in Table 2.

Point 1

Every patient is instructed to measure the pH value of her vagina once or twice a week. This is a very simple procedure in which she either introduces a test-paper with her finger or she uses a special device that she prepares by herself. The patient fixes a test paper by a plastic cap on a centrifugal tube, introduces this prepared device into her vagina, withdraws it shortly afterwards and then compares the color of the test paper with the enclosed special color scale and reads the pH value. If the pH level has increased to 4.7 or higher, measured by special test paper from Merck Co. (art.-No. 9542), she should see her practitioner immediately. If her doctor confirms the reduced acidification, we recommend application of *Lactobacillus* preparations to correct the vaginal acidity, but at the same time, examinations should be performed to determine the cause of the acidity disturbance.

Independent of the vaginal pH self-measurement, all expectant mothers should be made aware of the most important potential risk factors and how to recognize them if they occur.

Table 2   Basic guidelines of the prenatal care self-examination

(1) Recommended measures undertaken by the patient herself:
    (a) Vaginal pH self-measurement 1–2 times a week;
    (b) Paying attention for risk factors occurring between consultations

(2) Improvements expected through active participation of the patients:
    (a) Avoidance of time lags by earliest possible detection of pH increase and earliest possible detection of other risk factors not detectable by pH measurement;
    (b) Possibility of controlling the behavior of vaginal acidity

(3) Target group: motivate all pregnant women to take part if possible

(4) Initiation should take place as early as possible. In cases of poor history it is best to start before conception

If anything unusual happens at a later stage, also listed in our risk catalog, such as premature contractions, clearly increased discharge, or painful or frequent urination, the patient should consult her doctor.

Point 2

The main advantage achieved by the patient's active participation is that increases in vaginal pH or the manifestation of any other risk factors are noticed very early and this leads to the detection of a considerable number of disturbances connected with spontaneous abortions and prematurity. This enables us to avoid longer, critical periods of delay, sometimes of several weeks. What we mean in particular is that without this self-examination program, some symptoms remain concealed although they are in fact easily recognizable. Furthermore, there is also a possibility of controlling the behavior of vaginal acidity within short intervals, by following the effects of therapeutic measures.

Point 3

This concerns the target group. Since the program is fundamentally based on a screening principle, as many patients as possible should be motivated to take part; at best, every pregnant woman without any exception.

Point 4

This concerns the time to start with the self-examination. This should be chosen very early on, so as to detect the threat of irregularities in good time, i.e. at the earliest possible moment in the pregnancy. It would be even better, in the case of an unfavorable history, to choose a preconceptional moment, that is weeks or months before a planned pregnancy.

RESULTS

First results up to now justify the pH self-measurement by pregnant patients. In a study in our department[16], we confirmed that out of 100 women who had measured their vaginal pH themselves using test paper, 91% of the measurements corresponded with the results later measured by a physician with a pH meter. In 9% the results were false positive; this means that with the test paper an increased pH value was measured, but the value measured by pH meter was normal. This was not a grave error as no pathological findings were overlooked. Furthermore, we found that in about 70% of the patients who had increased pH values measured both by test paper and by the pH meter, evidence of pathogenic organisms was found in the vagina and/or the cervix, whereas the figure was only 8% when the pH values were normal.

The full prenatal care self-examination program was started in September 1993 and has been announced in special newspapers which are frequently read by pregnant women. Details about the information given to pregnant women interested in taking part were published in the German journal *Der Frauenarzt*[17]. Up to now about 5500 pregnant patients have participated or are still participating.

Of the 1359 women who have returned the papers to us up to now, 485 were pregnant for the first time and 874 had been pregnant before. The anamnestic information given by the group of women with previous pregnancies was particularly interesting. It can be seen that a high number of them, i.e. 30.4%, had miscarriages and about 20.3% had underweight infants during previous pregnancies. We can so far draw the conclusion that the participating women belong to a higher risk rather than to a lower risk group. According to the returned records, 60.5% of the patients reported 'disturbed courses' in their present pregnancy.

What we can today confirm with satisfaction is the fact that the rate of birth of underweight infants (Figure 1), in particular the very small ones (birth weight < 1500 g), is now clearly lower at 1.5% than in previous pregnancies, when it was 8.5%. The rate of extremely small infants (< 1000 g) amounts to 0.9% now, compared to 4.2% in previous pregnancies.

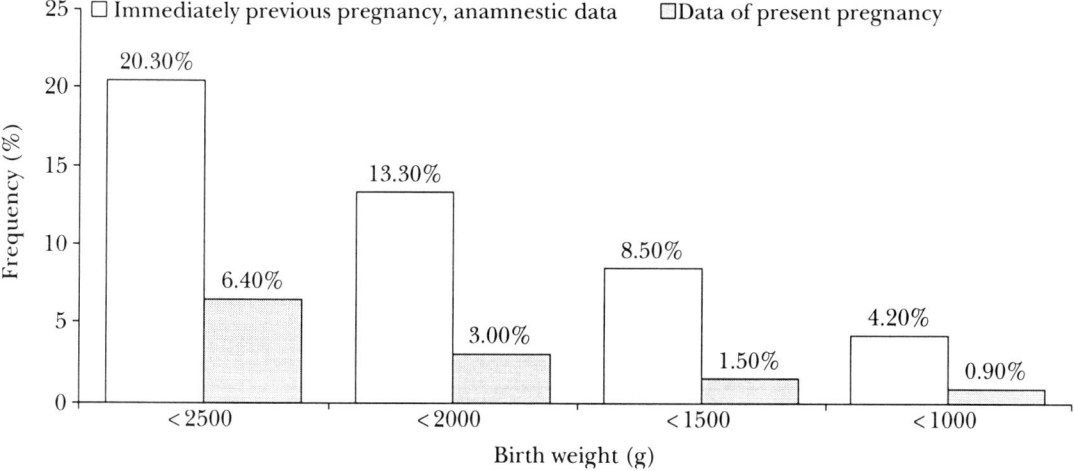

Figure 1 Frequency of low birth weight infants prior to and during the prenatal care self-examination study (multigravida, $n = 874$)

Another evaluation shows comparisons between the results of the immediately previous pregnancies and the present pregnancies, when women have participated in the prenatal care self-examination program. Here the only results evaluated were from those women who had suffered a premature birth in the immediately previous pregnancy. Of the 100 women, only 12 again gave birth a preterm baby (< 37 weeks of gestation). Of the 30 women who had given birth to a very early preterm infant (< 31 + 0 weeks of gestation) in the immediately previous pregnancy, only two (that is 7%) suffered the same misfortune again. Of the 20 who had given birth to an extremely early preterm infant (< 28 weeks of gestation), no recurrence happened in any case.

From a retrospective evaluation performed in our department, we have found that a direct correlation exists between the degree of prematurity and the increase in the vaginal pH levels of mothers upon admission to the hospital (Figure 2). In premature births at less than 32 + 0 weeks of gestation, all the 15 mothers had increased pH levels; between 32 + 0 and 36 + 6 weeks of gestation it was only 60%. From this one can conclude that ascending infections most frequently play a role in threatened prematurity, particularly in the cases with very early preterm birth.

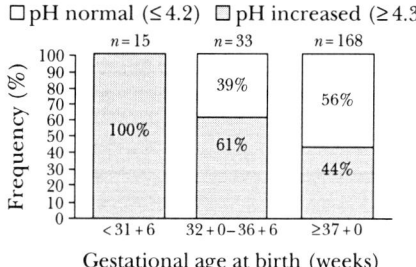

Figure 2 Vaginal pH in patients with symptoms of threatened prematurity measured on admission to the hospital and gestational age at birth

In another earlier evaluation the question was also examined of how many pregnant patients have normal and how many have pathological vaginal pH values. Normal pH levels were present in 67% of all women, while in 33% the levels were twice or more often increased, and in 7% they were permanently increased.

It is of particular interest to see how often one can successfully normalize the pH in cases with increased vaginal pH levels by using *Lactobacillus acidophilus* therapy. Success was achieved in 83% out of 75 such patients, and this is really an unexpectedly good result. The therapy has been carried out for 5 ± 3 days to achieve this success.

279

CONCLUSIONS

Of course there are still many questions concerning the origin of late abortion and prematurity that have not yet been explained and that cannot be answered today. We are also aware that our statistical evaluations are not fully satisfactory, and that randomized prospective studies would be more appropriate. However, the difficulties from the practical medical point of view in realizing such studies at a given time, should not be underestimated. To this end we have been trying to draw up a suitable, correct study concept in our country for some years now. It could not be realized due to ethical considerations, namely in the failure to give the already available preventive and/or therapeutic help to women at high risk of prematurity in the control group. Therefore we urgently recommend examiners in other countries, who have not as yet started employing the measures we recommend, to complete such prospective studies. however, due to our positive results we think that an important and, in our opinion, decisive step, as far as the practicability and efficiency of prematurity prevention is concerned, has been taken. There is now a real chance of making progress, as yet not achieved, in this essential field of our specialty.

References

1. Riegel, K., Ohrt, B., Wolke, D. and Österlund, K. (1995). Die Entwicklung gefährdet geborener Kinder bis zum fünften Lebensjahr. (Stuttgart: Enke)
2. Hack, M., Taylor, H. G., Klein, N., Eiben, R., Schatschneider, Ch. and Mercuri-Minich, N. (1994). School-age outcomes in children with birth weight under 750 g. *N. Engl. J. Med.*, **331**, 753–59
3. Papiernik, E. (1984). Proposals for a Programmed Prevention Policy of Preterm Birth. *Clin. Obstet. Gynecol.*, **27**, 614–35
4. Saling, E. (1971). Prämaturitäts- und Dysmaturitäts-Präventions-Programm (PDP-Programm). In Saling, E. and Dudenhausen, J. W. (eds.) *Perinatale Medizin III*, Proceedings of IVth Deutscher Kongreß für Perinatale Medizin, Berlin 1971. (Stuttgart: Thieme)
5. Saling, E. (1972). Prämaturitäts- und Dysmaturitäts-Präventions-Programm (PDP-Programm). *Z. Geburth. Perinat.*, **176**, 70–81
6. Saling, E., Brandt-Niebelschütz, S. and Schmitz, C. (1991). Vermeidung von Spätaborten und risikoreichen Frühgeburten – für die Routine geeignete Maßnahmen. *Z. Geburtsh. Perinat.*, **195**, 209–21
7. Saling, E. (1992). Current measures to prevent late abortion or prematurity. In Saling, E. (ed.) *Perinatology, Nestlé Nutrition Workshop Series*, Vol. 26, pp. 141–51. (New York: Raven Press)
8. Saling, E. (1991). Programme for prevention of prematurity. In Hirsch, H. A. (ed.) *Infection and Preterm Labor*, pp. 31–40. (Stuttgart, New York: Thieme)
9. Saling, E. (1992). Effective prevention of premature birth – some recent aspects and results. In Koppe, J. G., Eskes, T. K. A. B., van Geijn, H. P., Wiesenhaan, P. F. and Ruys, J. H. (eds.) *Care, Concern and Cure in Perinatal Medicine*, pp. 147–53. (Carnforth, New York: Parthenon Publishing Group)
10. Saling, E. (1981). Der frühe totale Muttermundverschluß zur Vermeidung habitueller Aborte und Frühgeburten. *Z. Geburtsh. Perinat.*, **185**, 259–261
11. Saling, E. (1993). Infektiologische Spätabortursachen und operativer Muttermundverschluß. *Arch. Gynecol. Obstet.*, **254**, 1265–71
12. Vogel, M. (1991). Das Amnioninfektionssyndrom. *Verh. Dtsch. Ges. Path.*, **75**, 418
13. Vogel, M. (1992). *Atlas der Morphologischen Plazentadiagnostik.* (Berlin, Heidelberg, New York, Paris, Tokyo: Springer)
14. Romero, R., Gomez, R., Baumann, P., Mazor, M. and Cotton, D. (1993). The role of the infection and cytokines in preterm parturition. In Chwalisz, K. and Garfield, R. E. (eds.) *Basic Mechanisms Controlling Term and Preterm Birth, Ernst Schering Research Foundation, Workshop*, 7. (Berlin: Springer)
15. Reidewald, S., Hanifi-Afshar, T. and Saling, E. (1992). pH-Selbstmessung in der Vagina durch die Schwangere (im Vergleich zu Kontrollmessungen durch den Arzt). *Z. Geburtsh. Perinat.*, **196**, 61–62

16. Saling, E., Raitsch, S., Placht, A., Fuhr, N. and Schumacher, E. (1994). Frühgeburten-Vermeidungs-Programm und Selbstvorsorge-Aktion für Schwangere. *Der Frauenarzt*, **35**, 84–92

17. Brandt-Niebelschütz, S., Saling, E., Uphoff, A., Raitsch, S., Schmolke, B., Vetter, K., Römisch, K. and Kaehler, H. (1995). Untersuchungen zur Immunitätslage Schwangerer insbesondere beim Vorliegen einer Frühgeburtsymptomatik. *Geburtsch. Frauenheilk.*, **55**, 456–63

Fetal and neonatal psychology: intrinsic motives and learning behavior
48

C. Trevarthen

FOUNDATION STRUCTURES FOR HUMAN PSYCHOLOGY

In the voluntary behavior of a conscious person, perceiving, thinking and acting respond to environmental stimuli, and learning. Information taken in changes brain activity and builds new skills and memories. But the process is far from passive. Anticipatory motives and emotions have a decisive role.

Concepts of the innate foundations for these fundamental processes of cognition in a human being have greatly changed in the past three decades. The idea that an infant is born with only physiological reactions and reflex responses without discriminating representations of objects outside the body has been disproved by experiments on how newborns orient to and interact with controlled events. They learn, but their learning is motivated in certain directions with defined goals. Observations of fetuses *in utero* and of prematurely born infants confirm the picture. Evidently, human intentions, attentions and feelings grow from structures and functions active in the brain at birth.

ACTIONS OF INFANTS IN THE FIRST WEEKS, ESPECIALLY IN COMMUNICATION

Newborn infants exhibit whole-body co-ordination of movements, directed awareness and preferences for certain stimuli. They act voluntarily to recover some experiences and avoid others. Their investigative activity perceives equivalent objects in different modalities, and is particularly receptive to expressions of human care and communication. Imitation and learning studies have tested these integrations and factors that change them.

It has been demonstrated that the regular rhythmic properties of adult human expressions are matched by rhythms of expression in a newborn. These matching time patterns of moving facilitate synchronized interactions. Furthermore, the emotions of neonates not only excite emotional responses; they react selectively to the emotions of attending adults. These features imply dynamic, causal, regulatory psychological principles (motives), and presuppose a coherent central intrinsic motive formation (IMF)[1] that arises in brain morphogenesis in anticipation of the building of cognitive representations of experience (Figures 1 and 2).

Expressions in videos and audio records of neonates interacting with care-givers show up the differentiated motives and emotions[2]. Vocalizations and breathing, facial expressions, eye movements, head orientations and postures and movements of the hands, feet, limbs and whole body of the infant together manifest brain activity that is both integrated and rich in emotional definition (Figure 1). The emotions show both sensory equivalence and motor equivalence at birth – they activate many parts of the baby's motor system synchronously in co-ordination, and they also pick up feelings in others by many senses[3]. Newborn infants are aware of other human beings and they seek communication; at first through olfaction, touch and hearing, then increasingly through seeing. They have intentional control over their auditory

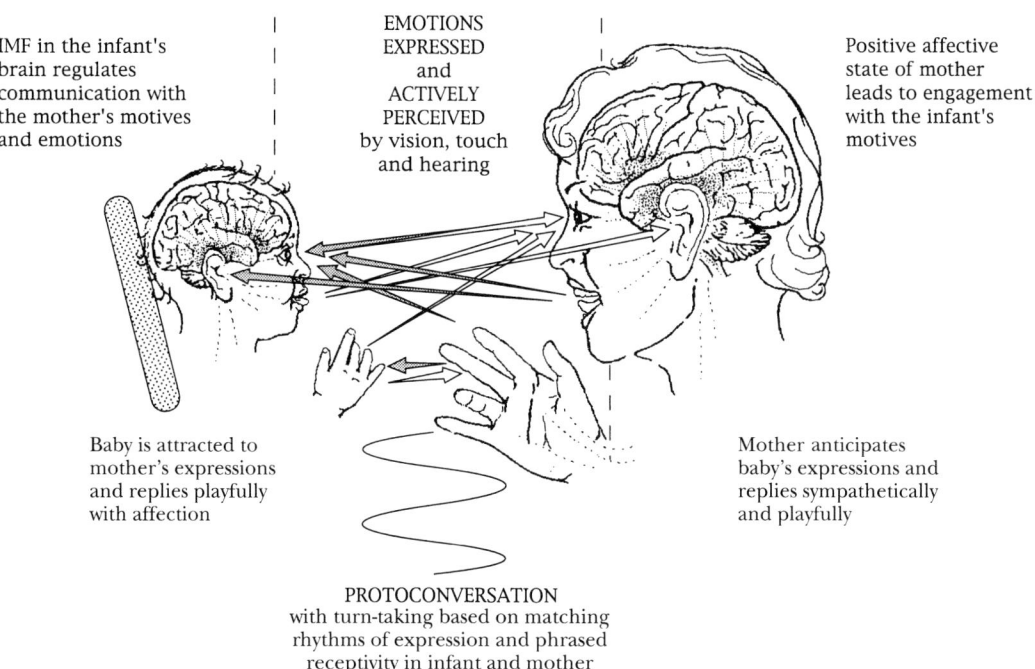

IMF in the infant's brain regulates communication with the mother's motives and emotions

EMOTIONS EXPRESSED and ACTIVELY PERCEIVED by vision, touch and hearing

Positive affective state of mother leads to engagement with the infant's motives

Baby is attracted to mother's expressions and replies playfully with affection

Mother anticipates baby's expressions and replies sympathetically and playfully

PROTOCONVERSATION
with turn-taking based on matching rhythms of expression and phrased receptivity in infant and mother

Figure 1 The many channels of expression by which an infant of 2 months can interact with the mother. IMF = intrinsic motive formation

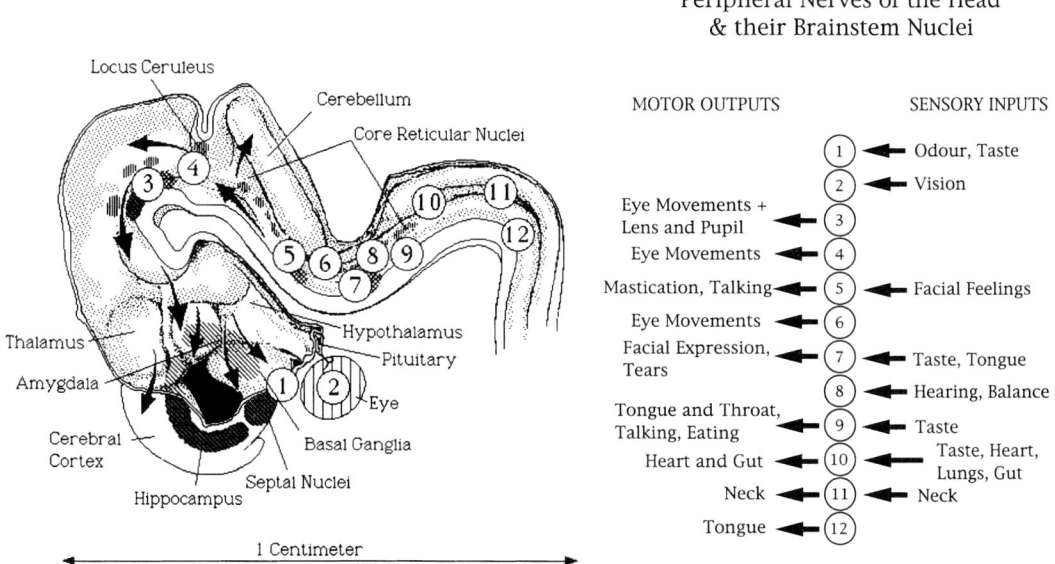

Peripheral Nerves of the Head & their Brainstem Nuclei

MOTOR OUTPUTS		SENSORY INPUTS
	1	Odour, Taste
	2	Vision
Eye Movements + Lens and Pupil	3	
Eye Movements	4	
Mastication, Talking	5	Facial Feelings
Eye Movements	6	
Facial Expression, Tears	7	Taste, Tongue
	8	Hearing, Balance
	9	Taste
Tongue and Throat, Talking, Eating		
Heart and Gut	10	Taste, Heart, Lungs, Gut
Neck	11	Neck
Tongue	12	

Locus Ceruleus
Cerebellum
Core Reticular Nuclei
Thalamus
Amygdala
Cerebral Cortex
Hippocampus
Septal Nuclei
Basal Ganglia
Eye
Pituitary
Hypothalamus

1 Centimeter

Figure 2 Human embryo brain (7 weeks) (adapted from reference 38). The cerebral hemispheres are in rudimentary condition, but the nuclei of the brainstem reticular formation and limbic system are clearly differentiated and project into the hemispheres (see intrinsic motive formation (IMF), reference 1). The locations of the nuclei of the twelve cranial nerves and their inputs and outputs are indicated

experiences of people[4,5] and feel preferences for audible or visible signs of human presence.

Imitations give startling proof of the correspondence between innate brain representations of the 'self' and 'other' as potentially equivalent or covalent partners in an exchange of expressions and states of motivation. In the first minutes or hours, infants may purposefully and communicatively reproduce adult partners' expressions of the mouth, vocalizations, eyebrow movements and hand opening and closing[6-11]. The newborns detect, through different senses, the emotional and intersubjective equivalence of expressive movements of different parts of another person's body. They can retain a representation of an expression made by another person and reproduce an imitated movement a day later in the absence of the model movement[11]. The movements are not imitated reflexly, but are used to negotiate a communicative exchange or dynamic interaction in which the partner, too, is imitating[8,12,13].

By making and breaking eye-contact, in conjunction with vocalizations and smiles, the infant can control the expressions of the partner, and it has been inferred that this serves in regulation of the infant's autonomic arousal or 'state'[14-16]. Touch and audition appear to be the principal senses through which mothers change neonatal state and brain activity[16,17]. However, the theory of 'state control' of neurohumoral activity[18] cannot explain the expressive range of infants' behaviors in playful encounters with parents, even in the neonatal period. These behaviors satisfy motives for intersubjective co-ordination of dynamic mental states, rather than physiological homeostasis[2].

Playful communicative encounters with 2-month-olds are described as 'proto-conversations'[19]. This term captures both the response-seeking subtlety of the infant's phases of animation in intense orientation to the partner, and the immediate acceptance by the parent that the child is trying to express messages of some kind – to make 'utterances' and negotiate an exchange (Figure 1). Microanalyses of face-to-face interactions between 2-month-old infants and adults prove that an infant can share in the generation of regular, patterned, turn-taking sequences, which are adapted to the eventual development of speech and language[3,20,21].

Analyses of what the adult does in proto-conversation confirms the impression of intuitive mutality between two brains that possess corresponding emotions and motives. A sympathetic adult will feel compelled to respond in a highly predictable way to the infant, using a unique, emotionally clear register of body-movement, touching, speech and facial expression with distinctive prosodic, poetic or musical dimensions[12,20,22-26]. Eye-to-eye contact is sought with the infant and the adult's modulated expressions of joy, concern, puzzlement, annoyance or surprise echo the rhythms of the infant's transforming mood[3,27,28]. The infant's body, hands or face are gently and rhythmically touched. The adult's speech becomes quiet, making short (c. 0.5 s) 'breathy' or 'lax' utterances with undulating intonation and an elevated pitch and pauses between. The mutual exchanges of expression settle around a common beat close to adagio (1/0.75 s) and regularities in the rhythms of articulation or gesture describe lifts or descents of motivation in phrases of 3–5 s. The speech has been described as 'intuitive motherese', 'intuitive parentese' or 'infant-directed speech'.

Thus infant communication, in spite of its cognitive and representational limitations, is manifestly inter-mental, inter-subjective or inter-personal[20,27]. It is based on shared 'dynamic affects'[28]. The adult partner approaches the infant with appropriate responsiveness as to a person who will react with affection, playfulness, etc., a fine rhythmic organization of mutual synchronous or alternating responses may be set up between them[3,29-31]. The efficiency of co-ordination between adult and infant in protoconversation proves that each is equipped to 'take account of' the other. They meet as mutually responsive agents, each of whom has a readiness for engagement with a 'virtual other', seeking 'dyadic closure' by exchange of expressions with an actual responsive other[32].

BEHAVIORS OF FETUSES *IN UTERO* AND CONTINUITY WITH EARLY INFANCY

Research since 1970 on activity, reactive states and learning of fetuses confirms that the above interpretation may be extended to the intrauterine period[33]. In the last months of gestation, psychological abilities develop in preparation for postnatal life and maternal care. Adaptive motor co-ordinations are emergent in the second trimester of gestation and elaborated in the last trimester[34,35]. The motor activities are framed rhythmically against a neurogenic time-base. Many of these co-ordinated activities are goal directed; they are ready to assimilate their specific environmental 'objects' into awareness at birth. The most remarkable are those that respond in selective ways to a living and expressive human presence. Expressions of infants correspond closely with expressed emotions of adults that transcend sophisticated social intentions or the conventions of different cultures. With ultrasound recordings, it can be confirmed that the same expressions are exhibited by fetuses *in utero*[36]. Four behavioral states of 'arousal' identified in the fetus – quiet sleep with startles, active sleep accompanied by periodic gross activity such as stretches, quiet awake with small movements including eye movements, and the active awake state with vigorous continual movements – are directly comparable with those already defined for neonates. Prenatal behavior serves in the sculpting of the central nervous system and can be exploited in the assessment of the state of health of the fetus and for the development of better environments for infants born before term.

In all mammals and humans, odor sensing follows the somesthetic and vestibular senses, and is active before audition and vision. Odor preferences are demonstrated immediately after birth for compounds encountered *in utero*, and with new odors preferences are similar to those of adults. A strong preference is shown for the odor of a lactating breast. Rapid postnatal learning of some stimuli may be triggered by genetic predispositions, but intrauterine experi-ence may determine postnatal acquisition by creating a chemical 'search image'.

Indications that the fetus has a meaningful auditory world come from observations that maternal heart beat is calming for premature infants, and that immediate postnatal recognition of the mother's voice helps attachment. Habituation tests of the perceptual capacities of fetuses demonstrate that the poetry or musicality of human speech can be heard, and learned, *in utero*. The fetus can distinguish syllables or phrases uttered in male or female voices, and newborns at 2–4 postnatal days show preferences for previously heard musical or speech sequences, and they can discriminate the mother's language. With fetuses at 26–34 gestational weeks, heart rate deceleration and respiratory changes of the 'orienting response' occur in quiet sleep, disproving the idea that sleep is used by the fetus to 'tune out' stimulation.

Handedness of fetuses can be detected early. A majority suck the right hand from 15 weeks, and this correlates with the head turning bias in the newborn and predicts which hand the infant will use to grasp a ball at 18 months after birth. Behavioral asymmetries that emerge in the first trimester could stimulate asymmetric growth of the cerebral hemispheres, but there is evidence from brain embryology that the trigger for asymmetry of the neocortex may come much earlier, from the reticular core of the brain[37] (Figure 3).

More than 95% of infants born 3 months early now survive. Their brains are developing more rapidly than at any other time, outside the environment to which they are adapted. Preterm birth is associated with increased reactivity, hypersensitivity and disorganized movement, and more dependence on human care to maintain state. It is also associated with brain abnormality, especially in frontal and right hemisphere regions. Preterm infants born very early can later show peaks of excellence in intelligence tests, which may indicate brain reorganization.

Nevertheless, premature infants are not entirely passive and helpless. They are capable of expressing their needs and states of discomfort

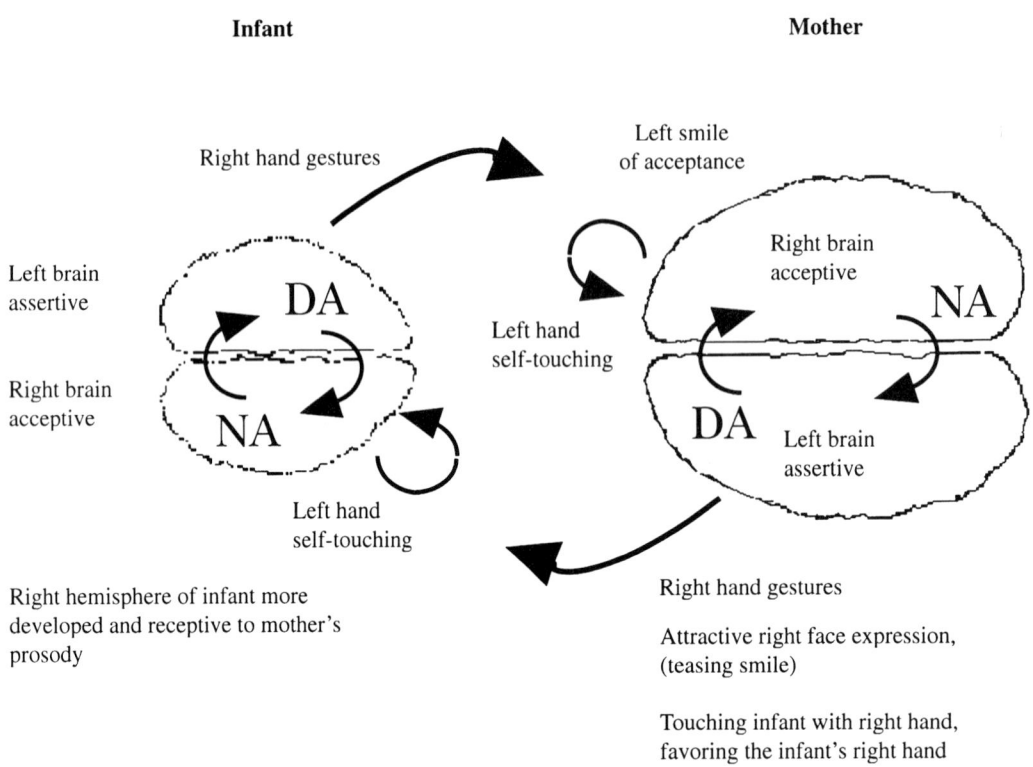

Figure 3 Proposed asymmetric tendencies of the motivating systems of the infant and mother when they are communicating, and their neurochemical correlates; NA = noradrenergic systems predominate; DA = dopaminergic systems more active (adapted from references 37 and 45)

or satisfaction, not just their degree of sleep or wakefulness. Above all, they show signs of readiness to engage in imitative or protoconversational contacts with human company. Individualized attention by carers trained to react to each infant's expressions of need, or skin-to-skin contact with parents who are offering solicitous tactile, auditory and visual responses and breast feeding can lead to improved development.

REGULATORY STRUCTURES OF THE EMBRYONIC AND FETAL BRAIN

We now have a description of human brain embryology that incorporates research information on other species[38]. This confirms that the core regulatory mechanisms of the autonomic nervous system, hypothalamus, reticular formation, basal ganglia and limbic system are laid down in the first trimester, before the cognitive structures of the cerebral cortex. The emotional and communicative precocity of human newborns indicates that emotions and emotional responses to caregivers play a crucial role in the regulation of brain development[16]. These same structures form a link between gene instructions and the developing mind that goes wrong in empathy disorders such as autism[1,13].

In the second half of the embryonic period, weeks 5–8, all the main components of the brain are formed and the body takes the appearance of a miniature human with relatively large head. The eyes, vestibular canals and cochlea, hands, nose and mouth are rapidly differentiating their dedicated forms. For most of this stage the nervous system has no electrical activity and it generates no movements. The cerebral hemispheres and cerebellum are rudimentary, but the brainstem regulatory and motivating structures are well-formed (Figure 2).

The basic layout of the cerebral cortex is visible about week 6. In the primordial plexiform layer (PPL) of the hemispheres, the primitive nursery tissue in which the mammalian neocortex emerges, afferents from the brain stem form some of the first synapses seen in human embryos, and then the first radially migrating neurons appear in the hemisphere wall, splitting the PPL and attaching themselves to the outer layer. The cell columns of the neocortex, which become local units of functional integration, arise from precursor stem cells in the proliferative zone adjacent to the ventricle[39]. Afferents entering the cortex are guided by position-specific molecules already in place before the afferents arrive, and before the cortical neurons finish migrating.

In week 7, cells from the generative zone migrate radially along glial stands to columns in the cortical plate[39]. The migrating cortical cells pass through a dense cellular lattice and 'subplate' of early neurons, axons, dendrites and glial fibers, which is larger in humans than in other primates and contains the waiting afferents from brainstem, basal forebrain, thalamus and ipse- and contralateral cortex. Input from subcortical regions, with influences from gonadal and adrenal hormones, can thus have a role in deciding the structure of the neocortex, including hemispheric asymmetries of emotional and cognitive function that become elaborated later.

A newborn infant's brain has considerable anatomical complexity, including innumerable somatotopic (body-charting) neural maps. These representations of the 'field of behavior' are interconnected by a system of axons that regulates states of motivation, balancing energetic action on the environment against passive self-maintenance or tentative exploration. The interconnected maps are extensively modified and refined by experience, but they are ready at birth to formulate and express motivated behaviors, including coherent emotions. Psychological evidence implies that the somatotopic neural arrays for self-maintenance and self-co-ordination (autonomic functions and proprioception) and those for regulating transactions with objects (exteroception) have evolved with a third system that can regulate self–other inter-co-ordination and 'alteroception'[40]. Brainstem motor nuclei concerned with uptake of visual information and the control of respiration, vocalization and biting in lower vertebrates have been adapted in humans to serve emotional expression and, eventually, language[41,42] (Figure 2).

An important output from the IMF controls the 'sensory-accessory motor systems' of the special receptors of the head and hands. The eyes, the ears and cochlea, the lips and tongue and the palms and fingers are separately aimable and tuneable. Movement of these structures dynamically and rhythmically 'gates' or 'directs' the uptake of perceptual information in different modalities of high sensitivity and resolution, and these motor adjustments occur in the exploratory and focussing phases of attention to the outside world, before the final commitment of a 'consummatory act'. They therefore exhibit *predictive information* to an observer about emerging intentions, and they have evolved into specialized expressive movements that offer advance information on the intrinsic regulation of awareness and preparations to act[3]. All the organs of human linguistic expression are recruited from this accessory motor set. In infancy, before the oral-vocal system is skilled in speech, or the hands are expressing symbols in a sign language or writing, eyes, hands, face and voice may be engaged in co-ordinated exchanges of feeling with an attentive partner (Figure 1). The mechanisms for vocal expression of emotion and those for speech that develop in the cerebral neocortex are organized around nuclei of the brain stem, and the basal ganglia, thalamus and limbic cortex[42] (Figure 2). Their co-ordinated action can be observed in mid-gestation[35,36]. Brainstem circuits would seen to be crucial to communication with neonates and the first imitations before visual awareness has undergone the rapid development that has been charted in the first 6 months[13].

Developments in the meso-limbic cortices of the temporal and frontal lobes in infants and toddlers transform functions of autonomic self-regulation, emotions in communication, and motives for action[16]. At all stages, the later maturing neocortical circuits emerge in reciprocal, dynamic and increasing involvement with the core regulatory systems of the IMF[1].

CEREBRAL ASYMMETRY OF MOTIVES FOR COGNITION AND COMMUNICATION

Adult speech, conversational gestures and the hand sign language of the deaf are unconsciously asymmetric, in most persons favoring the right half of the mouth and the right hand for the articulation of expressive 'declarative' messages. Hearing speech favors the right ear, and generally there is a shift of gaze to the right when an adult is making an utterance. These asymmetries indicate that expressions of referential communication are emitted and perceived by most persons with greater activity of the left half of the brain. The right hemisphere contributes to perception of the prosody of language and to narrative imagination, and is generally superior to the left in spatial awareness, in non-verbal paralinguistic emotional responses and in recognition of individuals. It integrates a system sensitive to dynamic-expressive features of emotions in all modalities[43]. This complements the language system in the left hemisphere, which is necessary for articulation and perception of the more subtle aspects of phonology and syntax, and for the decoding of rapid sequences of hand movement in a signing language[44]. The right side of the brain appears to be under the influence of sub-cortical motivating influences that maintain whole-body vigilance and self-referred cognitions. The left hemisphere is specialized for the initiation of action, and for focal perceptual guidance, especially of rapid sequences of oral or manual movement to be executed in specified order. Tucker[45] concludes that the left hemisphere has

stronger dopaminergic systems, while the right is relatively more involved with the norepinephrine system (Figure 3). Cognitive or neocortical asymmetries are now perceived to reflect intrinsic embryogenic differences in the left and right sides of the brain in its deeper levels[37,45].

Infants first prefer to hear music or maternal speech with the left ear, but they soon develop a right ear preference for speech. The right hand is usually raised higher than the left when the infant makes an utterance in a protoconversation and distressed or frightened babies may touch their bodies or clothes more with the left hand[37,46]. Evidently, as in adults, the right side of the body is more active in expressive communication and monitoring speech articulations while the left is more receptive of emotion transmitted in a partner's voice (Figure 3). In the second year, the emergence of clear hand dominance is correlated with the age of a baby's first words[47].

Asymmetry appears in recordings of infants' emotion-related frontal brain activity and expression[48]. Young infants hear the emotion in a mother's voice with the right hemisphere of their brains, which is more advanced in development than the left hemisphere[49]. Early postnatal growth is mainly in the right hemisphere which is believed to be responsible for the development of reciprocal relations in mother–infant regulatory systems. Frontal mouth areas develop first on the right of the brain when the infant is cooing and babbling, then on the left when speech articulation becomes mature.

In summary, the newborn infant's brainstem has the fundamental mechanisms of motivation coupled together to co-ordinate dynamic interactions of the body with the outside world, including those with other bodies and their moods. The forebrain cortex can learn from experience only by virtue of the integrations of these lower centers. The neocortex is reciprocally connected to every level of the prenatally organized motive apparatus of the brainstem that continues to impose motive asymmetry on consciousness in the adult.

THE CAUSES OF EMPATHY DISORDERS IN CHILDREN AND LINKS TO PROBLEMS OF INTELLIGENCE

The theory of innate motive processes helps explain pervasive developmental disorders of childhood that affect the integrity of the psychological subject and interfere with active orientation to the environment[51]. Most congenital disorders of brain function and their development are characterized by failure of motivation for relating to the psychology of people or 'intersubjectivity'. This has led Gillberg[50] to describe a spectrum of *empathy disorders*. Anomalies of development in the motivating and emotional systems in the embryo brain are mainly of genetic origin[52], but there is little evidence for simple, consistent effects of mutations in single genes. Disorders of psychology and behavior are the consequence of interactions between genes and complex epigenetic events, such as regulation of gene expression by sex hormones and monoamines transmitted between neurons, as well as effects from environmental stimulation[16], but evidence is accumulating that many originate very early in brain development. Core affective problems, including the autistic spectrum disorders and schizophrenia, frequently have a genetic component, and autism has associations with genetic disorders of brain development[53,54]. Autism, Asperger's syndrome, some forms of epilepsy and schizophrenia are associated with abnormal cell migration in early stages of the formation of the cerebral cortex or cerebellum[55].

Children with a cognitive handicap, as in the genetic disorders of William's syndrome, Down's syndrome and Rett syndrome, also have impairments in their social reactions, joint attention and communication about objects[1]. Non-verbal interpersonal communication, joint attention with sharing of spatial reference and affective exchange are crucial in the early development of both language and thinking. It is not surprising, therefore, that deficiencies in non-verbal communication[56] distinguish both empathic disorders and varieties of mental handicap.

Children with autism, like a majority of profoundly mentally handicapped children, including girls with Rett syndrome, respond positively to a basal level of human expression; in almost every case, their alertness and motivation can be captured by music or movement therapy[51]. This is evidence for retention of the subcortical system for co-ordination of motives with other persons which animates play between a mother and a young infant.

References

1. Trevarthen, C. and Aitken, K. J. (1994). Brain development, infant communication, and empathy disorders: intrinsic factors in child mental health. *Dev. Psychopathol.,* **6**, 599–635
2. Trevarthen, C. (1993). The function of emotions in early infant communication and development. In Nadel, J. and Camaioni, L. (eds.) *New Perspectives in Early Communicative Development,* pp. 48–81. (London: Routledge)
3. Trevarthen, C. (1993). The self born in intersubjectivity: an infant communicating. In Neisser, U. (ed.) *The Perceived Self: Ecological and Interpersonal Sources of Self-Knowledge,* pp. 121–73. (New York: Cambridge University Press)
4. De Casper, A. J. and Fifer, W. P. (1980). Of human bonding: newborns prefer their mother's voices. *Science,* **208**, 1174–6
5. De Casper, A. J. and Carstens, A. A. (1981). Contingencies of stimulation; effects on learning and emotion in neonates. *Infant Behav. Dev.,* **4**, 19–35
6. Field, T. M., Woodson, R., Greenberg, R. and Cohen, D. (1982). Discrimination and imitation of facial expressions by neonates. *Science,* **218**, 179–81
7. Heimann, M. and Schaller, J. (1985). Imitative reactions among 14–21-day-old infants. *Infant Ment. Health J.,* **6**(1), 31–9

8. Kugiumutzakis, G. (1993). Intersubjective vocal imitation in early mother-infant interaction. In Nadel, J. and Camaioni, L. (eds.) *New Perspectives in Early Communicative Development*, pp. 23–47. (London: Routledge)

9. Maratos, O. (1982). Trends in development of imitation in early infancy. In Bever, T. G. (ed.) *Regressions in Mental Development: Basis Phenomena and Theories*, pp. 81–101. (Hillsdale, NJ: Erlbaum)

10. Meltzoff, A. N. and Moore, M. H. (1977). Imitation of facial and manual gestures by human neonates. *Science*, 198, 75–8

11. Meltzoff, A. N. and Moore, M. K. (1992). Early imitation within a functional framework: the importance of personal identity, movement and development. *Infant Behav. Dev.*, 15, 479–505

12. Trevarthen, C. (1977). Descriptive analyses of infant communication behaviour. In Schaffer, H. R. (ed.) *Studies in Mother-Infant Interaction: The Loch Lomond Symposium*, pp. 227–70. (London: Academic Press)

13. Trevarthen, C., Kokkinaki, T. and Fiamenghi, G. A. Jr (1997). What infants' imitations communicate: with mothers, with fathers and with peers. In Nadel, J. and Butterworth, G. (eds.) *Imitation in Infancy*, in press. (Cambridge: Cambridge University Press)

14. Brazelton, T. B. (1979). Evidence of communication during neonatal behavioral assessment. In Bullowa, M. (ed.) *Before Speech: The Beginnings of Human Communication*, pp. 79–88. (London: Cambridge University Press)

15. Klaus, M. H. and Kennell, J. H. (1976). *Maternal-Infant Bonding: The Impact of Early Separation or Loss on Family Development*. (St Louis: C. V. Mosby)

16. Schore, A. N. (1994). *Affect Regulation and the Origin of the Self: The Neurobiology of Emotional Development*. (Hillsdale, NJ: Erlbaum)

17. Schanberg, S. M. and Field, T. M. (1987). Sensory deprivation, stress and supplemental stimulation in the rat pup and preterm human neonate. *Child Dev.*, 58, 1431–47

18. Hofer, M. A. (1990). Early symbiotic processes: hard evidence from a soft place. In Glick, R. A. and Bone, S. (eds.) *Pleasure Beyond the Pleasure Principle*, pp. 55–78. (Newhaven, CT: Yale University Press)

19. Bateson, M. C. (1979). 'The epigenesis of conversational interaction': a personal account of research and development. In Bullowa, M. (ed.) *Before Speech: The Beginnings of Human Communication*, pp. 63–77. (London: Cambridge University Press)

20. Trevarthen, C. (1979). Communication and cooperation in early infancy. A description of primary intersubjectivity. In Bullowa, M. (ed.) *Before Speech: The Beginnings of Human Communication*, pp. 321–47. (London: Cambridge University Press)

21. Trevarthen, C., Murray, L. and Hubley, P. (1981). Psychology of infants. In Davis, J. and Dobbing, J. (eds.) *Scientific Foundations of Clinical Paediatrics*, 2nd edn., pp. 235–50. (London: W. Heinemann Medical Books)

22. Fernald, A. (1989). Intonation and communicative interest in mother's speech to infants: is the melody the message? *Child Dev.*, 60, 1497–510

23. Grieser, D. L. and Kuhl, P. K. (1988). Maternal speech to infants in a tonal language: support for universal prosodic features in motherese. *Dev. Psychol.*, 24, 14–20

24. Papousek, M. and Papousek, H. (1981). Musical elements in the infants vocalization: their significance for communication, cognition and creativity. In Lipsitt, L. P. and Rovee-Collier, C. K. (eds.) *Advances in Infancy Research*, Vol. 1, pp. 163–224. (Norwood, NJ: Ablex)

25. Stern, D. N., Spieker, S. and MacKain, K. (1982). Intonation contours as signals in maternal speech to prelinguistic infants. *Dev. Psychol.*, 18, 727–35

26. Trehub, S. E., Trainor, L. J. and Unyk, A. M. (1993). Music and speech processing in the first year of life. *Adv. Child Dev. Behav.*, 24, 1–35

27. Stern, D. N. (1985). *The Interpersonal World of the Infant*. (New York: Basic Books)

28. Stern, D. N. (1993). The role of feelings for an interpersonal self. In Neisser, U. (ed.) *The Perceived Self: Ecological and Interpersonal Sources of Self-Knowledge*, pp. 205–215. (New York: Cambridge University Press)

29. Beebe, B., Jaffe, J., Feldstein, S., Mays, K. and Alson, D. (1985). Inter-personal timing: the application of an adult dialogue model to mother-infant vocal and kinesic interactions. In Field, F. M. and Fox, N. (eds.) *Social Perception in Infants*, pp. 217–48 (Norwood, NJ: Ablex)

30. Mayer, N. K. and Tronick, E. Z. (1985). Mothers' turn-giving signals and infant turn-taking in mother-infant interaction. In Field, F. M. and Fox, N. (eds.) *Social Perception in Infants*, pp. 199–216. (Norwood NJ: Ablex)

31. Stern, D. N., Beebe, B., Jaffe, J. and Bennett, S. L. (1977). The infant's stimulus world during social interaction: a study of caregiver behaviors with particular reference to repetition and timing. In Schaffer, H. R. (ed.) *Studies in Mother-Infant Interaction*, pp. 177–202. (New York: Academic Press)

32. Bråten, S. (1992). The virtual other in infant's minds and social feelings. In Wold, A. H. (ed.) *The Dialogical Alternative* (Festschrift for Ragnar

Rommetveit), pp. 77–97. (Oslo/Oxford: Scandanavian University Press/Oxford University Press)

33. Lecanuet, J.-P., Fifer, W. P., Krasnegor, N. A. and Smotherman, W. P. (eds.) (1995). *Foetal Development: A Psychobiological Perspective.* (Hillsdale, NJ: Lawrence Erlbaum)

34. Cioni, G. and Castellaci, A. M. (1990). Development of fetal and neonatal motor activity: implications for neurology. In Block, H. and Bertenthal, B. (eds.) *Sensory-Motor Organization and Development in Infancy and Early Childhood.* (Dordrecht: Kluwer)

35. de Vries, J. I. P., Visser, G. H. A. and Prechtl, H. F. R. (1984). Fetal motility in first half of pregnancy. In Prechtl, H. F. R. (ed.) *Continuity of Neural Functions from Prenatal to Postnatal Life,* pp. 46–64. (Oxford: Blackwell)

36. Piontelli, A. (1992). *From Fetus to Child.* (London: Routledge)

37. Trevarthen, C. (1996). Lateral asymmetries in infancy: implications for the development of the hemispheres. *Neurosci. Biobehav. Rev.,* **20**, 571–86

38. O'Rahilly, R. and Müller, F. (1994) *The Embryonic Human Brain: An Atlas of Developmental Stages.* (New York: Wiley-Liss)

39. Rakic, P. (1991). Development of the primate cerebral cortex. In Lewis, M. (ed.) *Child and Adolescent Psychiatry: A Comprehensive Textbook,* pp. 11–28. (Baltimore: Williams and Wilkins)

40. Trevarthen, C. (1986). Development of intersubjective motor control in infants. In Wade, M. G. and Whiting, H. T. A. (eds.) *Motor Development in Children: Aspects of Coordination and Control,* pp. 209–61. (Dordrecht: Martinus Nijhof)

41. Jürgens, U. (1979). Neural control of vocalization in non-human primates. In Steklis, H. D. and Raleigh, M. J. (eds.) *Neurobiology of Social Communication in Primates: An Evolutionary Perspective,* pp. 11–44. (New York: Academic Press)

42. Ploog, D. (1992). Neuroethological perspectives on the human brain: from the expression of emotions to intentional signing and speech. In Harrington, A. (ed.) *So Human a Brain,* pp. 3–13. (Boston: Birkhäuser)

43. Ross, E. D. (1993). Nonverbal aspects of language. *Neurol. Clin.,* **11**, 9–23

44. Kimura, D. (1982). Left-hemisphere control of oral and brachial movements and their relation to communication. *Phil. Trans. R. Soc. London, Series B,* **298**, 135–49

45. Tucker, D. M. (1992). Developing emotions and cortical networks. In Gunnar, M. R. and Nelson, C. A. (eds.) *Minnesota Symposium on Child Psychology,* Vol. 24, *Developmental Behavioral Neuroscience,* pp. 75–128. (Hillsdale, NJ: Erlbaum)

46. Murray, L. and Trevarthen, C. (1985). Emotional regulation of interactions between two-month-olds and their mothers. In Field, T. M. and Fox, N. A. (eds.) *Social Perception in Infants,* pp. 177–98. (Norwood, NJ: Ablex)

47. Trevarthen, C. (1986). Form, significance and psychological potential of hand gestures of infants. In Nespoulous, J.-L., Perron, P. and Lecours, A. R. (eds.) *The Biological Foundation of Gestures: Motor and Semiotic Aspects,* pp. 149–202. (Hillsdale, NJ: Erlbaum)

48. Davidson, R. J. and Fox, N. A. (1982). Asymmetric brain activity discriminates between positive and negative affective simuli in human infants. *Science,* **218**, 1235–7

49. Thatcher, R. W., Walker, R. A. and Giudice, S. (1987). Human cerebral hemispheres develop at different rates and ages. *Science,* **236**, 1110–13

50. Gillberg, C. (1991). The Emanuel Miller Memorial Lecture. Autism and autistic-like conditions: subclasses among disorders of empathy. *J. Child Psychol. Psychiatr.,* **33**, 813–42

51. Trevarthen, C., Aitken, K. J., Papoudi, D. and Robarts, J. (1996). *Children with Autism: Diagnosis and Interventions to Meet their Needs.* (London: Jessica Kingsley)

52. Lyon, G. and Gadisseux, J.-F. (1991). Structural abnormalities of the brain in developmental disorders. In Rutter, M. and Casaer, P. (eds.) *Biological Risk Factors for Psychosocial Disorders,* pp. 1–19. (Cambridge: Cambridge University Press)

53. Bauman, M. L. and Kemper, T. L. (eds.) (1994). *The Neurobiology of Autism.* (Baltimore: Johns Hopkins Press)

54. Rutter, M. (1991). Autism as a genetic disorder. In McGuffin, P. and Murray, R. (eds.) *The New Genetics of Mental Illness,* pp. 225–44. (Oxford: Butterworth-Heinemann)

55. Barth, P. G. (1992). Migrational disorders of the brain. *Curr. Opin. Neurol. Neurosurg.,* **5**, 339–43

56. Mundy, P., Kasari, C. and Sigman, M. (1992). Nonverbal communication, affective sharing, and intersubjectivity. *Infant Behav. Dev.,* **15**, 377–81

Neonatal psychology: system development

49

E. N. Adamson-Macedo

INTRODUCTION

The 1890 definition of psychology given by W. James defies improvement: 'the science of mental life, both its phenomena and of their conditions. The phenomena are such things as we call feelings, desires, cognition, reasoning, decisions and the like'. As a sub-discipline of medicine, neonatology is concerned with the newborn; of particular importance are the at-risk babies, including those likely to suffer developmental disabilities in the month after birth. Following James and the theories of Gottlieb[1], this paper defines neonatal psychology as 'the scientific study of the phenomena of mental life and the behavior of the preterm neonate as an emergent, coactional, hierarchical system'.

Precursory to mental life is *mind*, for which direct evidence is evasive because of different definitions of mind, as pointed out by Hepper and Shahidullah[2]. It is nevertheless clear that foundations of mind are laid down during fetal development with billions of neurons forming their connections, and with neural activity and stimulation crucial to completing this process[3]. A century ago, Preyer[4] emphasized that the fundamental activities of the mind, as they later become manifest, do originate before birth; this approach remains uncontested and Karmiloff-Smith[5] recently stated 'cognitive development starts in the womb. During the final 3 months of intrauterine life, the fetus is capable of extracting invariant patterns across the complex auditory input that is filtered through the amniotic fluid'.

For any developmental age, evidence continues to accumulate that the time spent in the womb is critical for normal development and function of the mind. In preterm cases, the abrupt interruption of womb experiences can be terminal for a few, whereas for others their normal rate of growth and development can be jeopardized. The recent emergence of neonatal psychology indicates that the time has come for psychology to make an effective contribution to both the theory and the care of the preterm neonate.

This paper presents an integrative approach in order to explain the psychoneurobiological development of the preterm neonate. The Equilibrium Model is proposed as a way of representing positive coactions; within this frame, Gottlieb's experiential canalization[6] contributes explanation of how the development of the preterm neonate can be facilitated.

PRETERMS: FETUSES OR UNDERDEVELOPED TERM INFANTS?

In the 1970s and early 1980s, two distinct views of the preterm were offered, each based on theories of preterm neurobehavioral development. In the first, preterms were seen as fetuses, each one expected to have the same developmental level as that of a fetus of equivalent gestational age; in the second, preterms were seen as underdeveloped term babies.

Investigators who held the first view sought to mimic the womb environment by providing tactile–kinesthetic or auditory stimulation[7]. Results suggested that simple changes in the physical environment could improve physical and neurobehavioral outcomes of the preterm baby;

as a consequence, oscillating waterbeds were introduced[8], lighting was reduced[9], heart beat recordings and other intrauterine sounds were used[10]. In Britain, a simple enhancement of the baby's environment, known as 'nursing the baby with lambswool', was investigated, and also showed an increase in growth rate of the infants[11].

Those who held the view of the preterm as an underdeveloped fullterm, exposed the babies to visual, auditory and tactile experiences which were appropriate for a normal newborn, e.g. bright shapes, faces, mobiles, recording of mother's speech, and so on[7,12]. Positive growth and developmental outcomes have been reported, including weight gain, decrease in the incidence of physical complications (especially respiratory difficulties), reduction of apnea attacks, decreased crying, and faster developmental progress.

A third approach was intermediate in that stimulation was advocated which was a mimic of both the womb and the environment of the term infants[13-18]. Whichever of these three viewpoints was adopted, early work always viewed the preterm infants as sensory-deprived, i.e. the so-called deficit model. In the 1980s suggestions were made, for example by Gottfried[19], that rather than being sensory-deprived the reality was that the preterms were sensory-bombarded. In consequence, Macedo[20] advocated an approach within which the preterm infant should experience adequate and appropriate sensory stimulation. In the late 1980s new disciplines of environmental neonatology were proposed by Gottfried and Gaiter[21], and environmental and developmental neonatology by Wolke[22].

The literature of this period shows outcomes only being reported, without attempts being made to explain any underlying mechanism(s). Moreover, both concurrent and immediately subsequent responses to stimulation were only sparsely reported[19]. One study carried out on infants nursed with lambswool did advance the thesis that the infant's increase in growth rate was due to less energy expenditure, since the babies investigated were shown to be calmer than controls; the authors also suggested addi-

tional positive effects such as improvement of the image of the baby in the eyes of the parents and other care-givers[11].

The meaning of a preterm baby's response had been recognized as problematic[23]. Although the observation and recording of how infants react, behaviorally and physiologically, to different types of stimulation has been firmly recommended[19], the use of response interpretations to argue for the benefits of interventions has hitherto been tenuous[24].

The state of the babies during treatment is very significant and should always be reported[25]; state is the first control of the newborn[26], and is capable of changing the environment[27-32]. As Thoman[33] has pointed out, 'state acts as a prelude, a mediator and an elicitor, as well as the context for any interaction that occurs between the infant and his mother'. Based on a combination of eye movements, body movements and heart rate, four behavioral states[34] have been identified in the newborn. These states have been observed from 36 weeks' gestation age (GA)[35], and it has been argued that they represent considerable integration between the various centers of the nervous system. The start of *mind* may coincide with this time, although it may well begin much earlier, e.g. 8 weeks' GA, as suggested from work carried out with the fetus[2].

The beginning of *mind* was considered by Carmichael[36] as being that time when the individual first responds to an external stimulus, and may range from 8 to 26 weeks' GA depending on the sense chosen. Taking into account studies on movements, sensory abilities and fetal learning, *mind* is here accepted as the ability to interact with either internal, external or with both stimuli. At birth, in the prematurely delivered baby, being neither a fetus nor an underdeveloped infant, the mind of the preterm baby has already emerged; moreover, the learning of preterms has recently been studied[37]. It follows that the sense of 'self' considered by Stern[38] to be a developmental organizing principle, is experienced by infants from birth. It has been pointed out by Gottlieb[39] that 'experience' is a relational term used for designating coactions, which are important to the regulation of the self.

THE CONCEPT OF SELF-REGULATION

Regulation implies adaptation of the organism from one to another stable level of order, subsequent to some change in the input. Whatever the input stimuli, a variety of messages are also generated within the organism and thereafter transmitted by physicochemical means and neural systems which may be regarded as the internal feedback loops. Viewed as a system, the successful organism is a complex adaptive system which selects, rejects, incorporates, or initiates responses. Such an organism operates with self-regulation and is rarely in a steady state, as noted by von Bertalanffy in 1934[40]. Later than this, a working definition of self-regulation[41] was given as 'a dynamic process of adaptive functioning operating through a large number of individually distinct mechanisms which may be hierarchically arranged or classified'.

Adaptive change ranges from self-regulation at the cellular level[42] to issues of child/care-giver communications; thus Krauss[43] recognized that self-regulatory principles are general characteristics common from the genome up to psychological behaviors and 'to be found in both organic and cognitive behaviors'. Other relevant viewpoints are those of Greenspan[44] on self-regulation relating to structure, Vygotsky[45,46] on function, Gedo[47] on developmental aim for a particular phase, Lichtenberg[48] and Stern[38] on relational processes, and Emde[49] on biopsychological principles.

Examples of relevant animal studies, which sought to elucidate the role of early sensory stimulation on self-regulation, or on the lack of it, may be quoted[50-63]. More intractable have been human studies with similar aims, but examples[11,20,64-71] can also be given from the last three decades. Self-regulatory constructs are now being used in many sub-disciplines of psychology, e.g. health psychology/behavioral medicine, and experimental psychology.

SYSTEMS APPROACH TO DEVELOPMENTAL PSYCHOLOGY

For a system of any degree of complexity to be studied, its envelope or boundaries must be defined; thereafter two elementary conditions are required in that the dynamical system's behavior must be both closed and single-valued. In principle, the system must be seen to be closed in order that an operator inducing change or transition in a set of operands produces detectable and unambiguous transformations; moreover, the system should have been so defined that these transformations are single-valued, i.e. the stable system cannot occupy two states simultaneously either before or after the operator causing change. It will be observed that such definition corresponds to the prior conditions for successful experimentation and, generally, subsequent analysis.

During the past decade, developmental psychology has witnessed a renaissance of interest in the study of the relations between genes and behavior. Corresponding system analysis in developmental psychology includes rationales and theories which have been called ecological[72], transactional[73,74], contextual[75], interactive[76,77], probabilistic–epigenetic[78], individual–sociological[79], and structural–behavioral[80].

As defined by Gottlieb, epigenesis is probabilistic, and his particular system view of development sees the individual as an 'emergent, coactional, hierarchical system'. This definition of epigenesis declares that 'individual development is characterized by an increase of complexity of organization, i.e. the emergence of new structural and functional properties and competencies – at all levels of analysis (molecular, subcellular, cellular, organismic) as a consequence of horizontal and vertical coactions among its parts, including organism–environment coactions'[39].

Horizontal coactions are those which occur at the same level, e.g. gene to gene, cell to cell; vertical coactions occur at different levels, e.g. gene–cytoplasm, behavioral activity–nervous system, and are reciprocal in that they can influence each other in either direction. Thus the sensory experience of a developing organism affects the differentiation of its nerve cells such that the more experience produces the more differentiation and vice versa. The more highly differentiated nervous system permits a greater degree of behavioral competency and the less differentiated nervous system permits a lesser degree of behavioral competency.

Gottlieb's system view[6,81] of individual development defends the principle that 'canalization can take place not only at genetic level, but at all levels of the developing system, ... including the developing organism's usually occurring experiences. What makes development happen is the relationship of the two or more components and not the components themselves'. Gottlieb's principal claim[6,81] is that genetic activity does not mediate behavior by itself but rather is part of a larger genes–behavior–environment grouping that interacts in complex ways to produce finished traits.

The bidirectionality of structure–function relationships is paramount. The hierarchical, reciprocal, and coactive definition of epigenesis holds for anatomical, physiological, behavioral and psychological functioning; according to Gottlieb[1,6,39,81], coactions or experiences can play different roles in anatomical, physiological and behavioral development, i.e. maintenance, facilitative and induction functions. Within this frame, positive coactions are here defined as those appropriate experiences of the preterm baby which are crucial in order that development should occur.

Since developing systems continually change, statements of causality involve time[39], with appropriate and positive coactions occurring when the stimulation is relevant to the needs and actions of the baby. On such occasions, the organism temporarily reaches equilibrium. Hitherto there has not been a conceptual model to illustrate the coactions between the various systems of the infant born too early, when viewed as 'an emergent, coactional and hierarchical developing system'.

THE EQUILIBRIUM MODEL

Origin and representation

In the case of the ventilated preterm infant, the opposing forces to be brought to equilibrium[82] are the organismic and psychological conditions, as well as the environmental constraints. The choices to be made of a particular sensory stimulating and its timing are critical: they are certainly not simple due to the controversy around intersensory perception. Yet it is these factors which maintain and enhance function integration, and support growth and development[83,84]. Consequently, the hypothesis is that an appropriate intervention, when offered to the infant at an optimum time, induces positive coactions:

(1) Horizontally, between the sensory stimulation–sensory system;

(2) Vertically, between the sensory stimulation–neuro-behavioral (NB), immunological (IM), and endocrinological/physiological (E/P) systems.

Three theories currently prevail to explain the phenomenon of intermodal perception. Two of these are: integration[85–88] which asserts that the senses are independent at birth; and differentiation or invariant detection[89,90] which advocates that the senses are unified at birth. The third is the intensity hypothesis[91–93], favored by the author of this paper, which draws elements from the previous two theories; it defends the proposition that multimodal relations can be detected early in development and that, with experience, infants can discern characteristics of stimulation ranging from the quantitative such as size, brightness, loudness, duration or rate of stimulation, to the qualitative such as rhythm, melody, texture or shape.

The positive coactions promoting temporary equilibrium are susceptible to representation on orthogonal axes. For example, should the sense of touch be the appropriate stimulation for the ventilated preterm infant, the vertical coactions consequently expected would be positive, i.e. the behavioral system would organize itself, the physiological system would stabilize, the endocrinological system would be balanced, and the immunological system would be 'enhanced'. It is thus helpful to display NB, IM and E/P geometrically, as shown notionally in Figure 1. It should be noted that the units in the three defined directions are not the same, but correspond to the specific measurements appropriate to the individual axes, the three scales being arbitrary but consistent.

Phenomena represented on these axes have been separately tested by using the sense of touch but with different types of stimuli such as handling, rubbing, massage, gentle human touch (GHT) or the gentle/light and systematic stroking known as touching and caressing–tender in caring (TAC–TIC) therapy. For infants born preterm, examples of studies which

demonstrate the occurrence of positive horizontal and/or vertical coactions are given below.

E/P axis

Endocrinological axes   In 1979[62], an enzymatic–hormonal mechanism was suggested as the mediator of physical benefits associated with tactile programs. More recently, de Roiste and Bushnell[68] measured stomach lipase concentration, i.e. lingual and gastric lipase before and after tactile stimulation; these researchers also measured gastric pH in order to determine the effect of tactile stimulation on hydrochloric acid (HCl) concentration. Overall results[68] suggested that gentle/light stroking improves gastro-intestinal functioning in preterm infants and that 'better digestion and greater nutrient absorption is facilitated by stroking prior to feeds'. References 11, 63, 64, 67 and 94 provide other examples.

Physiological axes   In 1996, it was reported that gentle human touch (GHT), when provided for 15 min daily, did not have adverse effects on the oxygen saturation of small preterm infants[95]; in 1994, 81 sessions of TAC–TIC therapy were administered to 11 ventilated small preterm infants; the results showed stabilization of oxygen saturation[69]. References 66, 67 and 96 provide other examples.

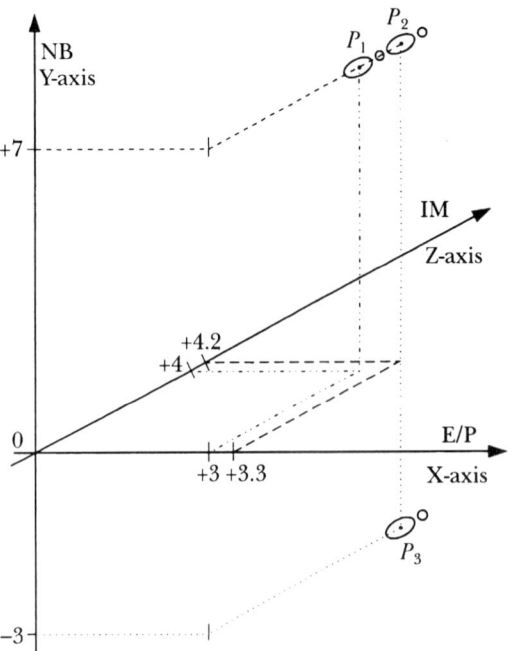

Figure 1   The Equilibrium Model, representing the positive coactions which promote temporary equilibrium in the ventilated preterm. NB, neurobehavioral; IM immunological; E/P, endocrinological/physiological; P_n, point representing condition of baby

IM axis

Immunological axes   Interest increases in investigating such coactions and in other organic and psychological systems; ongoing work conducted by Hayes, Adamson-Macedo and Perera[71] is showing that secretory immunoglobulin A (SIgA) can be detected during the first week of life of the very small ventilated preterm, and is suggesting that concentrations of SIgA are greater 3 min after intervention by gentle/light stroking, or TAC–TIC therapy. These results are being compared with baseline phase and a control condition in which the infants undergo spontaneous activities in their incubators.

NB axis

Neuro-behavioral axes Systematic studies which observe and record both behavior and behavioral state, prior to and during intervention, are rare. In the author's experience, gentle/light stroking tends to elicit a greater number of organizing rather than disorganizing behaviors, and this may indicate that positive coactions are occurring[97]. Other studies show negative coactions, i.e. disorganized behaviors as a consequence of other kinds of touch intervention[25,66,95]; these results are questionable, however, since the interventions employed do not appear to be systematic. In any event, the results of different studies are not directly comparable and the area remains controversial.

In studying the mediational role of sensory stimulation in promoting positive coactions, several variables need to be taken into account, such as gestational age (GA), birth weight (BW), gender, behavioral state or morbidity status, as well as quantitative and qualitative dimensions of the sensory stimulus itself. Systematic and well controlled studies which investigate intramodal (e.g. deep versus light stroking) variability have not hitherto been carried out.

There was no evidence that the 'touch' stimulation used by some of the authors above had deleterious effects such as increase in cortisol level[67], sharp fall in transcutaneous PO_2[66,67,69,95,96], decrease in secretory immunoglobulin A (SIgA)[71], or significantly higher frequency of disorganized behavior[97]; consequently, one can hypothesize that positive coactions are occurring within the sensory system of the preterm baby and between the sensory system and the baby's other systems. Current research by this author and associates is testing three axes simultaneously; this is sufficient for practical purposes, but a more complex way of representing the model is given in equation (4), below.

Geometric representation of the Equilibrium Model

In order to display the Equilibrium Model, the notation of three-dimensional co-ordinate geo-metry has been adapted. $P_n = n_1 X + n_2 Y + n_3 Z$, where n_1, n_2 and n_3 simply represent values on the three orthogonal axes $X (= E/P)$, $Y (= NB)$ and $Z (= IM)$; P_n is a point representing the condition of the baby on the diagram, as in Figure 1; $n_1 X$, $n_2 Y$, $n_3 Z$ are not algebraic products, but simply indicate positions or locations n_1, n_2, n_3, each to the measurement regime and scale adopted for its respective axis.

Equation (1) depicts a notional situation in arbitrary units where E/P response $= + 3$, behavior $= + 7$, and immunological resistance $= + 4$:

$$P_1 = 3X + 7Y + 4Z \tag{1}$$

As a further example, should the baby's behavior pattern remain at $+ 7$, but endocrinological/physiological and immunological responses improve by 10% and 5%, respectively, equation (1) would then become

$$P_2 = 3.3X + 7Y + 4.2Z \tag{2}$$

There is a conceptual problem whenever the baby is in a distressed condition before treatment, since this is represented by a negative value on the behavior axis; this is not a problem with adoption of the notation of the three-dimensional space equations (1) and (2). Thus, if the IM and E/P values remain as given in equation (2), but the behavioral index is poor (i.e. negative) at a value of -3, the graphical representation would become

$$P_3 = 3.3X - 3Y + 4.2Z \tag{3}$$

This geometric method of representation in the form of a space equation may be extended felicitously; its superiority is manifest whenever it is desired to represent four or more parameters. For example, data may be forthcoming from specific endocrinological as distinct from endocrinological/physiological measurements. This enables the E/P axis to be divided into two, the X-axis being retained for physiological phenomena, P.

The interaction of the endocrine system, E may now be given on a W-axis; effectively, there are now four axes in a four-dimensional space, a situation impossible to represent on orthogonal axes, as well as being conceptually difficult for the human mind. However, by extending the notation adopted above, the conceptual problem disappears and the geometrical representation of Figure 1 may be discarded; by adding a fourth term W to represent endocrinological effects E in, say, equation (3) and assigning an arbitrary value of + 2.5:

$$P_4 = 2.5W + 3.3X - 3Y + 4.2Z \qquad (4)$$

CONCLUSIONS AND OBSERVATIONS

The Equilibrium Model and its representations described here fulfill the requirements stipulated by Munro[98] who emphasized, 'although it is common to find diverse phenomena included in single formulations (e.g. the linking of immune function to mental effects, or social behavior to cognition), the nature of the linkage is typically obscure because, as Harré, Clarke, and de Carlo point out, there is no organizing conceptual framework such as one finds in the physical sciences'.

The model is compatible with Gottlieb's[6,81,99,100] theory of experiential canalization of behavioral development, with sociogenesis[44,101], and with Munro's[98] proposition of a model of integration rather than reduction in order to explain important phenomena of interest to psychology; it is supportive of the proposal of Wilson, Fel and Greenstein[102] for an integrative approach to self-regulation.

Sociogenesis holds that all higher psychological processes, such as learning, cognition, and personality are results of early social interactions. This concept has been recently used in the animal literature[100]. For example, social induction of malleability in ducklings has been studied; it was found that malleability was absent when ducklings were tactually isolated from one another. The experimental results indicated that tactile contact, even when provided by stuffed ducklings, is the sensory basis of malleability[100].

Careful and systematic observations of the incubated infant, which is temporarily his/her natural social ecological context, may lead to the acquisition of new ways of understanding human development within an integrative perspective. Interdisciplinary complexity of the phenomena of behavior and mentation requires a systematic approach which recognizes the interrelationships between the various non-independent variables; simplistic single stimulus/response models are quite insufficient and frequently erroneous. The hypotheses proposed in this paper should be further tested; the model could be extended to other phenomena such as measure of affect regulation[103] and intersubjective relatedness[104].

No single branch of neuroscience or of psychology, or other related discipline, can scientifically understand behavior and mentation; as Bunge[105] pointed out, 'the problem is a multi-level one, and this is because man exists on all levels'. To overcome such a difficulty, a systemic approach is manifestly necessary.

The aim of the Equilibrium Model is to establish a display and/or systematic format, as appropriate, for the interactive association of the individual self-regulatory mechanisms of the preterm infant, and so contribute to the theory and practice of neonatal psychology. The model is presently in use and fulfils two important functions:

(1) A method for illustrating self-regulatory phenomena in which the various relationships which contribute to self-regulation become easier to comprehend.

(2) An experimental framework from which further predictions and postulates may emerge more readily than would otherwise be the case, thereby leading to the design of systematically-formulated experiments, and towards a unified theory of development of the preterm neonate viewed as an emergent, coactional and hierarchical developing system.

References

1. Gottlieb, G. (1976). The roles of experience in the development of behavior and the nervous system. In Gottlieb, G. (ed.) *Neural and Behavioral Specificity*, pp. 25–50. (New York: Academic Press)

2. Hepper, P. G. and Shahidullah, S. (1994). The beginnings of mind – evidence from the behaviour of the fetus. *J. Reprod. Infant Psychol.*, **12**, 143–54

3. Shatz, C. J. (1992). The developing brain. *Scientif. Am.*, **267**(3), 35–41

4. Preyer, W. (1888). *The Mind of the Child. Part 1. The Senses and the Will.* (New York: Appleton)

5. Karmiloff-Smith, A. (1995). Annotation: the extraordinary cognitive journey from foetus through infancy. *J. Child Psychol. Psychiatry*, **36**(8), 1293–313

6. Gottlieb, G. (1991). Experiential canalization of behavioral development: theory. *Dev. Psychol.*, **27**(1), 4–13

7. Masi, W. (1979). Supplemental stimulation of the premature infant. In Field, T. M. (ed.) *Infants Born at Risk: Behavior and Development*, pp. 367–87. (New York: Spectrum Publications)

8. Korner, A. F., Rappel, E. M. and Rho, J. M. (1982). Effects of waterbeds on sleep and motility of theophylline-treated preterm infants. *Pediatrics*, **70**, 864–9

9. Als, H. (1986). Synactive model of neonatal behavioral organization: framework for the assessment and support of the neurobehavioural development of the premature infant and his parents in the environment of the neonatal intensive care unit. In Sweeney, J. K. (ed.) *The High-Risk Neonate: Developmental Therapy Perspectives*, pp. 3–55. (New York: The Haworth Press)

10. Wolke, D. (1987). Environmental and developmental neonatology. *J. Reprod. Infant Psychol.*, **5**, 17–42

11. Scott, S. and Richards, M. P. M. (1979). Nursing low-birthweight babies on lambswool. *Lancet*, **1**, 12 May, 1028

12. Field, T. M. (1980). Interactions of high-risk infants: quantitative and qualitative differences. In Sawin, D. B., Hawkins, R. C., Walker, L. O. and Penticuff, J. H. (eds.) *Psychosocial Risks in Infant–Environment Transactions*, 4, pp. 120–43. (New York: Brunner/Mazel)

13. Rice, R. D. (1977). Neurophysiological development in premature infants following stimulation. *Dev. Psychol.*, **13**(1), 69–76

14. Rice, R. D. (1979). The effects of the Rice infant sensorimotor stimulation treatment on the development of high-risk infants. *Birth Defects. Original Article Series*, **XV**(7), 7–26

15. Siqueland, E. R. (1973). Biological and experiential determinants of exploration in infancy. In Stone, L., Smith, H. and Murphy, C. (eds.) *The Competent Infant*, pp. 822–3 (New York: Basic Books)

16. Kramer, L. I. and Pierpont, M. S. (1976). Rocking waterbeds and auditory stimuli to enhance growth of preterm infants. *J. Pediatr.*, **88**, 297–9

17. Groom, G. (1973). Effects of perinatal factors and supplemental stimulation of premature infants upon measures of cognitive behavior. In Field, T. M. (ed.) *Infants Born at Risk*, p. 372. (New York: Spectrum Publications)

18. McNichol, T. (1975). Some effects of different programs of enrichment on the development of premature infants in the hospital nursery. In Field, T. M. (ed.) *Infants Born at Risk*, p. 373. (New York: Spectrum Publications)

19. Gottfried, A. W. (1981). Environmental manipulations in the neonatal period and assessment of their effects. In Smeriglio, V. L. (ed.) *Newborns and Parents: Parent-Infant Contact and Newborn Sensory Stimulation.* (Hillsdale, NJ: Erlbaum)

20. Macedo, E. N. (1981). The effects of a tactile stimulation programme on pre-term infants. Presented at the *Annual Conference of the British Psychological Society Postgraduate Psychology*, University of Durham. *BPS Bulletin* (1982), March, 121

21. Gottfried, A. W. and Gaiter, J. L. (1985). *Infant Stress Under Intensive Care.* (Baltimore: University Park Press)

22. Wolke, D. (1987). Environmental neonatology. *Arch. Dis. Child.*, **62**, 987–8

23. Lewis, N. (1967). The meaning of a response, or why researchers in infant behavior should be Oriental metaphysicians. *Merrill-Palmer Q.*, **13**, 7–18

24. Cornell, E. and Gottfried, A. (1976). Interventions with premature infants. *Child Dev.*, **48**, 152–7

25. Eckerman, C. O. and Oehler, J. M. (1992). Very-low-birthweight newborns and parents as early social partners. In Friedman, S. L. and Sigman, M. D. (eds.) *The Psychological Development of Low Birthweight Children – Annual Advances in Applied Developmental Psychology*, 6,

pp. 91–123. (Norwood, NJ: Able Publishing Corporation)

26. Brazelton, T. B. (1983). Precursors for the development of emotions in early infancy. In Plutchik, R. and Kellerman, H. (eds.) *Emotion, Theory, Research, and Experiences*, 2, pp. 35–55. (London: Academic Press)

27. Gregg, G. L., Haffner, M. E. and Korner, A. F. (1976). The relative efficacy of vestibular-proprioceptive stimulation and the upright position in enhancing visual pursuit in neonates. *Child Dev.*, **47**, 309–14

28. Escalona, S. (1984). Social and other environmental influences on the cognitive and personality development of low-birthweight infants. *Am. J. Ment. Def.*, **88**(5), 508–12

29. Brazelton, T. B. (1973). Neonatal behavioural scale. *Spast. Int. Med. Publ.*, No 50. (London: Heinemann)

30. Prechtl, H. F. R. (1968). Neurological findings in newborn infants after pre- and peri-natal complications. In Stratton, P. (ed.) *Psychobiology of the Human Newborn*, pp. 21–73. (New York: John Wiley)

31. Stern, N. D., Barnett, R. K. and Spieker, S. (1983). Early transmission of affect: some research issues. In Call, J. D., Galenson, E. and Tyson, R. L. (eds.) *Frontiers of Infant Psychiatry*, pp. 74–85. (New York: Basic Books)

32. Parker, M. and Rosenblatt, D. (1979). Issues in the study of social behaviour. In Schaffer, D. and Dunn, J. (eds.) *The First Week of Life*, pp. 7–36. (Chichester: John Wiley)

33. Thoman, E. B. (1975). Sleep and wake behaviors in neonates: consistencies and consequences. *Merrill-Palmer Q.*, **21**, 295–314

34. Prechtl, H. F. R. (1974). The behavioural states of the new-born infant (a review). *Brain Res.*, **76**, 1304–11

35. Nijhuis, J. G., Prechtl, H. F. R., Martin, C. B. and Bott, R. S. G. M. (1982). Are there behavioural states in the human foetus? *Early Hum. Dev.*, **6**, 177–95

36. Carmichael, L. (1941). The experimental embryology of mind. *Psychol. Bull.*, **38**(1), 1–27

37. de Roiste, A. and Bushnell, I. (1993). Tactile stimulation and preterm infant performance on an instrumental conditioning task. *J. Reprod. Infant Psychol.*, **11**, 155–63

38. Stern, D. N. (1985). *The Interpersonal World of the Infant: a View from Psychoanalysis and Development Psychology*. (New York: Basic Books)

39. Gottlieb, G. (1992). *Individual Development and Evolution: the Genesis of Novel Behavior*, pp. 159–60. (New York: Oxford University Press)

40. von Bertalanffy, L. (1934). Some aspects of system theory in biology. In von Bertalanffy, L.

(1979). *General System Theory*, pp. 164–9. (London: The Penguin Press)

41. Peters, D. L. (1971). The development of self-regulatory mechanisms: Epilog. In Walcher, D. N. and Peters, D. L. (eds.) (1971). *Early Childhood: the Development of Self-Regulatory Mechanisms*, p. 232. (New York and London: Academic Press)

42. Rosenzweig, M. R. (1971). Role of experience in development of neurophysiological regulatory mechanisms and in organization of the brain. In Walcher, D. N. and Peters, D. L. (eds.) *Early Childhood: the Development of Self-Regulatory Mechanisms*, pp. 15–37. (New York and London: Academic Press)

43. Krauss, R. M. (1971). The interpersonal regulation of behaviour. In Walcher, D. N. and Peters, D. L. (eds.) *Early Childhood: the Development of Self-Regulatory Mechanisms*, pp. 187–208. (New York and London: Academic Press)

44. Greenspan, S. (1979). Intelligence and adaptation: an integration of psychoanalytic and Piagetian developmental psychology. *Psychol. Iss.*, 47/48. (New York: International Universities Press)

45. Vygotsky, L. S. (1962). *Thought and Language*. (Cambridge, MA: The MIT Press)

46. Vygotsky, L. S. (1978). *Mind in Society*. (Cambridge, MA: The MIT Press)

47. Gedo, J. (1979). *Beyond Interpretation: Towards a Revised Theory for Psychoanalysis*. (New York: International Universities Press)

48. Lichtenberg, J. (1983). *Pscyhoanalysis and Infancy Research*. (Hillsdale, NJ: Analytic Press)

49. Emde, R. (1988). Development terminable and interminable I and II. *Int. J. Psychoanal.*, **69**, 23–42 and 283–96

50. Levine, S. (1962). The psychophysiological effects of infantile stimulation. In Bliss, E. L. (ed.) *Roots of Behavior*, pp. 246–53. (New York: Harper)

51. Denenberg, V. H. (1958). Effects of age and early experience upon conditioning in the C57BL10 mouse. *J. Psychol.*, **46**, 211–26

52. Denenberg, V. H. and Zarrow, M. X. (1971). Effects of handling in infancy upon adult behavior, and adrenocortical activity: suggestion for a neuroendocrine mechanism. In Walcher, D. N. and Peters, D. L. (eds.) *Early Childhood; the Development of Self-Regulatory Mechanisms*, pp. 39–64. (New York and London: Academic Press)

53. Denenberg, V. H. (1969). The effects of early experience. In Hafez, E. S. E. (ed.) *The Behavior of Domestic Animals*, pp. 95–130. (London: Bailliere, Tindall and Casell)

54. Denenberg, V. H. and Morton, J. R. C. (1962). Effects of environmental complexity and social

groupings upon modification of emotional behavior. *J. Comp. Physiol. Psychol.*, **55**, 242–6

55. Levine, S., Alpert, M. and Lewis, G. (1957). Infantile experience and the maturation of the pituitary adrenal axis. *Science*, **126**, 1347

56. Newton, G. and Levine, S. (eds.) (1968). *Early Experience and Behavior*. (Springfield, IL: Charles C. Thomas)

57. Solomon, G. F., Levine, S. and Kraft, J. K. (1968). Early experience and immunity. *Nature (London)*, **220**, 821–2

58. Raymond, L. N., Reyes, E., Tokuda, S. and Jones, B. C. (1986). Differential immune response in two handled inbred strains of mice. *Physiol. Behav.*, **37**, 295–7

59. Michaut, R.-J., Dechambre, R.-P., Doumerc, S., Lesourd, B., Devillechabrolle, A. and Moulias, R. (1981). Influence of early maternal deprivation on adult humoral immune response in mice. *Physiol. Behav.*, **26**, 189–91

60. Laudenslager, M. L., Reite, M. and Harbeck, R. (1982). Suppressed immune response in infant monkeys associated with maternal separation. *Behav. Neur. Biol.*, **36**, 40–8

61. Coe, C. L., Wiener, S. G., Rosenberg, L. T. and Levine, S. (1985). Endocrine and immune responses to separation and maternal loss in nonhuman primates. In Reite, M. and Field, T. M. (eds.) *The Psychobiology of Attachment and Separation*, pp. 162–99. (Orlando, FL: Academic Press)

62. Evoniuk, G. E., Kuhn, C. M. and Schanberg, S. M. (1979). The effect of tactile stimulation on serum growth hormone and tissue ornithine decarboxylase activity during maternal deprivation in rat pups. *Commun. Psychopharmacol.*, **3**, 363–70

63. Schanberg, S. M. and Field, T. M. (1987). Sensory deprivation and supplemental stimulation. *Dev. Psychol.*, **13**, 69–76

64. Rausch, P. B. (1981). Effects of tactile kinaesthetic stimulation on premature infants. *J. Obstet. Gynecol. Neonat. Nurs.*, **10**, 34–7

65. Adamson-Macedo, E. N. (1985). Effects of tactile stimulation on low and very low birth weight infants during the first week of life. *Curr. Psychol. Res. Rev.*, **6**, 305–8

66. Gorski, P. A., Huntington, L. and Lewkowicz, D. J. (1990). Direct computer recording of premature infant and nursery care: distress following two interventions. *Pediatrics*, **72**, 198–202

67. Acolet, D., Modi, N., Giannakoulopoulos, X., Bond, C., Weg, W., Clow, A. and Glover, V. (1993). Changes in plasma cortisol and catecholamine concentrations in response to massage in preterm infants. *Arch. Dis. Child.*, **68**, 29–31

68. de Roiste, A. and Bushnell, I. W. R. (1996). Tactile stimulation: short- and long-term benefits for pre-term infants. *Br. J. Dev. Psychol.*, **14**, 41–53

69. Adamson-Macedo, E. N., de Roiste, A., Wilson, A., de Carvalho, F. and Dattani, I. (1994). TAC–TIC therapy with high-risk, distressed, ventilated preterms. *J. Reprod. Infant Psychol.*, **12**(2), 249–52

70. Adamson-Macedo, E. N. (1996). The Equilibrium Model: understanding the psychoneuroimmunology of the preterm neonate. *Infant Behav. Dev.*, **19**, 6–9

71. Hayes, J. A., Adamson-Macedo, E. N. and Perera, S. (1996). Secretory immune responses of ventilated preterms to gentle/light systematic stroking. *Infant Behav. Dev.*, **19**, 7

72. Bronfenbrenner, U. (1979). *The Ecology of Human Development: Experiments by Nature and Design*. (Cambridge, MA: Harvard University Press)

73. Dewey, J. and Bentley, A. F. (1949). *Knowing and the Known*. (Boston: Beacon Press)

74. Sameroff, A. J. (1983). Developmental systems: contexts and evolution. In Mussen, P. H. (ed.) *Handbook of Child Psychology*, Vol. 1: W. Kessen (ed.) *History, Theory and Methods*, pp. 237–94. (New York: International Universities Press)

75. Lerner, R. M. and Kaufman, M. B. (1985). The concept of development in contextualism. *Dev. Rev.*, **5**, 309–33

76. Johnston, T. D. (1987). The persistence of dichotomies in the study of behavioral development. *Dev. Rev.*, **7**, 149–82

77. Magnusson, D. (1988). *Individual Development from an Interactional Perspective: a Longitudinal Study*. (Hillsdale, NJ: Erlbaum)

78. Gottlieb, G. (1970). Conceptions of prenatal behavior. In Aronson, L. R. *et al.* (eds.) *Development and Evolution of Behavior*. (San Francisco: W. H. Freeman)

79. Valsiner, J. (1987). *Culture and the Development of Children's Action*. (Chichester, UK: Wiley)

80. Horowitz, F. D. (1987). *Exploring Developmental Theories: Towards a Structural/Behavioral Model of Development*. (Hillsdale, NJ: Erlbaum)

81. Gottlieb, G. (1991). Social induction of malleability in ducklings. *Anim. Behav.*, **41**, 953–62

82. Onions, C. T. (ed.) (1968). *The Shorter Oxford English Dictionary on Historical Principles*, 3rd edn., revised with Addenda. (Oxford: Clarendon Press)

83. Turkewitz, G. and Devenny, D. A. (eds.) (1993). *Developmental Time and Timing*. (Hillsdale, NJ: Erlbaum)

84. Lickliter, R. (1993). Timing and the development of perinatal perceptual organization. In

Turkewitz, G. and Devenny, D. A. (eds.) *Developmental Time and Timing*, pp. 105–23. (Hillsdale, NJ: Erlbaum)

85. Birch, H. G. and Lefford, A. (1963). Intersensory development in children. *Monogr. Soc. Res. Child Dev.*, **28**, (5, Serial No 89), 1–47

86. Birch, H. G. and Lefford, A. (1967). Visual differentiation, intersensory integration, and voluntary motor control. *Monogr. Soc. Res. Child Dev.*, **32**, (1–2, Serial No 110)

87. Blank, M. and Bridger, W. H. (1964). Crossmodal transfer in nursery school children. *J. Comp. Physiol. Psychol.*, **58**, 277–82

88. Bryant, P. (1974). *Perception and Understanding in Young Children: an Experimental Approach.* (London: Methuen)

89. Gibson, E. J. (1969). *Principles of Perceptual Learning and Development.* (New York: Appleton-Century-Crofts)

90. Bower, T. G. R. (1974). *Development in Infancy.* (San Francisco: Freeman)

91. Schneirla, T. C. (1959). An evolutionary and developmental theory of biphasic processes underlying approach and withdrawal. In Jones, M. (ed.) *Nebraska Symposium on Motivation,* Vol. 7, pp. 1–42. (Lincoln: University of Nebraska Press)

92. Schneirla, T. C. (1965). Aspects of stimulation and organisation in approach/withdrawal processes underlying vertebrate behavioral development. In Lehrman, D. S., Hinde, R. A. and Shaw, E. (eds.) *Advances in the Study of Behavior,* Vol. 1, pp. 2–74. (New York: Academic Press)

93. Turkewitz, G., Lewkowicz, D. J. and Gardner, J. (1983). Determinants in infant perception. In Rosenblatt, J., Beer, C., Hinde, R. and Bushnell, M. (eds.) *Advances in the Study of Behavior,* pp. 39–62. (New York: Academic Press)

94. Scafidi, F. A., Field, T. M., Schanberg, S. M., Bauer, C. R., Tucci, K., Roberts, J., Morrow, C. and Kuhn, C. M. (1990). Massage stimulates growth in preterm infants: a replication. *Infant Behav. Dev.*, **13**, 167–88

95. Harrison, L. L., Leeper, J. and Yoon, M. (1991). Preterm infants' physiologic responses to early parent touch. *West. J. Nurs. Res.*, **13**(6), 698–713

96. Morrow, C. J., Field, T. M., Scafidi, F. A., Roberts, J., Eisen, L., Larson, S. K., Hogan, A. E. and Bandstra, E. S. (1991). Differential effects of massage and heelstick procedures on transcutaneous oxygen tension in preterm neonates. *Infant Behav. Dev.*, **14**, 397–414

97. Adamson-Macedo, E. N., Hayes, J. A. and Simcock, J. (1994). Distressed infant: early responses to gentle systematic touching therapy. *Infant Behav. Dev.*, **17**, 258

98. Munro, D. (1992). Process *vs.* structure and levels of analysis in psychology: towards integration rather than reduction theories. *Theory Psychol.*, **2**(1), 109–27

99. Gottlieb, G. (1976). Conceptions of prenatal development: behavioral embryology. *Psychol. Rev.*, **83**, 225–33

100. Gottlieb, G. (1993). Social induction of malleability in ducklings: sensory basis and psychological mechanism. *Anim. Behav.*, **45**, 707–19

101. Vygotsky, L. (1987). Thinking and speech. In Rieber, R. and Carton, A. (eds.) *The Collected Works of L. V. Vygotsky.* (New York: Plenum Press)

102. Wilson, A., Fel, D. and Greenstein, M. (1992). The self-regulating child: converging evidence from psychoanalysis, infant research, and sociolinguistics. *Appl. Prevent. Psychol.*, **1**, 165–75

103. Schore, A. N. (1994). *Affect Regulation and the Origin of the Self. The Neurobiology of Emotional Development.* (Hillsdale, NJ: Erlbaum)

104. Trevarthen, C. and Hubley, P. (1978). Secondary intersubjectivity: confidence, confiders and acts of meaning in the first year. In Lock, A. (ed.) *Action, Gesture and Symbol*, 183–229. (New York: Academic Press)

105. Bunge, M. (1989). From neuron to behavior and mentation: an exercise in levelmanship. In Pinsker, H. M. and Willis Jr, W. D. (eds.) *Information Processing in the Nervous System*, pp. 1–16. (New York: Raven Press)

Mother–fetal bonding

C. Niven, C. Wiszniewski and C. McVey

50

The processes underlying the attachment of the mother to her offspring have long been the subject of conjecture. However, more recent empirical research has centred on the hypothesized origins of maternal bonding in the early post-natal period. Klaus and Kennel's work has dominated this field and despite their own conclusion that 'at present there are no definitive studies to either confirm or refute the existence of a sensitive period for bonding'[1], the concept of an irreversible bond being formed immediately after birth, enhanced by skin-to-skin contact and time spent together is now enshrined in 'common knowledge', and often informs practice.

This 'knowledge' may not be soundly based. The methodologies which have been used to assess the existence of 'bonding' have been the subject of criticism, since they rely on a narrow range of observed behavior which may not accurately reflect the mother's actual feelings about her baby, nor her normal behavior towards it. Furthermore the emphasis on the importance of early post-natal contact has sometimes led to dangerous practice, for example in encouraging skin-to-skin contact between mothers and very sick infants, and in making damaging assessments of 'failure-to-bond' mothers.

Currently, the idea of mother–fetal bonding is receiving some attention. This may reflect the failure to establish a sensitive period for bonding after birth; hence the search for some pre-natal precursor. It is also in line with the current preoccupation within developmental psychology, with all things uterine. Advances in medical practice have a marked impact also, since the survival of extremely premature infants who are in essence 'extra-uterine fetuses' has become more common, and the intrauterine fetus has become visible through scanning. Anecdotal evidence has suggested that mothers of extremely premature babies appear to be bonded to their infants at birth, i.e. at a time when they should still be *in utero,* and that the sight of a scanned fetus leads to the development or enhancement of mother–fetal attachment. The status of the fetus is again a source of debate with issues related to abortion being highlighted by concerns over fetal reduction and research on pain perception in premature babies. Therefore the concept of mother–fetal bonding is of importance not only in theoretical terms, or merely in informing practice, but in helping to determine the status of the fetus. If we are not to run the risk of over-applying a potentially dangerous new 'bonding' concept, the existence and normal range of mother–fetal attachment needs to be established empirically. In order to do so, new assessment measures need to be developed, since behaviors such as eye-to-eye contact and fondling cannot be assessed between mother and fetus and are inappropriate measures to use when dealing with extremely premature babies.

One study which utilized alternative measures of attachment was carried out in Glasgow Royal Maternity Unit[2]. In this study 30 mothers of preterm babies were interviewed about their attachment to their babies during pregnancy, referring when necessary to experiences such as naming the fetus, talking to it, thinking of the fetus as a baby, etc. Seven mothers of full-term babies were also interviewed in an associated pilot study. The mother's reports of attachment feelings during pregnancy were scored on a numerical scale and correlated with attachment scores at birth, during the first post-natal days, during the remainder of the babies' stay in hospital (preterm babies only) and on return home. For ethical reasons all data were collected retrospectively except for a report of attachment at the time of interview.

The results showed that reported attachment during pregnancy was highly variable both in mothers of term babies and in those who subsequently gave birth prematurely. Twenty-one out of the 30 'preterm' mothers reported some degree of attachment, but strong attachment was rare. Three out of the seven 'term' mothers reported no attachment. Reasons which were given for non-attachment included unexpected or difficult pregnancies. Factors which were reported to encourage attachment included multiparity, scanning and fetal movement. Twelve subjects reported previous reproductive problems including infertility, recurrent miscarriage or stillbirth. Four of these subjects felt strongly attached to the fetus, while six consciously avoided attachment until the baby was born or until the pregnancy was viable.

Attachment scores during pregnancy were not significantly related to scores at any other time period sampled, including at the time of interview. In some subjects, fetal attachment did not smoothly transmute into maternal attachment. This was much more common in the preterm group, where 18 mothers reported no sense of attachment at all to their babies at birth and 11 were still reporting little attachment during the first post-natal days. Such an effect is not surprising given the shock and distress associated with a premature delivery and the self-protective distancing strategies some parents of premature babies attempt. However, these results emphasize that fetal attachment is not an irreversible process.

Mothers' comments about attachment during the period their premature baby was in hospital illuminated the complexity of 'bonding'. Many commented that while they loved their babies and were exceptionally anxious about their well-being, they had no sense that the baby belonged to them. Instead many felt that the baby 'was the nurses'' and only became 'theirs' after some time at home. This sense of ownership is often regarded as an intrinsic component of attachment, at least in western cultures, but may be an entirely separate dimension of mother–infant relations.

The results of this small study suggest that maternal–fetal bonding is not ubiquitous. When present, it apparently varies in strength and may, at least in exceptional circumstances, wax and wane. Thus, the origins of maternal bonding do not appear to be exclusively pre-natal.

The study described here offers only one method of assessing mother–fetal bonding. It depends not only on the accuracy of a mother's recall of her feelings of attachment but also on her honesty in reporting these. Given our culture's requirement to 'bond', the honesty of the mothers' reports of the absence of attachment, and of the factors which they perceived as interfering with attachment, is surprising and compelling. However, further prospective research, utilizing larger numbers of subjects and a variety of methodologies, is needed before we can reach any firm conclusions about the normal range of maternal–fetal attachment. Only then can we conclude whether attachment in humans is a complex, lengthy process akin to other forms of human development, or a rapid, irreversible bonding, akin to imprinting.

References

1. Klaus, K. and Kennel, J. H. (1983). Parent to infant bonding: setting the record straight. *J. Paediatr.*, **102**, 575–6

2. Niven, C. A., Wiszniewski, C. and AlRoomi, L. (1993). Attachment (bonding) in mothers of preterm babies. *J. Reprod. Infant Psychol.*, **11**, 175–85

The preterm responses to the environment – long-term effects?

51

D. Wolke

INTRODUCTION

Parents and professionals alike have wondered, speculated and phantasized about the long-term effects for preterm infants who spent the early months in an incubator, often attached to life support. The enquiry arises because the early world of the preterm infant in the Neonatal Intensive Care Unit (NICU) appears so different from that of a full-term infant delivered in hospital but raised at home from the early days. To explore the long-term effects of the early experience of preterm infants we need to know what the Special Care Baby Unit (SCBU) is like. What may very preterm or sick newborns experience and learn in the SCBU which is different from other infants? Do preterm infants develop differently to non-SCBU infants in the long-term? If no differences are found in long-term development then there is little practical reason to continue the enquiry about early environmental effects. If there are developmental differences then the most difficult question arises: is it possible to separate the long-term effects of early SCBU experience from the reasons for being there (e.g. immaturity, sickness)?

THE NICU/SCBU ENVIRONMENT

Those working daily in the NICU often forget how different the physical and care environment is from normal postnatal care[1]. Parents often report that the units are more like a space station than a nursery[2-4]. Some of these differences are reviewed briefly.

Noise

Preterm infants are exposed to moderate noise levels for weeks and months without having any control over the noise exposure[5]. Noise in the NICU is also one of the most concerning and disturbing worries of parents[6]. The noise levels outside the incubator are in the range of 55–75 dB(A) which resembles the noise pollution found in a busy office environment[7]. Incubators of the 90s generation comply with the British safety standards which require that the mean noise level inside an incubator should not exceed 60 dB(A) but this protection is not given in open thermo-controlled radiant heater cots.

Frequencies of less than 500 Hz easily penetrate the incubator but human voices which are in the 100–5000 Hz range are obscured, muffled or masked and the sound source is difficult to locate[7,8]. Impulse sound pressures of 114 dB(SPL) can be reached by opening and closing the incubator portholes in older type incubators[3]. Overall, noise pollution is mainly caused by staff talking and laughing, radios playing, abrupt porthole closing, the placing of bowls and other equipment on the incubator and inconsiderate placement of sound sources such as the telephone located near the incubator[3,9]. Noise levels are generally higher in intensive compared to special care nurseries[9].

There is little risk of permanent hearing loss due to SCBU noise levels[10]. In contrast, sudden loud noises often lead to adverse physiological and behavioral effects, including sleep disturbance, motor arousals such as startles and crying, hypoxemia, tachycardia and increased intracranial pressure[11,12]. The latter contribute to the development of intraventricular hemorrhage when associated with poor autoregulation of cerebral blood flow in the preterm infant's brain[13,14]. Meaningful sounds are masked by the incubator and make it unlikely that the infant will acquire recognition and integration of a particular sound (e.g. a voice) with a particular visual stimulus (i.e. face) and habituation to this noise exposure is unlikely[15].

Handling

The amount of handling received by the preterm infant has increased drastically from about 32 episodes/day in the early 1970s[16] to a mean of 132–234 handling procedures/day in the mid-1980s[17]. Very preterm infants in intensive care are handled, on average, as often as every 5–10 min and handling accounts for 4 h in a 24-h period. The main 'disturbers' are nursing and support staff, then the pediatricians and only lastly the parents. The sickest and most fragile infants are handled most frequently but not necessarily for the longest duration[18]. Social activities have been found to account for no more than a quarter of the total contact with the infant in intensive care and only up to one-third in the postintensive care nurseries[9,19].

Handling carried out by nursing and medical staff has consistently been found to disrupt the young infant's sleep pattern[20]. It is also associated with a significantly higher incidence of hypoxemia, bradycardia, apnea and behavioral distress, with between 40% and 93% of these episodes accounted for by handling only[12,17,21,22]. Handling most frequently precipitates adverse physiological consequences, with the most uncomfortable and adverse procedures (endotracheal suctioning and chest physiotherapy) leading to a marked increase in cerebral blood flow and intracranial pressure and increased catecholamine release[23,24]. In contrast to the handling by the nursing and pediatric staff, parental handling has been found to be mostly benign[17]. Parents often intuitively talk to and gently stroke their infants[25].

Summary

There is a bad fit between the NICU and SCBU environment and the infant's behavioral organization and developmental needs[3,4,26,27]. Current, often 'too intensive care'[28] for small babies can have adverse effects on their physiological and behavioral organization. Direct effects include, for example, retinopathy of prematurity due to high light exposure[29] and adverse physiological variations, for example, in oxygen saturation due to handling or noise which may contribute to bleedings into the brain. The NICU physical and caretaking environment is still mostly geared towards accommodating equipment and staff needs rather than the needs of the patient: the small newborn infant. Considerations for the infant have often only been afterthoughts[30].

LONG-TERM DEVELOPMENTAL OUTCOME

Very preterm infants

Neonatal mortality rates have reduced dramatically in most Western countries mainly due to the increased survival of very low birth weight (< 1500 g; VLBW) and very preterm (< 32 weeks gestation; VPI) infants. Despite decreased mortality, the rate of cerebral palsy (CP) has not increased in recent years[31] and may even have decreased slightly. Cerebral palsy is about 30 to 40 times more frequent for VLBW infants than full-term infants[32–35]. Even if there has been a slight decrease in CP rates for VLBW infants as speculated by some, because more VLBW infants survive, a higher absolute number of VLBW infants with major neurodevelopmental handicaps is to be found in the population today[31,36,37].

There have been more than 150 studies on the cognitive development of VLBW infants and children. Wolke and colleagues[38,39] and Wolke[40,41] recently demonstrated that, due to methodological shortcomings, the true rate of cognitive deficits has previously often been underestimated. Recent findings from multicenter or epidemiological longitudinal controlled

Table 1 GQ/IQ scores of a longitudinally studied sample of very preterm infants (VPI) ($n = 254$) and matched controls ($n = 273$). For reasons of comparability over time all scores were z-transformed and standardized according to same birth cohort normative sample as 100 ± 15 (mean $\pm$ SD)

Age	Test[†]	IQ (mean $\pm$ SD)		Major IQ deficits (% $<$ −2 SD)	
		VPI*	Controls	VPI	Controls
5 months	Griffiths (GQ)	88.3 ± 28.5	102 ± 14.5	22.8	1.1
1 year, 8 months	Griffiths (GQ)	69.8 ± 47.0	100.2 ± 14.9	28.3	1.5
4 years, 8 months	CMM	83.4 ± 26.2	99.3 ± 14.3	21.7	1.1
6 years, 3 months	K-ABC (MPC)	82.0 ± 21.9	100.2 ± 14.7	24.4	1.1
8 years, 5 months	K-ABC (MPC)	83.5 ± 26.3	100.4 ± 14.6	23.2	2.2

[†]Griffiths General Quotient[65] (German); CMM: Columbia Mental Maturity Scale[66] (German); K-ABC: Kaufman Assessment Battery for Children (Mental Processing Component)[67] (German); *all differences in VPI vs. controls significant at $p < 0.001$

samples such as the Bavarian Longitudinal Study (BLS)[38], indicate that the IQ scores of VPI or VLBW children, as a group, are more than one standard deviation (SD) below the mean compared to matched controls. As shown in Table 1, the risk of very preterm infants having an IQ more than 2 SD below the mean (i.e. IQ < 70) was 10–33 times greater than for term controls at each assessment point over the first 9 years of life (see also references 38 and 41).

Very low birth weight children have been found by us[33,42] and others[43,44] more often to have deficits in language, reading or writing. They more often have behavior problems than term controls[45]. Very low birth weight boys appear to be more frequently affected and the major behavior problems are difficulties with attention and hyperactivity[42,46–48]. Wolke[40] also reported poorer child–mother interaction at 6 years of age.

Schooling problems of VLBW infants have been reported previously but due to variable definitions and different school systems interpretation of rates has been difficult[25,49]. The Dutch Project on Preterm and Small for gestational age infants (POPS) study[50] and the BLS both recorded the early school career most systematically (i.e. special schooling, repeating a class or delayed school admission, special needs within the mainstream school). For the first time, the findings on schooling problems from the BLS study are presented here (Wolke and Leon-Villagra, in preparation) and are compared to the POPS study results[50] (Figure 1).

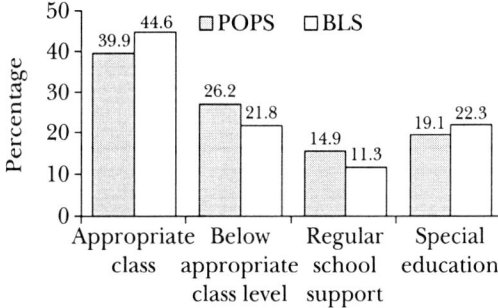

Figure 1 Schooling problems of very preterm infants (VPI; < 32 weeks gestation or < 1500 g): comparison of the Bavarian Longitudinal Study (BLS; $n = 390$) findings with the Dutch POPS study[50] ($n = 813$)

The BLS found a rate of 1.7% of special schooling in a representative Bavarian sample while special education was 22.3% in the VLBW/VPI group (Figure 1; POPS study 19.1%), a 13 times increased rate. Less than half of all VLBW children received schooling at the appropriate age level. The results of the POPS and BLS studies could hardly be more similar, underlining the generalizability of these findings. Children with a schooling problem are much more likely to encounter later difficulties, ranging from unemployment to lower social status and income.

Preterm infants

The majority of infants admitted to SCBUs are preterm (32–36 weeks gestation) and sick term infants. These infants usually remain in special care for much briefer periods. Riegel and associates[33] reported on the developmental progress of ex-SCBU infants until 4.8 years in the binational Bavarian-Finnish Longitudinal Study (BFLS). The study involved some 8421 infants in Germany and 2194 in Finland. Ex-SCBU infants, whether preterm (32–36 weeks gestation) or full-term (> 36 weeks gestation), only slightly more often had performance IQ deficits (more than 2 SD below the mean) and major verbal IQ deficits than controls matched for sociodemographic variables. Ex-SCBU preterm and term infants in comparison to term routine care infants experienced these cognitive deficits about 2–4 times more often. No differences were found in the number of minor deficits for ex-SCBU children in comparison. The shorter the gestation (and the higher the associated neonatal complications), the more behavior problems were apparent. Looking at the IQ mean scores over time (5, 20 and 56 months), excluding those with major congenital, motor or sensory handicap, it was apparent that the mean scores hardly differed between ex-SCBU preterm and term infants and term infants who received normal postnatal care.

DIFFERENTIAL IMPACT OF NEONATAL VS. SOCIO-ENVIRONMENTAL FACTORS

As part of the BLS we determined the influence of neonatal complications and treatment ('biological factors') and family and social risk factors ('social factors') on the IQ score at the ages from 5 months to 8.5 years of age. For this analysis, all infants with major neurosensory impairment (CP, blind, deaf, congenital abnormalities) were excluded. Figure 2b shows that already at 1.8 years of age more of the variance in the IQ scores of preterm (> 31 weeks gestation) and term ex-SCBU infants was explained by social factors than biological factors. There is evidence that social factors show increasing influence on IQ development for preterm and term ex-SCBU infants while biological risk effects decrease over time. In contrast (Figure 2a), although social factors also showed increasing influence over time in very preterm infants (< 32 weeks gestation), biological factors remained by far the best predictors of IQ until the 9th year of life. These findings indicate lowered plasticity for change and greater continuity of IQ deficits over time for VPI. There was more plasticity and thus a higher likelihood that environmental factors can compensate for IQ deficits over time in larger preterm and term SCBU infants.

These findings from our longitudinal observation study have received support from the

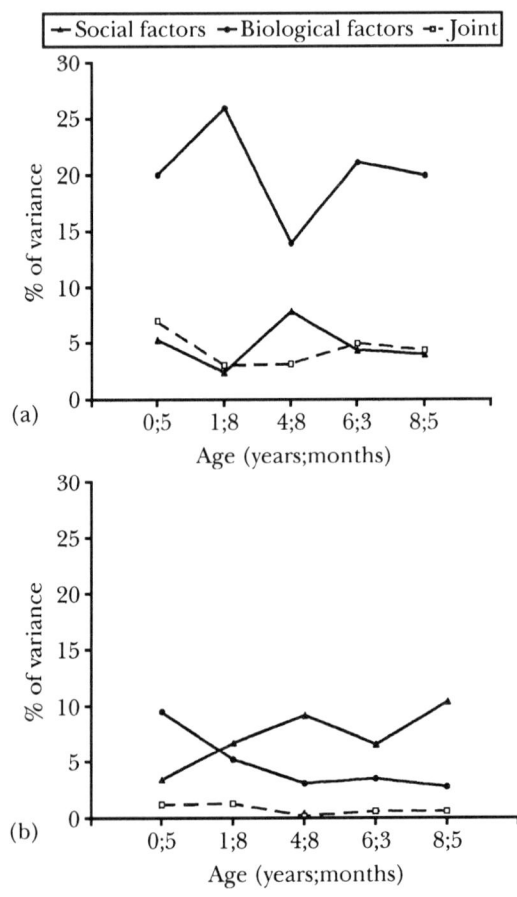

Figure 2 The influence of biological and social factors on IQ development of ex-Special Care Baby Unit infants over the first 9 years of life. (a) Very preterm infants (< 32 weeks gestation) without major neurodevelopmental disability ($n = 227$); (b) at risk infants (> 31 weeks gestation) without major neurodevelopmental disability ($n = 769$)

largest randomized controlled intervention study for LBW infants to date. The Infant Health and Development Program[51] implemented a regular home visiting program and day care educational program for LBW infants and their families from 0 to 3 years. While intervention effects were still found for larger LBW children (> 2000 g) 2 years after the intervention had ceased (i.e. 5 years of age), no intervention effects at all were detected at 5 years for infants < 2000 g[51]. The results indicate that smaller infants are less able to take advantage of environmental enhancements. The deficits detected in childhood appear to have their origin before their discharge home to their parents.

THREE WAYS OF INVESTIGATING THE LONG-TERM IMPACT OF THE NICU ENVIRONMENT

How can we separate the long-term impact of the NICU environment from the long-term effects of the reasons for being in the NICU?

Predicting specific long-term impacts

A first approach is to investigate predicted long-term consequences. For example, it has been

speculated that the lack of daily day–night cycles in lighting levels and activities in the NICU leads to long-term sleeping impairments[52,53]. Recent large-scale studies of the sleeping behavior of VPI found no evidence of more impaired sleeping behavior[54,55]. Rather, VPI were found to sleep better in early infancy at home. There is thus little evidence that early NICU experience impairs the development of circadian rhythms once discharged home.

Natural variations: comparisons between different NICUs

Comparative studies between different neonatal units indicate that medical care and success rates in terms of mortality tend to vary considerably[56]. As part of the BFLS[33], we compared initial peri- and neonatal complications and the intensity and duration of intensive treatment and developmental outcome at 4.8 years for all VPI survivors (without major neurodevelopmental disability (MND), mother tongue speaker) in South Germany vs. South Finland born in 1985. Table 2 shows the mortality, attrition, MND rates and cognitive developmental outcome of the survivors in both populations. No differences were found in mortality rates, MND and

Table 2 Sample characteristics, mortality, attrition and developmental outcome of very preterm infants (VPI; < 32 weeks gestation) in Germany and Finland

	South Germany	South Finland
Sample (n)		
Population born[†]	560 (100%)	93 (100%)
Died (0–4 years, 8 months)[†]	164 (29%)	31 (33%)
Not mother tongue speaker	43	2
Dropouts (tel. information only)	70	13
MND	29	3
Target sample[‡]	254 (80%)	44 (78%)
Neonatal (mean ± SD)		
Gestation (weeks)	29.7 ± 1.5	28.8 ± 2.3*
Birthweight (g)	1315 ± 344	1351 ± 404
Development (4 years, 8 months) (mean ± SD)		
Performance IQ (CMM)	86.2 ± 24.2	87.5 ± 19.4
Verbal IQ (AWST)	86.3 ± 22.1	96.4 ± 16.7**
Language comprehension (LSVT)	87.2 ± 21.0	96.7 ± 17.9**

MND = major neurodevelopmental disability; [†]% of all VPI born; [‡]% of survivors without MND and mother tongue speaker; CMM = Columbia Mental Maturity Scale[66]; AWST = Allgemeiner Wortschatztest[68]; LSVT = Logopädischer Sprachverständnistest[69]; *$p < 0.05$; **$p < 0.01$

performance IQ. However, VPI in Finland were significantly advanced in their language development compared to German VPI children. There were no differences in the birth weight of survivors but a small but significant tendency for Finnish survivors to be of slightly lower gestation. Table 3 shows that no differences were found between groups in neonatal complications encountered according to a detailed optimality scoring system[55]. Neonatal care procedures including respiratory treatment, oxygen supplementation, care level and neurological status were recorded daily and prospectively by specially trained staff[33,39,55]. The analysis indicated that VPI in Finland received less intensive and invasive care and for shorter periods. In particular, as shown in Table 3, Finnish VPI were less likely to be ventilated or given continuous positive airway pressure (CPAP) and if ventilated, to receive ventilation for shorter periods. Fewer Finnish infants ever received parenteral nutrition and if they received it, they terminated it sooner to graduate to oral (tube) feeding. The net result of less invasive care was that Finnish infants in 1985/86 were discharged sooner, suffered no more adverse outcome and even showed more advanced language development.

Changing the NICU environment: intervention programs

While evidence from studies comparing different treatment approaches of different NICUs provides important hints that less invasive care is beneficial, controlled studies provide a more rigorous test. Jacobsen and co-workers[57] and Porz and associates[58] reported on less invasive treatment in the first 2 h after birth. Jacobsen and co-workers[57] found that their 'minitouch' approach reduced mechanical ventilation rates to 35% compared to 76% of historical controls (i.e. those born in the 2 years before introduction of 'minitouch'). The incidence of intracranial hemorrhage was reduced from 49% to 25%. Reductions of nearly 40% in ventilation rates were also reported by Porz and associates[58]. Less mechanical ventilation means less need for parenteral nutrition, less handling and more rest.

Three studies, so far, have investigated an integrated individualized developmental approach to care, as advocated by Als[59] and Wolke[3,25,60]. In the first study, using historical controls, Als and colleagues[61] found that longer term complications (bronchopulmonary dysplasia) could be reduced by preventing inappropriate sensory input and providing individualized care, depending on the developmental and behavioral status of the very preterm infant. Infants in the experimental group had significantly shorter stays on the respirator, their feeding behavior was normalized earlier, behavioral regulation was more efficient in infancy and they obtained higher scores in the Bayley Developmental Test. Becker and co-workers[9] replicated this study, training nurses according to a modified version of Als's program, and

Table 3 Differences in neonatal treatment of very preterm infants (VPI) in South Germany vs. South Finland (mean ± SD)

	South Germany	South Finland
Number of neonatal complications	9.5 ± 2.7	9.0 ± 3.5
Intensity of treatment	12.3 ± 3.6	8.6 ± 3.1***
Duration of intensive treatment (days)	60.0 ± 35.2	40.0 ± 34.4**
Duration of neonatal hospitalization (days)	80.4 ± 38.0	62.9 ± 37.9**
Discharge weight (g)	2930 ± 691	2515 ± 607***
Specific treatments		
infants ventilated/CPAP	82.7%	65.9%**
if ventilated, duration (days)	25.2 ± 21.0	13.5 ± 7.4**
parenteral nutrition	91.7%	77.3%**
if parenteral, duration (days)	27.4 ± 20.4	10.8 ± 6.6***

**$p < 0.01$; ***$p < 0.001$; CPAP = continuous positive airway pressure

investigating whether individualized care actually led to reduced noise and light levels. They found that the physical changes (reduction of noise and light) in the environment were successfully implemented, however, a clear daily rhythm was not achieved in either the experimental or the control condition. Experimental infants had lower morbidity levels, were introduced to oral feeding sooner and had shorter stays in the hospital. Their overall behavioral organization at discharge was also better, as assessed by the Brazelton NBAS total score[62]. Similar positive effects on motor organization were reported by Mouradian and Als[63].

The first study using a randomized, controlled design comparing an individualized developmental care approach to traditional care within the same NICU was reported by Als and co-workers[64]. Subjects weighing less than 1250 g, born before 30 weeks gestation and mechanically ventilated within 3 h of delivery, were assigned randomly either to a control group (normal NICU care) or an experimental group (individualized developmental care). Experimental infants developed intraventricular hemorrhage less often, had bronchopulmonary dysplasia (chronic lung disease) less frequently, were ventilated or required oxygen for shorter periods, and had a shorter stay in the NICU and in hospital. The cost savings were large, with the average cost of treatment for the control infants amounting to 189 000 US$ vs. 98 000 US$ for the experimental group. Furthermore, electrophysiological differences in brain functioning were demonstrated between the groups and developmental outcome assessed with the Bayley Scales was significantly better for the experimental group at 9 months of age.

This review indicates that less invasive but medically closely monitored treatment is beneficial in reducing distress for infants, improving development and saving costs. Although the findings so far are impressive, they were obtained in small samples. The approach of Als[59] focuses on nursing and involves a lengthy and expensive training (i.e. NIDCAP[59]), making no reference to integrated changes in early medical care. For example, all infants in the study of Als

and co-workers[64] were routinely ventilated. The findings by Wolke[40], Jacobsen and associates[57] and Porz and colleagues[58], however, show that invasive medical treatments can be reduced in the initial hours and this alone is putting NICU infants on track for less invasive subsequent care. Further studies are needed to investigate the relative efficacy of changes in nursing and/or early medical care.

CONCLUSIONS AND FUTURE DIRECTIONS

Very preterm infants, representing 0.7–0.9% of all births, are at a much increased risk of requiring special education and of long-term handicap. There is an urgent need to prevent long-term sequelae and the high cost resulting from initial neonatal care, subsequent rehabilitation, community care, special education and loss of revenue.

Our longitudinal and recent intervention research suggests that long-term outcome for very preterm (but not preterm) infants is strongly predicted by neonatal complications and intensity of treatment. There is thus increasing evidence that for a large minority of very preterm infants the damage is present or done before discharge.

The initial question has been whether changes in the neonatal intensive care unit environment and the infant's responses to these could change the poor outcome for very preterm infants. The answer is a cautious 'Yes'. The review has indicated that soul or mind and physiological organization in preterm infants are difficult to differentiate – they are two sides of the same coin. Stress to the mind (e.g. noise) is reflected in physiological changes in the immature organism. Less 'iatrogenic' complications, quicker recovery and psychologically oriented care can lead to improved outcome. There is a need for more systematic and controlled evaluation research; however, there is enough accumulated evidence to suggest that initial less invasive and individualized developmental care is not any more an option but is likely to be the major component for enhancing the effectiveness of neonatal intensive care over the next decade.

ACKNOWLEDGEMENTS

I would like to thank Brigitte Söhne and Renate Meyer for their help in data analysis and the 17 clinics in Bavaria and six clinics in South Finland which participated in the research. The reported research was supported by the German Federal Government Ministry of Science and Education (BMBF) grants to K. Riegel, D. Wolke and B. Ohrt.

References

1. Wolke, D. and Eldridge, T. (1992). The environment of care. In Campbell, A. G. M. and McIntosh, N. (eds.) *Forfar and Arneill's Textbook of Paediatrics*, 4th edition, pp. 112–17 (Edinburgh: Churchill Livingstone)

2. Redshaw, M. E., Rivers, R. P. A. and Rosenblatt, D. B. (1985). *Born Too Early*. (Oxford: Oxford University Press)

3. Wolke, D. (1987). Environmental and developmental neonatology. *J. Reprod. Infant Psychol.*, **5**, 17–42

4. Wolke, D. (1987). Environmental neonatology (Annotation). *Arch. Dis. Child.*, **62**, 987–8

5. Saunders, A. N. (1995). Incubator noise: a method to decrease decibels. *Paediatr. Nursing*, **21** (3), 265–8

6. Redshaw, M. E. and Harris, A. (1995). Maternal perceptions of neonatal care. *Acta Paediatr.*, **84**, 593–8

7. Gottfried, A. W. (1985). Environment of newborn infants in special care units. In Gottfried, A. W. and Gaiter, J. L. (eds.) *Infant Stress Under Intensive Care: Environmental Neonatology*, pp. 23–54. (Baltimore: University Park Press)

8. Bess, F. H., Peek, F. B. and Chapman, J. J. (1979). Further observations on noise levels and infant incubators. *Pediatrics*, **63**, 100–6

9. Becker, P., Grunwald, P. C., Moorman, J. and Stuhr, S. (1991). Outcomes of developmentally supportive nursing care for very low birth weight infants. *Nursing Res.*, **40**, 150–5

10. Abramowich, S. J., Gregory, S., Slemick, M. and Stewart, A. (1979). Hearing loss in very low birthweight infants treated with neonatal intensive care. *Arch. Dis. Child.*, **54**, 421–5

11. Long, G. J., Lucey, J. F. and Philip, A. G. S. (1980). Noise and hypoxaemia in the intensive care nursery. *Pediatrics*, **65**, 143–5

12. Zahr, L. K. and Balian, S. (1995). Responses of preterm infants to routine nursing interventions and noise in the NICU. *Nursing Res.*, **44** (3), 179–85

13. Friis-Hansen, B. (1985). Perinatal brain injury and cerebral flow in newborn infants. *Acta Paediatr. Scand.*, **74**, 323–31

14. Volpe, J. J. (1989). Intraventricular hemorrhage in the premature infant: current concepts, part 1. *Ann. Neurol.*, **25** (3), 3–11

15. Philbin, M. K., Ballweg, D. D. and Gray, L. (1994). The effect of an intensive care unit sound environment on the development of habituation in healthy avian neonates. *Dev. Psychobiol.*, **27** (1), 11–21

16. Speidel, B. D. (1976). Adverse effects of routine procedures on preterm infants. *Lancet*, **1**, 864–6

17. Murdoch, D. R. and Darlow, B. A. (1984). Handling during neonatal intensive care. *Arch. Dis. Child.*, **59**, 957–61

18. Symon, A. and Cunningham, S. (1995). Handling premature neonates: a study using time-lapse video. *Nursing Times*, **91** (17), 35–7

19. Linn, P. L., Horowitz, F. D., Buddin, B. J., Leake, J. C. and Fox, H. A. (1985). An ecological description of a neonatal intensive care unit. In Gottfried, A. W. and Gaiter, J. L. (eds.) *Infant Stress Under Intensive Care: Environmental Neonatology*, pp. 83–112. (Baltimore: University Park Press)

20. Fajardo, B., Browning, M., Fisher, D. and Paton, J. (1990). Effect of nursery environment on state regulation in very-low-birth-weight premature infants. *Infant Behav. Dev.*, **13**, 287–303

21. Long, J. G., Philip, A. G. S. and Lucey, J. F. (1980). Excessive handling as a cause of hypoxaemia. *Pediatrics*, **65**, 203–7

22. Gorski, P. A., Huntington, L. and Lewkowicz, D. J. (1990). Handling preterm infants in hospitals. *Clin. Perinatol.*, **17**, 103–12

23. Lagercrantz, H., Nilsson, F., Redham, I. and Hjemdal, P. (1986). Plasma catecholamines following nursing procedures in a neonatal ward. *Early Hum. Dev.*, **14**, 61–5

24. Greisen, G., Frederiksen, P. S., Hertel, J. and Christensen, N. J. (1985). Catecholamine

response to chest physiotherapy and endotracheal suctioning in preterm infants. *Acta Paediatr. Scand.*, **74**, 525–9

25. Wolke, D. (1991). Supporting the development of low-birthweight infants (Annotation). *J. Child Psychol. Psychiatr.*, **32**, 723–41

26. Als, H., Lawhon, G., Gibes, R., Brown, E. and Duffy, F. H. (1985). Individualised behavioral and environmental care for the VLBW preterm at high risk for chronic lung disease. Presented at the *Biennial Meeting of the Society for Research in Child Development Conference*, Toronto, Canada, April 25–28

27. Wolke, D. (1997). The environment of care. In Campbell, A. G. M. and McIntosh, N. (eds.) *Forfar and Arneill's Textbook of Paediatrics*, 5th edition, (Edinburgh: Churchill Livingstone), in press

28. Silverman, W. A. (1992). Overtreatment of neonates? A personal retrospective. *Pediatrics*, **90** (No.6), 971–6

29. Glass, E., Avery, G. B., Subramaniou, K. N. S., Keys, M. P., Sostek, A. M. and Friendly, D. S. (1985). Effect of bright light in the hospital nursery on the incidence of retinopathy of prematurity. *N. Engl. J. Med.*, **313**, 401–4

30. Hodgman, J. E. (1985). Introduction. In Gottfried, A. W. and Gaiter, J. L. (eds.) *Infant Stress Under Intensive Care: Environmental Neonatology*, pp. 131–56. (Baltimore: University Park Press)

31. Hagberg, B. and Hagberg, G. (1993). The changing panorama of cerebral palsy in Sweden IV. *Acta Paediatr. Scand.*, **82**, 387–93

32. Hagberg, B., Hagberg, G. and Zetterström, R. (1989). Decreasing perinatal mortality – increase in cerebral palsy morbidity? *Acta Paediatr. Scand.*, **78**, 664–70

33. Riegel, K., Ohrt, B., Wolke, D. and Österlund, K. (1995). *Die Entwicklung gefährdet geborener Kinder bis zum fünften Lebensjahr*. Die ARVO-YLLPÖ Neugeborenen-Nachfolge Studie in Südbayern und Südfinnland. (Stuttgart: Enke Verlag)

34. de Vonderweid, U., Spagnolo, A., Corchia, Chiandotto, V., Chiappe, S., Chiappe, F., Colarizi, DeLuca, T., Didato, M. and Fertz, F. C. (1994). Italian multicentre study on very low birth weight babies. Neonatal mortality and two year outcome. *Acta Paediatr.*, **83** (4), 391–6

35. Escobar, G. J., Littenberg, B. and Petitti, D. B. (1991). Outcome among surviving very low birthweight infants: a meta-analysis. *Arch. Dis. Child.*, **66**, 204–11

36. Atkinson, S. and Stanley, F. J. (1983). Spastic diplegia among children of low and normal birthweight. *Dev. Med. Child Neurol.*, **25**, 693–708

37. Emond, A., Golding, J. and Peckhan, C. (1989). Cerebral palsy in two national cohort studies. *Arch. Dis. Child.*, **64**, 848–52

38. Wolke, D., Ratschinski, G., Ohrt, B. and Riegel, K. (1994). The cognitive outcome of very preterm infants may be poorer than often reported: an empirical investigation of how methodological issues make a big difference. *Eur. J. Pediatr.*, **153**, 906–15

39. Wolke, D., Söhne, B., Ohrt, B. and Riegel, K. (1995). Follow-up of preterm children: important to document dropouts. *Lancet*, **345** (No. 8947), 447

40. Wolke, D. (1995). Verhaltensprobleme und soziale Beziehungen ehemals sehr kleiner Fruehgeborener: Einfluesse des intensivmedizinischen Handlings. *Zeitschrift Geburtsh. Neonatol.*, **199**, 208

41. Wolke, D. (1997). Entwicklung Sehr Fruehgeborener bis zum 7. Lebensjahr (Development of very preterm infants until the seventh year of life). In Horstmann, T. and Leyendecker, C. (eds.) *Fruehforderung und Fruehbehandlung – wissenschaftliche Grundlagen, praxisorientierte Ansaetze unde Perspektiven interdisziplinarer Zusammenarbeit*, pp. 271–88. (Heidelberg: Universitatsverlag C. Winter)

42. Wolke, D. and Meyer, R. (1994). Psychologische Langzeitbefunde bei sehr Frühgeborenen. *Perinatal Med.*, **6**, 121–3

43. Klein, N. K., Hack, M. and Breslau, N. (1989). Children who were very low birthweight. Development and academic achievement at 9 years of age. *Dev. Behav. Pediatr.*, **10**, 32–7

44. Vohr, B. R., Garcia-Coll, C. and Oh, W. (1988). Language development of low-birthweight infants at two years. *Dev. Med. Child Neurol.*, **30**, 608–15

45. Buka, S. L., Lipsitt, L. P. and Tsuang, M. T. (1992). Emotional and behavioural development of low birthweight infants. In Friedman, S. L. and Sigman, M. D. (eds.) *The Psychological Development of Low Birthweight Children*, pp. 187–214. (New Jersey: Ablex)

46. Breslau, N., Klein, N. and Allen, L. (1988). Very low birthweight: behavioral sequelae at nine years of age. *J. Am. Acad. Child Adolesc. Psychiatr.*, **27**, 605–12

47. Sykes, D. H., Hoy, E. A., Bill, J. M., McClure, B. G., Halliday, H. L. and Reid, M. M. (1997). Behavioural adjustment in school of very low birthweight children. *J. Child Psychol. Psychiatr.*, in press

48. Weisglas-Kuperus, N., Koot, H. M., Baerts, W., Fetter, W. P. F. and Sauer, P. J. J. (1993). Behaviour problems of very low-birthweight children. *Dev. Med. Child Neurol.*, **35**, 406–16

49. Wolke, D. (1993). Langzeitprognose von Frühgeborenen: was wir wissen und was wir wissen sollten (Longterm prognosis of preterm infants: what we know and what we should know). In Lischka, A. and Bernert, G. (eds.) *Aktuelle Neuropädiatrie 1992*, pp. 99–121. (Wehr/Baden: Verlag Ciba Geigy)

50. Hille, E. T. M., Den Ouden, A. L., Bauer, L., van den Oudenrijn, C., Brand, R. and Verloove-Vanhorik, S. P. (1994). School performance at nine years of age in very premature and very low birthweight infants: perinatal risk factors and predictors at five years of age. *J. Pediatr.*, **125**, 426–34

51. Brooks-Gunn, J., McCarton, C. M., Casey, P. H., McCormick, M. C., Bauer, C. R., Bernbaum, J. C., Tyson, J., Swanson, M., Bennett, F. C., Scott, D. T., Tonascia, J. and Meinert, C. L. (1994). Early intervention in low-birth-weight premature infants: results through age 5 years from the Infant Health and Development Program. *J. Am. Med. Assoc.*, **272** (16), 1257–62

52. Mann, N. P., Haddow, R., Stokes, L. and Goodley, S. R. N. (1986). Effect of night and day on preterm infants in a newborn nursery: randomised trial. *Br. Med. J.*, **293**, 1265–7

53. McMillen, I. C., Kok, J. S. M., Adamson, T. M. and Deayton, J. M. (1991). Development of circadian sleep-wake rhythms in preterm and full-term infants. *Pediatr. Res.*, **29** (4), 381–4

54. Shimada, M., Segawa, M. and Higurashi, M. A. H. (1993). Development of the sleep and wakefulness rhythm in preterm infants discharged from a neonatal care unit. *Pediatr. Res.*, **33**, 159–63

55. Wolke, D., Meyer, R., Ohrt, B. and Riegel, K. (1995). The incidence of sleeping problems in preterm and fullterm infants discharged from special neonatal care units: an epidemiological longitudinal study. *J. Child Psychol. Psychiatr.*, **36**, 203–23

56. Hack, M., Horbar, J. D., Malloy, M. H., Tyson, K. J. E., Wright, E. and Wright, L. (1991). Very low birth weight outcomes of the National Institute of Child Health and human development neonatal network. *Pediatrics*, **87**, 587–97

57. Jacobsen, T., Gronvall, J., Petersen, S. and Andersen, G. E. (1993). 'Minitouch' treatment of very low-birth-weight infants. *Acta Paediatr.*, **82**, 934–8

58. Porz, F., von Schoenaich, P. and Bernsau, U. (1995). Auswirkungen eines neuen Erstversorgungskonzepts der 'individuellen Pflege' auf die Morbidität kleiner Frühgeborener. *Symposium der Deutsch-Österreichischen Gesellschaft für Neonatologie und Pädiatrische Instensivmedizin* 21, pp. 214–15. (München: Alete Wissenschaftlicher Dienst)

59. Als, H. (1992). Individualized, family-focused developmental care for the very low birthweight preterm infant in the NICU. In Friedman, S. L. and Sigman, M. D. (eds.) *The Psychological Development of Low Birthweight Children*, pp. 341–88. (New Jersey: Ablex)

60. Wolke, D. (1991). Psycho-biologische Aspekte der Pflege von Frühgeborenen. *Deutsche Krankenpflege-Zeitschrift (Schwerpunktthema Perinatalmedizin)*, **44**, 478–83

61. Als, H., Lawhon, G., Brown, E., Gibes, R., Duffy, F. H., McAnulty, G. and Blickman, J. G. (1986). Individualized behavioral and environmental care for the very low birth weight preterm infant at high risk for bronchopulmonary dysplasia: neonatal intensive care unit and developmental outcome. *Pediatrics*, **78**, 1123–32

62. Brazelton, T. B. and Nugent, K. (1995). *Manual of the Neonatal Behavioral Assessment Scale*, 3rd edition. (Oxford: McKeith Press)

63. Mouradian, L. E. and Als, H. (1994). The influence of neonatal intensive care unit caregiving practices on motor functioning of preterm infants. *Am. J. Occup. Ther.*, **48** (6), 527–33

64. Als, H., Lawhon, G., Duffy, F. H., McAnulty, G. B., Gibes-Grossman, R. and Blickman, J. G. (1994). Individualized developmental care for the very low-birth-weight preterm infant. *J. Am. Med. Assoc.*, **272**, 853–8

65. Brandt, I. (1983). *Griffith Entwicklungsskalen (GES zur Beurteilung der Entwicklung in den ersten beiden Lebensjahren)*. (Weinheim: Beltz)

66. Bondy, C., Cohen, R., Eggert, D. and Lüer, G. (1975). Testbatterie für geistig behinderte Kinder. *TBGB Manual* (3. Aufl). (Weinheim: Beltz)

67. Melchers, P. and Preuss, U. (1991). K-ABC: Kaufman Assessment Battery for Children. *Deutschsprachige Fassung*. (Frankfurt/Main: Swets & Zeitlinger)

68. Kiese, C. and Kozielski, P. M. (1979). Aktiver Wortschatztest für drei-bis sechsjährige Kinder. *Allgemeiner Wortschatztest 3–6*. (Weinheim: Beltz)

69. Wettstein, P. (1983). *LSVT: Logopädischer Sprachverständnis-Test*, Zürich Heilpädagogisches Seminar

Effects of major neonatal surgery on subsequent behavior

52

L. Ludman

INTRODUCTION

Over the last 35 years, rapid advances in medical and surgical techniques have led to significant changes in neonatal intensive care, and an impressive decrease in infant mortality and morbidity. This period was also a time of major expansion in development psychology. Advances in these two scientific disciplines gradually intermingled as scientists began to focus attention on the effects of hospitalization on young children and the consequences of high technology medicine on the quality of life of infants who survive medical problems in the perinatal or neonatal period.

Research into the effects of hospitalization on young children revealed that for children aged between 6 months and 4 years, a single hospital admission of more than one week and/or multiple hospital admissions, increased the risk for both short-term[1] and long-term psychological problems some years later[2,3]. However, the evidence as to whether hospitalization for infants under 6 months had any lasting negative effects was equivocal. For example, studies by Schaffer and Callender[4] and Douglas[2] clearly indicated that there were no adverse effects on the infant if admission to hospital was before the age of 6 months. Yet studies of low-birth weight babies treated in neonatal special and intensive care units suggested that early hospitalization could adversely effect the mother–infant bond and subsequently later parenting behavior[5,6]. Although other research failed to confirm an association between prematurity and later parental abuse[7], anxieties about the effects of separation on the mother–child relationship were very pervasive, especially in the 1970s and early 1980s. However, outcome studies of early intervention concentrated almost exclusively on the health and development of babies who were premature and of low birth weight. Newborn infants requiring major surgery were generally excluded from these studies.

In order to rectify this omission and to try to clarify the effects of hospitalization in the first few months of life, we have in the past decade at the Institute of Child Health and at Great Ormond Street Hospital for Children been carrying out innovative research aimed at obtaining information about the psychosocial effects of early surgical intervention. The first study was a 3-year prospective longitudinal study. The patients in this study all had major neonatal surgery at Great Ormond Street Hospital between November 1983 and December 1984[8–11]. The second study (1991–1993) was a large-scale cross-sectional study. The children in this study were all born with anorectal malformations and had neonatal surgery and primary definitive surgery for correction of their anomaly at Great Ormond Street Hospital between 1974 and 1987[12–14].

This paper presents an overview of the findings from both studies and focuses on the question of whether neonatal surgery and hospitalization has consequences for the emotional development of the child and whether this persists into adolescence. Previous publications include detailed descriptions of the characteristics of the study samples and methods of assessment. Only summaries will be presented here.

SUMMARY OF FINDINGS FROM STUDY 1

Methods

Subjects: surgical group

The study sample comprised a consecutive sample of 30 term newborn infants admitted for major surgery to the neonatal surgical unit at Great Ormond Street Hospital between November 1983 and December 1984. All the infants were admitted because of life-threatening developmental abnormalities: 19 had abnormalities of the alimentary and respiratory tracts, such as esophageal atresia, diaphragmatic hernia, gastroschisis, Hirschsprung's disease and malrotation of the gut; four had anorectal abnormalities, two had non-malignant tumours, one had a meningomyelocele, and four infants had developed necrotizing enterocolitis. Seven babies had multiple abnormalities including heart defects. With the exception of the baby with a meningomyelocele, all the infants were neurologically normal.

Control group

The control group consisted of 29 healthy term babies closely matched with the surgical group for sex, birth order, age of mother, marital status and social grouping of mother, and geographical location. The controls were collected over the period December 1983 to October 1985.

There was a further comparison group of babies admitted to special care baby units for medical reasons, but this presentation will be limited to comparisons between the surgical and control groups. Furthermore, only data about the children's emotional development as determined by their behavior and relationships with their parents, especially the mother, will be reported here.

Design

The infants and their families were seen four times during the first year of life and then followed up at 3 years of age. The first parental interview was carried out in the hospital but all subsequent interviews and child assessments were carried out in the family home.

Behavioral measures

The main outcome measures of behavior and mother–child relationships were obtained from standardized questionnaires and standardized semi-structured interviews. At each stage of the study the parents were asked to complete infant/child temperamental questionnaires and information about infant and child behavior was obtained from semi-structured interviews and questionnaires. In addition, at the 12 month stage, the mother–infant relationship was examined using a standardized behavioral observation and a standardized assessment of infant–mother attachment. At 3 years the mother–child relationship was examined using a standardized assessment of current parenting behavior[8]. Two important measures included in the assessment battery at each stage of the study, and which are relevant to this presentation, were standardized assessments of parental mental health and the parental relationship.

Assessment of behavior

First 12 months

At both the 6 and 12 month stages, a higher proportion of the infants in the surgical group were rated by their mothers as having a 'difficult' temperament compared with the controls (54 vs. 30% at 6 months, and 57 vs. 28% at 12 months; neither difference is significant). During the first year, a much higher proportion of the surgical parents had significant problems coping with the disturbed sleeping patterns of their babies. This was one of the factors which contributed to the significantly higher stress scores among the surgical families at the 6 week, 6 and 12 month stages. At the 6 week and 12 month stages, a significantly higher proportion of the surgical mothers were depressed compared with the controls. However, despite these factors, the quality of the relationships among the surgical group parents was similar to that of the control group parents.

The assessment of the mother–infant relationship at the 12 month stage showed that there were no important differences between the case-control pairs. In common with their healthy matched controls a majority of the surgical babies were classified as 'securely' attached. Moreover, in both groups, the proportions of secure relationships were similar to those in other groups of healthy 1-year-olds.

Three-year stage

A high follow-up rate was achieved. Assessments were carried out on 90% of both cases and controls. At this stage, in contrast to the earlier findings, fewer surgical children (26%) were rated as temperamentally difficult by their mothers compared with the controls (36%). However, comparisons of the behavioral assessments of the case-control pairs revealed that disturbed behavior tended to occur more frequently among the cases than among the controls ($z = -1.69$, $p = 0.09$). The proportions were 30% of the cases compared with 11.5% of the controls (rates reported in population studies of 3-year-olds range between 10 and 15%)[15–17].

The mental health scores of the surgical and control group mothers were similar. Just over two-thirds (68%) of the surgical group parents' relationships were rated as satisfactory compared with 76% in the control group.

Mother–child relationship: current parenting behavior

A higher proportion of the surgical group mothers had an overall rating of poor parenting (27%), compared with the control group mothers (11.5%). Similarly, more than twice as many surgical group mothers were rated as insensitive in their handling of their children, and their style of disciplinary control was rated as

'indulgent' as well as being more inconsistent than the control group mothers. Their control techniques were also less effective than those of the control group mothers.

Summary of results

At the age of 12 months, in the sample reported here, hospitalization in the early months of life, together with major surgical intervention and associated medical treatment, did not appear to have an adverse effect on the mother–infant relationship. However, by the time the children were 3 years old, there was evidence of an increased rate of emotional disturbance and difficulties in the mother–child relationships among cases compared with controls.

We examined the data to try to establish whether early mother–infant separation, hospitalization in the first 6 months of life, or repeat hospital admissions contributed to the 3-year outcome. We found no evidence that post-partum separation had any short or long term effects on the mother–child relationship. However, the length of a baby's first admission and repeat admissions appeared to be associated with behavioral problems and parenting difficulties at 3 years of age. However, further analyses of the data revealed that family factors such as the age of the mother, her educational attainments and whether the baby was her first child were also important factors contributing to poorer outcomes (see Table 1).

Conclusions

Our findings indicated that it is not a single factor such as hospitalization, or repeat admissions, or mother–child separation that leads to an increased rate of emotional disturbance and difficulties in the mother–child relationships, but that a combination of factors, both family and social may contribute to adverse outcome for babies requiring major surgical intervention in the neonatal period.

Table 1 Illustration of the pattern of relationships between social and family factors, length of initial admission, repeat hospitalization and outcome at 3 years. The mothers of the eight children who had been readmitted and who had few behavior problems (low behavior scores) were, with one exception, older than the mothers of the seven children with high behavior scores. Only three of these more mature mothers were first-time mothers, and a majority had formal educational qualifications. In contrast, readmitted children with disturbed behavior were all first babies of teenage mothers, three of whom were single at the time of the birth. The mothers' education levels tended to be low, the majority having left school without qualifications, and both parenting skills and marriage ratings were generally poor. When a lengthy first admission was not followed by repeat hospital admissions, however, none of the children had behavior problems and only one of the five mothers was rated as having poor parenting skills. There was also a suggestion that more of the mothers in this situation were supported by a good relationship with their partners

Mother's age < 25	Primiparous	Social group	Education level	1st admission ≥ 26 days	Repeat admissions (days)	Behavior problem scores	Parenting	Postpartum separation > 7 days	Marriage
	+	NM	A+	+	4	low	G		G
	+	U(ML)	NFQ		31	low	M		P
		NM	A+		8	low	G	+	M
		U(ML)	NFQ	+	1	low	P	+	G
		NM	O		1	low	M		P
+	+	U(ML)	A+		12	low	G		M
	+	NM	O		56	low	G	+	G
		NM	CSE		129	low	G		G
+	+	NM	O	+	11	high	G		G
+	+	SM	NFQ	+	183	high	M		M
+	+	NM	NFQ	+	5	high	P		P
+	+	U(ML)	NFQ		7	high	P		P
+	+	SM	NFQ	+	11	high	P		M
+	+	SM	NFQ	+	19	high	P		P
+	+	ML	CSE	+	6	high	P		SEP
		NM	CSE		0	high	M		P
	+	ML	O		0	low	G		G
		ML	CSE		0	low	G		G
		NM	A+		0	low	G		G
		NM	NFQ		0	low	G		G
		ML	A+	+	0	low	G		G
+	+	NM	CSE	+	0	low	M		G
+	+	SM	NFQ	+	0	low	M		—
+		NM	O	+	0	low	G	+	G
		NM	A+		0	low	G	+	G
+		ML	NFQ	+	0	low	P		P

NM, non-manual; ML, manual; U, unemployed; SM, single mother at time of birth; A+, educated to advanced levels and beyond; O, educated to ordinary levels; CSE, certificate of secondary education; NFQ, no formal qualifications; G, good; M, moderate; P, poor; SEP, separated

SUMMARY OF FINDINGS FROM STUDY 2 (1991–1993)

Methods

Subjects

The study sample comprised 160 children, 90 boys and 70 girls, aged between 6 and 18 years at the time of assessment (mean age 11.3, SD 3.4 years). All were born with anorectal malformations, and had primary definitive surgery for correction of their anomaly at Great Ormond Street Hospital between 1974 and 1987. All the children had surgery in the neonatal period. The infants with low anomalies will have had immediate definitive surgery in the newborn period, while those with high and intermediate anomalies will have had a staged procedure commencing with a colostomy in the newborn period followed by a pull-through procedure and closure of the colostomy within the first year of life. Many required repeat admissions and/or further surgical procedures.

Of all of the children, 32% had associated anomalies; 80% of the sample were born at term, 17% had low birth weight and 4% had very low birth weight.

Design and measures

The children and their parents were seen in the outpatient department at Great Ormond Street Hospital. The medical and physical status of each child was reviewed by the surgeons. This was followed by separate psychosocial interviews with the parents and the child/adolescent. The child's psychological state was assessed using a standardized interview, and the parental interview included questions aimed at assessing psychological symptoms in the child. The parents also completed a standardized behavioral questionnaire, as did the children's teachers. The children completed a standardized depression questionnaire and a questionnaire which provided measures of self-esteem. Once again, other important factors contributing to outcome such as parental mental health, educational levels and the parental relationship formed part of the assessment battery[13].

Psychological and behavioral assessment

Based on the standardized diagnostic psychiatric interview with 157 out of the 160 children, 46 (29%) were judged as having some psychiatric disorder. The severity of the disorder ranged from 'mild' in 16 cases (10%) to 'moderate' in 30 (19%) (someone with a moderate disorder has a disorder which is severe enough to influence their daily lives). This prevalence of 19% is significantly higher when compared with a rate of 10% in the general child population ($p < 0.001$)[18].

Based on the behavior questionnaire completed by the parents, 39 (27%) youngsters had scores indicating psychopathology. This prevalence is significantly higher than the populations norms ($p < 0.01$). A high proportion of the youngsters had scores indicative of depressive-like symptoms (31%), so-called internalizing symptoms, while the proportion with high 'externalizing' scores (19%) – conduct disorders such as antisocial, aggressive or delinquent behaviors, was close to the population norm. The questionnaire completed by the teachers indicated that 17% of the sample had scores indicating maladjustment – a prevalence rate very similar to the population norm.

The depression scale completed by the youngsters showed that 24% rated themselves as having depressive symptoms – this was higher than expected when compared to the general child population. The youngsters' ratings of self-worth were similar to the norm for the population.

Summary of results

The prevalence of clinically significant emotional problems was higher than expected in relation to the population norms, with a high proportion of the children showing internalizing behavior problems, as well as reporting depressive symptoms.

Overall summary

The results from these two studies indicate that children who require major surgical intervention and hospitalization in the neonatal period are at risk for behavioral maladjustment and psychological disorder in early childhood and adolescence.

DISCUSSION

What factors contribute to this higher prevalence of maladjustment among children born with surgically correctable anomalies? The first point I would like to make is that although there was evidence of a higher prevalence of disorder among these children compared to normative populations, the level of disorder was similar to that found among children with chronic health problems. However, although a relatively high proportion of these children have chronic health problems, emotional disturbance at 3 years of age, and among the older children with anorectal anomalies, was not related to severity of the condition. Parental factors and parenting skills, or possibly an interaction between these factors and repeat hospital admissions, had a stronger influence on outcome. This empirical evidence and the data I obtained from the in-depth interviews leads me to suggest that when discussing families who have children with medical problems (but no significant developmental delay), it is important to differentiate between those families with children who are *born* with congenital abnormalities, and those whose children develop health problems in childhood or adolescence. Although it may be stating the obvious, giving birth, usually at or near term, to a child with an abnormality, has a substantial impact on parents, and I believe this has a marked influence on their feelings towards that child. The majority of parents interviewed during the course of this research found it impossible to ignore or forget the fact that the child was born with a life-threatening abnormality. Even if the child or adolescent was functioning 'as normal', he or she continued to be very special and tended to be treated differently from other children in the family. So, from infancy onwards, sympathy for the child and parental feelings of guilt may lead parents to treat the child as especially 'vulnerable', and as they grow up, this results in over-indulgence, and over-involvement with the child. Additionally, as a relatively high proportion have long term health problems, the child may require frequent visits to hospital, repeat hospital admissions and operative procedures. The parents may also be involved in carrying out procedures which may be unpleasant and even painful for the child as well as seeming intrusive. These factors tend to exacerbate parental over-involvement with the child, and increases the child's dependence of the parent(s).

The second important issue was parenting behavior. A high proportion of the parents found it difficult to respond to the behavior of their growing child in a firm and consistent manner. If they were firm or tried to set limits, they did not persist or maintain their stance. This was apparent in the first study as well as among the 6- to 18-year-old age group. So, many of these youngsters manipulated the inconsistency in their parents' response. Patterns of behavior developed which had an adverse effect on their emotional and social development and consequently behavior. All these factors may also have an effect on overall family functioning which in turn has an important impact on children's social and emotional development.

In conclusion, difficult or disturbed behavior might be avoided, and the quality of life for the child and the family improved, both in the short and longer term, if informed psychological guidance and support were available to these families as part of the continuing care following surgery. In the 1990s these considerations are particularly important since many more survivors of major neonatal surgery reach adult life and their personal adjustment assumes a high priority.

References

1. Rutter, M. (1981). *Maternal Deprivation Reassessed*, 2nd edn. (London: Penguin Books)
2. Douglas, J. W. B. (1975). Early hospital admissions and later disturbances of behavior and learning. *Dev. Med. Child Neurol.*, **17**, 456–80
3. Quinton, D. and Rutter, M. (1976). Early hospital admissions and later disturbances of behaviour: an attempted replication of Douglas's findings. *Dev. Med. Child Neurol.*, **18**, 447–57

4. Schaffer, H. R. and Callender, W. M. (1959). Psychological effects of hospitalization in infancy. *Pediatrics*, **24**, 528–39

5. Elmer, E. and Gregg, G. S. (1967). Developmental characteristics of abused children. *Pediatrics*, **40**, 596–602

6. Lynch, M. A. and Roberts, J. (1977). Predicting child abuse: signs of bonding failure in the maternity hospital. *Br. Med. J.*, **1**, 624–6

7. Minde, K. K. (1980). Bonding of parents to premature infants: theory and practice. In Taylor, P. M. (ed.) *Parent–Infant Relationships*, pp. 291–313. (New York: Grune)

8. Ludman, L. (1990). *The psychological effects of major neonatal surgery on infants and their families.* PhD, University of London

9. Ludman, L., Spitz, L. and Lansdown, R. (1990). Developmental progress of newborns undergoing neonatal surgery. *J. Pediatr. Surg.*, **25**(5), 469–71

10. Ludman, L., Spitz, L. and Lansdown, R. (1993). Intellectual development at 3 years of age of children who underwent major neonatal surgery. *J. Pediatr. Surg.*, **28**(2), 130–4

11. Ludman, L., Lansdown, R. and Spitz, L. (1992). Effects of early hospitalization and surgery on the emotional development of 3-year-olds: an exploratory study. *Eur. Child Adolescent Psychiatr.*, **1**(3), 186–95

12. Ludman, L., Spitz, L. and Kiely, E. M. (1994). Social and emotional impact of faecal incontinence following surgery for anorectal anomalies. *Arch. Dis. Child.*, **71**, 194–200

13. Ludman, L. and Spitz, L. (1995). Psychosocial adjustment of children treated for anorectal anomalies. *J. Pediatr. Surg.*, **30**(3), 495–9

14. Ludman, L. and Spitz, L. (1996). Coping strategies of children with faecal incontinence. *J. Pediatr. Surg.*, **31**(4), 563–7

15. Richman, N., Stevenson, J. E. and Graham, P. J. (1975). Prevalence of behaviour problems in 3-year-old children: an epidemiological study in a London borough. *J. Child Psychol. Psychiatry*, **16**, 277–87

16. Earls, F. (1980). Prevalence of behaviour problems in three-year-old children. *Arch. Gen. Psychiatry*, **37**, 1153–7

17. Jenkins, S., Owen, C., Bax, M. and Hart, H. (1984). Continuities of common behaviour problems in preschool children. *J. Child Psychol. Psychiatry*, **25**(1), 75–90

18. Pearce, J. (1993). Child health surveillance for psychiatric disorder: practical guidelines. *Arch. Dis. Child.*, **69**, 394–8

Information technology in the neonatal unit

53

N. McIntosh

INTRODUCTION

Information of use in a neonatal unit may be demographic, or it may be specific to the babies' condition in either static or dynamic form.

Demographic data

Demographic data about an infant may be important for effective management, thus the parents' telephone number may be required in the middle of the night as a crisis develops or it may be essential to get in touch with the family doctor to appraise him of a baby's condition. A file of useful demographic data is essential on most patients in intensive care.

Static data

Any infant admitted to a neonatal unit (or child admitted to an intensive care unit) has a preceding history, both in terms of its environment, which in the context of the neonate is usually the mother's pregnancy, and in terms of the current problems. For instance, respiratory distress syndrome in the baby may already have been treated with surfactant at a referring hospital. Such data should be instantaneously available for optimal care. In many babies there will be relatively little static data, but in some there will be a complex maternal history and history of the baby before admission.

Monitoring data

Over the last 30 years monitors have developed for respiratory, cardiovascular, cerebral and thermoregulatory functions. Electronic monitoring does not exist to replace nurses but to complement their observation with a reliable alternative. Quite often the primary goal of electronic monitors is to draw attention to a deterioration in the patient's condition. The nurse or doctor has to act on this. For effective action, the staff must appreciate the physiology behind the monitoring so as to be able to discern artefacts from true physiological information. Monitoring consists of making observations or measurements on a repetitive basis. The information gained through monitoring indicates a patient's condition and from this evaluation appropriate courses of therapy are determined. There should thus be a link between the physiological variables being monitored and the patient's prognosis. The choices of signals for a particular illness are well established; it may be appropriate to measure the pO_2 in pneumonia or in a postoperative thoracotomy patient, but in addition to measure blood pressure if there is septicemia or if the thoracotomy involved cardiac surgery (many would consider that blood pressure measurement should be part of the monitoring in any significantly ill child). In all cases temperature monitoring would be useful.

The clinical objectives are to decrease neonatal mortality and also reduce morbidity. In relation to this, physiological monitoring identifies physiological concepts rather than diagnostic conditions. Thus monitoring the blood pressure is a way of looking at the effectiveness of cardiac activity related to cardiac output and peripheral resistance, not specific to ventricular septal defect or myocardial ischemia. Effective blood pressure ensures perfusion of organs, particularly the brain, and monitoring of pO_2 ensures that hypoxia and hyperoxia are avoided. A further goal with monitoring is to ensure that the response of a patient to treatment is adequate, thus the improvement in blood pressure with inotrope infusion reduces the likelihood of brain damage from ischemia, and the improvement in oxygen with increased ventilator mean airway pressure or surfactant makes cerebral hypoxia less likely. Any parameter believed to be associated with mortality or morbidity could legitimately be repeatedly or continuously measured with limit alarms set for each end of the normal range. Table 1 shows some physiological variables and their derivatives that may be seen monitored in a neonatal unit.

PHILOSOPHY OF MONITORING

The public expect monitoring, but it is worth asking why we do it. At present we might monitor a high-risk baby to reassure ourselves of normality; this may be undertaken by using limit alarms which indicate abnormality outside a particular range, or stability. Trend monitors looking at temporal patterns add a time dimension to current normality. If a trend has been constant and stable for a period of time, staff at a changeover can be very reassured about a high-risk infant. We may be attempting to diagnose abnormality, but with limit alarms this diagnosis may be at a very late stage with little time to rectify the underlying problem before lasting damage is done.

In contrast trend analysis, in detecting a steady change, may give warning before a reference range is exceeded, e.g. a fall in blood pressure. A trend monitor is designed to sense a change, ideally before damage occurs.

Reference ranges

Knowledge of reference ranges related to the baby's age and condition is appropriate when setting both limit alarms on monitors and in order to appreciate abnormal trends. Remarkably little data are available on reference ranges with regard to gestation and postnatal age, though blood pressure would be an exception to this[1-3].

Table 1 Physiological variables and their derivatives that are monitored in a neonatal unit

Measured parameters	Derived parameters
Central temperature	differential temperature
Peripheral temperature	
Incubator temperature	
Heart rate	cardiac output
Blood pressure (systolic, diastolic and mean)	
Venous pressure	
Respiratory rate	apnea
Arterial or transcutaneous oxygen tension	oxygenation index
Arterial or transcutaneous carbon dioxide tension	gas exchange
Arterial oxygen saturation	
Fraction of inspired oxygen	
Apnea	
Blood pH	base deficit/excess
Electroencephalogram	cerebral function
Cerebral function monitor	
Ultrasound examination	
Computed tomography and magnetic resonance	
Nuclear magnetic resonance spectroscopy	
Near infrared spectroscopy	cerebral perfusion pressure intracranial pressure

Display of data

Data should only be displayed when it reveals important physiology to the person observing the display. Thus it may be appropriate to have different displays for the nurse, doctor and respiratory therapist. Information should be presented about patients in a manner which is easily comprehensible. If the individual staff member has no ability to understand the displayed information, either he or she needs education or the information should be displayed in a different manner (if in the first place it is important enough to be recorded at all). Figure 1 shows how the decreasing trend in peripheral temperature over 8 hours is difficult to appreciate when displayed with other parameters on the screen. In Figure 2 there are an equal number of trend displays and the temperature displays are scaled the same. The plot of differen-

tial temperature displays easily to the eye that there is an increasing problem (probably cold stress).

Most commercially available neonatal monitors will provide only two types of display; a view of all signals monitored over 3–60 s, and a summary view of the data trended over a period of time from a few minutes to several days, through which the user can scroll. The display of only a proportion of the monitored data which is on line in real time, so important information may or may not be revealed to the clinician. A sick neonate may be monitored for weeks or occasionally months, so displaying a small proportion of the time in a scrolling window may not be ideal.

Who decides which parameters should be displayed and over what time base? Different display sets will be of interest to different people and over different time bases, but in addition

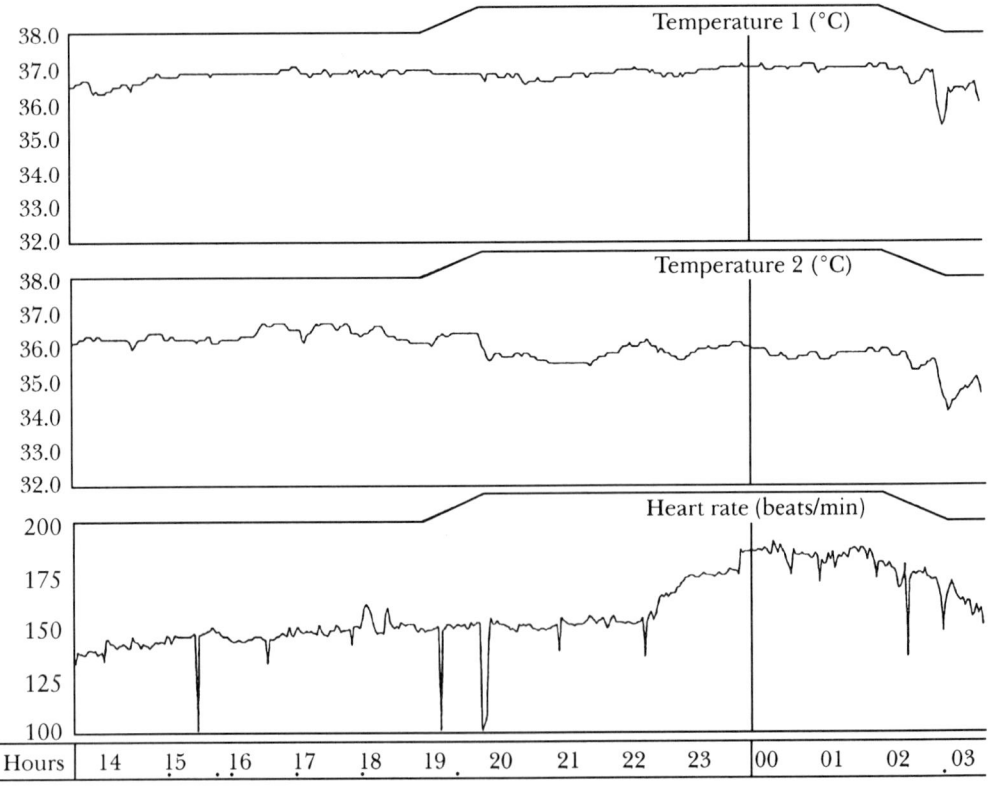

Figure 1 Falling peripheral temperature. The top trace shows the central temperature, the middle trace the peripheral temperature and the bottom trace the heart rate

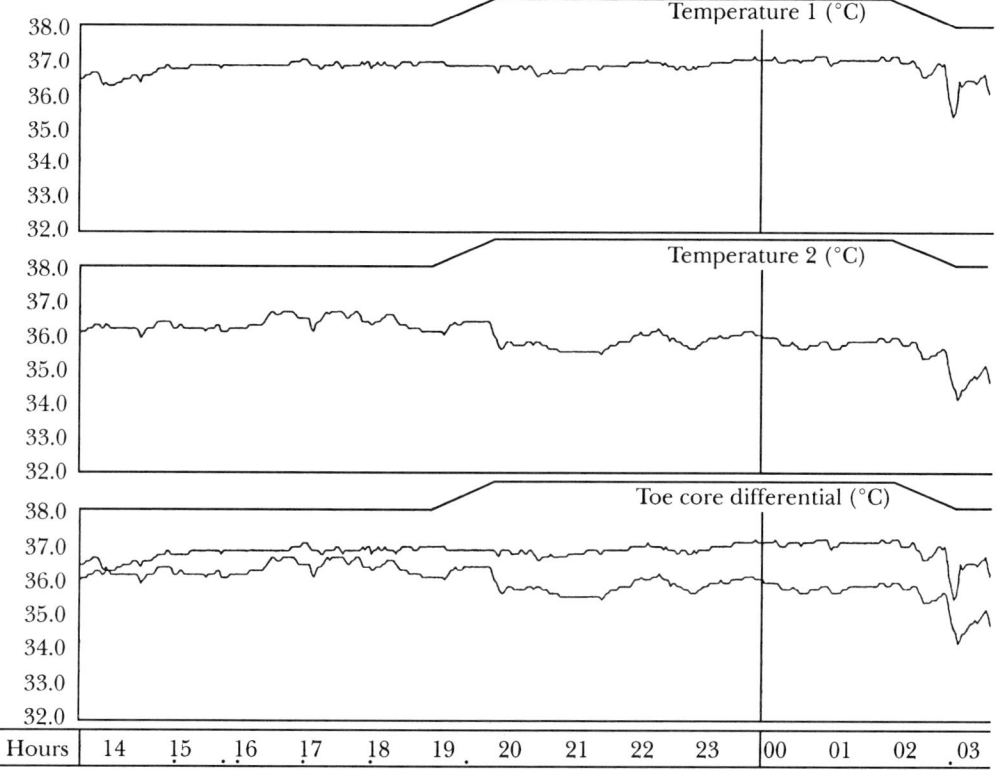

Figure 2 Increasing differential temperature. The top trace shows the central temperature, the middle trace the peripheral temperature and the bottom trace the differential temperature. The scaling is the same as in Figure 1, but the eye can now more easily appreciate the problem

different display sets will be appropriate for different patients with different problems.

Overload

Understanding of the parameters and their deviations by junior medical and nursing staff varies considerably, and this may be a powerful reason for decision support. Although data overlooked *per se* is unlikely, there may be display overload, and the more information that is displayed on the screen, the more likely it is that a critical item will be overlooked. This is more from cognitive or attentional overloading[4], where the attentional resource of the observer is swamped, leading to perceptual error. More attention is required to see the thermal problems displayed in Figure 1 than the same thermal problems in Figure 2. It is likely that attentional overload is common in junior staff and it could be said that only abnormal data should be placed on display. This however negates the usefulness and reassurance of a normal display.

Attentional overload is compounded by noise and artefacts, and although there has been considerable improvement in monitors over recent years, artefacts remain the commonest reason for staff switching off alarms.

Alarms and intelligence

The current alarms on monitors are limit alarms. These are activated late if the reference limits are widely set, or are frustrating in the high false-positive rate if set too closely. The setting of alarms is closely bound up with the detection of artefacts and it is an important consideration for the development of monitor intelligence and decision support in the future[5]. Trend alarms allow the possibility of pattern recognition, the rise in blood pressure associated with increased heart rate variability during a care procedure or cranial ultrasound may be characteristic of a physiological but iatrogenic abnormality. Pathologically, blockage or displacement of the endotracheal tube or the development of a pneumothorax may be associated with a pattern of increasing oxygen variability, heart rate and blood pressure variability and a rise in carbon dioxide. Patterns and pattern recognition are of particular importance for intelligent trend monitoring in the future but at this stage we do not know the consistency of patterns for a particular artefact,

physiological response or pathological process, i.e. what the sensitivity and specificity are for each pattern. When such data are available they can be built into the trend monitors which can also take account of the static data available on an infant. In this way, the knowledge that the baby is ventilated might indicate that a rising CO_2 level is due to blockage of an endotracheal tube. If, on the other hand, the monitor 'knew' that the baby was not ventilated, the rising CO_2 might indicate a respiratory drive problem or the development of a pneumothorax.

The development of intelligent monitoring and decision support in intensive care areas will lead to a more consistent knowledge of an infant which is less dependent on the individual knowledge of the staff member.

References

1. Cunningham, S., Deere, S. and McIntosh, N. (1993). Cyclical variation of blood pressure and heart rate in neonates. *Arch. Dis. Child.*, **69**, 64–7
2. Tan, K. L. (1988). Blood pressure in very low birth weight infants in the first 70 days of life. *J. Pediatr.*, **112**, 266–70
3. Cunningham, S. and McIntosh, N. (1992). Blood pressure monitoring in intensive care neonates. *Br. J. Int. Care*, **2**, 381–8
4. Coiera, E. W., Tombs, V. J., Higgins, G. J. and Clutton-Brock, T. H. (1994). *Real Time Clinical Decision Making. A Case Study in Anaesthesia.* (Bristol: Hewlett-Packard Laboratories)
5. Cunningham, S., Symon, A. G. and McIntosh, N. (1994). The practical management of artifact in computerised physiological data. *Int. J. Clin. Monit. Comput.*, **11**, 211–16

Medical rationale and current research in the nebulization of surfactant in newborns with respiratory distress syndrome

S. Bambang Oetomo and P. H. Dijk

Surfactant treatment for neonatal respiratory distress syndrome (RDS) has become a routine in most developed countries. The introduction of this therapy resulted in reduction of mortality and complications due to RDS. However, the surfactant instillation procedure has raised some concerns about safety. Rapid fluctuations in blood pressure and cerebral blood flow during and after surfactant treatment have been described. Furthermore, not all babies respond to surfactant treatment, in terms of sustained improvement of lung function, so that they can be weaned off the ventilator without development of chronic lung disease. Among other factors, non-uniform distribution of surfactant could be one of the explanations for the incomplete success of this therapy. We hypothesized that surfactant nebulization could be a reasonable alternative, since theoretically a more gradual administration would avoid fluctuations in blood pressure and would probably result in a more uniform distribution to the lung. Therefore we tested several jet-nebulizers and assessed the efficiency and safety of the devices and we studied the surface lowering properties of the surfactant after nebulization. We found that the MiniNEB (Vortran) had the highest efficiency and that surfactant (Alveofact®, Boehringer Ingelheim, Germany) function was not impaired following nebulization. In rabbits with respiratory failure induced by multiple lung lavage we compared surfactant instillation and surfactant nebulization with respect to cerebral blood flow and blood pressure in the carotid artery. We found that surfactant instillation resulted in an instantaneous drop in blood pressure and a more pronounced drop in cerebral blood flow. In the rabbits that were treated by surfactant nebulization these parameters only decreased gradually over time. Differences in surfactant distribution were assessed by labelling the surfactant before administration with ^{99m}Tc-nanocoll. Distribution histograms were obtained of the radioactivity of the ^{99m}Tc-nanocoll in 200 lung pieces from each animal. A more uniform distribution was found in the lungs of the rabbits that had been treated by surfactant nebulization.

In subsequent experiments we compared surfactant nebulization and surfactant instillation with respect to effects on lung function in rabbits with severe respiratory failure. In contrast to the instantaneous rise in arterial pO_2 that is well known for surfactant instillation, we found that during and following surfactant nebulization the arterial pO_2 gradually increased, reaching a maximum 90 min after the onset of the nebulization. After the physiological measurements, the lungs were isolated and pressure volume curves were obtained and static compliance and stability index were calculated. We found lower values for these parameters in the animals that underwent surfactant nebulization compared to surfactant instillation.

We conclude that nebulization is a safe procedure for administering surfactant and leads to a more uniform distribution than surfactant instillation. Lung function of subjects with severe respiratory failure is improved following surfactant nebulization, but so far the effects of surfactant instillation in these animals are more pronounced.

Alteration of pulmonary surfactant in adult respiratory distress syndrome: effects of a transbronchial surfactant application

A. Günther, D. Walmrath, F. Grimminger and W. Seeger

Pulmonary surfactant is a lipoprotein complex covering the alveolar surface. By profoundly reducing the surface tension at the air–liquid interface, it prevents alveoli from collapse, in particular during expiration. It is composed of ≈ 90% lipids (mostly phospholipids and minor percentages of neutral lipids) and 10% proteins. Phosphatidylcholine (mostly dipalmitoylated, DPPC) accounts for ≈ 80% and phosphatidyl-glycerol (PG) for ≈ 10% of the phospholipids. Among the protein fraction, four surfactant-specific apoproteins have so far been discovered and are called surfactant protein (SP)-A, SP-B, SP-C and SP-D. The major cellular source of pulmonary surfactant is the alveolar type II cell. Upon exocytosis of the surfactant-containing lamellar bodies, which is physiologically triggered by the inspiratory stretch of the alveolar cell layer, the surfactant is reorganized into tubular myelin and large multilamellar vesicles, also comprising large surfactant aggregates. Presentation of the hydrophobic compounds, in particular DPPC, from these aggregates to the air–liquid interface results in the formation of a stable phospholipid film, which, upon compression, can reduce the surface tension to near zero mN/m. Next to DPPC and PG, the hydrophobic surfactant apoproteins SP-B and SP-C, in particular, seem to represent essential constituents for fulfillment of this function. The periodic compression and re-expansion of the interfacial phospholipid film provokes its permanent refinement, with squeeze-out and re-entry of single components. Thus, via the interfacial monolayer, the large surfactant aggregates are converted into unilamellar vesicles (small surfactant aggregates), which represent the 'degradation' products of the lining layer subjected to the fate of re-uptake and recycling by the type II cell (triggered by the hydrophilic SP-A), phagocytosis by alveolar macrophages or loss along the mucociliar escalator. By reducing the alveolar surface tension, pulmonary surfactant additionally influences the alveolar liquid homeostasis. Any increase in alveolar surface tension will further lower the hydrostatic pressure in the alveolar lining layer and the interstitial compartments and thus favour fluid flux into these spaces. Finally, although the details are far from clear, pulmonary surfactant has an effect on host-defense mechanisms within the alveolar compartment. In particular, SP-A and SP-D, both being C-type lectins, have been suggested to opsonize microbial agents and thereby to favour their phagocytosis by alveolar macrophages.

Lack of surface active material is the primary cause of the infant respiratory distress syndrome (IRDS), and surfactant therapy (50–100 mg/kg body weight) now represents the 'gold standard'. However, in the acute respiratory distress syndrome (ARDS), both in adults and infants, which is characterized by overwhelming inflammatory processes at the gas exchange unit, surfactant deficiency does not seem to be of major importance, but a broad pattern of biochemical and biophysical abnormalities of the pulmonary surfactant system is observed, which, together favor alveolar collapse with ventilation/perfusion-mismatch and in particular, shunt flow. Analysis of bronchoalveolar lavage fluids (BALF) from ARDS patients consistently demonstrated a decrease of the surface tension reducing properties, with minimum surface tension values being increased to > 15–20 mN/m, instead of near zero in healthy controls. Several biochemical alterations were encountered in these patients and included:

(1) Alteration of the phospholipid profile with a reduction of the relative percentages of phosphatidylcholine and phosphatidylglycerol and an increase in the relative percentages of phosphatidylinositol, phosphatidylethanolamine and sphingomyelin.

(2) Alteration of the fatty acid composition with a marked reduction of the relative content of saturated, especially palmitic acid, species among the phospholipid fraction.

(3) Decreased levels of surfactant apoproteins, as shown for the hydrophilic SP-A in native BALF and for SP-B among the large surfactant aggregate fraction.

(4) Reduced content of large surfactant aggregates: several experimental studies suggested that induction of an acute lung injury would result in a higher abundance of the small surfactant aggregates at the expense of the large surfactant aggregates. Accordingly, a reduction in the relative content of large surfactant aggregates could be demonstrated in ARDS.

(5) Inhibition of surfactant function by leaked plasma proteins: leakage of plasma proteins into the alveolar space is a common finding in ARDS. The BALF phospholipid to protein ratio normally lies in the region of 0.5 (wt/wt) but reaches mean values as low as 0.05 in ARDS. Strong surfactant inhibitory capacity could be demonstrated *ex vivo* for the total BALF proteins and *in vitro* for albumin, hemoglobin, fibrinogen and especially fibrin, the latter known to be easily generated in the alveolar space of

ARDS patients due to increased procoagulant and antifibrinolytic activities.

(6) Inhibition by inflammatory mediators, in particular proteases and oxygen radicals released by inflammatory cells, which may primarily attack the functionally important hydrophobic apoproteins SP-B and SP-C. A corresponding scenario of complex surfactant disturbances, as described for ARDS primarily triggered by diseases remote from the lung (e.g. sepsis, polytrauma, pancreatitis), was also observed under conditions of severe pneumonia demanding mechanical ventilation.

Against this background, improvement of alveolar surfactant function appears to be a reasonable approach to improve gas exchange in ARDS patients. Such attempts may include pharmacological approaches to stimulate the secretion of intact surfactant material from type II pneumocytes, but clear evidence that this approach may be effectively used under conditions of acute respiratory failure is still missing. In addition, transbronchial administration of exogenous (natural) surfactant preparations, commonly used in IRDS, may also be employed in ARDS, but will clearly demand larger quantities of material to overcome the surfactant inhibitory capacities in the alveolar space under these conditions. The publication of two pilot studies in this field is under way. Performing repetitive intratracheal application of Survanta® with cumulative doses between 300 and 800 mg/kg body weight, T. Gregory and colleagues noted some improvement of gas exchange and even obtained some preliminary evidence for an increase in survival in adults with acute respiratory failure[1]. Our group investigated the safety and efficacy of a bronchoscopic application of a natural surfactant extract (Alveofact®) in patients with severe ARDS[2]. All patients fulfilled extracorporeal membrane oxygenation (ECMO) criteria (mean Murray lung injury score ≈ 3.3) and were treated within the first 5 days of disease, i.e. before the onset of major fibrotic processes. Underlying diseases were mostly sepsis and severe pneumonia; at the present time, the study includes 21 patients. Alveofact 300 mg/kg was delivered bronchoscopically in divided doses to each segment of both lungs (total dose 22.5 ± 1.4 g in 375 ml saline), followed by a second application of 200 mg/kg (total dose 15.5 ± 1.05 g in 260 ml saline) 18–24 h later in selected patients. Measurements of gas exchange, including ventilation-perfusion characteristics, hemodynamic measurements and bronchoalveolar lavage (BAL) were performed before and after surfactant application. The first surfactant application resulted in an immediate increase of mean PaO_2/FiO_2 from < 90 mmHg to ≈ 200 mmHg, mainly due to a decrease in shunt-flow (from $\approx 40\%$ to $\approx 20\%$). Approximately two-thirds of the patients 'responded', with a PaO_2/FiO_2 increase of at least 25%. The effect was partially lost within the following hours in some of the responders, but was restored with prolonged improvement of arterial oxygenation by the second application. Initial BAL showed severe alteration of surfactant composition and impairment of biophysical surfactant function. Surfactant application resulted in a marked, but still incomplete, restoration of surfactant properties, with a profound improvement of the phospholipid (PL) : protein ratio (0.04 pre, 0.27 post, healthy controls 0.58); relative content of large surfactant aggregates (38.6% pre, 74.2% post, control 76%, as percentage of total PL); relative content of phosphatidylcholine (70.5 pre, 85.3 post, control 83.1%, as percentage of total PL); minimum surface tension in the absence (23.3 mN/m pre, 13 mN/M post, control 0.25 mN/m) as well as in the presence of the BALF proteins (34 mN/m pre, 23.3 mN/m post, control 0.3 mN/m). Analysis of the ventilation/perfusion characteristics revealed that in response to the bronchoscopic surfactant application, formerly collapsed alveoli were reaerated, yielding a reduction of the intrapulmonary shunt flow and an increase in regions with low and normal ventilation/perfusion ratios.

In conclusion, profound alterations of the alveolar surfactant system are encountered in ARDS. There is now good evidence that these abnormalities contribute to the severe impairment in gas exchange under these conditions. Transbronchial surfactant application, performed by bronchoscopy by our group, may offer a feasible and safe approach to improve the biochemical and biophysical properties of the endogenous surfactant pool and, by this, the gas exchange conditions in most severe early-stage ARDS. However, a high and/or repetitive dosage regimen appears to be necessary to overcome inhibitory capacities in the alveolar space of these patients and to achieve sustained alveolar recruitment. Forthcoming studies will have to define the optimum timing and dosage regimen of such interventions and will have to address the question as to whether this therapy is capable of reducing the high mortality of patients with very severe ARDS.

References

1. Gregory, T. *et al.* (1994). *Am. J. Resp. Crit. Care Med.*, Abstr.
2. Walmrath, D., Ghofrani, H. A., Grimhinger, F. and Seeger, W. (1996). Synergism of alveolar endotoxin 'priming' and intravascular exotoxin challenge in lung injury. *Am. J. Resp. Crit. Care Med.*, **154**, 460–8

Surfactant in the treatment of secondary respiratory failure in preterm and term infants

56

J. C. Möller, M. Herkenhoff, M. Kohl, I. Reiss, T. F. Schuible and L. Gortner

INTRODUCTION

New concepts in the treatment of respiratory disorders introduced to neonatal medicine are frequently used in adult medicine later on, and *vice versa*. For example, intermittent mandatory ventilation was introduced for preterm neonates and was later on used successfully in all age groups[1].

A causative treatment for respiratory distress syndrome, in which there is a relative surfactant deficiency state, is intratracheal exogenous surfactant supplementation, as first described by Fujiwara and associates in 1980[2]. Adult respiratory distress syndrome (ARDS) is an end-stage disease of many different etiologies; in adults sepsis and trauma are the major underlying conditions for ARDS. Proteins, prostaglandins, adhesion molecules, blood components and other inflammation-associated factors which are produced in the alveoli during ARDS inactivate surfactant. Supplementation of surfactant in these secondary surfactant deficiency situations in ARDS is based on these considerations[3]. Over the last years many small series on surfactant treatment in ARDS have been published, most of them reporting an improved oxygenation, lung compliance and outcome[3].

Acute severe respiratory failure in infants, and children beyond neonatal age is not very different from adult ARDS[4]. Underlying diseases might be different, barotrauma and oxygen toxicity might be more important, and therefore basic treatment strategies may be different, for example ventilation. However, new techniques to improve the poor outcome of ARDS in adults, such as high frequency ventilation, nitric oxide, liquid ventilation and surfactant, are being discussed in relation to and have already been applied to children after the neonatal period[4–7].

We demonstrated a significant increase in oxygenation, i.e. the oxygenation index (partial pressure oxygen/fraction inspired oxygen) in 19 children between 2 and 50 months of age, from 56 before surfactant administration to 84 at 4 h and 98 at 24 h after 80–250 mg/kg bovine surfactant (Alveofact, Boehringer, Germany). None of our patients died because of respiratory failure, although four died due to their underlying disease[6] (Figure 1).

ARDS is frequently associated with pulmonary hypertension, the more so the younger the patients are. We observed an additional beneficial effect of inhaled nitric oxide on the treatment of non-neonatal pediatric ARDS patients[7]. Nitric oxide was the primary therapy if pulmonary hypertension was detected by echocardiography, and surfactant was the secondary treatment. A substantially different technique used predominantly in children is extracorporeal membrane oxygenation, where lung rest reducing the amount of alveolar hyperoxia and barotrauma is the fundamental rationale[5]. This therapy was first successful, however, in neonates with pulmonary hypertension of the newborn of different origin[8]. Neonatal severe respiratory failure is usually not associated with the term ARDS, especially because pulmonary hypertension is so much more predominant in

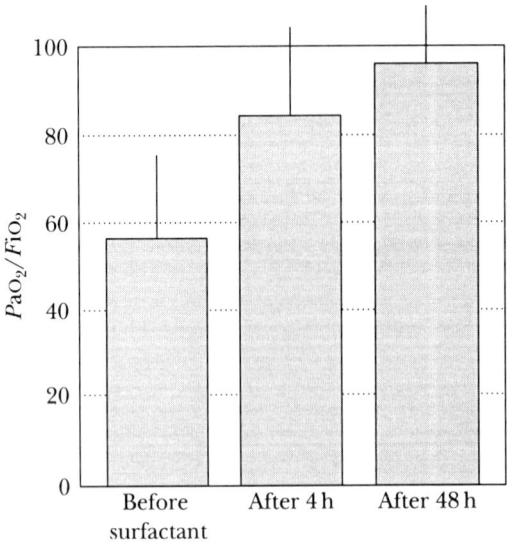

Figure 1 Partial pressure oxygen (PaO_2)/fraction inspired oxygen (FiO_2) ratio in non-neonatal adult respiratory distress syndrome (ARDS) before and after therapy with 50–250 mg bovine surfactant, as studied by our group. Mean data from 19 patients (2–50 months of age), bars represent standard deviation from mean

neonates, characterizing severe neonatal respiratory failure.

RATIONALE FOR SURFACTANT USE IN RESPIRATORY FAILURE OF TERM NEONATES

ARDS in its original concept is defined by histological, radiographical, oxygenation and compliance characteristics[4]. Based on this concept ARDS can be found in term neonates, especially the radiographical picture of diffuse alveolar infiltrates[9]. The underlying diseases are many: congenital pneumonia, meconium and blood aspiration syndrome, sepsis, hypoxia, etc. The overlapping with etiologies of secondary pulmonary hypertension, as the original extracorporeal membrane oxygenation (ECMO) indication, is nearly 100%[8–10]. Perhaps only primary pulmonary hypertension of the newborn with totally clear lungs is not an 'ARDS-like disease'. So neonatologists, having become used to surfactant in the treatment of preterm infants

with RDS on the one side, asked whether surfactant could be a treatment of choice in pneumonia, meconium aspiration and persistent fetal circulation (synonymous with secondary pulmonary hypertension of the newborn) in term babies[10]. Similarly adult specialists looked at the similarities between ARDS and respiratory failure in term neonates[11].

As ECMO has been proven to be of benefit to neonates with severe respiratory failure[12], therapeutical strategies with surfactant should not exclude the possibility of ECMO as a rescue therapy and be concentrated in institutions offering ECMO. Nitric oxide, which is efficacious in pulmonary hypertension of the newborn, should also be available[4,7].

RESULTS IN TERM NEWBORN PATIENTS WITH RESPIRATORY FAILURE

To study the effects of surfactant and a combined surfactant/nitric oxide therapy in term neonates with severe respiratory failure we introduced a treatment algorithm with a strict time frame using the Hallman oxygenation index (OI = $FiO_2 \times 100 \times$ MAWP (mean airway pressure)/PaO_2) and the echocardiographically determined degree of pulmonary hypertension as parameters for choosing treatment options (Figure 2). If a neonate transferred to our institution had $PaO_2 < 35$ mmHg, ECMO was immediately started. In other children with an oxygenation index > 40 over 4 h, we tried to optimize ventilation and hemodynamics with conventional means; if after that the OI did not decrease by 10, exogenous surfactant was given (50–250 mg/kg as tolerated); if the pulmonary artery pressure was determined to be suprasystemic 4 h after surfactant therapy we added 10–20 ppm of nitric oxide.

We have treated a total of 32 patients since introducing this algorithm. Only four patients required ECMO based on the above-mentioned rapid entrance criteria (two long-term survivors). Nine patients were treated with surfactant alone, all of which had a remarkable decrease of their OI from a mean of 52 before

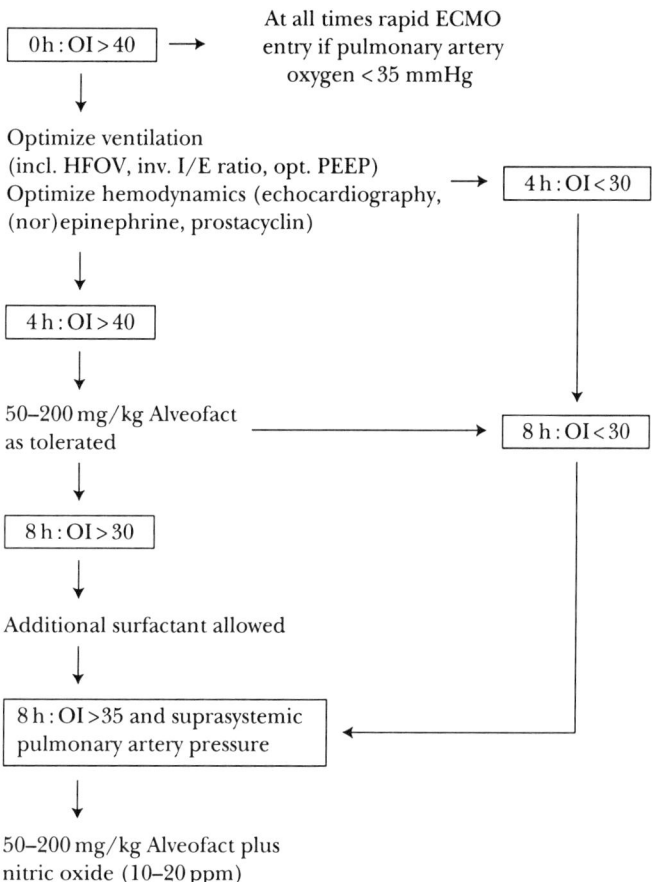

Figure 2 Treatment algorithm as used in the treatment of adult respiratory distress syndrome-like disease in term neonates at the Medical University of Lübeck. OI, oxygenation index = fraction inspired oxygen × 100 × mean airways pressure/partial pressure oxygen; ECMO, extracorporeal membrane oxygenation; HFOV, high-frequency oscillatory ventilation; I/E, inspiratory/expiratory time ratio; PEEP, positive end expiratory pressure

surfactant to 34 only 1 h after surfactant therapy. Adding nitric oxide in 18 patients (group of combined surfactant/NO therapy) who had a suprasystemic pulmonary artery pressure did not significantly alter the rate of OI decrease; there was only a trend towards an additive effect of nitric oxide (Figure 3). The underlying diseases in our patients were: pneumonia ($n = 4$), posthypoxic respiratory failure ($n = 7$), congenital diaphragmatic hernias ($n = 3$), meconium aspiration syndrome ($n = 9$), sepsis ($n = 4$), blood aspiration ($n = 2$) and severe wet lung ($n = 3$).

DISCUSSION OF OUR RESULTS IN TERM NEONATES

Meconium aspiration syndrome, pneumonia, sepsis and many other conditions causing ARDS-like disease in newborn infants, are characterized by secondary surfactant inactivation, and tracheal aspirates contain significantly less phospholipids in these children[13,14]. Surfactant therapy in a sepsis pig model was shown to correct the endotoxin-induced secondary surfactant deficiency, but lung function, i.e. oxygenation, is only moderately influenced by

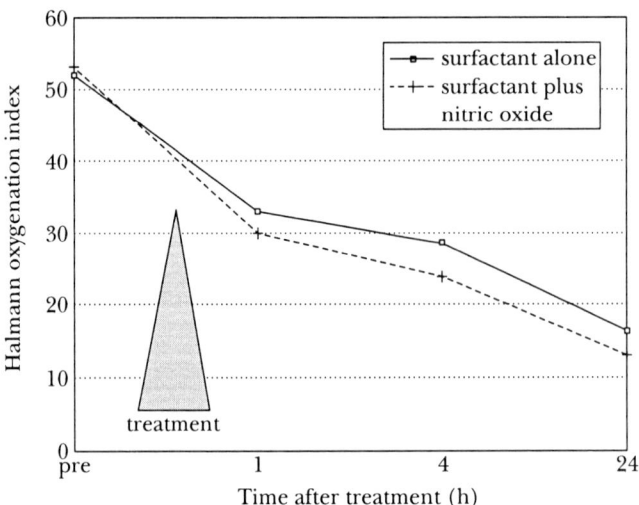

Figure 3 Halmann oxygenation index in term infants treated either with surfactant alone ($n = 9$) or with surfactant plus nitric oxide ($n = 18$). Differences between the two groups are not significant (t-test) at any time. In each group the oxygenation index drops significantly from before treatment to 1 h after treatment, and from 4 h after to 24 h after treatment ($p < 0.01$)

surfactant treatment[15,16]. In a small observational study, Fetter and colleagues, however, demonstrated a remarkable increase in oxygenation after surfactant therapy in septic newborns in the clinical situation[15]. The clinical study was performed based on positive results in septic ARDS in animals[16]. In cases of meconium aspiration both in animal models and in clinical case reports a substitution of secondarily inactivated surfactant could either improve lung function or oxygenation[17–20].

Our observation that, based on the introduced algorithm, a sustained improvement of oxygenation by surfactant therapy with 50–250 mg/kg bovine surfactant could be achieved in a group of neonates with respiratory failure of different etiologies is comparable with smaller previously published series of surfactant-treated term neonates[21–23]. Case reports exist claiming a benefit of surfactant in blood aspiration and congenital diaphragmatic hernia[24,25].

We do not have an explanation for the minimal additional therapeutic benefit of nitric oxide. As pulmonary hypertension is a universal finding in severe term neonatal respiratory failure, nitric oxide should be of benefit. The hypothesis of a genetically determined malfunction of surfactant (surfactant protein B mutants) in these responders is very speculative[26]. The finding, however, that lysophosphatidylcholine, a constituent of the bovine surfactant preparation we used, is a vasodilator might give a hint as to why surfactant as primary therapy was so effective in our patients without a remarkable additional effect of nitric oxide[27].

As under continuous positive airway pressure (CPAP), surfactant helps to open alveoli[28], this primary effect could also as a secondary effect induce vasodilatation and so improve ventilation, perfusion and the ventilation/perfusion mismatch quickly. Nitric oxide is then not of much additional therapeutic value.

Adjustment of ventilation after surfactant therapy is essential, as a surfactant-treated neonatal lung is much more sensitive to barotraumatization than that of an older patient[29]. Surfactant could induce neutrophil granulocyte activation, but for bovine surfactant compared to synthetic preparations this activation seems to be minimal[30]. Using bovine surfactant with a careful ventilation strategy with minimal tidal volumes, permissive hypercapnia and limited inspiratory pressures is a treatment with few side-effects[31].

As ECMO is still the best-evaluated life-saving therapy in severe neonatal respiratory failure, this has to be instantaneously available, and surfactant and or nitric oxide therapy should be limited to ECMO centers. These alternative treatments will reduce the need for ECMO, as has been demonstrated already in Japan[32].

SURFACTANT NON-RESPONDERS AS A MODEL FOR ARDS-LIKE DISEASE IN PRETERM INFANTS

It is speculative whether an 'ARDS-like' disease exists in preterm infants. Tracheal aspirate analysis for cells and interleukins suggests that some preterm infants with respiratory distress syndrome (RDS), especially those who develop bronchopulmonary dysplasia later on, have indeed signs of early inflammation similar to those in ARDS[30]. It could be speculated that especially those preterm infants with surfactant deficiency RDS who do not respond favorably to several doses of surfactant, and do still require more than 40% oxygen, could have some ARDS-like disease. As data from our group indicates[33], 15–20% of preterm infants are 'surfactant non-responders'.

A frequently used argument for the hypothesis of 'non-responders' as preterm infants with ARDS-like inflammatory lung disease is the finding of improved lung condition after treatment with inhaled or systemic steroids[34,35]. In addition to steroid treatment, liquid ventilation and high-frequency oscillation have been proposed for these 'non-responders'[36,37].

Table 1 summarizes different approaches which have been published in small series. For nitric oxide in preterm infant surfactant non-responders, for liquid ventilation, hemodynamic optimization and combined NO/surfactant therapy, controlled clinical studies are under way.

PRELIMINARY DATA ON ADDITIONAL SURFACTANT, NITRIC OXIDE, AND SYSTEMIC STEROIDS IN SURFACTANT NON-RESPONDERS

Over 2 years we have analyzed our surfactant non-responders, i.e. preterm infants < 1500 g birth weight who required an $FiO_2 > 0.4$ at 48 h age to achieve arterial oxygen saturation > 87%[33]. All these patients had had two or more surfactant doses totalling more than 150 mg/kg. The following strategy was followed for these infants:

(1) Up to three more surfactant doses of 50 mg/kg each;

(2) (Nor)epinephrine to achieve mean arterial blood pressures > 40 mmHg;

(3) 0.5–1 mg dexamethasone, first dose 1 h before additional surfactant therapy, and as a last-line therapeutic option; and

(4) 1–10 ppm nitric oxide, if pulmonary hypertension was documented by echocardiography

All non-responders were compared with surfactant responders during the same period in respect of prenatal history (premature rupture of membranes, intrauterine ischemia documented by Doppler, abnormal cardiotocography, maternal signs of infection, anticardiolipine antibodies, eclampsia etc.), postnatal variables indicating hypoxia or infection (ratio of immature to total granulocytes, C-reactive protein, granulocyte elastase, creatine kinase, MB isozyme of creatine kinase, blood pressure, Apgar scores, etc.), and birth weight and gestational age. In all deceased patients,

Table 1 Published treatment options for surfactant non-responding very-low-birth-weight infants (older than 72 h, > 2 applications of surfactant)

Additional surfactant[32,33]
Systemic steroids[34]
Inhaled steroids (budesonide)[35]
Nitric oxide[33]
Perflubrone associated gas exchange[37]
Hemodynamic optimization[33]
Combined surfactant and nitric oxide[33]

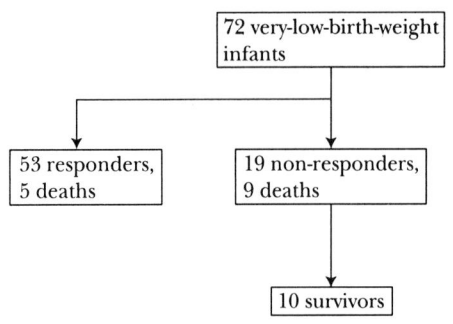

Figure 4 Data on the surfactant non-responding respiratory distress syndrome infants with birth weight < 1500 g at the Medical University of Lübeck 1995–96. Non-responders are defined as those with fraction inspired oxygen (FiO_2) > 0.4 after 48 h, despite 1–3 surfactant doses

postmortem examinations of the lung, looking for lung hypoplasia indicated by a low radial cell count, were performed.

The results are shown in Figure 4. Of 72 infants with RDS , i.e. with radiographic signs plus FiO_2 > 0.4 required to achieve saturation readings > 87% during the first 4 h of life, 53 were responders (less than 0.4 FiO_2 at 48 h age), and of these five patients died (two of severe intracranial hemorrhage, one of sepsis and two after the neonatal period). We identified 19 non-responders, of whom nine patients died; in five of these severe lung hypoplasia was found, and four died of severe respiratory and hemodynamic problems after 6–18 days of ventilation. In the ten surviving patients, the FiO_2 could be reduced to < 0.4 after the 5th day of life, and seven patients improved with additional surfactant, catecholamines and dexamethasone, while three improved with nitric oxide.

We could not detect any differences in the non-responders in respect of the prenatal and postnatal parameters and variables mentioned. However, the non-responders had a significantly lower gestational age (mean of 25.4 compared with 28.7 weeks) and birth weight compared with responders. Studies analyzing tracheal aspirates for interleukins, cells and adhesion molecules give some hints, however, that in 'non-responders' a more intense inflammatory reaction is going on.

The hypothesis that surfactant non-responders are predominantly posthypoxia or sepsis patients rather than 'healthy' RDS infants could not be verified. Non-responders were just significantly more immature. Whether nitric oxide is of benefit in these non-responders will be studied in a Central European co-operative study which is just under way, as are co-operative studies for high frequency ventilation in this patient group[38–40].

CONCLUSIONS

Term infants

In term infants with ARDS-like disease, independent of its etiology, surfactant therapy is beneficial. Inhalation of nitric oxide in those patients with obvious pulmonary hypertension only improves oxygenation marginally. Co-operative studies comparing surfactant with other options for alveolar recruitment, like high frequency oscillation, should be performed. These therapeutic strategies should only be followed in institutions which offer ECMO as rescue therapy.

Preterm infants

Surfactant non-responders do not give much evidence that they have an ARDS-like disease. However, additional surfactant, systemic or inhaled steroids and nitric oxide might be beneficial and reduce the high mortality (in other studies 60–80%) of these infants. Caution is recommended until the studies which are under way have led to conclusions.

References

1. Herman, S. and Reynolds, E.O.R. (1973). Methods for improving oxygenation in infants mechanically ventilated for severe hyaline membrane disease. *Arch. Dis. Child.*, **48**, 612–17

2. Fujiwara, T., Chida, S., Watabe, H., Maeta, T., Morita, T. and Abe, T. (1980). Artificial surfactant therapy in hyaline membrane disease. *Lancet*, **1**, 55–9

3. Richman, P.S., Spragg, R.G., Robertson, B., Merritt, T.A. and Curstedt, T. (1989). The adult respiratory distress syndrome: first trials with surfactant replacement. *Eur. Resp. J.*, **2** (Suppl. 3), 109s–111s

4. Paulson, E., Spear, R.M. and Peterson, B.M. (1995). New concepts in the treatment of children with acute respiratory distress syndrome. *J. Pediatr.*, **127**, 163–73

5. Möller, J.C., Gilman, J.T., Sussmane, J., Raszynski, A. and Wolfsdorf, J. (1993). Changes in plasma levels of oxygen radical scavenging enzymes during extracorporeal membrane oxygenation in a lamb model. *Biol. Neonate*, **64**, 134–9

6. Möller, J.C., Reiss, I., Schaible, T., Tegtmeyer, F.K. and Gortner, L. (1995). Surfactant treatment in children with acquired respiratory distress syndrome. *Monatsschr. Kinderheilkd.*, **143**, 685–90

7. Möller, J.C., Schaible, T.F., Reiss, I., Artlich, A. and Gortner, L. (1995). Treatment of severe non-neonatal ARDS in children with surfactant and nitric oxide in a 'pre-ECMO' situation. *Int. J. Artif. Organs*, **18**, 598–602

8. Möller, J.C., Vardag, A.M., Sussmane, J.B., Raszynsik, A. and Wolfsdorf, J. (1990). Extracorporeal membrane oxygenation in the treatment of persistent pulmonary hypertension of the newborn. *Int. Pediatr.*, **5**, 337–43

9. Faix, R.G., Viscardi, R.M., DiPietro, M.A. and Nicks, J.J. (1989). Adult respiratory distress syndrome in full-term newborns. *Pediatrics*, **83**, 971–6

10. Martin, R.J. (1991). Neonatal surfactant therapy – where do we go from here? *J. Pediatr.*, **118**, 555–6

11. Lachmann, B. and Gommers, D. (1994). Surfactant treatment for neonatal lung diseases other than the respiratory distress syndrome. *Lung and Respiration*, **9**, 35–9

12. UK Collaborative ECMO Trial Group (1996). UK collaborative randomised trial of neonatal extracorporeal membrane oxygenation. *Lancet*, **348**, 75–82

13. LeVine, A.M., Lotze, A., Stanley, S., Stroud, C., O'Donnell, R., Whitsett, J. and Pollack, M.M. (1996). Surfactant content in children with inflammatory lung disease. *Crit. Care Med.*, **24**, 1062–7

14. Zimmerman, J.J. (1996). Surfactant is a target during acute lung injury inflammation. *Crit. Care Med.*, **24**, 916–17

15. Fetter, W.P.F., Baerts, W., Bos, A.P. and van Linge, R.A. (1995). Surfactant replacement therapy in neonates with respiratory failure due to bacterial sepsis. *Acta Paediatr.*, **84**, 14–16

16. Nieman, G.F., Gatto, L.A., Paskanik, A.M., Yang, B., Fluck, R. and Picone, A. (1996). Surfactant replacement in the treatment of sepsis induced adult respiratory distress syndrome in pigs. *Crit. Care Med.*, **24**, 1025–33

17. Sun, B., Curstedt, T., Guo-Wei, S. and Robertson, B. (1993). Surfactant improves lung function and morphology in newborn rabbits with meconium aspiration. *Biol. Neonate*, **63**, 96–104

18. Sun, B., Curstedt, T. and Robertson, B. (1993). Surfactant inhibition in experimental meconium aspiration. *Acta Paediatr.*, **82**, 182–9

19. Sun, B., Herting, E., Curstedt, T. and Robertson, B. (1994). Exogenous surfactant improves lung compliance and oxygenation in adult rats with meconium aspiration. *J. Appl. Physiol.*, **77**, 1961–71

20. Findlay, R.D., Taeusch, H.W. and Walther, F.J. (1996). Surfactant replacement therapy for meconium aspiration syndrome. *Pediatrics*, **97**, 48–52

21. Khammash, H., Perlman, M., Woijtulewicz, J. and Dunn, M. (1993). Surfactant therapy in full-term neonates with severe respiratory failure. *Pediatrics*, **92**, 135–9

22. Gortner, L., Pohlandt, F. and Bartmann, P. (1993). Bovine surfactant in full-term neonates with adult respiratory distress syndrome-like disorders. *Pediatrics*, **92**, 538

23. Marraro, G. (1994). Emploi du surfactant dans la pathologie respiratoire du noveau-né et du nourisson. *Cahiers d'Anesthesiologie*, **42**, 159–66

24. Pandit, P.B., Dunn, M.S. and Colucci, E.A. (1995). Surfactant therapy in neonates with respiratory deterioration due to pulmonary hemorrhage. *Pediatrics*, **95**, 32–6

25. Bos, A.P., Tibboel, D., Hazebroek, F.W.J., Molenaar, J.C., Lachmann, B. and Gommers, D. (1991). Surfactant replacement therapy in high risk infants with congenital diaphragmatic hernia. *Lancet*, **337**, 1279

26. Nogee, L.M., Garnier, G., Dietz, H.C., Singer, L., Murphy, A.M., De Mello, D.E. and Colten, H.R. (1994). A mutation in the surfactant protein B gene responsible for fatal neonatal respiratory disease in multiple kindres. *J. Clin. Invest.*, **93**, 1860–3

27. Duncan, J.E., Hatch, G. and Belik, J. (1994). Is surfactant a pulmonary vasodilator? *Pediatr. Res.*, **35**, 223A

28. Lutz, C., Picone, A., Gatto, L.A., Nieman, G., Paskanik, A. and Landas, S. (1996). Exogenous surfactant and positive end-expiratory pressure act synergistically to improve pulmonary function in endotoxin-induced lung injury. *Crit. Care Med.*, **24**, A98

29. Coker, P.J., Hernandez, L.A., Peevy, K.J., Adkins, K. and Parker, J.C. (1992). Increased sensitivity to mechanical ventilation after surfactant inactivation in young rabbit lungs. *Crit. Care Med.*, **20**, 635–40

30. Reiss, I., Tegtmeyer, F.K., Ziesenitz, S., Möller, J.C., Schaible, T. and Gortner, L. (1995). Modulation of N-formyl-methionin-leucin-phenylalanin induced elastase release from PMN by surfactant and pentoxiphyllin. *Eur. Respir. J.*, **8**, 543S

31. Burchardi, H. (1996). New strategies in mechanical ventilation for acute lung injury. *Eur. Respir. J.*, **9**, 1063–72

32. Ito, Y., Kawano, T., Miyasaka, K., Katayama, M. and Sakai, H. (1994). Alternative treatment may lower the need for use of extracorporal membrane oxygenation. *Acta Paediatr. Jpn.*, **36**, 673–7

33. Herkenhoff, M., Schaible, T., Reiss, I., Kandzora, J., Möller, J. and Gortner, L. (1996). Ursachen and Risiken von Surfactant Non-Respondern. *Monatsschr. Kinderheilkd.*, **144**, S50

34. Yeh, T.F., Torre, J.A., Rastogi, A., Anyebuno, M.A. and Pildes, R.S. (1990). Early postnatal dexamethasone therapy in premature infants with severe respiratory distress syndrome: a double blind, controlled study. *J. Pediatr.*, **117**, 273–82

35. LaForce, W.R. and Brudno, S. (1993). Controlled trial of beclamethasone dipropionate by nebulization in oxygen and ventilator dependent infants. *J. Pediatr.*, **122**, 285–8

36. Leach, C.L., Holm, B., Morin, F.C., Fuhrman, B.P., Papo, M.C., Steinhorn, D. and Hernan, L. (1995). Partial liquid ventilation in premature lambs with respiratory distress syndrome: efficacy and compatibility with exogenous surfactant. *J. Pediatr.*, **126**, 412–16

37. Hirschl, R.B., Pranikoff, T., Gauger, P., Schreiner, R.J., Dechert, R. and Bartlett, R.H. (1995). Liquid ventilation in adults, children, and full-term neonates. *Lancet*, **346**, 1201–2

38. Keszler, M., Donn, S.M., Bucciarelli, R.L., Alverson, D.C., Hart, M., Lunyong, V., Modanlou, H.D., Noguchi, A., Pearlman, S.A., Puri, A., Smith, D., Stavis, R., Watkins, M.N. and Harris, T.R. (1991). Multicenter controlled trial comparing high-frequency jet ventilation and conventional mechanical ventilation in newborn infants with pulmonary interstitial emphysema. *J. Pediatr.*, **119**, 85–93

39. Sjöstrand, U.H., Lichtwark-Aschoff, M., Nielsen, J.B., Markström, A., Larsson, A., Svensson, B.A. and Nordgren, K.A. (1995). Different ventilatory approaches to keep the lung open. *Intensive Care Med.*, **21**, 310–18

40. Godin, P.J. and Buchman, T.G. (1996). Uncoupling of biological oscillators: a complementary hypothesis concerning the pathogenesis of multiple organ dysfunction syndrome. *Crit. Care Med.*, **24**, 1107–16

Changes in cerebral oxygenation and electrical activity following surfactant treatment in preterm neonates with respiratory distress syndrome

57

F. Mosca, M. Lattanzio, M. Bray, M. R. Colnaghi, G. Compagnoni, L. Pastorino, M. Fumagalli and A. Marini

INTRODUCTION

Surfactant replacement treatment of respiratory distress syndrome (RDS) in the preterm infant improves pulmonary function and decreases mortality. However, the effects of this therapy on the incidence of periventricular–intraventricular hemorrhage or periventricular leukomalacia are less certain[1]. Acute changes in pulmonary compliance, vascular resistance and pressure, and on arterial blood pressure caused by bolus surfactant administration, could have major effects on cerebral circulation and oxygenation which could explain the depression of cerebral electrical activity that has been observed in some studies after rapid instillation of natural[2] and synthetic[3] surfactant. To clarify the effect on the brain of surfactant administration, several studies of cerebral hemodynamics, based on Doppler ultrasonography[4–6], the xenon-133 clearance technique[7] and near-infrared spectroscopy (NIRS) have been performed, yielding contrasting results. In particular, one NIRS study of rapid porcine surfactant administration reports highly variable effects on cerebral blood volume and no significant change in cerebral blood flow or cerebral oxygen delivery[8], while two other reports indicate a rapid-onset, short-lasting increase in cerebral blood volume and a transient reduction in cerebral oxyhemoglobin, concomitant to the brief desaturation which occurs during surfactant instillation[9,10]. Data on cellular oxygen availability, evaluated from the oxidation state of the mitochondrial enzyme cytochrome-c oxidase, are lacking. The purpose of our study was to investigate the effects on cerebral blood volume and cytochrome-c oxidase oxidation state, measured by NIRS, and on cerebral electrical activity of bolus bovine surfactant administration in preterm infants with respiratory distress syndrome (RDS).

MATERIALS AND METHODS

Subjects

Initially cerebral hemodynamics and oxygenation were studied by NIRS, and cerebral electrical activity recorded and analyzed, in 14 preterm infants receiving 100 mg/kg bovine surfactant. Subsequently, the effects of 50 mg/kg surfactant administration were studied in five more infants, to evaluate the possibility of a dose-related effect. The criteria for surfactant therapy were clinical and radiologic features of RDS, mechanical ventilation with synchronized intermittent mandatory ventilation (SIMV) (Babylog 8000, Drägerwerke, Lübeck), mean airways pressure (MAP) $\geq 7\,cmH_2O$ and/or fraction of inspired oxygen (FiO_2) $\geq 40\%$[11]. None of the studied infants was paralyzed. Infants with known major congenital abnormalities, history of maternal amnionitis or clinical evidence of infection were excluded from the study. Informed parental consent for the study was obtained for all infants.

Surfactant administration

Bovine surfactant (Alveofact, Boehringer, Ingelheim) was administered at a dose of 100 mg/kg (2.4 ml/kg) in 14 infants and at a dose of 50 mg/kg (1.2 ml/kg) in five infants. Administration involved disconnection of the supine infant from the ventilator, insertion of a catheter down the endotracheal tube to a premeasured distance, corresponding to the end of the endotracheal tube, followed by bolus surfactant instillation in approximately 15 s, with the patient's head resting on the midline. The infant was then ventilated manually with the same FiO_2 as before surfactant treatment for 15–20 s to enhance surfactant distribution. After this procedure, mechanical ventilation was resumed, initially with unmodified ventilatory settings, except for a rapid reduction of FiO_2 aimed at avoiding hyperoxic peaks. Subsequent ventilatory management was aimed at maintaining blood gases within the normal range. Table 1 shows mean airway pressure and FiO_2 changes.

General monitoring

Heart rate was continuously recorded by electrocardiogram, arterial oxygen saturation was monitored by a pulse oxymeter (OXImeter, Radiometer, Copenhagen) placed on the right hand, and oxygen and carbon dioxide tensions were monitored by a calibrated transcutaneous electrode (TCM3, Radiometer, Copenhagen). Arterial blood pressure was measured by a transducer connected to an umbilical artery catheter.

Near-infrared spectroscopy

Relative changes in cerebral blood volume and cerebral oxygenation were detected by near-infrared spectroscopy. The principle of NIRS is based on the characteristic absorption of near-infrared radiation (700–900 nm) by oxyhemoglobin (HbO_2), deoxyhemoglobin (Hb) and oxidized cytochrome-c oxidase ($CytO_2$). Relative changes in the concentrations of each of these molecules can be derived from algorithms of the transmittance-reflection relationship at these wavelengths according to the Beer-Lambert law[12]. Changes in the concentrations of HbO_2 and Hb reflect changes in cerebral oxygen supply; HbO_2 concentration increases when there is a rise in arterial blood oxygen saturation or an increase in arterial blood flow to the monitored portion of the brain. The opposite conditions cause a decrease in HbO_2 concentration. Hb concentration increases with the inflow of desaturated blood and with obstruction to outflow of venous blood[13]. Changes in the concentration of $CytO_2$ reflect changes in cellular oxygen availability. Changes in the concentration of total hemoglobin are calculated as the sum of changes in concentrations of HbO_2 and Hb; changes in cerebral blood volume, expressed in ml/100 g are calculated from changes in concentration of total hemoglobin[14].

For this study the instrument NIRO 500 (Hamamatsu Photonics KK, Hamamatsu, Japan) was employed. Near-infrared radiation at four wavelengths (774, 826, 845 and 908 nm) was carried to the infant's head through a fiberoptic bundle, terminating in an optode that was applied to the parietal region. Transmitted light emerging from the opposite parietal region was collected by another optode and carried to the photomultiplier. The distance between the optodes was measured by callipers and multiplied by 4.4 to obtain the optical pathlength[15]. Absorption at the four wavelengths was continuously sampled at a rate of 0.5 Hz.

Cerebral electrical activity

Parietal and occipital electrodes were connected by a bipolar longitudinal recording system. The signal was sent simultaneously to a cerebral function monitor, to analyze the amplitude of cerebral electrical activity, and to the electroencephalogram and from the latter to a Berg Fourier analyzer, to analyze the frequency distribution of cerebral electrical activity. Qualitative analysis of electroencephalogram recordings was performed according to the criteria of Tharp[16]; analysis of cerebral function monitor recordings involved quantification each hour, of percentage continuous activity of amplitude above 3 μV and of the number of bursts of amplitude above 15 μV. Analysis of Berg Fourier analyzer recording involved assessment of percentage cerebral electrical activity at frequencies between 2 and 16 Hz. Values for the one-hour period before surfactant administration were compared to values for the one-hour period immediately after surfactant administration.

Data analysis

All recorded parameters were transferred to a computer and stored for later analysis. Physiological and NIRS data were evaluated at time 0 (baseline value before deconnection from ventilator for surfactant administration) and at 1, 5, 15, 30 and 60 min from reconnection after the end of the procedure. All data were analyzed by repeated-measures ANOVA, followed by the Student-Newman Keuls test when significant differences were found. The association between mean arterial blood pressure and carbon dioxide tension and cerebral blood volume changes was determined by multiple regression analysis.

RESULTS

Fourteen infants of median gestational age 29 weeks (range 24–35), birth weight 880 g (600–1840), and receiving 100 mg/kg Alveofact (first dose) at a median age of 4 h (2–6.5) were studied by cerebral NIRS and simultaneous recording of cerebral electrical activity. Subsequently, cerebral NIRS was performed in five infants of 29 weeks (26–31) gestational age, 1060 g (660–1650) birth weight, and receiving a 50 mg/kg dose at a median age of 3.8 h (2–5). No significant difference in clinical features (gestational age, birth weight, age, severity of RDS) was present between the two treatment groups. Table 1 shows values of mean airway pressure and FiO_2 before surfactant administration and 30 and 60 min thereafter in the infants of the two groups.

100 mg/kg group

Mean arterial oxygen saturation was significantly higher than baseline at 1 and 5 min after surfactant instillation; mean oxygen tension was significantly higher after 1, 5, 15 and 30 min; mean carbon dioxide tension did not change significantly, although a marked reduction was observed in one infant who had high pre-surfactant levels; mean heart rate was significantly reduced 1 min after surfactant administration but recovered after 5 min; no significant change

Table 1 Mean airway pressure and fraction of inspired oxygen before treatment (baseline) and 30 and 60 min after administration of 100 mg/kg ($n = 14$) and 50 mg/kg ($n = 5$) surfactant. Values are given as means ± SD

| | Surfactant dose | |
	100 mg/kg	50 mg/kg
Mean airway pressure (cmH$_2$O)		
baseline	12.4 ± 4.5	8.8 ± 2.3
30 min	11.1 ± 3.4*	8.2 ± 2.1
60 min	10.3 ± 2.9*	7.3 ± 2.0
Fraction of inspired oxygen (%)		
baseline	66 ± 24	59 ± 22
30 min	44 ± 19*	33 ± 9*
60 min	35 ± 14*	35 ± 11*

*, $p < 0.05$ compared with baseline

in mean arterial blood pressure was observed (Table 2).

Near-infrared spectroscopy

After surfactant administration we observed a progressive increase in cerebral blood volume in 13 of 14 patients and an initial decrease, with return to baseline by 15 min and a small increase by 60 min, in one patient in which the initial fall in cerebral blood volume was associated with decreasing transcutaneous carbon dioxide partial pressure (P_{CO_2}) from a high pre-treatment level; overall, however, no significant correlation between cerebral blood volume changes and P_{CO_2} ($r^2 = 0.032$, NS) or mean arterial blood pressure ($r^2 = 0.012$, NS) was found. Changes in HbO_2 concentrations were not significant. Mean Hb concentrations decreased initially, then showed a gradual increase which was significant at 60 min, when deoxyhemoglobin represented the main contributor to the increase in cerebral blood volume. A gradual decrease in $CytO_2$ concentration following surfactant administration, with maximal change ranging from −0.74 to −5.92 μmol/l, was observed in 11 of 14 patients; mean $CytO_2$ concentration was significantly decreased at 60 min (Table 3). Comparing infants who had received antenatal steroids ($n = 4$) with those who had

not ($n = 10$), a slight trend towards smaller changes in the antenatal steroids group was seen, although not significant (cerebral blood volumes at 60 min: antenatal steroids 526 ± 328 μl/100 g, non-antenatal steroids 604 ± 319 μl/100 g; $CytO_2$ concentration 60 min: antenatal steroids −1.9 ± 1.8 μmol/l, non-antenatal steroids −2.5 ± 2.2 μmol/l).

Cerebral electrical activity

No significant difference in either number of bursts/hour (103 ± 28/h pre-surfactant vs. 103 ± 25/h post-surfactant) or percentage continuous activity (65.4 ± 23 pre- vs. 66.7 ± 26 post-surfactant) was observed as a result of surfactant administration. Frequency distribution of cerebral electrical activity was not modified by surfactant administration. Regression analysis failed to demonstrate any correlation between individual changes in arterial pressure and any of the investigated correlates of cerebral electrical activity. No correlation between the severity of RDS (F_{iO_2}, MAP) and modifications of cerebral electrical activity was observed.

50 mg/kg group

Mean values for arterial oxygen saturation, oxygen tension, carbon dioxide tension, heart rate

Table 2 Arterial oxygen saturation (SaO_2, %), transcutaneous P_{O_2} (mmHg) and P_{CO_2} (mmHg) heart rate (HR, (beats/min)) and mean arterial blood pressure (MABP, mmHg) before (baseline) and 1, 5, 15, 30 and 60 min after 100 mg/kg ($n = 14$) or 50 mg/kg ($n = 5$) surfactant administration. Values are given as means ± SD

Parameter	Surfactant dose (mg/kg)	*Time after administration of surfactant*					
		Baseline	*1 min*	*5 min*	*15 min*	*30 min*	*60 min*
SaO_2	100	93 ± 4	98 ± 3*	96 ± 3*	95 ± 3	95 ± 3	95 ± 2
	50	94 ± 1	96 ± 2	96 ± 3	95 ± 2	94 ± 2	94 ± 2
P_{O_2}	100	66 ± 22	88 ± 24*	89 ± 22*	85 ± 21*	90 ± 26*	78 ± 18
	50	92 ± 31	97 ± 35	95 ± 27	94 ± 25	95 ± 23	94 ± 20
P_{CO_2}	100	39 ± 12	40 ± 11	39 ± 10	39 ± 8	36 ± 8	37 ± 7
	50	45 ± 9	45 ± 12	48 ± 13	47 ± 12	45 ± 9	44 ± 10
HR	100	156 ± 15	132 ± 36*	154 ± 22	151 ± 19	153 ± 27	158 ± 18
	50	148 ± 16	138 ± 25	151 ± 21	147 ± 23	149 ± 20	151 ± 19
MABP	100	43 ± 9	41 ± 9	40 ± 12	39 ± 11	44 ± 5	45 ± 10
	50	41 ± 4	40 ± 5	41 ± 5	40 ± 5	45 ± 4	39 ± 9

*, $p < 0.05$ compared with baseline

and mean arterial blood pressure are shown in Table 2. No significant differences from baseline were seen, probably due to large inter-patient variability and small sample size.

Near-infrared spectroscopy

A small cerebral blood volume increase was observed in three of five patients in which both carbon dioxide tension and mean arterial blood pressure remained constant. A decrease, associated with decreasing PCO_2, was seen in two infants. Overall, mean cerebral blood volume increase was not significant. Deoxyhemoglobin, HbO_2 and $CytO_2$ concentrations showed trends similar to the 100 mg/kg treatment group (Table 3), although of smaller magnitude; again, no statistical significance was seen.

DISCUSSION

The main findings of our study are a marked and sustained increase in cerebral blood volume and a progressive decrease in cerebral oxidized cytochrome-c oxidase concentration, following bolus administration of 100 mg/kg bovine surfactant in preterm infants with RDS. Such an effect appears to be dose-related since similar but smaller changes were seen following a 50 mg/kg dose. Antenatal steroidal treatment also appeared somehow to reduce these modifications. In comparison with the results of Skow and colleagues[9], who reported an increase in

cerebral blood volume lasting for 2–10 min, and with those of Dorrepal and associates[10], who confirmed a transient elevation of cerebral blood volume following surfactant administration, the cerebral blood volume increase observed in our study is of significantly greater duration. Initially HbO_2 represented the main contributor to the observed cerebral blood volume increase in the 100 mg/kg treatment group, suggesting an increased cerebral flow of well oxygenated arterial blood[13] as previously observed in some Doppler studies[3,4]. However, neither modifications in arterial blood pressure not in blood gases could explain the observed cerebral blood volume increase, since in our study neither mean arterial blood pressure nor PCO_2 increased. A recent study in surfactant-deficient newborn piglets[17] shows that cerebral vasodilation is induced by surfactant instillation and that nitric oxide synthase inhibition prevents this effect. Thus, nitric oxide mediated cerebral vasodilation could potentially underly the increase in cerebral blood volume observed after surfactant administration, but the mechanism leading to the activation of this pathway remains to be established. The sustained cerebral blood volume rise, continuing after the first minutes following surfactant administration, resulted predominantly from an increase in Hb concentration, occurring in spite of elevated PO_2, suggesting increased cerebral venous pressure[13]. Impaired cerebral venous drainage could result from partially obstructed

Table 3 Changes in cerebral blood volume (ΔCBV, $\mu l/100\,g$), oxyhemoglobin concentration ($\Delta[HbO_2]$ $\mu l/100\,g$), deoxyhemoglobin concentration ($\Delta[Hb]$, $\mu l/100\,g$) and oxidized cytochrome-c oxidase concentration ($\Delta[CytO_2]$, $\mu mol/l$ measured 1, 5, 15, 30 and 60 min after either 100 mg/kg or 50 mg/kg surfactant administration. Values are given as means ± SD

Parameter	Surfactant dose (mg/kg)	Time after administration of surfactant				
		1 min	5 min	15 min	30 min	60 min
ACBV	100	153 ± 167	259 ± 235 *	254 ± 290*	373 ± 315*	565 ± 325*
	50	−119 ± 203	2 ± 120	125 ± 175	173 ± 226	234 ± 321
A[HbO₂]	100	240 ± 194	291 ± 309	178 ± 405	231 ± 388	301 ± 319
	50	−41 ± 254	122 ± 245	156 ± 223	149 ± 180	138 ± 198
A[Hb]	100	−86 ± 153	−33 ± 264	76 ± 329	142 ± 326	264 ± 346*
	50	−54 ± 81	−129 ± 175	−29 ± 118	24 ± 104	96 ± 187
A[CytO₂]	100	−0.09 ± 0.45	−0.60 ± 0.85	−0.85 ± 1.24	−1.26 ± 1.34	−2.20 ± 1.91*
	50	−0.1 ± 0.64	0.49 ± 0.90	−0.33 ± 0.55	−0.56 ± 0.43	−0.61 ± 0.63

*, $p < 0.05$ compared with baseline

intrathoracic circulation, due to increased transmission of ventilatory pressures as lung compliance improves. Although after surfactant administration, MAP was significantly reduced, an increase in intrathoracic pressure, leading to partial obstruction of cerebral venous return, cannot be ruled out. We further tested this possibility by measuring cardiac blood volume changes after head elevation and temporary reduction of MAP in a few other intubated infants. We did not, however, observe any significant reduction of cerebral blood volume, making the hypothesis quite doubtful.

The decrease in CytO2 concentration is quite striking; it was observed in 11 of 14 studied infants and was of greater magnitude, in some cases, than that previously reported to occur following indomethacin administration in preterm infants[18]. Studies of the relation between oxygen delivery and cytochrome oxidation state have shown a reduction of CytO2 concentration with graded hypoxemia in the human adult brain[19]. CytO2 concentration has also been shown to decrease as a result of ischemia[18,20] and

of hypocapnia[21] which reduces cerebral blood flow. Interestingly, CytO2 concentration has been found to decrease in critically ill preterm infants following movements, coughing or breath-holding, which increase intrathoracic pressure leading to a rise in cerebral blood volume, resulting solely or predominantly from an increase in cerebral deoxyhemoglobin[22]. The lack of modification of cerebral electrical activity in our study raises doubts about the negative clinical significance of these changes; such observations, however, warrant further research in an experimental setting for the evaluation of neural tissue metabolism. In fact, a similar dissociation between cerebral hemodynamical changes and oxygen consumption on one side, and cerebral electrical activity on the other, has recently been described after treatment with cAMP and pentoxifylline in dogs with experimentally induced cerebral ischemia[23,24]. The smaller magnitude of the changes seen with the 50 mg/kg dose indicates a dose-related effect, suggesting a possible advantage of fractionated dosage.

References

1. Reynolds, E.O.R., Edwards, A.D. and McCormick, D.C. (1995). Effects of surfactant replacement on cerebral hemodynamics and oxygenation. In Robertson, B. and Taeusch, H.W. (eds.) *Surfactant Therapy for Lung Disease,* Vol. 84. (New York: Marcel Dekker, Inc.)
2. Hellstroem-Westas, L., Bell, A.H., Skow, L., Greisen, G. and Svenningsen, N.W. (1992). Cerebroelectrical depression following surfactant treatment in preterm neonates. *Pediatrics,* 89, 643–7
3. Saliba, E., Nashashibi, M., Vaillant, M.-C., Nasr, C. and Laugier, J. (1994). Instillation rate effects of Exosurf on cerebral and cardiovascular haemodynamics in preterm neonates. *Arch. Dis. Child.,* 71, F174–8
4. Van de Bor, M., Ma, E.J. and Walther, F.J. (1991). Cerebral blood flow velocity after surfactant instillation in preterm infants. *J. Pediatr.,* 118(2), 285–7
5. Cowan, F., Whitelaw, A., Wertheim, D. and Silvermann, M. (1991). Cerebral blood flow

velocity changes after rapid administration of surfactant. *Arch. Dis. Child.,* 66, 1105–9
6. Jorch, G., Rabe, H., Garbe, M., Michel, E. and Gortner, L. (1989). Acute and protracted effects of intratracheal surfactant application on internal carotid blood flow velocity, blood pressure and carbon dioxide tension in very low birth weight infants. *Eur. J. Pediatr.,* 148 , 770–3
7. Bell, A.H., Skow, L., Lundstrom, K.E., Saugstad, O.D. and Greisen, G. (1994). Cerebral blood flow and plasma hypoxanthine in relation to surfactant treatment. *Acta Pediatr.,* 83, 910–14
8. Edwards, A.D., McCormick, D.C., Roth, S.C., Elwell, C.E., Peebles, D.M., Cope, M., Wyatt, J.S., Delphy, D.T. and Reynolds, E.O.R. (1992). Cerebral hemodynamic effects of treatment with modified natural surfactant investigated by near infrared spectroscopy. *Pediatr. Res.,* 32(5), 532–6
9. Skow, L., Hellstroem-Westas, L., Jacobsen, T., Greisen, G. and Svenningsen, N.W. (1992). Acute changes in cerebral oxygenation and cere-

bral blood volume in preterm infants during surfactant treatment. *Neuropediatrics,* **23**, 126–30

10. Dorrepal, C.A., Benders, M.J.N.L., Steendijk, P., van de Bor, M. and van Bel, F. (1993). Cerebral hemodynamics and oxygenation in preterm infants after low- vs. high-dose surfactant replacement therapy. *Biol. Neonate,* **64**, 193–200

11. Fujiwara, T., Konishi, M., Chida, S. *et al.* (1990). Surfactant replacement therapy with a single postventilatory dose of a reconstituted bovine surfactant in preterm neonates with respiratory distress syndrome: final analysis of a multicenter, double blind, randomized trial and comparison with similar trials. *Pediatrics,* **86**, 753–64

12. Joebsis-Vandervliet, F.F. (1977). Noninvasive infrared monitoring of cerebral and myocardial oxygen sufficiency and circulatory parameters. *Science,* **198**, 1264–7

13. Brazy, J.E. (1991). Near infrared spectrophotometry. In *Clinics in Perinatology. Newer Technologies and the Neonate,* September, Vol. 18(3), pp. 519–34. (W. B. Saunders)

14. Wyatt, J.S., Edwards, A.D., Cope, M., Delpy, D.T., McCormick, D.C., Potter, A. and Reynolds, E.O.R. (1991). Responses of cerebral blood volume to changes in arterial carbon dioxide tension in term and preterm infants. *Pediatr. Res.,* **30**, 570–3

15. Wyatt, J. S., Cope, M., Delpy, D. T. et al. (1990). Measurement of optical path length for cerebral near-infrared spectroscopy in newborn infants. *Dev. Neurosci.,* **12**, 140–4

16. Tharp, B. R., Scher, M. S. and Clancy, R. R. (1989). Serial EEGs in normal and abnormal infants with birth weight less than 1200 grams. A prospective study with long-term follow-up. *Neuropediatrics,* **20**, 64–72

17. Yu, X.O., Moen, A., Feet, B.A. and Saugstadt, O.D. Nitric oxide (NO) synthase inhibition prevents surfactant-induced cerebral vasodilation in newborn piglets with surfactant deficiency. *Pediatr. Res.,* **39(4)**, 356(A)

18. McCormick, D.C., Edwards, A.D., Brown, J.S., Wyatt, J.S., Potter, A., Cope, M., Delpy, D.T. and Reynolds, E.O.R. (1993). Effect of indomethacin on cerebral oxidized cytochrome oxidase in preterm infants. *Pediatr. Res.,* **33**, 603–8

19. Hampson, N.B., Camporesi, E.M., Stolp, B.W., Moon, R.E., Shook, J.E., Griebel, J.A. and Piantadosi, C.A. (1990). Cerebral oxygen availability by NIR spectroscopy during transient hypoxia in humans. *J. Appl. Physiol.,* **69(3)**, 907–13

20. Hampson, N.B. and Piantadosi, C.A. (1988). Near infrared monitoring of human skeletal muscle oxygenation during forearm ischemia. *J. Appl. Physiol.,* **64(6)**, 2449–57

21. Chance, B. and Williams, G.R. (1965). The respiratory chain and oxidative phosphorylation. *Adv. Enzymol.,* **17**, 65–134

22. Brazy, J.E. and Lewis, D.V. (1986). Changes in cerebral blood volume and cytochrome aa3 during hypertensive peaks in preterm infants. *J. Pediatr.,* **108**, 983–7

23. Toung, T.J., Kirsch, J.R. and Traystman, R.J. (1996). Enhanced recovery of brain electrical activity by adenosine 3′,5′-cyclic monophosphate following complete global cerebral ischemia in dogs. *Crit. Care Med.,* **24(1)**, 103–8

24. Toung, T.J., Kirsch, J.R., Maruki, Y. *et al.* (1994). Effects of pentoxifylline on cerebral blood flow, metabolism and evoked response after total cerebral ischemia in dogs. *Crit. Care Med.,* **22**, 273–81

Section III   Controversies

347

The short-term benefits of epidural anesthesia for delivery outweigh long-term detriments

THE CASE IN FAVOR

P. Jouppila and S. Alahuhta

58

INTRODUCTION

Effective pain relief during labor using modern anesthetic techniques is unique in medicine because invasive and potentially hazardous methods are used in generally healthy women during a physiological process. Why should we use these procedures, are they necessary, should we limit their use to extremely painful labor only and is it possible that the mother loses some valuable experiences of the natural course of labor through these methods?

It can be said that the labor process is one of the most painful events experienced by the majority of women in their lifetime and according to questionnaires it is comparable with other sources of acute severe pain such as bone fracture or deep lacerations[1]. In prospective studies, over 80% of both primi- and multiparous women describe their labor pains as severe or intolerable[2]. Many variables have been found, which seem to correlate with the level of labor pain. These include primiparity, obesity, poor childbirth training and a low socioeconomic status.

The main indications for pain relief are purely humanitarian considerations and individual demands. The avoidance of long-term psychological and emotional problems after intolerably painful labor is also reflected in these considerations. Obstetric reasons include the avoidance of the negative effects of exacerbated levels of many stress hormones, such as cortisol and catecholamines, on uterine contractility and hemodynamics. The avoidance of maternal hyperventilation and concomitant disturbances in maternal and fetal acid–base balance are also practical indications for labor analgesia.

Modern childbirth training must also include realistic information on labor pains and the local potential for their relief. One important point in daily practice on the labor ward is that the level of pain cannot be objectively calculated by an observer, but only by the sufferer herself. In the selection of methods for obstetric pain relief, universal goals include the safety of the technique for the wellbeing of both the mother and the fetus. Minimal interference in the natural labor process and the rate of operative deliveries is also required. Epidural analgesia provides the only truly effective method for pain relief during labor today. Other available methods (psychoprophylaxis, parenteral opioids, nitrous oxide/oxygen inhalation, paracervical block, etc.) play an important role in this field as a whole, but have only supplementary value in severe pains.

ARGUMENTS IN FAVOR OF THE RATIONAL USE OF EPIDURAL ANALGESIA DURING LABOR

The main clinical and humanitarian fact when comparing epidural analgesia with other analgesic methods is the real effect of epidural block on pain intensity. According to the prospective study by Ranta and co-workers[2], its efficiency was regarded by mothers as excellent or good in

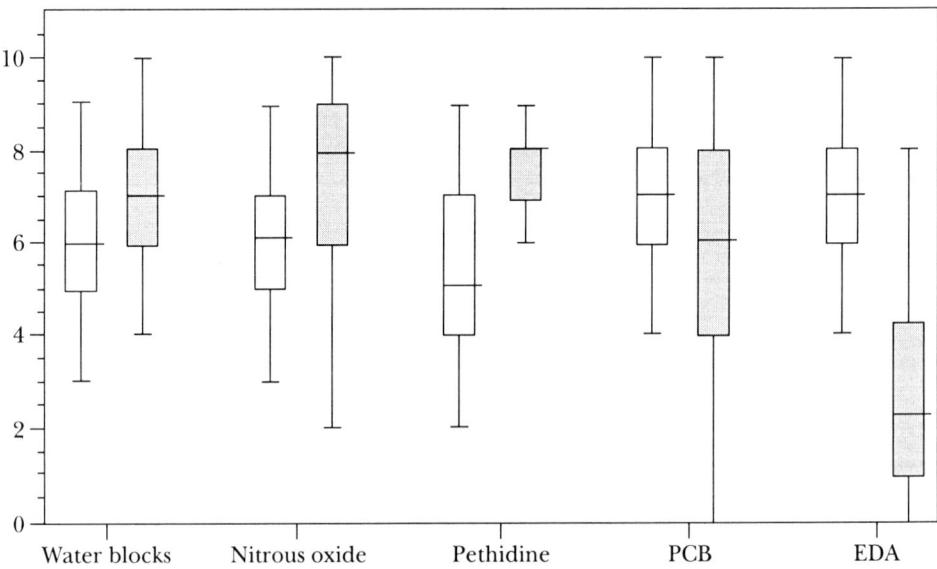

Figure 1 Visual pain scale scores (0–10) before (open columns) and after (hatched columns) pain management in the first stage of labor in the various pain relief groups. Minimum, lower (25%) quartile; median; upper (75%) quartile, maximum. PCB, paracervical block; EDA, epidural analgesia

94% of cases and the relief was significant as opposed to all other analgesic methods used (Figure 1). It is well-known that increased levels of cortisol and catecholamines during labor reflect a decreased uterine perfusion and increased blood pressure[3]. Important evidence of the positive effects of epidural analgesia is the decreased or stable levels of stress hormones during the first stage of labor. One example of these studies is the observation by Grenman and colleagues[4] that epidural analgesia decreased the serum levels of adrenaline during the first stage of labor. The vascular resistance in the uterine and umbilical circulation seems to be unchanged after epidural block using bupivacaine and sufentanil, in spite of the tendency of maternal blood pressure to decrease[5]. No detrimental effects on the fetal or neonatal acid–base status[6], fetal oxygen saturation[7], fetal heart rate pattern[8] or neurobehavioral responses of the newborns[9] have been documented.

Despite its obvious benefits, epidural analgesia has some potential side-effects, which must be recognized and can mostly be prevented. Maternal hypotension due to sympathetic block may occur in 15–20% of mothers. By using a preloading infusion of 500–1000 ml of Ringer lactate solution and the laterally tilted position, its rate is less than 5% and is rapidly and safely corrected with vasopressors such as ephedrine. Many analgesic agents may also be toxic to the cardiovascular system. Thus, the unintentional intravascular injection of bupivacaine, for example, may lead to vasoconstriction of the uterine arteries, leading to fetal asphyxia and, rarely, to maternal convulsions. These complications are largely avoidable by employing an advanced technique and low concentrations and through the development of new anesthetic agents, such as ropivacaine.

One of the most controversial subjects in the evaluation of the positive and negative points of epidural analgesia during labor is its effect on the course of labor and on the number of instrumental deliveries. It seems that a lumbar epidural block with sufficient perineal analgesia prolongs the duration of the second stage of labor. Also, the number of instrumental vaginal deliveries increases by using this type of extended block and frequency of Cesarean sections has been increased in many series[10]. The obstetric and cultural traditions in many countries and the economic facts do not justify these extra activities. Fortunately, by using new modifications of anesthetic techniques, they can be mainly avoided. One example is the use of segmental epidural block, in which the analgesia is only in effect for the first stage of labor, the volume and concentration of analgesic agents can be decreased, and no effect on the course of labor, fetal malpositions and instrumental deliveries has been observed[11]. This difference between wide and segmental block regarding effect on assisted vaginal deliveries has been documented by meta-analysis[10]. One must remember, however, that epidural analgesia during labor is not a generic procedure. Therefore, conclusions regarding the effect of one technique on, for example, the progress of labor cannot be applied to other methods and materials. The occurrence of a primarily dysfunctional labor before analgesia often has more influence on the rate of operative deliveries than the epidural block *per se*.

Another controversial point is the occurrence of postpartal long-term backache, which has been attributed to the epidural block. Many factors, such as the use of a large needle, the occurrence of hematomas and maternal position have been suggested as etiological factors. The first retrospective studies indicated a significant increase of back pain in epidural mothers compared with control parturients[12]. In later, prospective studies, the results can be regarded as more reliable due to better differentiation between ante- and postnatal backaches, and the occurrence of new backache after delivery seems to be similar in epidural and non-epidural groups[13].

The recent methodological development of epidural analgesia for labor pains has also greatly improved its clinical applications. The combination of opioids, such as fentanyl and sufentanil, with bupivacaine minimizes motor block of the legs caused by local analgesic agents. This enables the ambulation of the mother during the opening stage and the number of operative vaginal deliveries may be lower using this technique compared with the 'normal epidural'. The faster onset and longer duration of analgesia are also benefits. Recently, patient-controlled epidural analgesia and the initiation of analgesia by spinal opioid or a very small dose of local anesthetic have also provided a rapid onset and sufficiently long-term effects of epidural analgesia.

CONCLUSION

Epidural analgesia is the most and often the only effective form of intrapartum analgesia currently available. It has many additional benefits such as the possibility to quickly extend a pre-existing epidural block for Cesarean section surgery. In most cases, the maternal request for effective pain relief represents a sufficient indication for the administration of epidural analgesia and therefore it should be universally available in obstetric units.

The costs of this activity are mainly due to the need for anesthetic staff with good experience of epidural practice around the clock. Therefore, the availability of this method is not adequate and is not equally distributed even in developed countries. For instance, in Finland the mean frequency of epidural analgesia in 1995 was 21.6% but the range was 2.1–41.3% in different hospitals.

In spite of practical problems, the benefits of epidural analgesia greatly outweigh the mostly very controversial negative considerations. In my opinion, it is unethical and inhumane to leave the parturient, during one of the greatest experiences of her life, without relief if she experiences intolerable pain. We have a good method, why not use it when necessary! Natural processes, such as labor and delivery, are not always easy and positive events and due to the extreme pain may be terrible experiences with severe, long-term sequelae. Nowadays we can modify undesirable courses and allow the positive experience of these events. The goal is not a painless labor, with a block of the natural sensations during delivery and the irrational extension of epidural analgesia to all parturients, but rather an effective, smooth and safe response to the individual wishes for pain relief, which often cannot be predicted before labor nor calculated by an outsider.

References

1. Melzack, R., Kinch, R., Dobkin, P., Lebrun, M. and Taenzer, P. (1984). Severity of labour pain: influence of physical as well as psychologic variables. *Can. Med. Assoc. J.*, **130**, 579–84
2. Ranta, P., Spalding, M., Kangas-Saarela, T., Jokela, R., Hollmén, A., Jouppila, P. and Jouppila, R. (1995). Maternal expectations and experiences of labor pain – options of 1091 Finnish parturients. *Acta Anaesthesiol. Scand.*, **39**, 71–8
3. Shnider, S. M., Wright, R. G., Levinson, G., Roizen, M. F., Wallis, K. L., Rolbin, S. H. and Craft, J. B. (1979). Uterine blood flow and plasma norepinephrine changes during maternal stress in the pregnant ewe. *Anesthesiology*, **50**, 524–7
4. Grenman, S., Erkkola, R., Kanto, J., Scheinin, M., Viinamäki, O. and Lindberg, R. (1986). Epidural and paracervical blockades in obstetrics. Catecholamines, arginine vasopressin and analgesic effects. *Acta Obstet. Gynecol. Scand.*, **65**, 699–704
5. Alahuhta, S., Räsänen, J., Jouppila, P., Jouppila, R. and Hollmén, A. I. (1993). Epidural sufentanil and bupivacaine for labor analgesia and Doppler velocimetry of the umbilical and uterine arteries. *Anesthesiology*, **78**, 231–6
6. Jouppila, R. and Hollmén, A. (1976). The effect of segmental epidural analgesia on maternal and foetal acid-base balance, lactate, serum potassium and creatine phosphokinase during labour. *Acta Anaesthesiol. Scand.*, **20**, 259–68
7. Johnsson, N., van Oudgaarden, E., Montague, I. A. and McNamara, H. (1996). The effect of maternal epidural analgesia on fetal oxygen saturation. *Br. J. Obstet. Gynaecol.*, **103**, 776–8
8. Jouppila, P., Joupilla, R., Käär, K. and Merilä, M. (1977). FHR patterns and uterine activity after segmental epidural analgesia. *Br. J. Obstet. Gynaecol.*, **84**, 481–4
9. Kangas-Saarela, T., Jouppila, R., Jouppila, P., Hollmén, A., Puukka, M. and Juujärvi, K. (1987). The effect of segmental epidural analgesia on the neurobehavioural responses of newborn infants. *Acta Anaethesiol. Scand.*, **31**, 347–51
10. Howell, C. J. and Chalmers, I. (1992). A review of prospectively controlled comparisons of epidural with non-epidural forms of pain relief during labour. *Int. J. Obstet. Anesth.*, **1**, 93–110
11. Jouppila, R., Jouppila, P., Karinen, J.-M. and Hollmén, A. (1979). Segmental epidural analgesia in labour: related to progress of labour, fetal malposition and instrumental delivery. *Acta Obstet. Gynecol. Scand.*, **58**, 135–9
12. MacArthur, C., Lewis, M., Knox, E. G. and Crawford, J. S. (1990). Epidural anaesthesia and long term backache after childbirth. *Br. Med. J.*, **301**, 9–12
13. MacArthur, A. J., MacArthur, C. and Weeks, C. (1993). Epidural anesthesia and postpartum back pain. *Anesthesiology*, **79**, 973–8

The case against the provision of epidural analgesia to all mothers: the costs

59

THE CASE AGAINST

J. Thorburn

The enthusiasm with which epidural analgesia has been adopted throughout the developed world is a tribute to its efficacy. Like many of the most important advances in medicine, its introduction has not been based on scientific evaluation but on one aspect of its activity, its ability to completely relieve the pain of labor. In the United Kingdom it was introduced and administered to specific patients in the post-war era, but this use was very limited and it was not until 1964 that epidural analgesia first became available 24 h, 7 days a week at the Queen Mothers Hospital in Glasgow. The quality of the pain relief was vastly superior to anything that was or is available and its use rapidly spread[1,2]. At first only a few patients were selected to receive it, such as patients with concomitant obstetric problems like hypertension and severe pain, but as it became obvious that in skilled hands, complications were acceptable, most obstetric hospitals of any pretension offered an epidural service to patients in labor. This type of creeping spread of a service, particularly when the spread is rapid, often means that the technique is inadequately researched.

The benefits of epidural analgesia were obvious, what was less clear was the cost of this analgesia to the mother. Many research studies were initiated and proved beyond doubt that the analgesic efficacy was unmatched. Studies from the 1960s and early 1970s demonstrated how complete pain relief can be obtained in over 80% of patients[3], the stress of labor was reduced to both the mother and the baby, mothers could now 'enjoy' labor and pain had been effectively banished from the labor room. In 1977 a landmark paper was published by Hoult, MacLennan and Carrie[4], which suggested that fetal malposition was increased when epidural analgesia was given to mothers, and the use of rotational forceps was more common in the mothers who had received epidural analgesia. In 1981 we undertook a study of differing concentrations of epidural bupivacaine to assess the effects of less concentrated solutions and the use of differing volumes[5]. The results of this study are not relevant to this paper, but at the time of the study we looked at the method of delivery and the duration of labor in patients who did not receive an epidural (Table 1). The proportion

Table 1 Outcome of labor in patients who received an epidural and those who did not (from reference 5)

	Non-epidural	Epidural
Primigravida (%)	28.6	66
Duration of labor (h)	4.8	11
Spontaneous delivery (%)	86	32
Cesarean section delivery (%)	1.9	17
Average duration of block (h)	—	5.3

of primigravid patients receiving epidural analgesia was much greater than those who did not, the labors were longer and the incidence of instrumental delivery was considerably greater in those given an epidural block.

Of course, this was only to be expected; mothers who had longer and more difficult labors were most likely to be given an epidural for pain relief. The contribution which the block played in complicating the labor and delivery could not be assessed from this type of study. Many studies of the benefits of epidural analgesia have been published, but analysis of the results is confusing as a result of the many variables which are potentially conflicting and which must include the obstetric management. Many of the immediate complications were recognized and accepted. It was accepted that 1% of mothers might have a dural puncture with a resultant severe headache which might prevent her from looking after her baby. This was a small price to pay for the benefits that epidural analgesia provided, and the headache could be easily treated with a blood patch which was effective in over 80% of patients. The leg weakness which accompanied an effective block might be reduced in incidence and severity if more dilute solutions were used. In Belgium, Van Steenberge and colleagues showed that good pain relief could be provided for women if a 0.125% solution of bupivacaine was used[6]. The incidence of forceps delivery was low and the duration of labor was short, certainly shorter than that experienced in the United Kingdom. The use of this solution in the UK proved disappointing and it was not until the opioids were introduced that perhaps a new way forward had been identified which would provide good pain relief and reduce the severity of the motor paralysis which had hitherto accompanied a successful epidural block. Unfortunately, despite many studies, the results of using dilute concentrations of bupivacaine combined with a low dose of an opioid, usually fentanyl, in terms of effect on labor and delivery remain unclear.

The overall safety of epidural analgesia also remained unclear until a study by Scott and Hibbard[7] which demonstrated the relative safety of the technique. Of the 506 000 patients in the study (Table 2), 108 suffered serious but non-fatal complications; three were cardiac arrests, 20 convulsed from acute toxicity and 39 had severe neuropathy. The incidence is low, but it is not inconsiderable. Recently there have been a number of publications from the USA in which the mothers have been randomly allocated to receive epidural analgesia or non-epidural pain relief in labor. This is the only type of study which can supply the missing information about the effects of an epidural block on normal labor. The results from these studies are not reassuring, as they suggest that epidural analgesia has an adverse effect on labor and the complications which occur. To date there

Table 2 Serious but non-fatal adverse events in a large series of epidural blocks (adapted from reference 7)

Adverse event	Number
Cardiac arrest	3
Neuropathy	39
Urinary problems	6
Severe backache	5
Dural tap severe headache	16
Acute toxicity	20
Total number of complications	108
Total number of epidurals	506 000

Table 3 Prospective clinical trials which demonstrate the relationship between epidural analgesia and Cesarean section (CS)

Study		Sample size	Relative risk of CS with epidural analgesia
Thorp 1993[8]	nulliparous	93	11.4 (5.8–16.9)*
Ramin 1994[10]	nulliparous	693	2.6 (1.5–4.3)*
	parous	637	3.8 (1.3–11)*

*$p = < 0.05$

have been three clinical trials which have prospectively randomized patients to epidural *vs.* narcotic analgesia in early labor and in all these studies epidural analgesia is associated with a two- to three-fold increase in Cesarean section from dystocia[8-10] (Table 3). Of course, it might be argued that aspects of the design of such studies are flawed, particularly with the need for escape groups, and one of the studies has been the subject of heated debate in the American obstetric literature in which more heat than light was exhibited.

The hypothesis that epidural analgesia contributes to maternal morbidity must remain as one which is supported by the only available objective and ramdomly controlled studies. The studies that have been published to date have been too small to show that the frequency of fetal malposition and instrumental deliveries is increased, as suggested by Hoult, MacLennan and Carrie in 1977[4].

Maternal complications which have followed instrumental delivery have also been in the news recently and in a study of 8000 deliveries the incidence of recognized third degree tears was estimated to be 0.5%, and despite immediate repair, 47% of women with a recognized tear remained incontinent of faeces 1 year after delivery. Prolonged labor, induced labor, the presence of a large baby and forceps delivery were found to be risk factors[11]. It must be emphasized that, so far, epidural analgesia has not been implicated directly, but we are aware that of the mothers who receive epidural analgesia, the incidence of instrumental delivery is high; in our institute it is over 50%. Rectal incontinence is a very high price to pay.

Similarly, urinary complications follow forceps delivery and epidural usage; urinary retention and overflow are increased, but do not influence genuine stress incontinence[12].

In summary, it is clearly evident that epidural analgesia offers the most effective form of pain relief, but it is not without cost. Mothers must be informed of the possible complications of epidural analgesia before the onset of labor. This will enable them to choose the form of pain relief which they feel would be most appropriate. When assessing the risk/benefit of epidural analgesia, it is important to remember that, in addition to pain relief, the ease of conversion to provide satisfactory operating conditions for Cesarean section and the avoidance of general anesthesia must not be overlooked. Meantime, as anesthetists, we should attempt to optimize the control of pain and tailor it to the patient in an attempt to minimize the risks of instrumental delivery and Cesarean section.

References

1. Crawford, J. S. (1972). Lumbar epidural block in labour: a clinical analysis. *Br. J. Anaesth.,* **44**, 66–74
2. Holdcroft, A. and Morgan, M. (1974). An assessment of the analgesic effect in labour of pethidine and 50% nitrous oxide in oxygen (Entonox). *J. Obstet. Gynaecol. Br. Commonw.,* **81**, 603–7
3. Moir, D. D., McLaren, R. and Slater, P. (1974). Experience with carbonated lignocaine in obstetric epidural analgesia. *Anaesthesia,* **29**, 305
4. Hoult, I. J., MacLennan, H. and Carrie, L. E. S. (1977). Lumbar epidural in labour: relation to fetal malposition and instrumental delivery. *Br. Med. J.,* 14–16

5. Thorburn, J. and Moir, D. D. (1981). Extradural analgesia: the influence of volume and concentration of bupivacaine on the mode of delivery. *Br. J. Anaesthesia,* **53**, 933–9
6. Vanderick, G., Greerinkx, K., Van Steenberge, A. L. and De Muylder, G. (1974). Bupivacaine 0.125% in epidural block analgesia during childbirth: clinical evaluation. *Br. J. Anaesthesia,* **46**, 838–41
7. Scott, D. B. and Hibbard, B. M. (1990). Serious non fatal complications associated with extradural block in obstetric practice. *Br. J. Anaesthesia,* **64**, 537
8. Thorp, J. A., Meyer, B. A., Cohen, G. R., Yeast, J. D. and Hu, D. (1994). Epidural analgesia in

labour and Caesarean delivery for dystocia. *Obstet. Gynecol. Surv.*, **49**, 362

9. Morton, S. C., Williams, M. S., Keeler, E. B., Gambone, J. C. and Kahn, K. L. (1994). Effect of epidural analgesia for labor on the Cesarean delivery rate. *Obstet. Gynecol.*, **83**, 1045–92

10. Ramin, S. M., Gambling, D. R., Lucas, M. J., Sjarma, D. K., Sidawi, J. E., and Leveno, K. J. (1995). Randomized trial of epidural versus intravenous analgesia during labor. *Obstet. Gynecol.*, **86**, 783–9

11. Sultan, A. H., Kamm, M. A., Hudson, C. N. and Bartram, C. I. (1994). Third degree obstetric anal sphincter tear: risk factors and outcome of primary repair. *Br. Med. J.*, **308**, 887–91

12. Ramsay, I. (1996). Effect of mode of delivery on urinary incontinence. Presented at the *Obstetric Anaesthetist's Association Meeting, Glasgow*

60

Prophylaxis versus rescue surfactant

THE CASE IN FAVOR

C. J. Morley

INTRODUCTION

Randomized trials have shown that surfactant therapy reduces the mortality and morbidity of very premature babies. However, there is controversy about whether surfactant should be given as soon as the baby is born, or withheld until respiratory distress syndrome (RDS) is diagnosed. This chapter sets out the arguments for and against treating babies with surfactant at birth or a few hours later.

REASONS FOR SURFACTANT TREATMENT AT BIRTH

The lung epithelium of very premature babies is damaged within minutes of ventilation[1]. This causes protein to leak on to the surface and interferes with surfactant function[2,3]. Animal studies have shown that surfactant treatment, as soon as possible after birth, reduces the severity of RDS and airway damage[4], improves blood gases, lung function and survival[5,6]. Clinical trials have shown that surfactant treatment for very premature babies is very beneficial and remarkably safe[7]. For example, the Ten Centre Trial of artificial lung expanding compound (ALEC, Britannia Pharmaceuticals Ltd., Redhill, UK), used prophylactically[8], showed a 30% reduction in the incidence of RDS compared with untreated controls and a 48% reduction in neonatal mortality. It is not possible to identify which baby will develop RDS and therefore benefit from surfactant. The shorter the gestation the more likely that RDS will develop but older babies, compromised in some way, are also at high risk of RDS and its complications. Good neonatal practice is to anticipate and try to prevent problems. To wait until a baby is requiring ventilation and a high level of inspired oxygen[9] before giving a treatment which has been proven to reduce the severity of RDS and save lives, is counter-intuitive.

REASONS FOR NOT GIVING SURFACTANT AT BIRTH

If surfactant is given at birth, some babies will be treated who do not need it[10]. Surfactant might be harmful or destabilize the baby and therefore should only be given to babies who obviously need it. If surfactant is administered without knowing the endotracheal tube position, it may be delivered into one area of the lung[11]. Surfactant is expensive and should only be used when the babies really need it. If surfactant treatment is equally effective if it is given when RDS is established, there is no point in early administration.

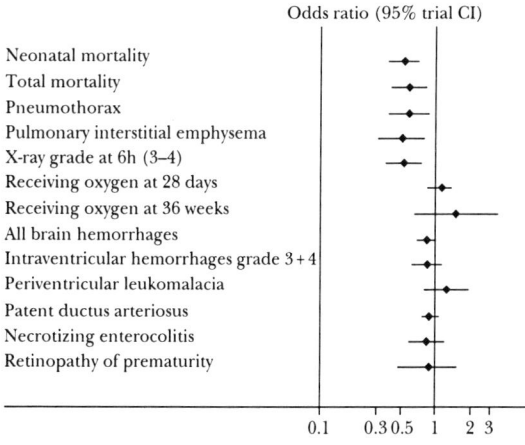

Figure 1 Comparisons and outcomes of prophylactic vs. rescue treatment

META-ANALYSIS OF THE CLINICAL TRIALS

Six trials[10-15] studied prophylactic vs. rescue treatment and met criteria for inclusion in meta-analysis. The results are summarized in Figure 1. The neonatal mortality was significantly reduced by prophylactic surfactant with an odds ratio (OR) and 95% confidence interval (CI) of 0.55 (0.41–0.73). This was a reduction in neonatal deaths from 139/1251 (11.1%) to 86/1269 (6.8%). The mortality was also significantly reduced, with an OR and 95% CI of 0.59 (0.42–0.82). However, this was only reported for the four trials with the smallest babies. The trial not reporting overall mortality enrolled babies from 29 to 32 weeks[13]. There was a reduction in deaths from 101/498 (20%) to 66/506 (13%). Therefore prophylaxis would save about seven more lives than rescue treatment for every 100 babies treated. The pneumothoraces were significantly reduced, with an OR and 95% CI of 0.60 (0.40–0.88), a reduction from 68/1250 (5.6%) to 32/1031 (3.1%). The incidence of severe RDS graded from chest X-rays[15] was only reported in two trials[12,14]. This was a significant reduction, with an OR and 95% CI of 0.54 (0.38–0.77).

There were no differences in the incidence of chronic lung disease, intraventricular hemorrhage (IVH), periventricular leukomalacia, patent ductus arteriosus, necrotising enterocolitis, retinopathy of prematurity.

The trials recorded different information about the effect on oxygenation, ventilation and the severity of RDS. Therefore it is not possible to compare these in meta-analysis. However, all trials showed improvements in gas exchange and the severity of RDS with prophylactic surfactant. These were all short-term studies but there was no evidence of any harm from prophylactic surfactant.

Table 1 Total number of doses of surfactant given to each group

Trial	Prophylaxis	Rescue
Dunn et al.[10]	112	81
Kendig et al.[11]	322	248
Egberts et al.[12]	83	23
Kattwinkel et al.[13]	661	321
Walti et al.[14]	234	161
Bevilaqua[15]	142	53
Doses per baby enrolled	1.2	0.7
Doses per baby treated	1.2	1.5

COST/BENEFIT RATIO

The prophylactic group received about 60% more doses of surfactant than the rescue group Table 1. However, babies in the rescue group treated with surfactant had an average of 1.5 doses compared with 1.2 in the prophylactic group.

If 100 babies less than 32 weeks' gestation were treated prophylactically, about 148 doses would be used. If they had rescue treatment, about 100 doses would be needed. Therefore, prophylactic treatment of 100 babies uses 48 more doses. However, prophylaxis saves about seven extra lives for every 100 babies treated. Therefore prophylactic surfactant used about seven more doses of surfactant but saved one extra life. The cost of extra surfactant for each life saved would be approximately: ALEC £1050 (£150 per vial), Exosurf (Wellcome UK, Middlesex, UK) and Survanta (Abbott Laboratories (UK) Ltd., Kent, UK) £2142 (£306 per vial) and Curosurf (Serono Laboratories (UK) Ltd., Hertfordshire, UK) £2800 (£400 per vial).

It is recommended that all babies born at less than 32 weeks' gestation should, if possible, be treated with surfactant at birth. Pragmatically, they should be given surfactant whenever they are intubated.

References

1. Gandy, G., Jacobson, W. and Gairdner, D. (1970). Hyaline membrane disease. I. Cellular changes. *Arch. Dis. Child.*, **45**, 289–310
2. Robertson, B., Berry, D., Curstedt, T. *et al.* (1985). Leakage of protein in the immature rabbit lung; effect of surfactant replacement. *Resp. Physiol.*, **61**, 265–76
3. Seeger, W., Stohr, G., Wolf, H. R. D. and Heuhof, H. (1985). Alteration of surfactant function due to protein leakage: special interaction with fibrin monomer. *J. Appl. Physiol.*, **58**, 326–38
4. Nilsson, R., Grossmann, G. and Robertson, B. (1980). Bronchiolar epithelial lesions induced in the premature neonate by short periods of artificial ventilation. *Acta Pathol. Microbiol. Scand.*, **88**, 359–67
5. Lachmann, B., Grossmann, G., Nilsson, R. and Robertson, B. (1981). Effect of supplementary surfactant on the *in vivo* lung mechanics in the premature rabbit neonate. *Eur. J. Pediatr.*, **136**, 173–9
6. Enhorning, G., Hill, D., Sherwood, G., Cutz, E., Robertson, B. and Bryan, C. (1978). Improved ventilation of prematurely-delivered primates following tracheal deposition of surfactant. *Am. J. Obstet. Gynecol.*, **132**, 529–36
7. Soll, R. F. and McQueen, M. C. (1992). Respiratory distress syndrome. In Sinclair, J. C. and Bracken, M. B. (eds.) *Effective Care of the Newborn*, pp. 325–52. (Oxford: Oxford University Press)
8. Ten Centre Study Group (1987). Ten centre trial of artificial surfactant (artificial lung expanding compound) in very premature babies. *Br. Med. J.*, **294**, 991–6
9. Collaborative European Multicenter Study Group (1988). Surfactant replacement therapy for severe noenatal respiratory distress syndrome: an international randomized clinical trial. *Pediatrics*, **82**, 683–91
10. Dunn, M. S., Shennan, A. T., Zayack, D. and Possmeyer, F. (1991). Bovine surfactant replacement therapy in neonates of less than 30 weeks' gestation – a randomized controlled trial of prophylaxis versus treatment. *Pediatrics*, **87**, 377–86
11. Kendig, J. W., Notter, R. H., Cox, C. *et al.* (1991). A comparison of surfactant as immediate prophylaxis and as rescue therapy in newborns of less than 30 weeks' gestation. *N. Engl. J. Med.*, **324**, 865–71
12. Egberts, J. E., de Winter, P., Sedin, G. *et al.* (1993). Comparison of prophylaxis and rescue treatment with Curosurf in neonates less than 30 weeks' gestation: a randomized trial. *Pediatrics*, **92**, 768–74
13. Kattwinkel, J., Bloom, B. T., Delmore, P. *et al.* (1993). Prophylatic administration of calf lung surfactant extract is more effective than early treatment of respiratory distress in neonates of 29 through 32 weeks' gestation. *Pediatrics*, **92**, 90–8
14. Walti, H., Paris-Llado, J., Breart, G., Couchard, M. for the French Collaborative Multicenter Study Group (1995). Porcine surfactant replacement therapy in newborns of 25–31 weeks' gestation: a randomized, multicentre trial of prophylaxis versus rescue with multiple low doses. *Acta Paediatr.*, **84**, 913–21
15. Bevilaqua, G., Parmigiani, S. and Robertson, B., on behalf of the trial participants (1996). Prophylaxis of respiratory distress syndrome by treatment with modified porcine surfactant at birth: a multicentre prospective randomized trial. *J. Perinat. Med.*, **24**, 609–20
16. Bomsel, F. (1970). Contribution of l'etude radiologique de la maladie des membranes hyalines: a propos de 110 cas. *J. Radiol. Electrol.*, **51**, 259–68

Prophylactic surfactant for preterm infants

61

THE CASE AGAINST

H. L. Halliday

INTRODUCTION

There are now more than 30 randomized controlled trials demonstrating that surfactant administered prophylactically or as treatment for respiratory distress syndrome (RDS) reduces the risk of air leaks and death. Meta-analyses have shown that the risk of air leak is reduced by between 30% and 70% depending upon the type of surfactant used, and that the odds of neonatal death are decreased by about 40%[1,2].

Accepting that surfactant therapy is effective both in the prevention and treatment of RDS, seven trials comparing these two treatment strategies have been reported[3-9]. All of these trials have used natural surfactants of bovine, porcine or human origin and most have enrolled very immature babies of less than 32 weeks' gestation. A meta-analysis of these trials is reported below.

Prophylactic surfactant replacement has potential theoretical advantages[10]:

(1) Facilitation of initial lung aeration;

(2) Improved distribution of surfactant at the alveolar air–liquid interfaces;

(3) Decreased alveolar–capillary leakage of inhibitory serum proteins[11]; and

(4) Decreased barotrauma[12], possibly reducing the risks of bronchopulmonary dysplasia (BPD).

However, without knowledge of lung maturity, a significant proportion of babies in the gestational age group of less than 32 weeks will be treated unnecessarily if all are given prophylactic surfactant[10]. The percentage of babies not developing RDS varies between 20% and 70%[3,5,6]. In a randomized trial of more mature infants of 29 to 32 weeks' gestation, the need for surfactant treatment for mild RDS varied from 32% to 63% (Table 1)[6].

Routine prophylaxis of all preterm infants with a gestational age below 32 weeks would therefore constitute significant overtreatment, the consequences of which would be:

(1) Unnecessary intubation of some babies;

(2) Unnecessary exposure to possible adverse effects of surfactant; and

(3) Increased costs due to surfactant.

In addition, the prophylactic instillation of relatively large volumes of surfactant could complicate the resuscitation and stabilization of small preterm babies. Indeed, one small trial with

Table 1 Need for endotracheal intubation and surfactant treatment for mild respiratory distress syndrome in infants not randomized to have prophylaxis in a large randomized controlled trial. Adapted from Kattwinkel *et al.*, 1993[6]

Gestation (weeks)	Number needing (%)	
	Intubation	*Surfactant*
29	81/101 (80)	64/101 (63)
30	96/134 (72)	70/134 (52)
31	86/161 (53)	58/161 (36)
32	107/225 (48)	72/225 (32)
Total	370/621 (60)	264/621 (43)

human surfactant found lower Bayley scores of developmental assessment in babies treated prophylactically compared to rescue treatment (Table 2)[13]. The unexpected results of this trial may have been due to chance or to the increased incidence of chronic lung disease in the prophylactically treated group. However, a similar trend in developmental outcome has been noted in studies with a bovine surfactant (Dunn, M. and Shennan, A., personal communication, 1992) quoted in the paper of Vaucher and colleagues[13]. It is possible that physiological factors associated with surfactant administration, including bradycardia, oxygen desaturation, changes in blood pressure and reduction in cerebral blood flow velocities, could adversely affect brain function in these immature, high risk babies[13].

RANDOMIZED CONTROLLED TRIALS COMPARING PROPHYLAXIS WITH TREATMENT OF RDS

There have been seven trials, all using natural surfactants[3–9] (Table 3). Three trials used calf lung surfactant extract (CLSE) or Infasurf® (Ony Inc., New York)[3,4,6], three used Curosurf® (Chiesi Farmaceutica, Italy) (a porcine lung extract)[7–9], and one used human surfactant derived from amniotic fluid[5]. Most of the infants enrolled had gestational ages of 31 weeks and less but one trial recruited more mature infants of 29 to 32 weeks' gestation[6] (Table 3). In each case the prophylaxis group was treated in the delivery room but the time after birth until surfactant was administered ranged from a few seconds[3–5] to 10–15 min[7–9]. The treatment groups received surfactant when or if they fulfilled certain and varied criteria (Table 3). Age at treatment in this group was usually less than 24 h[3,5,7,9] but the severity of RDS varied from the presence of clinical signs[3] to an inspired oxygen fraction (FiO_2) of ≥ 0.60, constituting quite severe RDS[7]. Thus these seven trials showed considerable heterogeneity, making a

Table 2 Outcome at 12 months of adjusted age of babies treated with human surfactant: prophylaxis vs. rescue. Adapted from Vaucher et al., 1993[13]

	Prophylaxis (n = 34)	Rescue (n = 29)
Number assessed	25	25
Chronic lung disease (%)	68	25
Normal (%)	28	48
Mild delay (%)	24	32
Moderate or severe delay (%)	48	20
Bayley MDI (mean ± SD)	78 ± 25	96 ± 16*
Bayley PDI (mean ± SD)	73 ± 20	87 ± 22†

*$p = 0.02$; †$p = 0.04$; MDI = mental development index; SD = standard deviation; PDI = psychomotor development index

Table 3 Randomized controlled trials of prophylactic surfactant vs. surfactant treatment of respiratory distress syndrome (RDS)

Author	Year	Surfactant	Gestation (weeks)	Prophylaxis	Treatment
Dunn et al.[3]	1991	CLSE	< 30	ASAP	Clinical RDS, age < 6 h
Kendig et al.[4]	1991	CLSE	24–29	ASAP	$FiO_2 \geq 0.40$ MAP ≥ 7 cmH$_2$O
Merritt et al.[5]	1991	human	24–29	ASAP	IPPV, $FiO_2 \geq 0.50$ MAP < 7 cmH$_2$O, age 2–12 h
Kattwinkel et al.[6]	1993	CLSE	29–32	< 5 min	CXR, RDS, $FiO_2 \geq 0.30$
Egberts et al.[7]	1993	Curosurf	25–31	< 10 min	RDS, IPPV, $FiO_2 > 0.60$, age 6–24 h
Walti et al.[8]	1995	Curosurf	25–31	< 15 min	$PaO_2/FiO_2 < 20$ kPa at MAP = 8 cmH$_2$O
Bevilacqua et al.[9]	1996	Curosurf	24–30	< 10 min	RDS, IPPV, age < 24 h

CLSE = calf lung surfactant extract; ASAP = as soon as possible; MAP = mean airway pressure; IPPV = intermittent positive pressure ventilation; CXR = chest X-ray; FiO_2 = fractional inspired oxygen concentration; PaO_2 = arterial oxygen tension

meta-analysis of their outcomes somewhat difficult[14,15]. It was felt that timing of surfactant administration in the prophylactic group was of greatest importance and in order to comply with the concept of prophylaxis, 15 min from birth was taken as the longest permissible time. Another study where surfactant was given within 30 min of birth[16] has been included in the meta-analysis of early vs. late trials (see below). The most important outcomes were adjudged to be:

(1) Neonatal mortality;

(2) Bronchopulmonary dysplasia; and

(3) Death or bronchopulmonary dysplasia.

These were defined as: neonatal mortality, death within 28 days of birth; and bronchopulmonary dysplasia, oxygen needed after 28 days[3,4,6,8,9] and characteristic chest radiographic appearance as described by Edwards and co-workers[17] (study reference 5) or Bancalari and associates[18] (study reference 7).

Odds ratios (OR) and 95% confidence intervals (CI) for pooled data were calculated using the method of Altman and Gardner[19]. Typical estimates for each of the outcomes were calculated using the Mantel-Haenszel method[20]. Event rate differences (ERD) and their 95% CI were calculated as described by Sinclair and Bracken[21]. The number needing to be treated (NNT) to obtain an effect was estimated as the inverse of the absolute risk reduction.

Results

In Table 4 the results of the meta-analysis for bronchopulmonary dysplasia (BPD) is shown. There was considerable variation in the incidence of BPD in these seven studies (14 groups of infants) with a range of 2–50%. Not surprisingly, the incidence of BPD was lowest in the study of Kattwinkel and co-workers[6] who enrolled the most mature infants in their large study performed in 1993. In three studies[3,6,7] the incidence of BPD was greater in the prophylactic group but the ERD were not significant except for the trial of Dunn and associates[3] in which there was a 23% increase, 95% CI 7–40% (Table 4). However, the typical estimate for OR was 1.12 and the 95% CI of 0.59–1.40 indicated no overall significance of this difference. At worst, prophylactic therapy would be associated with a 4% increase in the rate of BPD, and the number needing to be treated to reduce this risk in the late treatment group would be 50 (95% CI 25–100) (Table 5).

In Table 6 the effect of prophylactic surfactant vs. surfactant treatment of RDS on neonatal mortality is shown. Here the outcomes were more homogeneous, with a range of 0–35% but there was still considerable variation. Two studies showed insignificant increases in neonatal mortality with prophylaxis[3,5] but the others showed decreases [4,6–9] so that the typical estimate was significant with OR 0.63 (95% CI

Table 4 Effect of prophylactic surfactant vs. surfactant treatment of respiratory distress syndrome on bronchopulmonary dysplasia

		Prophylaxis		Treatment				ERD	95% CI
Author	Year	n	%	n	%	OR	95% CI	(%)	(%)
Dunn et al.[3]	1991	31/62	50	16/60	27	2.75	1.29–5.87	23	7 to 40
Kendig et al.[4]	1991	85/235	36	89/244	36	0.99	0.68–1.43	0	−9 to 8
Merritt et al.[5]	1991	8/102	8	8/101	8	0.99	0.36–2.75	0	−7 to 7
Kattwinkel et al.[6]	1993	29/627	5	14/621	2	2.10	1.10–4.02	3	0 to 4
Egberts et al.[7]	1993	22/75	29	17/72	24	1.34	0.64–2.81	5	−8 to 20
Walti et al.[8]	1995	38/134	28	43/122	35	0.73	0.43–1.23	−7	−18 to 4
Bevilacqua et al.[9]	1996	12/136	9	17/132	13	0.65	0.30–1.43	−4	−11 to 3
Typical estimate						1.12	0.89–1.40	2	0 to 4

OR = odds ratio; 95% CI = 95% confidence interval; ERD = event ratio difference

0.49–0.82) and ERD a 3% reduction (95% CI 1–5% reduction). The number needing to be treated with prophylaxis to save one extra life is 33 (95% CI 20–100) (Table 5).

To determine if the slightly increased risk of BPD was offset by a lower risk of death in the prophylaxis group a meta-analysis of the combined outcome of death and BPD was performed (Table 7). There was considerable heterogeneity in this outcome, with a range of incidence of 5–64%. Two studies showed an increased risk with prophylaxis[3,5] and in one study this was significant[3]. However, the other trials all showed reductions in risk so that the typical estimate of OR was 0.76 (95% CI 0.63–0.92). The ERD was −4% (95% CI −2% to −6%) corresponding to a number needing to be treated of 25 (95% CI 17–50) (Table 5).

Table 5 Effect of prophylactic surfactant vs. surfactant treatment of respiratory distress syndrome

| | Number | | | | | | | |
| | Trials | Babies | | | | | | |
Outcome	Trials	Babies	OR	95% CI	ERD (%)	95% CI (%)	NNT	95% CI
Death	7	2723	0.63	0.49–0.82	−3	−5 to −1	33	20–100
BPD	7	2723	1.12	0.89–1.40	2	0 to 4	50	25–100
Death or BPD	7	2723	0.76	0.63–0.92	−4	−6 to −2	25	17–50

OR = odds ratio; 95% CI = 95% confidence interval; ERD = event ratio difference; BPD = bronchopulmonary dysplasia; NNT = number needing to be treated

Table 6 Effect of prophylactic surfactant vs. surfactant treatment of respiratory distress syndrome on neonatal mortality

| Author | Year | Prophylaxis | | Treatment | | OR | 95% CI | ERD (%) | 95% CI (%) |
		n	%	n	%				
Dunn et al.[3]	1991	9/62	14	8/60	13	1.10	0.39–3.08	1	−11 to 13
Kendig et al.[4]	1991	29/235	12	49/244	20	0.56	0.34–0.92	−8	−14 to −1
Merritt et al.[5]	1991	29/102	28	23/102	23	1.35	0.71–2.54	5	− 6 to 18
Kattwinkel et al.[6]	1993	3/627	0	11/621	2	0.27	0.07–0.96	−2	−2 to 0
Egberts et al.[7]	1993	9/75	12	14/72	19	0.56	0.23–1.40	−7	−19 to 4
Walti et al.[8]	1995	15/134	11	23/122	17	0.54	0.27–1.10	−6	−16 to 1
Bevilacqua et al.[9]	1996	28/136	21	46/132	35	0.48	0.28–0.84	−14	−25 to −4
Typical estimate						0.63	0.49–0.82	−3	−5 to −1

OR = odds ratio; 95% CI = 95% confidence interval; ERD = event ratio difference

Table 7 Effect of prophylactic surfactant vs. surfactant treatment of respiratory distress syndrome on bronchopulmonary dysplasia or death

| Author | Year | Prophylaxis | | Treatment | | OR | 95% CI | ERD (%) | 95% CI (%) |
		n	%	n	%				
Dunn et al.[3]	1991	40/62	64	21/60	35	3.38	1.61–7.10	29	12 to 47
Kendig et al.[4]	1991	108/235	46	129/244	53	0.76	0.53–1.09	−7	−16 to 2
Merritt et al.[5]	1991	35/102	34	29/101	29	1.30	0.72–2.35	5	−7 to 18
Kattwinkel et al.[6]	1993	32/627	5	54/621	9	0.56	0.36–0.89	−4	−6 to −1
Egberts et al.[7]	1993	31/75	41	31/72	43	0.93	0.48–1.79	−2	−18 to 14
Walti et al.[8]	1995	53/134	39	66/122	54	0.55	0.34–0.91	−15	−27 to −2
Bevilacqua et al.[9]	1996	40/136	29	63/132	48	0.46	0.28–0.75	−19	−30 to −7
Typical estimate						0.76	0.63–0.92	−4	−6 to −2

OR = odds ratio; 95% CI = 95% confidence interval; ERD = event ratio difference

Discussion

Meta-analysis of these seven trials suggests that prophylaxis (treatment within 15 min of birth) is superior to delayed selective treatment once moderate to severe RDS has developed (Table 3). A small potential risk of increased incidence of BPD is offset by a reduction of neonatal mortality for this heterogeneous group of infants of less than 33 weeks' gestation. However, it is not clear if all babies in this gestational age group should be treated with prophylaxis for at least two reasons. The first is that long-term follow-up studies are not available except for one small trial with human surfactant[13] discussed above. The second is that subgroups of infants are more likely to achieve greater benefit from prophylactic surfactant with reduced risk of long-term complications. These subgroups would include infants at increased risk of developing RDS and exclude infants with a low risk who would be treated unnecessarily with a strategy of routine prophylaxis.

GROUPS AT INCREASED RISK OF RDS

These groups include boys, absence of prenatal steroids, lower gestational age and confirmed biochemical pulmonary immaturity[7]. In one trial using Curosurf, prophylactic administration was most effective in male babies and/or those of less than 28 weeks' gestation[7]. In this study prenatal steroid treatment was also confirmed to be very effective in reducing the incidence of severe RDS[7] and this benefit has been emphasized in the overview of Crowley and colleagues[23]. It is likely that prenatal steroid treatment is as effective as prophylactic surfactant and it is considerably cheaper[7,24,25].

In one study using human surfactant, infants in whom analysis of amniotic fluid for surfactant phospholipids within 24 h of delivery showed a lecithin/sphingomyelin ratio of ≥ 2.0 and the presence of phosphatidylglycerol were not enrolled[5] because they were unlikely to develop RDS[26]. However, a difficulty remains in that these tests take time and may not be readily available at all times to guide pediatricians in the management of RDS from birth. Recently, the stable microbubble test has been developed as a rapid predictor of pulmonary maturity[27]. When tested prospectively in 105 preterm babies it gave positive predictive values of between 96% and 100% and negative predictive values of between 84% and 91%[28]. It is likely that the stable microbubble test could be used as a bedside test to define a population of neonates with surfactant deficiency in whom prophylactic surfactant could be most effectively and economically administered[7,28].

Surfactant administration to neonates without surfactant deficiency could theoretically cause problems from lipid overload of the terminal air spaces and alveolar macrophages[29], although this has not been reported in human studies.

In conclusion, it has been recommended that if certain risk factors are present (such as short gestational period, low birth weight, male sex, and especially the absence of prenatal corticosteroid treatment), prophylactic surfactant administration should be given[7]. However, as an alternative approach, early (in contrast to delayed) rescue treatment also seems to lower mortality rate[16,30–31] by preventing progression of the disease[7].

EARLY VS. DELAYED TREATMENT

What constitutes early treatment as opposed to prophylaxis is not generally agreed. One group has suggested that the need for endotracheal intubation should be used as a criterion for surfactant administration[30]. Others have suggested that careful clinical assessment over the first few hours of life allows those babies who clearly have normal lungs to be identified and avoid treatment[11]. In one small study, early surfactant treatment reduced mortality rates in babies with severe RDS when the results were examined by multiple discriminant analysis[32]. This study and others like it[35,36] did not provide information on the optimal timing of early surfactant therapy. In the very large OSIRIS trial of Exosurf® (Burroughs-Wellcome, Research Triangle Park, North Carolina) it was found that treatment at a median age of 2 h led to an improved outcome as regards death and/or BPD compared to treatment at a median age of 3 h[30].

There have been three studies that compared early and delayed selective treatment of preterm babies with RDS (Table 8)[16,30,31]. All three studies were randomized but they used different approaches in defining early and late treatment. The Japanese trial of Surfactant-TA® (Tokyo Tanabe, Japan) was similar to the prophylaxis vs. rescue studies discussed above except that the early group of infants was treated before 30 min and the late group at 6 h[16]. However, since some infants were treated up to 30 min after birth, I have not included this study with the others that attempted true prophylaxis[3-9], and this decision could be open to criticism. Babies in the late treatment group received surfactant if they had RDS and needed at least 40% oxygen and/or had a mean airway pressure of > 7 cmH$_2$O[16]. In the OSIRIS trial of Exosurf, 2690 babies were enrolled in a study to compare early and delayed selective treatment[30]. The entry criteria for this study were less strict in that infants of any gestational age could be enrolled if the clinician judged that the risk of RDS was sufficiently high to consider immediate administration of surfactant, the age was less than 2 h and the baby needed endotracheal intubation for respiratory assistance[30]. The mean gestational age of babies enrolled in this study was 27.9 weeks and birth

weight 1120 g. Babies received late surfactant treatment if after 2 h of age they needed mechanical ventilation and had an arterial to alveolar oxygen tension ratio[35] of < 0.22. The third trial compared two treatment regimens using Curosurf, a porcine surfactant[31]. Babies enrolled in this study had moderately severe RDS (FiO_2 0.40–0.59). The timing of surfactant was based upon oxygen requirement rather than age. The early treatment babies were treated as soon as they reached the entry criteria at a median age of 7.5 h, whilst the late treatment group only received surfactant at $FiO_2 \geq 0.60$ which occurred at a median age of 17 h[31].

Results

The meta-analysis of the effect of early vs. delayed surfactant on BPD is shown in Table 9. Although one study showed a striking reduction in risk of BPD with early treatment[16], this was not confirmed by the meta-analysis (OR 0.94, 95% CI 0.80–1.09; ERD –2%, 95% CI –5% to 1%). There was, however, a significant reduction in the risk of neonatal mortality (Table 10) with an ERD of –4% (95% CI –7% to –1%). As a result, the meta-analysis for death or BPD also showed a significant reduction in the early treated group (Table 11) with ERD –5% (95% CI –8% to –2%). The reduction in the risk of severe intraventricular hemorrhage (Papile grades III and IV)[36] was not significant (Table 12). For pulmonary air leaks the reduced risk in the early treated group was quite striking (Table 13), with

Table 8 Early vs. delayed surfactant treatment

Author	Year	n	Surfactant	Entry criteria	Early	Late
Konishi et al.[16]	1992	32	Surfactant-TA	500–1500 g; surfactant deficiency; IPPV	< 30 min	at 6 h; RDS; $FiO_2 \geq 0.40$ and/or MAP > 7 cmH$_2$O
OSIRIS[30]	1992	2690	Exosurf	Any gestation; RDS; IPPV	< 2 h (med. age 2 h)	> 2 h; IPPV; a/APO$_2$ < 0.22 (median age 3 h)
Bevilacqua et al.[31]	1993	182	Curosurf	600–2000 g; 2–24 h; RDS; IPPV; FiO_2 0.40–0.59	At entry (med. age 7.5 h)	$FiO_2 \geq 0.60$ (med. age 17 h)

IPPV = intermittent positive pressure ventilation; FiO_2 = fractional inspired oxygen concentration; RDS = respiratory distress syndrome; MAP = mean airway pressure; a/APO$_2$ = arterial/alveolar oxygen tension ratio

Table 9 Effect of early vs. delayed surfactant on bronchopulmonary dysplasia

Author	Year	Early		Delayed		OR	95% CI	ERD (%)	95% CI (%)
		n	%	n	%				
Konishi et al.[16]	1992	1/16	6	7/16	44	0.09	0.01–0.81	−38	−65 to 11
OSIRIS[30]	1992	483/1344	36	497/1346	37	0.96	0.82–1.12	−1	−5 to 3
Bevilacqua et al.[31]	1993	7/86	8	12/96	12	0.62	0.23–1.66	−4	−13 to 5
Typical estimate						0.94	0.80–1.09	−2	−5 to 1

OR = odds ratio; 95% CI = 95% confidence interval; ERD = event ratio difference

Table 10 Effect of early vs. delayed surfactant on neonatal mortality

Author	Year	Early		Delayed		OR	95% CI	ERD (%)	95% CI (%)
		n	%	n	%				
Konishi et al.[16]	1992	1/16	6	2/16	12	0.47	0.04–5.73	−6	−26 to 14
OSIRIS[30]	1992	359/1344	27	404/1346	30	0.85	0.72–1.01	−3	−6 to 0
Bevilacqua et al.[31]	1993	8/86	9	22/96	23	0.34	0.14–0.82	−14	−27 to −1
Typical estimate						0.82	0.70–0.98	−4	−7 to −1

OR = odds ratio; 95% CI = 95% confidence interval; ERD = event ratio difference

Table 11 Effect of early vs. delayed surfactant on death or bronchopulmonary dysplasia

Author	Year	Early		Delayed		OR	95% CI	ERD (%)	95% CI (%)
		n	%	n	%				
Konishi et al.[16]	1992	2/16	12	9/16	56	0.11	0.02–0.66	−44	−73 to −15
OSIRIS[30]	1992	779/1344	58	834/1346	62	0.85	0.72–0.99	−4	−8 to 0
Bevilacqua et al.[31]	1993	15/86	17	32/96	33	0.42	0.21–0.85	−16	−28 to −4
Typical estimate						0.81	0.69–0.94	−5	−8 to −2

OR = odds ratio; 95% CI = 95% confidence interval; ERD = event ratio difference

Table 12 Effect of early vs. delayed surfactant on severe intraventricular hemorrhage

Author	Year	Early		Delayed		OR	95% CI	ERD (%)	95% CI (%)
		n	%	n	%				
Konishi et al.[16]	1992	4/16	25	4/16	25	1.00	0.20–4.95	0	−30 to 30
OSIRIS[30]	1992	234/1344	17	246/1346	18	0.94	0.77–1.15	−1	−4 to 2
Bevilacqua et al.[31]	1993	6/86	7	17/96	18	0.35	0.13–0.93	−11	−20 to −2
Typical estimate						0.91	0.75–1.10	−2	−5 to 1

OR = odds ratio; 95% CI = 95% confidence interval; ERD = event ratio difference

an ERD of −9% (95% CI −12% to −6%). The overall results are summarized in Table 14. The numbers needing to be treated for an additional favorable outcome were lowest for pulmonary air leaks at 11 (95% CI 8–17) and highest for neonatal mortality at 25 (95% CI 14–100).

Discussion

It is clear that early surfactant treatment from 0.5 to 7 h after birth has considerable benefits when compared to later treatment at 3–17 h for babies with moderate or severe RDS. The crucial question, however, is whether treatment just

Table 13 Effect of early vs. delayed surfactant on pulmonary air leaks

Author	Year	Early n	%	Delayed n	%	OR	95% CI	ERD (%)	95% CI (%)
Konishi et al.[16]	1992	1/16	6	4/16	25	0.20	0.02–2.03	–19	–43 to 5
OSIRIS[30]	1992	286/1344	21	394/1346	29	0.65	0.55–0.78	–8	–11 to –5
Bevilacqua et al.[31]	1993	10/86	12	27/96	28	0.34	0.15–0.74	–16	–27 to –5
Typical estimate						0.63	0.53–0.75	–9	–12 to –6

OR = odds ratio; 95% CI = 95% confidence interval; ERD = event ratio difference

Table 14 Early vs. delayed surfactant – all outcomes

Outcome	Number Trials	Babies	OR	95% CI	ERD (%)	95% CI (%)	NNT	95% CI
Air leaks	3	2904	0.63	0.53–0.75	–9	–12 to –6	11	8–17
Severe IVH	3	2904	0.91	0.75–1.10	–2	–5 to 1	NA	NA
BPD	3	2904	0.94	0.80–1.09	–2	–5 to 1	NA	NA
Death	3	2904	0.82	0.70–0.98	–4	–7 to –1	25	14–100
Death or BPD	3	2904	0.81	0.69–0.94	–5	–8 to –2	20	12–50

OR = odds ratio; 95% CI = 95% confidence interval; ERD = event ratio difference; NNT = number needing to be treated; IVH = intraventricular hemorrhage of grade III/IV; BPD = bronchopulmonary dysplasia; NA = not applicable

after birth confers any additional benefits. Unfortunately there are no randomized trials comparing prophylaxis and early treatment that could answer this question.

Early studies with preterm rabbits suggested that prophylaxis before the first breath was necessary to obtain maximum benefit from surfactant treatment[37,38] and indeed it was suggested that delayed treatment would not prevent lung damage from a short period of mechanical ventilation[39]. However, one of the authors of these papers has since admitted that immediate treatment is not necessary for the optimal effects of surfactant replacement[40]. 'Yet another postulate that fortunately turned out to be wrong was the claim that, in order to be effective in a baby with surfactant deficiency, the exogenous substitute would have to be given very soon after birth, preferably before the first breath[40,41].

CONCLUSIONS

Routine prophylaxis with surfactant cannot be recommended on the basis of gestational age alone. Gestational age, however, is important in determining the risk of developing respiratory distress syndrome. It can be used, along with other information such as use of prenatal steroids, lung maturity studies, sex and need for endotracheal intubation during resuscitation, to develop guidelines on the optimal timing of surfactant therapy (Figure 1). If prophylaxis is not used then early rather than late treatment should be employed for infants developing respiratory distress syndrome. As a guideline, early treatment could be considered when inspired oxygen needs exceed 30–40% and certainly within 2 h of birth for those infants with more severe disease. These guidelines may need revision in the light of new research. For example, in utero surfactant replacement is effective in the preterm baboon[42], although the quantity of surfactant needed for a response is very large. Also, new developments in the administration of surfactant such as aerosolization[43], instillation followed by continuous positive airway pressure[44] or high frequency ventilation[45], and the introduction of inhaled nitric oxide therapy[46] may further modify these guidelines.

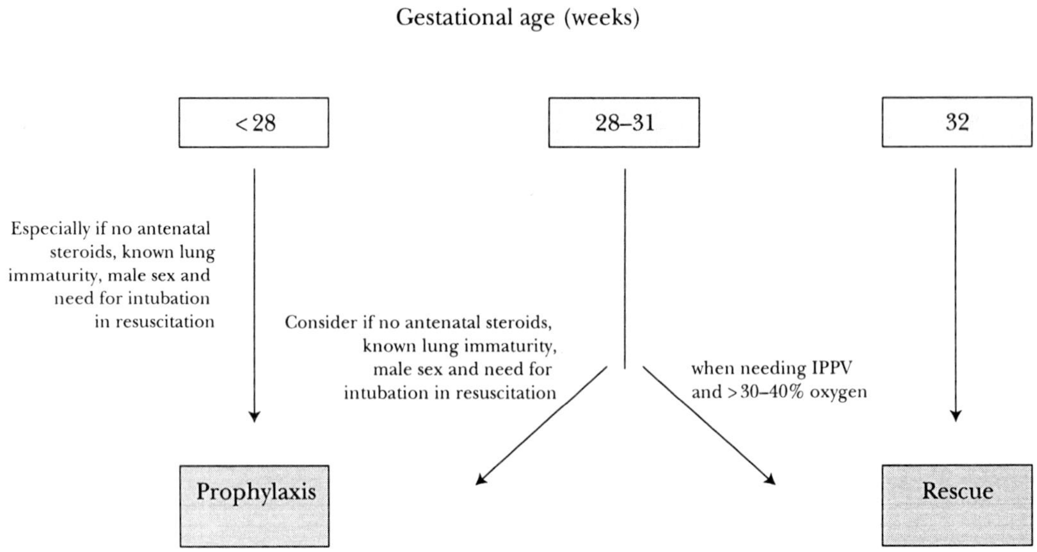

Gestational age (weeks)

Figure 1   Flow chart to guide timing of surfactant treatment. IPPV = intermittent positive pressure ventilation

There is an urgent need for follow-up studies of babies enrolled in randomized studies of the timing of surfactant administration. The use of prenatal corticosteroids should be encouraged in all pregnancies likely to end before 35 weeks' gestation[25,47]. Early surfactant treatment rather than late should be the aim for most preterm babies with respiratory distress syndrome, so that prophylaxis can be reserved for very immature babies at the highest risk of developing this disease. This has sound clinical and economic support as savings in costs per survivor and non-survivor have been shown to be greatest with prophylaxis and early treatment and these are also the most cost-effective strategies for surfactant replacement[48].

This overview has not considered which surfactant preparation is best and the Controversy Session at the XIVth European Congress of Perinatal Medicine in Helsinki concluded that natural surfactants had the edge over their synthetic counterparts[49,50]. The debate at the XVth Congress in Glasgow is likely to be a closer call with a compromise conceding that both prophylaxis and rescue treatment have their roles in the management of preterm babies.

ACKNOWLEDGEMENT

I would like to thank Mrs Samantha Jameson for typing the manuscript.

References

1. Soll, R. H. and McQueen, M. C. (1992). Respiratory distress syndrome. In Sinclair, J. C. and Bracken, M. B. (eds.) *Effective Care of the Newborn Infant,* pp. 329–58. (Oxford, New York and Tokyo: Oxford University Press)

2. Halliday, H. L. (1992). Other acute lung disorders. In Sinclair, J. C. and Bracken, M. B. (eds.) *Effective Care of the Newborn Infant,* pp. 359–84. (Oxford, New York and Tokyo: Oxford University Press)

3. Dunn, M. S., Shennan, A. T., Zayack, D. and Possmayer, F. (1991). Bovine surfactant replacement therapy in neonates of less than 30 weeks' gestation: a randomized controlled trial of prophylaxis versus treatment. *Pediatrics*, **87**, 377–86

4. Kendig, J. W., Notter, R. H., Cox, C., Reubens, L. J., Davis, J. M., Maniscalco, W. M., Sinkin, R. A., Bartoletti, A., Dweck, H. S., Horgan, M. J., Risemberg, H., Phelps, D. L. and Shapiro, D. L. (1991). A comparison of surfactant as immediate prophylaxis and as rescue therapy in newborns of less than 30 weeks' gestation. *N. Engl. J. Med.*, **324**, 865–71

5. Merritt, T. A., Hallman, M., Berry, C., Pohjavuori, M., Edwards, D. K., Jaaskelaninen, J., Grafe, M. R., Vaucher, Y., Wozniak, P., Heldt, G. and Rapola, J. (1991). Randomized, placebo-controlled trial of human surfactant given at birth versus rescue administration in very low birth weight infants with lung immaturity. *J. Pediatr.*, **118**, 581–94

6. Kattwinkel, J., Bloom, B. T., Delmore, P., Davis, C. L., Farrell, E., Friss, H., Jung, A. L., King, K. and Mueller, D. (1993). Prophylactic administration of calf lung surfactant extract is more effective than early treatment of respiratory distress syndrome in neonates of 29 through 32 weeks' gestation. *Pediatrics*, **92**, 90–8

7. Egberts, J., de Winter, J. P., Sedin, G., de Kleine, M. J. K., Broberger, U., van Bel, F., Curstedt, T. and Robertson, B. (1993). Comparison of prophylaxis and rescue treatment with Curosurf in neonates less than 30 weeks' gestation: a randomized trial. *Pediatrics*, **92**, 1–7

8. Walti, H., Paris-Llado, J., Breart, G., Couchard, M. and the French Collaborative Multicentre Study Group (1995). Porcine surfactant replacement therapy in newborns of 25–31 weeks' gestation: a randomized, multicentre trial of prophylaxis versus rescue with multiple low doses. *Acta Paediatr.*, **84**, 913–21

9. Bevilacqua, G., Parmigiani, S. and Robertson, B., on behalf of the Italian Collaborative Multicentre Study Group (1996). Prophylaxis of respiratory distress syndrome by treatment with modified porcine surfactant at birth: a multicentre prospective randomized trial. *J. Perinat. Med.*, **24**, 609–20

10. Speer, C. P. and Halliday, H. L. (1994). Surfactant therapy in the newborn. *Curr. Paediatr.*, **4**, 5–9

11. Dunn, M. S. (1993). Surfactant replacement therapy: prophylaxis or treatment? *Pediatrics*, **92**, 148–50

12. Robertson, B. (1980). Surfactant substitution: experimental models and clinical applications. *Lung*, **158**, 57–68

13. Vaucher, Y. E., Harker, L., Merritt, T. A., Hallman, M., Gist, K., Bejar, R., Heldt, G. P., Edwards, D. and Pohjavuori, M. (1993). Outcome at twelve months of adjusted age in very low birth weight infants with lung immaturity: a randomized, placebo-controlled trial of human surfactant. *J. Pediatr.*, **122**, 126–32

14. Sacks, H. S., Berrier, J., Reitman, D., Ancona-Berk, V. A. and Chalmers, T. C. (1987). Meta-analysis of randomized controlled trials. *N. Engl. J. Med.*, **316**, 450–5

15. Bulpitt, C. J. (1988). Meta-analysis. *Lancet*, **1**, 93–4

16. Konishi, M., Fujiwara, T., Chida, S., Maeta, H., Shimada, S., Kasai, T., Fujii, Y. and Murakami, Y. (1992). A prospective, randomized trial of early versus late administration of a single dose of surfactant-TA. *Early Hum. Dev.*, **29**, 275–82

17. Edwards, D. K., Hilton, S. W., Merritt, T. A., Hallman, M., Mannino, F. and Boynton, B. R. (1985). Respiratory distress syndrome treated with human surfactant: radiographic findings. *Radiology*, **157**, 329–34

18. Bancalari, E., Abdenour, G. E., Feller, R. and Gannon, R. N. (1979). Bronchopulmonary dysplasia: clinical presentation. *J. Pediatr.*, **95**, 819–23

19. Gardner, M. J. and Altman, D. G. (1989). *Statistics with Confidence*. (London: British Medical Journal)

20. Mantel, N. and Haenszel, W. (1959). Statistical aspects of the analysis of data from retrospective studies of disease. *J. Natl. Cancer Inst.*, **22**, 719–48

21. Bracken, M. B. (1992). Statistical methods for analysis of effects of treatment in overviews of randomized trials. In Sinclair, J. C. and Bracken, M. B. (eds.) *Effective Care of the Newborn Infant*, pp. 13–18. (Oxford, New York and Tokyo: Oxford University Press)

22. Cook, R. J. and Sackett, D. L. (1995). The number needed to treat: a clinically useful measure of treatment effect. *Br. Med. J.*, **310**, 452–4

23. Crowley, P., Chalmers, I. and Keirse, M. J. N. C. (1990). The effect of corticosteroid administration before preterm delivery: an overview of evidence from controlled trials. *Br. J. Obstet. Gynaecol.*, **97**, 11–25

24. Mugford, M., Piercy, J. and Chalmers, I. (1991). Cost implications of different approaches to the prevention of respiratory distress syndrome. *Arch. Dis. Child.*, **66**, 757–64

25. Halliday, H. L. (1993). Current views of the use of surfactant. *Contemp. Rev. Obstet. Gynaecol.*, **5**, 65–70

26. Amenta, J. S., Brocher, S. and Serenko-Aber, A. L. (1987). Evaluating the clinical effectiveness of amniotic fluid assays in predicting respiratory

distress syndrome in the neonate. *Clin. Chem.*, **33**, 647–52

27. Chida, S. and Fujiwara, T. (1993). Stable micro-bubble test for predicting the risk of respiratory distress syndrome: I. Comparisons with other predictors of fetal lung maturity in amniotic fluid. *Eur. J. Pediatr.*, **152**, 148–51

28. Chida, S., Fujiwara, T., Konishi, M., Takahashi, H. and Sasaki, M. (1993). Stable microbubble tests for predicting the risk of respiratory distress syndrome: II. Prospective evaluation of the test on amniotic fluid and gastric aspirate. *Eur. J. Pediatr.*, **152**, 152–6

29. Ziegler, H. W. and Albermann, K. (1988). Efficacy and tolerability of sufactant-substitution with SF-R1. 1. A histopathological study of rat and rabbit lungs. *Naunyn-Schmiedeberg's Arch. Pharmacol.*, **337**, R87

30. The OSIRIS Collaborative Group (1992). Early versus delayed neonatal administration of a synthetic surfactant: the judgement of OSIRIS. *Lancet*, **340**, 1363–9

31. Bevilacqua, G., Halliday, H. L., Parmigiani, S. and Robertson, B. (1993). Randomized multicentre trial of treatment with porcine natural surfactant for moderately severe neonatal respiratory distress syndrome. *J. Perinat. Med.*, **21**, 3–9

32. Lang, M. J., Hall, R. T., Reddy, N. S., Korth, C. G. and Merritt, T. A. (1990). A controlled trial of human surfactant replacement therapy for severe respiratory distress syndrome in very low birth weight infants. *J. Pediatr.*, **116**, 295–300

33. Collaborative European Multicentre Study Group (1991). Factors influencing the clinical response to surfactant replacement therapy in babies with severe respiratory distress syndrome. *Eur. J. Pediatr.*, **150**, 433–9

34. Charon, A., Taeusch, H. W., Fitzgibbon, C., Smith, G. B., Treves, S. J. and Phelps, D. S. (1989). Factors associated with surfactant treatment response in infants with severe respiratory distress syndrome. *Pediatrics*, **83**, 348–54

35. Gilbert, R. and Keighley, G. F. (1974). The arterial/alvoelar oxygen tension ratio: an index of gas exchange applicable to varying inspired oxygen concentrations. *Am. Rev. Resp. Dis.*, **109**, 142–5

36. Papile, L.-A., Burstein, J., Burstein, R. and Koffler, H. (1978). Incidence and evolution of subependymal and intraventricular hemorrhage: a study of infants with birthweights less than 1500 gm. *J. Pediatr.*, **92**, 529–34

37. Enhorning, G., Grossmann, G. and Robertson, B. (1973). Trachael deposition of surfactant before the first breath. *Am. Rev. Resp. Dis.*, **107**, 921–7

38. Enhorning, G., Grossmann, G. and Robertson, B. (1973). Pharyngeal deposition of surfactant in the premature rabbit fetus. *Biol. Neonate*, **22**, 126–32

39. Nilsson, R., Grossmann, G. and Robertson, B. (1978). Lung surfactant and the pathogenesis of neonatal bronchiolar lesions induced by artificial ventilation. *Pediatr. Res.*, **12**, 249–55

40. Halliday, H. L. and Robertson, B. (1992). Surfactant replacement. In Hanson, M. A., Spencer, J. A. D., Rodeck, C. H. and Walters, D. (eds.) *Fetus and Neonate: Physiology and Clinical Applications*, pp. 265–302. (Cambridge, New York and Melbourne: Cambridge University Press)

41. Enhorning, G. and Robertson, B. (1972). Lung expansion in the premature rabbit fetus after tracheal deposition of surfactant. *Pediatrics*, **56**, 58–66

42. Galan, H. L., Cipriani, C., Coalson, J., Bean, J. D., Collier, G. and Kuehl, T. J. (1993). Surfactant replacement therapy *in utero* for prevention of hyaline membrane disease in the preterm baboon. *Am. J. Obstet. Gynecol.*, **169**, 817–24

43. Lewis, J. F., Ikegami, M., Jobe, A. H. and Tabor, B. (1991). Aerosolized surfactant treatment of preterm lambs. *J. Appl. Physiol.*, **70**, 869–76

44. Verder, H., Robertson, B., Greisen, G., Ebbesen, F., Albertsen, P., Lundström, K. and Jacobsen, T. (1994). Surfactant therapy and nasal continuous positive airway pressure for newborns with respiratory distress syndrome. *N. Engl. J. Med.*, **331**, 1051–5

45. Heldt, G. P., Merritt, T. A., Golembeski, D., Gilliard, N., Bloor, C. and Spragg, R. (1992). Distribution of surfactant, lung compliance, and aeration of preterm rabbit lungs after surfactant therapy and conventional and high-frequency oscillatory ventilation. *Pediatr. Res.*, **31**, 270–5

46. Kinsella, J. P., Neish, S. R., Shaffer, E. and Abman, S. H. (1992). Low dose inhalational nitric oxide therapy in persistent pulmonary hypertension of the newborn. *Lancet*, **340**, 819–20

47. Robertson, B. (1993). Corticosteroids and surfactant for prevention of neonatal RDS. *Ann. Med.*, **25**, 285–8

48. Egberts, J. (1995). Theoretical changes in neonatal hospitalisation costs after the introduction of porcine-derived lung surfactant ('Curosurf'). *Pharmacoeconomics*, **8**, 324–42

49. Halliday, H. L. (1996). Controversies: synthetic or natural surfactant. The case for natural surfactant. *J. Perinat. Med.*, **24**, 417–26

50. Halliday, H. L. (1996). Natural vs. synthetic surfactants in neonatal respiratory distress syndrome. *Drugs*, **51**, 226–37

World Health Organization attitudes to modern perinatal practice: a debate

The case in favor

M. Wagner

INTRODUCTION

I have worked for 15 years as the Regional Officer for Women's and Children's Health at the European Regional Office of the World Health Organization (WHO). I left the United Nations at mandatory retirement age and have since been working as an independent consultant. So I am able to speak about WHO attitudes to perinatal practice without the constraints I might otherwise have as part of an organization.

When I wrote to a professor of obstetrics in Rostock inquiring why he had made statements in the press about the use of perinatal technology for which there was no scientific basis, he replied that he was perfectly justified since his statements were consistent with the standard of practice of the German Society of Obstetricians and Gynecologists. His standard was determined not by science but by peers. Using the standard of practice of peers means that the individual practitioner is secure because the knowledge used, whether or not based on scientific evidence, is approved by the leading practitioners.

To understand the conflict between practice based on science and that based on peers, and between the recommendations of the WHO and the recommendations of organizations of clinicians, we must go back to 1979, the International Year of the Child. In that year, the governments of Europe, concerned by rapidly increasing use of high-technology interventions in obstetrics, and rapidly rising costs, asked the WHO to evaluate perinatal services. The WHO organized the European Perinatal Study Group, containing representatives from all interested disciplines, including obstetrics, neonatology, midwifery, nursing, perinatal epidemiology, health administration, economics, psychology and sociology, as well as service users. The emphasis of the WHO European Perinatal Study Group was not on how best to manage complications of pregnancy and birth but rather on what constitutes appropriate care for the 80% or more of women with normal pregnancy and birth. Although it was the beginning of the 1980s and the term 'evidence based practice' did not yet have the widespread agreement it has today as the essential criterion for practice, the Perinatal Study Group looked at perinatal practices using scientific evidence as their criterion to determine what should and should not be part of routine practice.

The Perinatal Study Group commissioned a study of the world's literature, which showed that only around 10% of all routine obstetrical interventions have a satisfactory evidence basis[1]. The group conducted surveys which showed great variation in obstetrical practices with little or no relationship to perinatal outcome[2]. The variation was among countries, within countries, within districts and between hospitals, demonstrating that much of perinatal practice is not necessarily based on the best scientific evidence but rather based on the opinions and beliefs of the local physicians, especially chief physicians. The result of this study was the WHO publication *Having a Baby in Europe*[3]. The WHO then organized three international conferences on appropriate perinatal technology, in Washington DC, Forteleza, Brazil and Trieste, Italy[4].

These consensus conferences, following a thorough review of the best scientific evidence and consensus from all interested parties, resulted in the WHO publications 'Appropriate Technology for Birth'[5] and 'Appropriate Technology Following Birth'[6].

These WHO publications were often at odds with current standards of practice. In 1986 the President of the British Royal College of Obstetricians and Gynaecologists (RCOG) wrote in a letter to the Regional Director of the European Office of the WHO, 'The WHO guidelines used in *The Lancet* (WHO 1985) are mostly unacceptable and represent a very radical view which is not reflected in general British obstetric practice.' Similar comments were made by obstetric societies in other European countries. However, a more recent paper comparing these same WHO recommendations (guidelines) one by one with the concluding recommendations from a book that reviewed randomized controlled trials of perinatal practices[7] concludes: 'The recommendations of the WHO for appropriate technology at birth, developed through survey research, discussions and debate, are strongly endorsed by the findings of carefully controlled and critically evaluated randomized controlled trials'[8]. What is going on? Why is there a gap between evidence and practice – that is, between the WHO recommendations proven to be evidence-based and the obstetric practice endorsed by obstetrical

organizations? Why did the RCOG so vigorously oppose the WHO effort? Why does the European Association of Perinatal Medicine, by holding this debate, imply that the work of the WHO on perinatal issues may be less than helpful?

PUBLIC HEALTH OR CLINICAL APPROACHES?

The answer to these questions lies in a fundamental difference in perspective between what the WHO recommends as routine practice and what is actually practiced in European countries. Essentially the public health approach used by the WHO to formulate recommendations is different to the clinical approach used by practicing physicians (Table 1). Whereas the public health approach uses scientific evidence as its basis and then combines the best of the medical model with the best of the social model in making recommendations for health policy, the clinical approach uses standards of practice as its base with the medical model as its sole perspective.

The origins of the standards of practice used by clinicians are multifactorial. Some of the standards of practice are indeed based on scientific evidence. If the evidence reveals a particular practice to have extreme risk (thalidomide, diethylstilbestrol), that practice is likely to be

Table 1 The clinical and public health models of health services

Clinical model	Public health model
Standards of practice	scientific evidence
Medical model	medical and social models
Individual patients	community
Curing sickness	promoting wellness
Health equals medical care	health equals social and economic conditions
Doctors are most important health care providers	women are most important health care providers
Doctors decide	self-determination based on human rights
Authoritarian hierarchy	democratic
top down	bottom up
experts	all interested parties
exclusive knowledge	shared knowledge
Technology equals progress	appropriate use of technology
Goal: prevent pain and death	goal: optimal benefit to individual and society

dropped as standard practice. If the evidence supports a practice which is doctor-friendly (the electronic fetal monitor used with induction and epidural block), that practice is likely to become standard practice. If the evidence in favor of a practice is incontrovertible but not doctor-friendly (vertical birth positions preferable to lithotomy position), that practice is much less likely to become standard practice and there will remain a gap between evidence and standard practice.

Standards of practice is an important issue because several non-medical factors come into play (Table 2). Whereas clinicians often give 'experience' as the basis for a particular practice, the truth is probably closer to 'habit' – the way it has always been done. This is illustrated by the way operative vaginal birth practices vary internationally: in Britain and in some former British colonies (Canada, Australia, New Zealand) forceps predominate, while in Continental Europe vacuum extraction predominates. Convenience is another non-medical factor underlying standard practice. Since the advent of induction, scientific studies have shown birth to be more common on weekdays[9–11]. Other studies show *emergency* Cesarean section to be more commonly performed on weekdays[12,13].

Because 85% of British obstetricians have been sued at least once, and 65% have been sued twice[14–16], British obstetricians themselves give fear of litigation, or so-called defensive obstetrics, as their second most common reason for the unnecessarily high Cesarean section rates. Thus we have another non-medical influence on standards of practice. Even the American College of Obstetricians and Gynecologists now has written policy against routine use of the electronic fetal monitor on all women in labor[17], but its routine use is still standard practice in many places because of the fear that a doctor who does not have an electronic fetal monitor tracing in the patient's record will be vulnerable in court.

In those countries such as the USA, where the income of the obstetrician and the hospital, at least in part, is determined by how many interventions are performed, scientific data show significantly higher hospital-specific rates of Cesarean sections in private profit-making hospitals than in public and private non-profit-making hospitals[18]. Other studies from the USA show that women with private health insurance have significantly higher rates of Cesarean section than women without insurance and women with publicly-provided health insurance[19–21]. Such excessive Cesarean section rates remain a concern because data suggests they carry higher mortality and morbidity rates than vaginal birth both for the woman and the baby, even including elective repeat Cesarean sections[4].

What about the role of commercial interests? Their role in determining perinatal standards of practice is subtle but pervasive. Universities, hospitals and physicians co-operate closely with industry. Industry gains access to patients and to highly skilled researchers (physicians). Industry also gains by the communication of research – regarding use of a technology – in medical journals and at conferences. Hospitals or universities (sometimes physicians) may receive royalties and patent rights. More importantly, physicians and others may further their research careers through industry-funded research, which in turn is the avenue to promotion and status.

Table 2 Non-medical determinants of perinatal standards of practice

Non-medical determinants	Examples of practice
Habit	forceps vs. vacuum extraction
Convenience	induction, Cesarean section
Fear of litigation	routine electronic fetal monitoring, Cesarean section
Money	Cesarean section
Commercial interests	routine electronic fetal monitoring

As a less subtle example of how commercial interests can influence standards of practice, a meeting was organized by the International Federation of Gynaecology and Obstetrics (FIGO) to develop guidelines for the use of the electronic fetal monitor during labor. The WHO participant discovered on arrival that most of the cost of the meeting, including bringing obstetricians from all over the world, was borne by the manufacturers of the monitors to be evaluated. The participants had to pass through a manufacturers' display of monitors to get to the room in which the value of the monitors was to be discussed. Ultimately the WHO could not endorse the report from the meeting because it recommended the global use of routine electronic fetal monitoring on all women during labor, and the scientific evidence supporting this position was (and is) inadequate.

Since a basic principle of medical practice is that whatever is done must always be for the benefit of the patient and not the doctor, these non-medical factors – convenience, profit motive, fear of litigation and commercial interests – which are clearly for the benefit of the doctor, should never influence standards of practice. As a leading perinatal scientist has written, 'the increasing prominence (of legal influences) as determinants of clinical practice is not in the best interests of either present or future users of the maternity services'[22]. But the reality is that the standard of practice in any given place is the compilation and legitimization of what the influential doctors are doing. Unfortunately practices are very often not evidence-based and are strongly influenced by non-medical factors.

CHALLENGING AUTHORITY

The power of the knowledge used by those in authority is not that it is correct but that it counts[23]. Because of the authority of the WHO, if the orthodox standards of perinatal practice were to maintain their ascendancy, it was necessary for the WHO recommendations to be devalued, hence the letter from the RCOG to the WHO. In other words, 'to legitimize one way of knowing as authoritative, it is necessary to devalue or dismiss all other ways of knowing'[23]. A variety of strategies have been used to try to devalue or dismiss the WHO publications. I know of no attempt to challenge directly the scientific validity or 'truth' of the WHO publications – no articles that I have seen take on specific recommendations to show why they are not scientifically justified. Rather it is the relevance and authority which is challenged. For example, a professor of obstetrics in Austria declared publicly that the WHO recommendations on perinatal technology were for the third world (i.e. they may be valid but do not apply to us), although in fact the recommendations were directed primarily to highly industrialized countries.

Another way to challenge the authority of the WHO and to dismiss the WHO publications is to discredit the individuals promoting the recommendations. 'Those who espouse alternative knowledge systems tend to be seen as backward, ignorant or naive trouble-makers. Whatever they might have to say about the issues up for negotiation is judged irrelevant, unfounded, and not to the point'[23]. In other words, if you don't like the message, shoot the messenger. This helps explain why attempts have been made to separate me from the WHO and claim that the recommendations are my idea. In this way the authority is removed and the publications can be dismissed.

HEALTH POLICY FOR PERINATAL SERVICES

From a public health perspective, today's modern perinatal practice includes extensive, intensive, often invasive, very costly, often unnecessary interventions. The list of obstetrical interventions with a gap between the evidence and what is practiced is long, and includes routine ultrasound scanning during pregnancy, routine electronic fetal monitoring during birth, induction, lithotomy position during labor, operative vaginal birth, Cesarean section and episiotomy[4]. One might be forgiven for wondering what the efficacy of all this obstetrical intervention can be and why it continues when data on perinatal outcomes in industrialized countries show that the cerebral palsy rate has not decreased in 30 years, the low birth weight rate has not decreased in 20 years, the maternal mortality rate has not decreased in 10 years and the commendable slight fall in the perinatal mortality rate in the past 10 years is due essentially to a slight fall in the neonatal mortality rate and not to a fall in the fetal death rate. In addition, certain obstetric fads come along from time to time – every dogma has its day. At the moment, the active management of labor is popular dogma in some places, in spite of the fact that it has never had an adequate scientific basis[24]. Similarly an epidemic of epidural block for labor pain is occurring, in spite of a lack of adequate scientific assessment[25,26], and serious risks for both woman and baby which are rarely included in the informed consent[17,27].

There is also widespread reaction to such excesses in perinatal practices, brought on by four fundamental changes taking place today in health care policy. First, the realization that no country can any longer afford to pay for all possible health care interventions has resulted in an emphasis on cost-effectiveness, which is driving decisions about what to reimburse. Secondly, governments are realizing that the best criterion in choosing which interventions to support is evidence-based practice. Thirdly, the understanding that choices about which health interventions to endorse are more social and ethical than medical is leading governments in the direction of placing health care decisions in the hands of patients, as well as doctors, and at a more local level. The fourth and perhaps most important change taking place in perinatal health policy is that governments are realising that decisions about human reproduction are part of human rights. At the United Nations Conferences in Cairo and Beijing it was decided that women have 'The right to make decisions concerning reproduction, free of discrimination, coercion and violence as expressed in human rights documents. The promotion of the responsible exercise of these rights for all

people should be the fundamental basis for government- and community-supported policies and programmes in the area of reproductive health'[28]. In other words, governments must insure that the woman and family have the right to freedom in having the experience of their choice, free of coercion (even subtle coercion) and with full respect for the integrity of the person, during one of the most important events in their lives, namely pregnancy and birth. The nature of perinatal services must be such as to empower the woman and family to have the resources, ability and freedom to make such decisions.

Unfortunately some clinicians are blind to the ways in which these political and social changes are impacting on health services, gradually forcing changes in health care delivery and shifts in control. It is happening more rapidly and more obviously in health services for birth and death where it is most clear that the issues are primarily social and not medical. This explains the struggle taking place in perinatal services. Public health agencies and public health professionals have a duty to bring the public health perspective to this struggle. Following the WHO international consensus conferences on appropriate perinatal technology, the consensus process demands a final step: presenting the recommendations to all relevant parties, including the public and governments, for consideration and discussion so that a general community consensus can evolve. Such debate must take place at the national and local levels and in public – not behind closed medical doors – to become part of the political process that determines health policy. This is what the WHO has been doing.

CONCLUSION

Every sports team needs players (clinicians) and a coach or trainer (public health scientist, such as a perinatal epidemiologist) working together, and we need a combination of both the clinical approach and the public health approach for optimal health care[29]. Until now there has not been a healthy balance in the two approaches as the predominant role of the clinical approach and the attempts to discredit the public health approach have steered us off the right track. The WHO has been working to correct the balance between the two approaches.

Even today in every industrialized country, it is men who control birth and women who give birth. All the efforts at the WHO European Regional Office have been directed at using the public health approach to expand the body of knowledge in perinatology which is recognized as authoritative, and opening it up to include, in addition to the viewpoint of clinicians, the viewpoints of midwives, scientific researchers, public health professionals and women generally. These efforts are part of the global struggle for control of perinatal services, which, in turn, is part of the much larger struggle for control of women and control of all health services.

As part of this struggle, the WHO European Regional Office, as a public health agency, has been bringing to the attention of the public and governments two serious problems brought about by the present hegemony of the clinical approach. The first problem is the reliance on standards of practice rather than scientific evidence leading to gaps between the evidence and the practice. While some clinicians still fear uncertainty and resist change, more and more clinicians are accepting evidence-based practice and the standards of practice are gradually changing.

The second problem is having doctors deciding health policy, leading to the failure to honor the self-determination of the individual and family and basic human reproductive rights. The medical profession is used by society to control women's reproductive health[30]. There is no place in modern perinatal practice for doctors deciding such issues as where babies can be born and who can be present at birth, or for using coercion such as court-ordered Cesarean section or, more subtly, trying to frighten a family out of choosing out-of-hospital birth[31].

As someone with many years in clinical practice, I understand that clinicians in general need to feel certain in what they are doing, even when that certainty is sometimes based on shared beliefs in a standard of care rather than evidence. But when I later trained as a perinatal scientist, I learned that science means uncertainty and scepticism and asking difficult questions. We in public health are like the little boy in the Hans Christian Andersen fairy tale who was the only one able to say 'The emperor has no clothes'. This is not always a popular role but an absolutely essential one. Sadly, it must be added that there are some scientists and public health professionals, including some in the WHO, who are afraid to go publicly against the power and authority of the medical profession.

By bringing the public health approach to maternity services, the WHO has created controversy and occasionally even conflict. While this may make some people uncomfortable, it is important to remember that progress does not occur without disagreement, controversy and debate. Perinatal services have progressed and clinicians can be given credit for working to close the gap between evidence and practice. But however far we have come, we can always go further. By holding this debate the European Association of Perinatal Medicine is helping to move things forward in maternity services through open, honest airing of differing points of view among clinicians, scientists and public health professionals. This will lead to better understanding on all sides, to the benefit of women.

References

1. Fraser, C. (1983). Selected perinatal procedures. *Acta Obstet. Gynecol. Scand., Suppl.* 117

2. Bergsjo, P., Schmidt, E. and Pusch, D. (1983). Differences in the reported frequencies of some

obstetrical interventions in Europe. *Br. J. Obstet. Gynaecol.*, **90**, 629–32

3. WHO (1985). *Having a Baby in Europe.* Public Health in Europe Series, no. 26. (Copenhagen: European Regional Office)

4. Wagner, M. (1994). *Pursuing the Birth Machine: the Search for Appropriate Birth Technology.* (Sydney, Australia and Sevenoaks, Kent, UK: ACE Graphics)

5. WHO (1985). Appropriate technology for birth. *Lancet*, **2**, 436–7

6. WHO (1986). Appropriate technology following birth. *Lancet*, **2**, 1387–8

7. Chalmers, I., Enkin, M. and Kierse, M. (eds.) (1989). *Effective Care in Pregnancy and Childbirth.* (Oxford: Oxford University Press)

8. Chalmers, B. (1992). WHO Appropriate Technology for Birth revisited. *Br. J. Obstet. Gynaecol.*, **99**, 709–10

9. Macfarlane, A. (1978). Variations in numbers of births and perinatal mortality by day of the week in England and Wales. *Br. Med. J.*, **2**, 1670–3

10. Macfarlane, A. (1984). Day of birth. *Lancet*, **2**, 695

11. Paccaud, F. (1984). Weekend births. *Lancet*, **2**, 470

12. Phillips, R., Thornton, J. and Gleicher, N. (1982). Physician bias in cesarean sections. *J. Am. Med. Assoc.*, **248**, 1082–4

13. Evans, M., Richardson, D., Sholl, J. and Johnson, B. (1984). Cesarean section: assessment of the convenience factor. *J. Reprod. Med.*, **29**, 670–3

14. Capstick, J. and Edwards, P. (1990). Trends in obstetric malpractice claims. *Lancet*, **336**, 931

15. Editorial (1991). Worried obstetricians. *Lancet*, **337**, 1597

16. Editorial (1991). Obstetric litigation. *Br. Med. J.*, **302**, 1487

17. American College of Obstetricians and Gynecologists (1995). Fetal heart rate patterns: monitoring, interpretation and management. *Technical Bulletin*, **207**

18. Stephenson, P. (1992). *International Differences in the Use of Obstetrical Interventions.* (Copenhagen: WHO Regional Office for Europe)

19. Stafford, R. (1990). Alternative strategies for controlling rising cesarean section rates. *J. Am. Med. Assoc.*, **263**, 683–7

20. Haynes, R., Minkoff, H., Feldman, J. and Schwartz, R. (1986). Relation of private or clinic care to the cesarean section rate. *N. Engl. J. Med.*, **315**, 619–24

21. Gould, J., Davey, B. and Stafford, R. (1989). Socioeconomic differences in rates of cesarean section. *N. Engl. J. Med.*, **321**, 233–9

22. Chalmers, I. (1985). Schizophrenia in obstetric practice: not intervening is negligence, intervening is assault. *Italian Perinatal Society*, Milan, June

23. Jordan, B. (1993). *Birth in Four Cultures.* (Prospect Heights, Illinois: Waveland Press)

24. Thornton, J. and Lilford, R. (1994). Active management of labour: current knowledge and research issues. *Br. Med. J.*, **309**, 366–9

25. Howell, C. and Chalmers, I. (1992). A review of prospectively controlled comparisons of epidural with non-epidural forms of pain relief during labour. *Int. J. Obstet. Anaesth.*, **1**, 93–110

26. Chalmers, I. (1992). Ethics, clinical research, and clinical practice in obstetric anaesthesia (letter to the editor). *Lancet*, **330**, 498

27. Thorp, J., Hu, D. *et al.* (1993). The effect of intrapartum epidural analgesia on nulliparous labor: a randomized, controlled prospective trial. *Am. J. Obstet. Gynecol.*, **169**, 851–8

28. United Nations (1994). International Conference on Population and Development, Cairo

29. Wagner, M. (1989). *Playing Football: Paediatric and Perinatal Epidemiology*, Vol. 3, pp 4–10

30. Stephenson, P. and Wagner, M. (1993). Reproductive rights and the medical care system: a plea for rational health policy. *J. Public Health Policy*, **14**, 174–82

31. Wagner, M. (1995). A global witchhunt. *Lancet*, **346**, 1020–2

Waterbirth – a safe alternative to conventional birth

63

THE CASE IN FAVOR

G. Eldering and K. Selke

INTRODUCTION

Waterbirth is a fact. Since 1982 we have performed about 2000 waterbirths and about 12% of the 2000 deliveries per year take place in water. Although humans have a lot of relationships with water, I do not want to participate in the ideological discussion about waterbirth. Rather, I will record the physiological background – what makes waterbirth work – and our clinical experience with it.

PHYSIOLOGY

The prejudices against waterbirth are based on physiological ignorance. One of the main pitfalls is the suggestion of Karlberg (1960, 1962) that during normal delivery the effect of vaginal squeezing expells the amniotic fluid from the lungs, thereby creating an intrathoracic vacuum with an enormous inspiration or aspiration force. Therefore when a child is born in water it must inevitably aspirate. Today, the facts are agreed as follows. The newborn does not aspirate because it already has water in its lungs. This lung fluid is not identical with amniotic fluid. This lung fluid is formed by the lung epithelium by an active, energy-dependent process, from early gestation. This lung fluid creates a net efflux through the larynx and contributes to the amniotic fluid (one can find a pulmonary hypoplasia in a case of oligohydramnios). The hormonal changes during birth promote the reabsorption of lung liquid. With catecholamine infusion one can stop the fluid formation and support the reabsorption. The reabsorption process is not accomplished until 6 h after delivery. This reabsorption of lung fluid into the pulmonary vasculature is essential for the newborn. When the pulmonary circulation opens after birth, there is a demand for 20% extra volume to perfuse the lungs. One can therefore have more problems with a child born through a primary Cesarean section.

Another fact to be considered is the diving reflex – that means an apnea in expiration with glottal stop. The diving reflex has been described as a protection, which is elicited in humans by water touching receptors of the facial skin around the mouth and nose. This is mediated via sensory fibers of the trigeminal nerve. The vagus nerve plays the efferent part. Comparable to other reflexes, the diving reflex underlies a higher control, in this case a so-called proportional-differential regulation. When the reflex is elicited, the response is overwhelming. Then if a constant stimulus persists, there is an adaptation, and the control and response decrease to a lower level. Despite this there are fetal breathing movements in early pregnancy. The English physiologist Dawes described these fetal activities in 1970, during the recording of a low voltage electrocorticogram, that represents the REM (rapid eye movement) phase[3]. The fetal breathing movements can be influenced by several factors, for example by high CO_2 tension, that promote breathing movements. Low oxygen tension abolishes breathing movements. With high oxygen tensions, breathing movements will be continuous.

Pharmacological agents, such as indomethacin, pilocarpine, 5-hydroxytryptophan and morphine induce continuous breathing for a variable duration.

In summary, already *in utero* the fetus practices breathing. During this time no amniotic fluid gets aspirated into the lung, but on the contrary a net efflux of lung fluid from the trachea takes place. This mechanism is crucial for the normal growth and differentiation of the lung. The final reabsorption of the fluid is completed within 6 h of birth. The vaginal squeezing effect can be neglected. On the contrary, the newborn needs the lung fluid for its vascular system. It uses it to fill up its intravascular volume, which has to be increased by 20% through opening of the lung system.

Postpartum, therefore, the newborn crucially depends on the absorption of lung fluid into his vascular system. When a child is born into water, the diving reflex works completely. When the umbilical supply is adequate, no reflex bradycardia commences. The lung fluid does not get squeezed out and it does not leave behind a vacuum, but it does get reabsorbed as the breathing starts. With asphyxia, other conditions apply. These are premature fluid absorption and increased breathing activity, which leads to aspiration *in utero*.

FROM THEORY TO CLINICAL PRACTICE

In our hospital we compared retrospectively the labor and the neonatal parameters of vitality of the first 1000 waterbirths since 1982, as a controlled study in a matched pairs system. The control group was formed by the subsequent spontaneous births of the same parity.

The aim of this research was to exclude increased risk to mother or child during an uncomplicated spontaneous birth in water. Only the pregnant woman's wish was used in determining whether to allow a waterbirth, according to the fetal condition. Further complicating factors, like breech, twins and pathological pregnancy (e.g. placental insufficiency, premature labor) were excluded from delivery in water.

The first 50 births were monitored by continuous cardiotocograph (CTG), via scalp electrodes. Since then the intermittent monitoring of the fetal heart rate has been used via external CTG, as is common for normal spontaneous births. The following parameters were compared between the two groups: age, education, residence, course of pregnancy, history of complications of pregnancy, length of contractions, dilatation of cervix at time of entering the water tub, length of stay in water, use of analgesics during labor, rate of episiotomies/trauma to the birth canal, placental stage, neonatal Apgar scoring and cord pH, neonatal morbidity (infections, transfers etc.) and mortality, as well as length of hospital stay postpartum and other minor factors.

Results

Both groups were homogeneous regarding age, residence, length of the present pregnancy, education, previous pregnancy complications and course of the present pregnancy. Only a small increase of numbers of women with a history of previous Caesarean sections was seen in the waterbirth group (4% vs. 1%). Most of the women were between 26 and 30 years old. This is in accordance with the statistical age distribution of women giving birth in Germany. The majority of women who delivered in water were giving birth to their second child. The newborn of both groups were not different regarding birth weight and length. The maximum of the distribution graph for the body weight in both groups was around 3500 g, and that for the head circumference was around 35 cm.

Some of the women entered the pool during labor for relaxation, but not all of them gave birth in water. Only a small proportion considered a waterbirth from the beginning. Of the women who delivered in water, 31.5% stayed in the pool for less than 1 hour, and the majority – 33.9% – between 1 and 2 hours. This means that two-thirds of the women had delivered after having been in the water for 2 hours.

According to Lenstrup[4], the second stage of labor in water is considered to be shorter than during a usual birth. However, in our study, the length of the expulsion phase was not significantly different between the two groups. Forty-eight per cent of the waterbirths needed less than 20 minutes, compared with 43% of the control group births.

According to our understanding, relaxation in warm water has a positive effect on the pelvic floor. We assume a mental relaxation as well. The vicious circle of tension – anxiety, more tension, increased pain – seems to be interrupted more easily in water; we found a significant difference regarding the need for analgesics – 1.1% in water compared with 20.1% outside water. The two groups showed a significant difference regarding the necessity for episiotomy; 16% in water vs. 33% outside water.

The fear of increased hemorrhage during the placental stage caused by dilatation of the blood vessels through increased warmth was not substantiated. Our women determined the comfortable temperature of the water themselves, but we made sure that the temperature was kept between 32 and 36°C, which is tolerated by the newborn. The rate of increased hemorrhage was equal in the two groups, being 12%.

The fetal outcome did not show a significant difference between the groups. The distribution of Apgar scores at 1, 5 and 10 min was nearly identical. The arterial cord pH values were between 7.20 and 7.29 in 51% of the waterbirths and 46% of the control group. Clinical assessment of the newborn did not show significant differences. The number of neonatal transfers to the neonatal intensive care unit was low in both groups: 1.1% for the waterbirths and 1.3% for normal births. There was neither a maternal nor a neonatal death in either group.

There was no profound redistribution of volume in the cardiovascular system of the babies born in water. The babies were brought to the surface and to their mothers' breasts within 5 to 40 seconds. The hospital stay after a waterbirth was shorter than average, and the percentage of domino deliveries was higher than average for normal births.

CONCLUSIONS

In summary, I want to emphasize the safety of a waterbirth. In water the consumption of analgesics was significantly lower – 1.1% compared to 20.1% – and the rate of episiotomies less than half (16% versus 33%) that in normal births. The described cases of morbidity and mortality in connection with waterbirth are due to incorrect obstetric management, which could also take place outside the water. Some deleterious waterbirths have been performed without midwives or physicians.

Waterbirth has a strong place in the whole concept of enabling the mother actively to find her own personal way to give birth. This choice is watched by skillfull midwives and obstetricians, taking into account state of the art techniques. They must be able to use the whole range of clinical medicine when necessary.

Water birth debate – against

64

THE CASE AGAINST

J. J. Walker

WHAT IS WATER BIRTH?

When discussing water birth, it is important to state what exactly water birth is. Laboring under water is not new. For generations, women have been advised to lie in a warm bath during the early stages to help ease the pain and allow labor to establish[1]. The relaxing qualities of warm water bathing have been widely recognized since ancient times. It was thought to have healing properties and its ability to relax and relieve aches and pains is well proven. However, the demand for birth under water is relatively new[2] but is becoming more common[3]. The recent report quotes many units laboring women under water in the United Kingdom (UK)[3] but, in most, women come out of water to deliver. It would appear that no more than 30% of women actually deliver there after laboring in the birthing pool. In the birthing centers in Australia, pools are provided for labor but women are not expected to deliver in them.

The author accepts that laboring under water has advantages to the mother and is to be encouraged. It is delivery underwater where he considers that there is concern and this should be offered with caution.

WHAT IS KNOWN?

In the UK, there have been only a few thousand water births, hardly a wide experience and far too small to calculate the safety or benefit associated with water birth[4]. If this were a new medical treatment, it would not yet have passed the scrutiny of the Committee of Safety of Medicines[5]. There is a desperate need for more information. When documenting water birth it is important that the actual place of delivery is noted clearly, as most risks to the baby are related to delivery under water rather than to the labor itself. Before we embrace this new method, safety evaluation is required so that women embarking on this mode of delivery can give informed consent. At present most of the information given is anecdotal because so little is known.

IS IT NATURAL?

It is claimed that water birth is natural, but, unlike alternative birth positions where support for them can be found both in anthropology and nature, there is no such support for water birth. No primitive people deliver under water, although some deliver close to a lake or river, allowing them to bathe themselves and their baby soon after birth. More particularly, no primate delivers under water. If it were seen as an advantage, surely some primate would have practised this.

We are told that whales and dolphins deliver under water, which is certainly true but they have little choice. There are several reasons why it is safer for them (Table 1). Whales deliver

Table 1 Factors influencing underwater delivery by whales and dolphins

They have little choice and have evolved to do so
They are designed for it with no shoulders for easy delivery
They deliver close to the surface
The baby usually comes tail first
The cord is severed soon after birth
The baby starts swimming immediately
The baby is pushed to the surface

close to the surface and the baby usually comes tail first. If it comes head first, it can drown because of its inability to breath air. The dolphin is designed in a streamlined way which allows easier deliver, unlike a baby human who would appear to have been designed to get stuck. The mother whale whips her tail soon after birth to sever the cord. The baby starts swimming immediately and is pushed to the surface to allow it to breathe. There are often midwife whales there to help in this nuzzling process. Other mammals that live in water, such as seals, all come out of water to deliver on land. Baby seals cannot swim at birth and need to be taught to do so after delivery. One of the few animals which chooses to deliver under water is the giant hippopotamus – hardly an attractive mammal to use in support of human birth under water but one that shows us the only potential advantage to underwater birth and that is buoyancy. So underwater birth is not natural.

WHAT IS THE HUMAN EXPERIENCE?

Experience of human birth under water is increasing. Charkovsky, a Russian obstetrician, is quoted as having wide experience of underwater birth since the 1960s[2]. His experience is not well documented. The worldwide experience of underwater birth outside Russia now numbers the tens of thousands. The survey recently carried out in the UK demonstrated that there are many units using this method but few could accurately quote numbers or adverse outcomes except to say that they did not think they were due to the water birth itself[3]. Although this is slightly reassuring, it will need far better documentation to prove safety[4]. The person with the best documented experience is Rosenthal in the Upland Birthing Center, California. Here, mothers enter the pool between 5 and 7 cm cervical dilatation and aim to deliver the baby under water[6]. They follow fairly rigid rules and bring the newborn to the surface immediately. In over 400 deliveries (now nearer a thousand), there was no overall medical benefit found,

although there were no complications. So the human experience is limited and the information inadequate to declare safety.

ARE THERE MATERNAL BENEFITS?

Much of the benefit claimed for underwater labor is to the mother[2,7]. Warm water soothes and reduces pain during labor and there is evidence from some studies that there is shortening of the labor with faster dilatation of the cervix[8]. One of the biggest advantages is the support the water gives the pregnant woman, allowing her to change position on a regular basis within the water bath. This may help the progression of labor, allowing descent of the baby's head within the pelvis. Therefore, it would appear that if a woman wishes to labor underwater, some advantages may occur. Intermittent fetal monitoring is even possible by bringing her abdomen to the surface for auscultation or by putting the sonar probe in a plastic bag.

These are all labor benefits. This makes our experience different from that in the United States where the aim is to deliver under water rather than to labor there. The baths used are similar to domestic baths[9], unlike the large 'paddling pools' used in the UK. It is interesting to note that these pools in the UK are still being developed as there is no historical precedent from which to derive the design.

There is no evidence of any delivery benefits, such as reduction of soft tissue damage, although this has also been claimed[5]. There is also no evidence that there is any harm, such as infection[10], for the mother but the numbers are small and the true risk is still unknown.

It must be accepted that, if underwater labor is to be allowed, deliveries will occur as the timing of exiting the bath may not be optimal. However, since the risks (and none of the benefits) of water delivery are to the baby, coming out of the bath for a dry land delivery should be planned. So there are labor benefits for the mother but no delivery benefits.

WHAT ABOUT THE BABY?

In contrast to the potential benefits to the mother, there is no evidence of any for the baby. It has been stated that because the baby is within water in the womb, it is attractive for the baby to deliver into water[2]. Within the womb the liquor is relatively isotonic, whereas the water used in birthing pools is fresh water. It is thought that the baby will not breathe under water, although there is little evidence to support this. It is known that if a baby is hypoxic in the uterus, there is an increase in respiratory movements, hence the presence of meconium below the vocal cords in babies with fetal distress.

It is suggested that the baby has a dive reflex and we all have seen babies swimming under-water in gas advertisements. What is clear is that they are a different shape from a dolphin. These are also older babies who have air breathed. The dive reflex is only present after the baby has air breathed. Although a baby delivered into warm water will not have a stimulus to breathe in the short term[11], there will be a certain amount of lung expansion after delivery. During passage through the birth canal, the lungs are com-pressed and about 25% of fluid from the lungs expelled. If the baby is then allowed to expand its lungs under water, or gasps, fresh water from the bath will return. This can be quickly absorbed into the circulation causing fluid over-load. Also, fecal material from the mother can be inhaled, causing obvious infective risk as has been documented.

It is stated that the baby will not become hypoxic in the water bath as it will continue to receive oxygen via the umbilical cord. This is untrue. After delivery, the uterus contracts down around the placenta and the maternal blood supply into it will virtually stop. There is no new oxidation of fetal blood occurring even though the cord still pulsates. This is the situation in uterine rupture. The baby delivered into the abdomen is still attached to the umbilical cord but hypoxic damage occurs leading to death within minutes. The baby born under water will get little more oxygen from the mother and has a limited amount of time to get to the surface and breathe normally.

This is where the major danger to the baby occurs. If all is straightforward and the baby, well oxygenated at birth, is brought to the surface reasonably quickly, all will be well. But if the baby is hypoxic at birth or there is a difficult delivery, the access to the baby is further re-duced under water and quick delivery into air impossible. The hypoxic risk to the baby is in-creased.

In a retrospective trial in Stockholm, 89 women who took a warm bath after spontaneous rupture of the membranes at term were com-pared with 89 women who had the same interval from spontaneous membrane rupture to delivery and who did not bathe[10]. There was no increase in infections, asphyxia or respiratory problems in the newborn infant, or maternal signs of amnionitis. However, there were more complications in the bathing group, with babies born more than 24 h after rupture of mem-branes more likely to have a significantly lower Apgar score at 5 min. As a result of the sparse literature on water births and the data from their study, the unit has modified the bathing policy at the birth center from a rather enthusi-astic to a more cautious approach. Recommen-dations about the use of a warm bath in labor will require further investigations, such as ran-domized trials with large numbers of subjects. So there are no benefits for the baby and some potential risks.

HUMANS DO SURVIVE UNDER WATER

Many of us enjoy underwater swimming using subaqua equipment, but we are warned that, although this experience is wondrous, it is potentially very dangerous. There is much pre-paration and training that is required before you are allowed to dive without close super-vision. You must learn all the safety techniques, be aware of the potential problems, learn to check your oxygen supply, return to the surface if the oxygen supply is low, learn to communi-cate your distress to your 'buddy' and never dive alone. So humans can survive under water but not without preparation and continued risk. If women wish to deliver under water, they should know that although it may give much pleasure, it is also increasing the risk to the baby. Any deviation from normal must be dealt with immediately and coming out of the bath early may be life-saving. The baby must not be allowed to run out of oxygen and must be brought to the surface early, while oxygen reserves are still in place.

WHAT IS DISCUSSED WITH THE MOTHER?

The above factors, however, are not usually discussed with the mother (Table 2). There is much misleading information which can lead to increased expectations for the mother and her partner. Karen Daniels states that water birth is the 'newest form of safe, gentle, joyous birth' and its description as one of wonder is extremely attractive[2]. However, there is no evidence that it is safe, there is nothing to support the claim that it is any more gentle than normal birth and why it should be any more joyous than the normal birth that mothers and their babies have enjoyed for generations. These raised expectations can lead to disappointment. They also put pressure on maternity hospitals to provide this service so that they are not seen as being intransigent. There has been no proper assessment of the risk of water birth, which would have been demanded if this were a medically desired change of practice. Further well documented information is required[4].

CONCLUSIONS

The vast majority of women who wish to labor under water, plan to leave the bath for delivery. Most of the maternal benefit is in the first stage of labor and leaving the water allows safer delivery of the baby. There is no benefit for the baby in underwater labor except the possibility of reducing the need for narcotics. Delivery under water is potentially dangerous for the baby if there is any complication of the delivery itself. It may be that we should provide good size domestic baths in every delivery room to allow people to labor under water if they so desire, and also for washing and relaxing with their baby after delivery.

However, much is unknown. We do not know the optimum temperature for the water, how long the mother should remain under water or the best design of the birthing pool. Until more information is available, water birth should be approached with great caution[4,11].

These thoughts are best summed up by an American woman who answered some of my queries concerning water birth in my research for this article and stated, 'My youngest sister was born under water and it wasn't worth it. It was a nicer entry into the world but she is still a demon and it had no effect on her as a baby. My best guess is that if they want one, let them pay the money and do it but don't advertise it as the greatest thing to hit this planet'.

Table 2 Issues which should be discussed with women who inquire about under water birth

There is little worldwide experience
It is joyous but all births can be
Safe if all goes well, but if complications occur, they can be aggravated
There is no benefit to the baby and little to the mother
Current knowledge should be given, not biased information
Do not compare humans with dolphins
Discuss the unknowns as well as the joys
Discuss the complications and what can be done

References

1. Brown, C. (1982). Therapeutic effects of bathing during labor. *J. Nurse Midwifery*, **27**, 13–16

2. Daniels, K. (1989). Water birth: the newest form of safe, gentle, joyous birth. *J. Nurse Midwifery*, **34**, 198–205

3. Alderdice, F., Renfrew, M., Marchant, S., Ashurst, H., Hughes, P., Berridge, G. and Garcia, J. (1995). Labor and birth in water in England and Wales. *Br. Med, J.*, **310**, 837

4. McCandlish, R. and Renfrew, M. (1993). Immersion in water during labor and birth – the need for evaluation. *Birth-Issues Perinat. Care*, 20, 79–85

5. Zimmermann, R., Huch, A. and Huch, R. (1993). Water birth – is it safe? *J. Perinat. Med.*, **21**, 5–11

6. Church, L. K. (1989). Water birth: one birthing center's observations. *J. Nurse Midwifery*, **34**, 165–70

7. Odent, M, (1983). Birth under water. *Lancet*, **2**, 1476–7

8. Lenstrup, C., Schantz, A., Berget, A., Feder, E., Roseno, H. and Hertel, J. (1987). Warm tub during delivery. *Acta Obstet. Gynecol. Scand.*, **66**, 709–12

9. Daniels, K. (1988). Water baby: experiences of water birth. *Birth*, **15**, 106–12

10. Waldenstrom, U. and Nilsson, C. A. (1992). Warm tub bath after spontaneous rupture of the membranes. *Birth-Issues Perinat. Care*, **19**, 57–63

11. Harned, H. S., Herrington, R. T. and Ferreiro, J. I. (1970). The effects of immersion and temperature on respiration in newborn lambs. *Pediatrics*, **45**, 598–604

A universal right to assisted reproduction?

65

THE CASE AGAINST

J.-P. Relier

INTRODUCTION

In vitro fertilization (IVF), gamete intrafallopian transfer (GIFT), zygote intrafallopian transfer (ZIFT), intracytoplasmic spermatid injection (ICSI) and related procedures are technologies intended to make life better. In and of themselves, technologies are neither good nor evil. The application of technology can be said to be appropriate or inappropriate. It should be acknowledged that medical technologies can, and often are, either over-used or misused in practice. To determine what is and is not an appropriate application of medical technology, information is required on the effectiveness, safety, costs and benefits of the technology in question. Most governments in the industrialized world have developed elaborate systems for evaluating drugs before their introduction on the market, but not for medical technologies (IVF, GIFT, ZIFT, ICSI), despite the fact that these technologies are now in widespread use. Their true value has not been determined, nor have the risks associated with such treatment been assessed adequately.

The aim of this chapter is to discuss the different categories of risks: physical and psychosocial for the parents, the fetus, the newborn and finally the human being and the society.

COMPLICATIONS OF OOCYTE RETRIEVAL

It is not my responsibility to go into details on the different complications arising from laparoscopy, anethesia, and even with ultrasonically directed oocyte retrival. These techniques carry a risk of infection, urinary disturbance, visceral injury and even later intrapelvic adhesions which can exacerbate pre-existing infertility or even cause infertility in normal women seeking treatment for male factors.

RISKS OF OVULATION INDUCTION

Besides these technical risks, one should consider the side-effects induced by ovulation induction by ovarian hyperstimulation. The literature reports the consequences due to marked increase in vascular permeability and the rapid accumulation of fluid in the peritoneal, pleural and pericardial cavities. While there are several case reports of severe ovarian hyperstimulation syndrome with clomiphene citrate, this syndrome is more common, severe and protracted with human menopausal gonadotropin (hMG) or hMG combined with other drugs.

Just for information, it is necessary to recall cases of extra-uterine pregnancy and ovarian cancer which have been widely reported in the literature with no clear pathophysiological explanations.

The main risks, however, concern the embryo, fetuses and neonates.

COMPLICATIONS OF EMBRYO OR EGG TRANSFER

Although infections are rare, it has been established that bacteria or viruses may be introduced

386

by contaminated equipment, contaminated cell-culture media, or through sperm, donor sperm and donor eggs.

The direct complication of egg transfer is multiple pregnancy. Every country recognizes that the introduction of IVF, GIFT and other techniques has dramatically increased the rate of multiple pregnancy with all the complications: embryo reduction, prematurity and intrauterine growth retardation (IUGR).

Recent studies in the UK demonstrated that from 1980 to 1985 more than one-third of all mothers of triplets and nearly three-quarters of all mothers of quadruplets had taken fertility drugs.

In France, FIVNAT bulletins have demonstrated that the rate of twins has been multiplied by *nine* and the rate of triplets and higher order by *forty*. Also documented by FIVNAT, the rate of live births after IVF and embryo or egg transfer is between 10 and 15%. The rate of congenital anomalies does not exceed 3%.

However, the two main complications are prematurity and IUGR and not only for multiple pregnancies. For single births, twins and higher order, the rate of prematurity (below 37 weeks) is 10%, 34% and 83%, respectively, vs. 6%, 25% and 70% in the general population.

The rate of severe IUGR (below the 5th percentile) is 16%, 54% and 69%, respectively, vs. 4%, 25% and 40% in the general population.

Perinatal mortality in IVF is much higher than expected. According to FIVNAT, the perinatal mortality rate is 17, 21 and 71 per 1000 for single, twins and triplets of IVF vs. 9, 15 and 60 per 1000 for the general population.

Cesarean section for IVF births is also elevated: 27% and 60% for single and twin IVF pregnancies vs. 11% and 30% for spontaneous pregnancies. For triplets and higher, percentage values are inaccurate due to the low rate of triplets and higher in spontaneous pregnancies.

Transfer into the neonatal intensive care unit is also significantly higher in IVF neonates. The rate of transfer is 11%, 39% and 91% for one, two or three IVF fetuses vs. 5%, 20% and 80% after spontaneous pregnancies.

After these considerations of perinatal complications one could say that perhaps IVF and other procreative methods do not increase the risk of fetal malformations. The two main types of complications are prematurity and IUGR. These are not due only to multiple pregnancies since the rate is still higher in single births. One could discuss the pathogenicity of these complications due to the procreative methodology itself.

COMPLICATIONS IN NEONATES ADMITTED TO NEONATAL INTENSIVE CARE UNITS

These have been extensively studied at the Port-Royal neonatal unit for the last 10 years. From January 1987 to December 1995, 400 newborns after IVF were admitted to our neonatal intensive care unit (NICU). These 400 neonates came from 208 pregnancies: 55 single, 112 twin (224 newborns), 40 triplet (120 newborns) and one quadruplet. In 1987 there were only ten neonates from five pregnancies (one single, three twin, one triplet). In 1989 there were 66 newborns admitted to the NICU. Since that time, the proportion has been about the same, with 63 in 1992, but only 44 in 1994–1995, perhaps due to the new law which prohibits the transfer of more than three eggs.

The rate of prematurity and IUGR is the same in our population as in the French population reported by FIVNAT, that is to say, much higher than in the normal population.

Complications due to prematurity are about the same as in the general population, although respiratory distress and bronchopulmonary dysplasia are twice as great as in prematures from spontaneous pregnancy (14% vs. 6%). This might be due to the fact that IVF prematures are also very often severely growth retarded (30% vs. 9%). Enteropathies, necrotizing enterocolitis and mainly parenteral nutrition (35% vs. 13%) are also higher in IVF newborns.

On the other hand, brain complications are about the same: peri- and/or intraventricular hemorrhage (28% vs. 22%) and leukomalacia (9% vs. 11%).

Survival rate is exactly the same, i.e. 88% vs. 86%. This rate has been even better during the last 2 years (94%).

MID- AND LONG-TERM FOLLOW-UP STUDIES

To my knowledge, there has been no organized long-term follow-up study in children after assisted reproduction. Two years ago, in Helsinki, we published the first data of a 6-year follow-up study, showing a striking difference mainly in the evolution of families with IVF children. I do not have time to describe extensively the results of this study. In summary, from January 1st 1987 to December 31st 1992, 200 neonates were admitted to Port-Royal NICU. Only 174 were followed for 3 years or more. The main outcome estimates were neurological sequelae (minor, moderate or major), developmental quotients, school level, behavioral disturbances, and family conditions.

From 21 singletons (two deaths, one lost), 18 survivors were followed; 17 were normal over 2 years of age (ten over 3 years old went to school) and one had a severe cerebral palsy with low IQ.

From 57 twin pregnancies (seven fetal and nine neonatal deaths), the 98 survivors were followed: 78 were normal over 2 years of age (65 over 3 years of age went to school); 20 had some neurodevelopmental deficits (of 14 over 3 years of age, 12 went to school); 25 families have or still have problems (death and/or anomalies (nine cases) and/or sequelae); three mothers were single parents (two divorced, and one separated).

From 20 triplet pregnancies (one fetal and three neonatal deaths), 54 of 56 survivors were normal over 2 years of age (33 over 3 years of age went to school); three siblings (one deaf and one with cataract) were put in foster care after severe maternal beating; two mothers were single parents (one divorced, one separated); four mothers had repeated breakdowns (one father tried suicide).

From one quadruplet pregnancy (one fetal and one neonatal death), two survivors were normal over 3 years of age and went to school.

These summarized data require some comments. Most sequelae involved very-low-birth-weight babies in association with a number of sleep and behavioral disturbances. From 98 mothers, 16 had 18 spontaneous pregnancies (11 full-term newborns, five miscarriages, one extrauterine pregnancy, one abortion) and three mothers had another IVF pregnancy (a few others had IVF failure).

Of interest is the specific early outcome of triplets compared to twins. The data indicate a high rate of sequelae and deaths in the group of twin births in contrast to a low rate of sequelae or death in the group of triplets in which pregnancies were carefully prolonged. However, families with triplets are highly dissatisfied in the first 3 years after birth mainly from fatigue and permanent stress. Other factors to be considered concern the cost and the psychological consequences.

COST OF *IN VITRO* FERTILIZATION

In addition to the cost of ovarian stimulation and care of pregnancy, the cost of IVF should include the cost of neonatal care and the cost of longterm care for sequelae.

A majority of IVF newborns stay for less than a month in the Port-Royal NICU. A few, such as full-term babies and few infants weighing over 1500 g, stayed for only 1 or 2 days and were rapidly transferred to level one or level two neonatal units. Over one-third of the IVF infants (38%) stayed for a month or longer and, of these, 10–15% stayed 1–2 months, 10% stayed between 2 and 3 months and 8% stayed 4 months. Five neonates stayed more than 9 months. In 1981 the average cost of initial care for neonates with a birth weight below 1500 g was estimated at 250 000 FF, but this cost reached 350 000 FF in patients with broncho-pulmonary dysplasia and 400 000 FF in those with necrotizing enterocolitis. Concerning the daily fee of 6500 FF in 1990 and 10 000 FF in 1995 or 1200 US$ in 1990 and 2000 US$ in 1995, this multiplies by almost three or four times the 1981 cost! This will give an average cost for an IVF child of around 650 000 FF in 1995, which is a little more than a heart transplantation in a neonate.

Of course the care of long-term sequelae should be added to this initial perinatal cost, especially the cost for care of pulmonary complications and neurological sequelae. These include the costs of home care programs, rehospitalization, physical therapy, special education, and sometimes institutionalization. When both the initial and later cost are combined, it is clear that the financial costs are extremely important for a significant proportion of IVF infants.

PSYCHOLOGICAL CONSEQUENCES

Physicians-in-charge and a psychoanalyst conduct routine interviews of parents of IVF babies at the Port-Royal NICU. These interviews provide some indication of the immediate reactions to the birth and subsequent hospitalization of these children. Fathers were usually quite happy; very often they were not really conscious of the potential underlying tragedy. In contrast, every mother was satisfied with finally having this most wanted baby, but they compared their experience to a rigorous military training camp. Their initial happiness quickly turned to distress when there were several premature, sick neonates, obtained at great personal cost and often after four, five or sometimes more attempts at IVF (one had 21 attempts).

When three, four, or five children survive the perinatal period, it is likely that the care they will require places such extraordinary demands on their parents that they cannot cope alone for any length of time. Families may need to either move their home or build additional rooms onto existing structures. Ordinary domestic life must be organized with military precision as well. Having a child, or several children, with physical or mental handicaps or both poses additional problems for families; these children may require special schooling appliances, and attention from both their parents and teachers.

Selective reduction of excess fetuses has been presented as a solution to the problem of multiple pregnancies. This invasive and ethically dubious procedure should be considered as yet another risk to women undergoing IVF, GIFT or ICSI. The legality of this procedure may rely on an interpretation of abortion law. It has been claimed as legal because the pregnancy as such is not terminated. Abortion generally is thought of as a procedure for the termination of unwanted or damaged pregnancies; therefore, the idea that a wanted and perhaps normal fetus would be aborted does not sit well with many ethicists. The long-term consequences of fetal reduction are unknown for the mother as well as for the other fetus who will become a child and adult.

CONCLUSION

The neonatal risks increase in IVF pregnancies. Much of this increase is caused by the higher incidence among IVF pregnancies of multiple gestation, which is an important risk factor for low birth weight, prematurity, intrauterine growth retardation and perinatal mortality. Single IVF births, however, also have a higher incidence of prematurity, low birth weight, and perinatal mortality compared with the general population, so the problem is not solely one of multiple births.

The increased perinatal mortality among IVF births is well documented, but the neonatal or long-term morbidity resulting form complications of prematurity and low birth weight is not. Multiple births, low birth weight, and prematurity are risk factors for long-term central nervous system handicap. This finding is consistent with other research on extremely low birth weight newborns which found long-term morbidity to be most severe in infants from multiple pregnancies.

Estimates of the cost to society for one IVF baby must include the cost of NICU care. Because over one-third of French neonatal intensive care IVF babies remained in the NICU for over 1 month, these initial costs are high, and the long-term costs of more frequent hospitalization and rehabilitation for handicapping conditions must be added to this. Similarly, the costs of IVF must include the drain on health service resources. If, as is the case in our NICU, close to one in every five babies is an IVF baby, then the demand on pediatric manpower and hospital facilities by the newer reproductive technologies is considerable. In addition, the psychological and social costs of these technologies to the family and the society must be included, and we know almost nothing about this type of cost. It may be greater than we realize.

At least to some extent, neonatology is rescue medicine – trying to help babies who are born too small and too soon. It has not, however, taken long to appreciate the importance of preventing these problems in the first place, if at all possible. In collaboration with the obstetrics and public health specialties, neonatology has worked to prevent low birth weight, congenital anomalies and genetic disorders and, in this way, has helped to lower perinatal mortality. Now, we suddenly find our NICU filled with high-risk newborns posing problems of our own making.

The implications of IVF for neonatal medicine were previously unclear; consequently, neonatologists stood by while IVF clinicians in France argued that the tragedy of infertility warrants the expansion of IVF services. Today, confronted with new information regarding the risks of IVF and the increasing admissions of such babies to NICUs, the neonatologist must argue that the tragedy of perinatal death, the suffering of extremely ill neonates, and the devastation of long-term handicaps is by comparison a good deal worse.

The way in which IVF is carried out must be considered in the light of newer information on these babies. Should the indications for IVF include (as we have found among our IVF parents) teenage mothers and mothers with children born following natural pregnancy? Should IVF clinicians be allowed to continue simultaneously transferring three or more eggs or embryos (a practice associated with the occurrence of multiple births) to improve IVF success rates? From our perspective, these practices should not continue.

Most importantly, we recommend that prospective IVF clients be informed fully regarding the immediate risk of multiple gestation as well as the long-term special problems associated with raising twins or higher-order multiple births, including such major stresses as financial worries, physical and mental exhaustion, and isolation. In addition, people suffering from infertility, health policy makers and the public must be made aware of the pediatric consequences of IVF and related technologies.

I would like to finish this discussion by recalling a very old adage which appeared in an atharva veda 5000 years ago. It was said that the 'best environment for conception is made of Beauty, Love and Harmony'. Where are these important qualities when conception occurs in the anonymity and the coldness of a test tube, surrounded by such aggressive technologies for the mother, far away from what this starting human being could have felt in the wonderful beauty of its parents' *love*?

Necessity for routine pain relief for ventilated infants: a debate

THE CASE IN FAVOR

N. McIntosh

THE CASE FOR PAIN RELIEF FOR VENTILATED INFANTS

We will never know whether newborn infants or those in the first year of life have the emotional experience we know of as pain, as this is a personal experience based on verbal report and such infants are preverbal. Nevertheless there is no reason to believe that ventilation in infancy is a procedure any less distressing than ventilation is at any other age. Why therefore should we invoke the double standards of analgesia for older children and adults but no analgesia for infants? At this level, however, the argument is emotional. Can we be any more specific in believing that such ventilated infants are in fact in pain?

There is no doubt that *acute* painful procedures in the newborn are acutely distressing – such infants wriggle and cry. Analysis of facial expression would also indicate that the procedures are painful[1-3]. This indicates that the state of being 'in pain' is at least probable in the infant. There is also data to suggest that all the neural connections necessary for pain reception and transmission are present by 24 weeks gestation[4]. Physiological data examining the flexor withdrawal reflex threshold to Von Frey hair stimulation suggest that preterm infants are more sensitive than term infants, which are themselves more sensitive than children[5]. The relevance of this is that the transmission of this stimulation is believed to be at least partly along pain fibers, and in older patients can be affected by opiates in a dose-dependent way. Whether this hypersensitivity is related purely to a peripheral hyperalgesia or reflects lack of spinal inhibition is now known[6].

Data from behavioral, anatomical and physiological studies indicate that there is no reason to believe that the pain and distress of ventilation in infants is different, and unless there is an overwhelming contraindication they should be treated routinely like older patients.

References

1. Grunau, R. V. E. and Craig, K. D. (1987). Pain expression in neonates: facial action and cry. *Pain*, **28**, 395–410
2. Johnston, C. C., Stevens, B., Craig, K. D. and Grunau, R. V. E. (1993). Developmental changes in pain expression in premature, full term, two- and four-month-old infants. *Pain*, **52**, 201–8
3. Rushforth, J. A. and Levene, M. I. (1994). Behavioral response to pain in healthy neonates. *Arch. Dis. Child.*, **70**, f174–6
4. Anand, K. J. S. and Hickey, P. R. (1987). Pain and its effects in the human fetus and neonate. *N. Engl. J. Med.*, **317**, 1321–9
5. Fitzgerald, M., Millard, C. and McIntosh, N. (1988). Hyperalgesia in premature infants. *Lancet*, **1**, 292
6. Fitzgerald, M., Millard, C. and McIntosh, N. (1989). Cutaneous hypersensitivity following peripheral tissue damage in newborn infants and its reversal with topical anaesthesia. *Pain*, **39**, 31–6

Index